ENCOUNTERS
WITH CHILDREN

Pediatric Behavior and Development

FOURTH EDITION

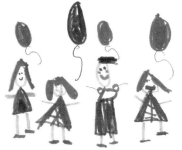

Suzanne D. Dixon, MD, MPH

Emeritus Professor of Pediatrics, University of California, San Diego
La Jolla, California

Clinical Professor, University of Washington
Seattle, Washington

Behavioral and Developmental Pediatrics, Great Falls Clinic
Great Falls, Montana

Martin T. Stein, MD

Professor of Pediatrics
Director, Developmental and Behavioral Pediatrics
University of California, San Diego
Children's Hospital, San Diego
La Jolla, California

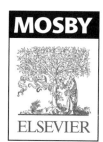

MOSBY

ELSEVIER

MOSBY
ELSEVIER

1600 John F. Kennedy Blvd.
Suite 1800
Philadelphia, PA 19103-2899

ENCOUNTERS WITH CHILDREN: PEDIATRIC BEHAVIOR AND DEVELOPMENT   ISBN 0-323-02915-9
Copyright © 2006, Mosby Inc.

Previous editions copyrighted 2000, 1992, 1987 by Mosby Inc.

Library of Congress Cataloging-in-Publication Data
Dixon, Suzanne D.
    Encounters with children: pediatric behavior and development/Suzanne D. Dixon,
Martin T. Stein.—4th ed.
      p. ; cm.
    Includes bibliographical references and index.

    ISBN 0-323-02915-9

    1. Child development. 2. Child development—Testing. 3. Behavioral assessment of children.
4. Adolescence. I. Stein, Martin T. II. Title.
    [DNLM: 1. Child Development. 2. Adolescent Behavior. 3. Child Behavior.
4. Growth—Adolescent. WS 105 D621e 2006]
RJ131.D59 2006
305.231—dc22   2005041591

Acquisitions Editor: Todd Hummel
Publishing Services Manager: Frank Polizzano
Senior Project Manager: Peter Faber
Design Direction: Gene Harris
Cover Art: Summer Morkrid

Printed in the United States of America

Last digit is the print number: 9 8 7 6 5 4 3 2 1

Contributors

SUZANNE D. DIXON, MD, MPH
Emerita Professor of Pediatrics, University of California, La Jolla, California;
Clinical Faculty, University of Washington, Seattle, Washington;
Behavioral and Developmental Pediatrics, Great Falls Clinic, Great Falls, Montana;
Editor, *Journal of Developmental Behavioral Pediatrics*

MARTIN T. STEIN, MD
Professor of Pediatrics; Director, Developmental and Behavioral Pediatrics,
University of California, La Jolla, California, Children's Hospital, San Diego

MARIANNE E. FELICE, MD
Professor and Chair, Pediatrics, University of Massachusetts Medical School, Worcester,
Massachusetts; Physician-in-Chief, Children's Medical Center,
UMass Memorial Medical Center, Worcester, Massachusetts

LAWRENCE S. FRIEDMAN, MD
Professor of Pediatrics; Chief, Division of Adolescent Medicine,
University of California, San Diego, San Diego, California

MICHAEL J. HENNESSY, MD
Orthopedic Surgeon, Great Falls Clinic, Great Falls, Montana

SUSAN L. INSTONE, DNSc, CPNP
Associate Professor of Nursing, Hahn School of Nursing and Health Science,
University of San Diego, San Diego, California

JENNIFER MAEHR, MD
Medical Director, Prince George's County School-Based Wellness Program

LORI TAYLOR, MD
Associate Professor of Pediatrics, University of California, San Diego,
La Jolla, California

MARIA TROZZI, M.Ed
Assistant Professor of Pediatrics, Boston University School of Medicine, Boston
Medical Center, Boston, Massachusetts

YVONNE E. VAUCHER, MD, MPH
Clinical Professor of Pediatrics and Director, Special Care Follow-Up Program,
University of California, San Diego, School of Medicine, San Diego, California

ROBERT D. WELLS, PhD
Associate Professor of Pediatrics and Psychiatry, University of California, San Francisco,
San Francisco, California

JOHN B. WELSH, MD*
Professor of Pediatrics, University of California, San Diego, San Diego, California

LYNDIA WILLIES–JACOBO, MD
Associate Professor of Pediatrics; Director, Pediatric Clerkship Program,
University of California, San Diego, La Jolla, California

---

*deceased

Foreword to the First Edition

This is a wonderful, timely book. Written for primary care practitioners who care for children and their families, it will meet an increasing need in pediatric care. At a time when the Task Force of the American Academy of Pediatrics has recommended a knowledge of child development for all pediatricians, when the American Nursing Association has developed a career for graduate nurses in primary care (the Pediatric Nurse Practitioner), and at a time when the public is for more support and guidance in parenting roles, the Committee on Psychosocial Development of Children and Families of the Academy of Pediatrics has published a series of guidelines for primary care physicians to enhance their attention to child and family development on routine visits to their caregiver. These guidelines are a help, but they need just such a volume as this to enhance their meaning and their value. The "lists" of items to be identified at these routine visits will be of no value to either pediatrician or targeted family unless they form a bridge for communication between the physician and parents and child. If the questions are asked simply as questions, the parents will feel bombarded by a new set of demands to answer in a relatively meaningless fashion. The already-too-pathological model of looking for and identifying failures in the parent will be made into a longer list by developmental questions aimed at looking for failure in the child and in the parent. If, on the other hand, with this textbook as a backdrop, the primary caregiver can participate in the enormous richness of the child's and parent's development as his or her area to share with families, he or she will feel the excitement of the developing child and family. If he or she can understand and participate in the emotional and cognitive development of the child as well as in his* physical development, the caregiver will feel the rewards of a deepening relationship with the parents in his or her care, for the child's development is the language of the parent. If the caregiver demonstrates a real understanding and gives a sense of caring for these aspects of the child's development, every parent will feel supported and cared for. In these days, new parents are no longer backed up by extended families, by strong cultural belief systems, or by support systems which are meaningful in the area about which they care the most—becoming a successful parent. As women must go to work (and over half of mothers of young children are in the work force now), their need for backup, for information, and for guidance in their precious job of childrearing is even greater. It is a time when we, as caring physicians and PNPs, can play a vital role in advocacy for the child and in enhancing the joy and assurance of the parenting role. Our opportunity to play a vital role in the family with attention to anticipatory guidance is out of proportion to the time and effort it will take from us. Each routine visit will become valued and valuable to us, as well as to parents. If we indeed transmit a sense of caring, of joining in each parent's job of parenting, we can establish rewarding roles for ourselves.

Having been in pediatric practice for 35 years now, I know that I personally would have "burned out" 25 years ago if I had not shared the child's development as a mutual goal with parents in my care. The quest for physical disease and for physical milestones is too sparse and unrewarding for most active minds at routine visits. They all too quickly become "routine." But the kind of shared knowledge and the kind of relationships with each family which this book will enhance at each visit can make the practice of primary care an act and a pleasure.

In Stein's chapter on interviewing, he displays the respect for children which underlies each subsequent chapter. He and Dixon give one a real sense of "how" to make and keep a working relationship with each set of parents at each visit. For it is within the context of relationships that a caregiver can be of any meaningful help to parents. Also, as the relationship deepens over time, the shared values deepen. I find that I no longer need to search for meaningful questions with the patients with whom I have developed a relationship. They bring me the important questions all too readily. Hence, each visit should be seen as an opportunity to strengthen and deepen the relationship between you and the parents. This is the reason why the child's development is such a critical ground for shared understanding.

Enhancing your relationship is also a reason for being sure that you hit "paydirt" in at least one area at each visit. You can recognize "paydirt," for the parent will lean forward, her face will become intense as her involvement with what you are saying becomes more and more obvious. I always try to be sure that I touch on one meaningful area for each parent and that I provide an opportunity for her (and him) to share the intensity of her own feelings as we approach such an area. With this concept of paydirt in mind, the concept of anticipatory guidance is a powerful one, because every parent will recognize her need for information and support you are offering as she approaches a new developmental phase in her child. If she can share her own feelings and anxiety with you as you share your developmental knowledge with her, you will be of real value to her.

Coincident with our capacity for conquering and preventing physical disease, we are becoming more sensitized to our capacity for the prevention of psychological disorders and for improving the quality of life for the children in our care. Prevention, intervention, and quality of life are becoming catchwords in pediatrics. Plasticity, the capacity of a developing organism to find pathways around a deficit or to recover from an insult, is a concept we can all utilize in pediatrics if we are aware of its forces and have a deeper understanding of its mechanisms in development. This book can provide such an understanding for pediatricians and for nurse practitioners.

The format of each chapter is economical and helpful. The theoretical base for the developmental processes which can be profitably addressed at each stage of development is excellent. The attention to deepening the relationship with parents and child is accompanied by specific questions which will help the practitioner. The section on what to observe, how to observe is followed by specific suggestions of how to share this with parents at each visit in infancy and toddlerhood. Sharing the developmental exam with parents is the most powerful way of achieving an effective working relationship to improve the child's outcome that I have found. I can then couch advice and anticipatory guidance without threat to our relationship or to the parent's feeling of competence because we have shared this mutually satisfying observation. I need this kind of communication at each visit. These chapters by Dixon, Stein, and Kaiser are rich in these values for all those involved in primary care.

Stein prepares us in the perinatal period for preventing the "vulnerable child syndrome." Dixon says "parents of premature infants are premature, too." Kaiser addresses the important issue of mothers dealing with sibling rivalry in the postpartum period. Each chapter addresses the cognitive and social progress of the child and the appropriate parental responses, which one can elicit at each well baby visit. The meaning and use of stranger anxiety at 8 months, of magic and fantasies in the third and fourth years are beautiful essays and should be read by all who are interested in small children.

Putnam and Nader address the issues of the preschool and school-aged child in the same valuable format. Pediatric practitioners will not only better understand the developmental issues, but the practical questions and observations of each area which should be addressed are clear and helpful.

Marianne Felice outlines the issues of preadolescence and adolescence for practitioners in a sympathetic way which will allow us to respect the adolescent's turmoil and need for privacy, but which will also help us to enhance our relationship with him and to address his issues in a straightforward, helpful manner. I find that adolescents with whom I've grown up are extremely grateful for my continued deep involvement with them. Although they may guard themselves from me from time to time, they use me in crises—drugs, sex, and other acting out periods—and remember my caring relationship later by bringing their own children to me. I now have more grandchildren than children in my practice. A real reward for all these years!

The last two chapters are as helpful as any in the book. The chapter on which books to have available by Felice, Caffery and Kaiser is very good. The marvelous chapter on children's drawings—their meaning and their use in enhancing a pediatrician's relationship with the parents—is by John Welsh, a pediatrician practicing for 35 years, and Susan Instone and Martin Stein. It is not only delightful but also insightful and wonderful in presenting a whole new system for communication for diagnostic work with children.

I wish I'd written this book, for it is sure to be a classic for pediatric practitioners. In their famous longitudinal study of the development of temperament, Thomas and colleagues found that the relationships of families with the observer pediatricians proved to be amazingly effective in alleviating potential psychological problems: 68% of the patients with mild or moderate symptoms improved markedly and 50% with real psychopathology improved with their team's preventive approach. I believe that pediatricians and pediatric nurse practitioners are in a unique position to provide the kind of relationship, insight, and therapeutic support which most parents will utilize to prevent disorders in their children. But pediatricians will need an understanding of normal development and of establishing supportive relationships in working with families to do that. This volume will go a long way toward providing that for primary caregivers.

T. Berry Brazelton, M.D.
Professor of Pediatrics
Harvard School of Medicine
Chief, Child Developmental Unit
Children's Hospital Medical Center
Boston, Massachusetts

BIBLIOGRAPHY

Brazelton TB: Anticipatory guidance. *Pediatr Clin North Am* 1975;22:553.
Brazelton TB: Developmental framework of infants and children: A future for pediatric responsibility. *J Pediatr* 1985;27:14.
Brazelton TB: Developmental framework of infants as an opportunity for early intervention for pediatricians. In Green M (ed): *The Psychosocial Aspects of the Family*. Skillman, NJ, Johnson and Johnson Publishers, Lexington Books, 0000 pp 53-65.
Committee on Psychosocial Development of Children and Families. *Guidelines for Health Supervision*. Evanston, Ill, American Academy of Pediatrics, 1985.
Thomas A, Chess S, Brick HG: *Temperament and Behavior Disorders in Children*. New York, University Press, 1968.

Preface

As much as things change, the more they stay the same.

The 4th edition of ***Encounters with Children: Pediatric Behavior and Development*** does bring much that is new. The developmental course of this text reflects the growth of this area of pediatric health care over the last quarter century. And that growth has been phenomenal. The scientific world of developmental psychology continues to flood us with new insights into infants, children and adolescents and we have been pleased to add these to all chapters as modifications and updates. The theoretical thinking from that core discipline has called for an expansion of the chapter dealing with theories and perspectives. These new insights give us an even broader understanding of the ways that children develop, strengthening our professional lives and our care of children.

The neurosciences have made major advances in helping us understand the brain/behavior interface so the reader will find much more from neurology in this edition, probably just the leading edge of all that will become known in the 21st century. We see a trend toward closer alignment between the behavioral and neurologic sciences and this volume moves in that direction.

We have responded to another trend as well: the populations we serve have become more culturally diverse and are likely to become even more so. One cannot be a good health care provider without a strong sense of culture and have considerable cultural competency. Our colleagues in anthropology, sociology and comparative psychology have given us more understanding of these core psychological dimensions that are at the heart of all children and families. This edition includes a whole chapter devoted to culture. This should add sparkle to practice by giving a framework in understanding this important aspect of families. It should add practice skills through providing both insights and management approaches to the challenges that culture adds to our lives. Child health professionals who work with diverse populations will find new insights about those families and about themselves—we all have a cultural dimension that shapes every action and interaction.

In addition, contemporary health issues that are mediated by behavioral issues are presented for all developmental ages. Exposure to violence, the omnipresence of media in children's lives and even the catastrophic events of 9/11/2001 have affected the life course for all. We have tried to give child health professionals ways to handle these issues as they present in practice, infused in several chapters and prominently in the chapter on stress and loss. We have also provided more direction on how to give parents resources, on the bookshelf, on the web and in the community. A health care office has become a community center of sorts, a place where parents go for direction. More is asked and more is expected of child health professionals these days. We have tried to help with that task by suggesting how to set up the office (See Chapter 3), what ideas to have available (See Chapter 28) and in all we do, how to be a source of guidance and direction.

Each chapter has two new features in this edition. Reflecting the suggestions of the residents, community pediatricians and academic faculty, we have added a "Quick Check" feature that is a brief listing of the main developmental milestones for the age in each chapter.

We have always resisted making professionals into check list technicians; we have always believed that professionals should have a professional level of knowledge and background on child development so that they can actually understand what they see in children every day. When we started writing this text (and perhaps even more today) there were too many stand alone check lists. We hope that the "Quick Check" provides a convenient review for the educated professional who still wants to understand in depth the main developmental processes of a given age, as presented in the main body of each chapter.

The other new feature is called "Heads Up". This helps the reader identify problems or high risk situations as they might present themselves at a given age. This is not meant to be a comprehensive presentation of developmental disability, behavioral pathology or mental health conditions; readers will need to look elsewhere to get that. This book remains an in-depth discussion of *normal child development*. However, this feature alerts the practitioner to concerns that require another look, another professional's input or further evaluation. Liken it to the shoulder bumps on a freeway that tell you that you are getting close to the edge, that you are off track.

But much has remained the same...

This is a book that teaches normal child development to the health care professional. The topics are not arranged with a theoretical, topical or historical point of view. Rather they have been shuffled to come out as they commonly occur during health supervision for children and adolescents. *When taken in its entirety, this is a full course in child development.* This volume allows our patients and our encounters with them to teach us what we as professionals need to know about those children, families, cultures and other influences on the lives of young people. This book allows the professional to set the stage to allow children to tell us what they are about, to prompt families to bring forward the issues and concerns they have, to get at the things that really matter to them. It allows the child health care professional to bring her knowledge in this area on a par with the other core sciences that touch pediatric practice.

If anything, the mandate to address issues of child development and mental health broadly has been strengthened significantly since the first edition of this book eighteen years ago. And the education of child health professionals in child development and behavior during residency training, in subspecialty fellowship and in continuing medical education courses has been increased over this interval. The first edition of **Encounters With Children; Pediatric Behavior and Development** required a big justification for the presentation of this material to clinicians; we had to do a lot of dancing to make the case for its publication. That is no longer the situation; no dancing was done for the 4th edition. Educational programs at all levels require inclusion of behavioral material and continuing education courses are oversubscribed. The hunger for more relevant material on child development is there; we hope this work satisfies that appetite. So the core ideas are here, pretty much unchanged from the 1st edition.

The target for this work is primarily the professional, in training and in clinical practice, in need of additional knowledge and skills in this area of pediatrics. Since adult learners, particularly clinicians, learn best from case examples, we have tried to strengthen this component of our work, with examples as they present in real clinical settings. With age comes experience so this was not hard to do for this edition. Some of these cases nail down a point of development, some illustrate the theme of the chapter and some highlight the complex crossroads of behavioral normalcy and pathology. We hope these clinical inserts will sustain and provide relevance for the reader through the text material that is the heart of the developmental discussion.

The children's drawings remain as a key element of this book. The children tell us what is on their minds through these drawings so we use them to reveal those thoughts and feelings throughout this book. We hope that readers will be enticed to use drawings in the same way in practice. The use of drawings sets up a wholly different dynamic—where children become important contributors to the visit, where psychological issues are clearly part of the territory of concern and where the clinician allows the issues to come from children and families. The chapter on the drawings has been moved forward as so many clinicians have found their use to be so valuable. The drawings have always served to illustrate the main developmental point of a chapter and they continue to do so. Readers have informed us that they remember a major theme or issue because they can recall the drawing that went with it. It was a struggle to get the drawings even included in the first edition (What kind of medical text has children's drawings?); now they are regarded as essential. Although the drawings do give this volume a lightness and, we hope, a sense of accessibility, we also hope that readers will see beyond the scribbles to the core of what children are about as they grow and develop.

Work with children and families should be fun and we hope that this book adds to a sense of delight, mystery and curiosity that that work brings to the child health professional. And that wish is the same as it always has been. We have been pleased to see this work grow and mature with time. This is the best edition ever.

Suzanne Dixon

Martin Stein

Acknowledgments

Many people have contributed to this work over the last 22 years and we are indebted to them and their contributions along the way. We are enriched by the insights they have given us. For this 4th edition we want to especially thank our wonderful colleagues, Drs. Lane Tanner and Pamela High. These two experienced teachers and scholars in this field gave us fresh insights and new ideas for this revision. We would also like to thank the anonymous residents and fellows who reviewed this work and gave us good direction for revision while providing us reassurance that this work is still helpful, easy to read and covers most bases for child health care professionals in training. We hope we have lived up to their expectations with this edition. We also appreciate the help of fellows—Drs. Eustratia Hubbard, Nerissa San Luis Bauer, and Yi Hui Liu—who assisted with the literature review, to be sure we are as up to date now as when we started lo these many years ago. Laura Lartch and Andi Baur assisted with manuscript preparation—we could not do without them. We appreciate the continuing support of Mary Caffery and Mike Hennessy. Finally to all the patients who have crossed our paths and taught us what child development is really all about—thanks. These encounters continue to intrigue, amaze and delight us.

Suzanne Dixon

Martin Stein

Contents

Encounters with
CHILDREN

Pediatric Behavior and Development

CHAPTER 1

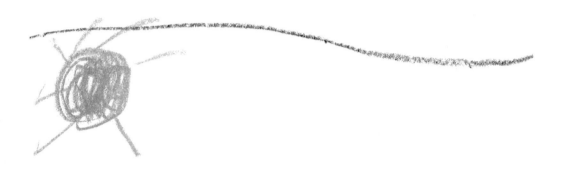

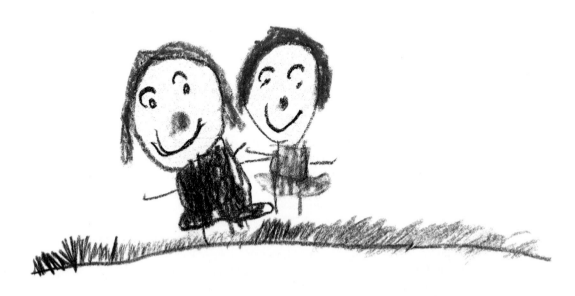

"Me and My Sister." By Meike Messick, age 6.

Perspectives on Child Development in Child Health Care

SUZANNE D. DIXON and MARTIN T. STEIN

This book is about normal child development. It presents material on the usual course of child, adolescent and family development across the age ranges seen by child health care providers. Because surveillance of a child's development is a vital part of pediatric health care, it is important to have a foundation in what is expected, what the range of typical development is and what can be done to support development. The book seeks to lay out the foundation for that work. It is a course in normal child development and behavior for clinicians who care for children. As child health care professionals, we think that clinicians should have a basic understanding of normal developmental processes.

This course is presented in a manner not seen in the usual texts of developmental psychology, where material is presented in a topical format. In this work, the topics are arranged as they usually come up in the practice of pediatric medicine. Although a child's development evolves along several dimensions at any one time, we have found that some strands of development emerge as prominent at particular, predictable times. The immediate clinical relevance of a topic allows the clinician to review the full range of a specific developmental theme across the ages. The foundations of the developmental process that have occurred earlier and the anticipated rollout of this process in the future are reviewed at each stage in the context of this specific developmental theme. This expanded discussion of a topic allows the clinician to see the matter in context, to see how it changes over time. It also allows for a review of the theoretical and research background that is relevant to the topic. As one goes through the entire book, a full course in child development is presented in a way that is relevant to the child health care provider.

For readers interested in pursuing even more in-depth knowledge of child development, we would recommend one of several general texts that have been used in the writing of this volume, listed at the end of this chapter. Other "classic" writings in child development and behavior are found in the Appendix (Section III). We would also encourage learners of every age and stage of professional development to access texts that look at developmental disabilities, psychopathology, neurological problems and behavioral concerns. This book provides prompts at the end of each chapter, under the "Heads Up" feature, to be aware of clinical clues in order to recognize early signs of delay and problems at particular ages. It is beyond the scope of this book to provide detailed discussions of pathology. However, we hope to provide the reader with solid grounding in what is normal so that pediatric counseling and anticipatory guidance can be carried out with a strong knowledge base and problems can be recognized and evaluated at an early stage.

The material in this book is designed to create an internal map of normal child development, with its multiple themes and overlapping processes. This task would be daunting were it not for the ability of individual children and families to so eloquently lay out these processes as they evolve and change over time. The mental map is built on the learning that can occur at each health care visit. By reading a chapter before an office visit and then seeing a child and family at a particular age, the clinician builds a full picture of the developmental processes over time. These new encounters can then be met with an in-depth understanding of how development is progressing in a particular child.

Child development is a foundation of child health care. The importance of evaluating developmental changes over time distinguishes pediatric medicine from adult health care. We believe that professionals delivering child health care should have knowledge in this area on a par with other sciences that touch their work. This text allows the clinician to lay the foundation for knowledge of child development in the course of practice, clinical encounter by clinical encounter. In this book, the science has been repackaged so that each visit opens up new information and perspective at a time when a particular developmental or behavioral theme is prominent, important to the family and easy to see in the child. When the foundation is set, the clinician is ready to take on parental concerns, problems, observed deviations from typical development and the issues of children and families in unusual circumstances.

We do not think it sufficient or even advisable to work from checklists of milestones, to council families from rote lists of guidance points or to see children in a normal/not normal dichotomy. That approach is not professional, and we would hope to avoid fostering this mentality in clinicians in training and practice. A broader perspective on a child sets the clinician up for a more educated and enlightened approach to the work of everyday practice. Checklists can be used, either mailed ahead of time or presented for completion at check-in, and reviewed by office personnel (see Appendix for examples of checklists). This practice will free up time for identifying the real concerns of families, for seeing the developmental processes unfold and for providing individualized guidance and support. In this edition, each chapter ends with a brief list of achievements that we expect to see at a given age, the "Quick Check" feature. We hope that this is not the focus of the visit, but rather a quick refresher of specific elements of developmental issues at that age. The educated clinician will have more knowledge and understanding of these items through thoughtful reading and synthesis of the expanded discussions of topics found in that or other chapters. This list of expected achievements should just jog the memory on topics not specifically discussed in the chapter.

The everyday encounters with children and parents in pediatric medicine offer a course in child development. All of us, young and old, experienced or on our first clinical rotation, can learn from each patient who comes in the door. Through focused observations, questions and a few interactions, a child will teach us what we need to know. Aiming these clinical probes correctly allows for easy access to understanding what a child and family are about. It also guides us in our understanding of and responses to a parent's main concerns at a particular age. This approach allows for a very efficient learning process, one that stays with us as the concepts and theories become real when we see them in the behavior of a child or the questions of a family. The format of this book allows the clinician to immediately apply the lessons learned to the laboratory of real practice and thus easily and painlessly develop a solid understanding of normal child development. Only then will the clinician be ready to evaluate problems, deviations and distortions of these processes.

The presentations of developmental skills and behavior at each age are necessarily short. Busy clinicians cannot devote the time to wade through volumes of source material; we've done that for them. Each chapter is a condensation of the large body of material that exists in the worlds of developmental psychology, psychiatry, developmental and behavioral pediatrics and, to some extent, neurology, public health and counseling. In the type, length, format and relevance of material, we have kept the child health care professional in mind. Adults learn best by real case examples and real life application. This text is designed to foster that type of learning.

Every chapter presents material on the child's environment, both physical and interpersonal. This is the proper territory for involvement of the child health care clinician because this interface, between the child and his surroundings, is where developmental change occurs. The old models of the child marching along in a preset course of development, unaffected by environmental conditions, have been completely debunked. New models see the child's development intricately evolving through the interaction between the child and the whole of his environment. It's not a question of nature or nurture as the prominent force in development. It's "all of the above"—what George Engle called "the biopsychosocial framework for development through the life cycle."

The child's nature plays a great role in how he acts on his world and how his world responds to him. Conversely, the very architecture of the child's brain is altered by his experiences. Early events determine a child's response to subsequent stressors, adverse events and even successes. Because of this interplay of forces that fuel the developmental processes, the job of the clinician is located at the crossroads of these forces. Summarizing the complexities of the developmental processes as we know them in the 21st century, Shonkoff and Phillips present us with the scope of our work as clinicians—"from neurons to neighborhoods." Care is not comprehensive if the scope of surveillance is not this broad. Intervention and guidance will not be effective unless they go across this whole gamut. New work on the complexity of brain development only intensifies the mandate to look at a child's environment carefully. Part of this book's goals are to lay out ways to look at the child in context, with precision, direction and focus.

BASIC TENETS

The following perspectives guide this work and inform the clinician as one approaches a child and family.

- **Most children are normal.** Although this statement is statistically obvious, clinicians are often so trained to look for abnormality that they rarely embrace the fact that *most children most of the time are developing broadly within the expected range.* However, without a solid grounding in exactly what is normal at a given age and around a specific theme, there is a danger of one of two extremes: either becoming too glib and blasé in one's approach to a situation or seeing every little variation as a disorder. Neither approach is healthy. The first is demeaning to a family and usually means that the clinician doesn't have a clue as to what's up. The second is a negative model that isn't what families want or need. Even within the range of normal development there are hurdles, problems, concerns and individual differences that have a serious impact on a child and family. It is at these junctures that the child health care clinician can be of tremendous help in providing support and guidance for families. We believe we have the chance to support optimal development for each child through recognition of strengths within a normal range of expectations. If you start from an assumption of normalcy but then look at the individual issues, you are most likely to be on target for the families you serve. If you only look for disease, you will rarely find it, you will miss most of what people want from you and your clinical encounters will be very sterile. There is wondrous individuality to unravel in every normal child, and there is a story to discover in every normal family.

- **Most unusual behavior is understandable.** Virtually all unusual behavior is both explainable and adaptive if one sees beyond the behavior to the core issues confronting a child and family and to the context in which such behavior occurs. This tenet is based on the premise that *behavior has meaning and it is up to the clinician to discover what that behavior is saying about the child and the family.* Even the most unusual behavior usually has some adaptive worth and persists in the child and family because there is some benefit derived from it. The clinician should be intrigued to discover those adaptive forces that merge with developmental processes in a given circumstance. They often have their origins in cross-cultural differences, temperament differences in the child and family and social stressors of a variety of types. Children do what they can to get what they need from their environment, even if their behavior seems strange on surface review. Unusual behavior often supports and reflects resiliency in children growing up in challenging circumstances. A solid grounding in normal development and a review of the child's physical and interpersonal environments will lead to an explanation of what at first seems strange or even bizarre.

- **Most families do their best for their children within their own range of resources. They will make good decisions if they have knowledge, skills, empathy and support.** No matter the situation, parents around the globe want their children to do well and apply whatever resources they have to forward that agenda. These include not only physical resources but also knowledge, their individual life experiences, the support systems available to them and the cultural understanding of what a good parent is and what good child rearing is. Child priorities are lined up with other family and personal demands on attention and energy. If bad choices are made, they usually have their origin in poor information, reduced energy or resources or failure to appreciate the child's needs and perspectives. Although a very few families purposely do harm to their children, most try their best, sometimes in the face of amazing adversity. With this perspective, the clinician positions himself as an ally, not an adversary to the family. With an analysis of what is missing in the situation, intervention is no longer simplified or standardized advice. This is a level of professionalism that goes beyond a cookbook approach to advice and counsel. The clinician can be a source of information, an interpreter of the child's needs and behavior or an observer of the child's strengths. He can mobilize resources that are lacking and can coach a family over the tough spots. With a shared goal of what is the best for the child, a therapeutic alliance is set in place. The specifics are then negotiated in the context of a shared commitment to a given child.

- **Development is not an even process.** Developmental progress is one of gains and plateaus in one area. Then another area becomes the prominent issue. Forward progression in one area may be accompanied by a seeming short-term decline in another. Periods of plateau are not ones of lack of progress but are times of consolidation and refinement

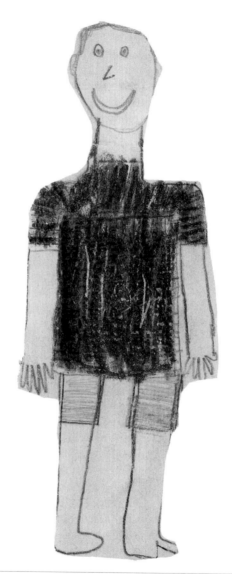

"A self portrait." By Neil Hennessy, age 8 (original in pencil and red and blue crayon).

of skills. The big shifts seem to be triggered by predictable neurological maturation that sets the child up to act on the environment in a new and exciting way. Child development is more like climbing a series of peaks rather than ascending one big mountain. Some skills seem to fall into place overnight, whereas other gains are made one baby step at a time. A linear mentality will make the clinician confused over the expected ups and downs in watching children mature. An undulating, interweaving model is more appropriate and, in fact, more interesting.

- **A child's approach to life and its challenges has some remarkable consistencies.** Temperamental differences have a profound effect on how an individual child approaches developmental work. Some children charge ahead and have lots of falls; others are cautious and thoughtful. The way that a child weaves the developmental processes together into his own story is almost more interesting than the story itself. We hope that this book inspires clinicians to look at and enjoy variation in development—the "how," not just the "what." *To be comfortable with variation, however, one must know the boundaries of normal.* In a long-term relationship with a family, one can see the different ages of a specific temperamental profile. The colicky baby becomes the toddler sleep problem, becomes the preschool dropout and eventually becomes the argumentative captain of the debate team! It is also fun to see how the personality and traits of family members show up in children. These family tapestries are woven over time and admirably decorate our clinical practice. Marvel and enjoy.

- **Developmental gains in a child always have a cascade effect on the family and the child's environment.** With each new skill, the child's view of himself and his effect on the world changes. His sense of himself is changed, and he becomes somewhat of a new child to those around him. Changes in care are needed to keep pace with this new and improved version of the child. These shifts can be unanticipated, painful and sometimes not even recognized. The clinician's role is to anticipate the change and identify what the new abilities will mean and what alterations in care will be required. This is real anticipatory guidance, beyond the checklist. For example, when a child is sitting comfortably, you know that mobility is not far behind because he is mapping the space around him and getting ready to go. He will need room to roam and a big review of safety around the house. He will start to get anxious about separations as he understands coming and going a lot better. He will soon demand more of a role in feeding. This means that the placid, quiet, just-feed-me-and-sleep-me baby is gone and a new energetic infant has come on the scene. The ripple effect is that the parents need to be a different kind of parent for this "new" infant.

- **Children will do their own developmental assessment if you just give them a chance.** Children always practice the leading edge of their developmental competency, work at an emerging or newly acquired skill and delight in a toy or activity that is just a little new and challenging. Through knowledge of developmental sequences, a wise clinician will set up toys or ask questions aimed at that developmental edge. The office visit should be orchestrated so that the assessment occurs automatically, seemingly incidentally through the process of checking in, weighing, measuring, playing in the waiting room and being observed in the exam room. The clinician should lay the agenda, set the stage and then let the drama unfold. With this proactive, playful and easy approach, rich information is gathered with no extra time or ongoing effort. However, this process depends on the clinician knowing what to look for, what to ask and what simple maneuvers can be done quickly with a child and family.

- **Developmental surveillance is the foundation of each health supervision visit.** It can be easy if one knows what is likely to be the biggest developmental or behavioral issue for the child and family and then sets things up to demonstrate or monitor these processes. Surveillance is not exhaustively testing each child but rather providing professional oversight to the developmental sequences as they unfold. By setting things up, the child with provide all the raw material for that surveillance. Children who are not ill, hungry or distressed will readily engage in what you do with them.

- **Parents almost always know what a child can do if asked.** This is true even if they do not always volunteer such information or may not be aware of its significance. A parent's recall of development and behavior is very poor except for broad milestones such as walking. That means that parents need to be asked in an ongoing manner about the new changes in their child, and these new changes need to be recorded at this time. The record needs to be accurate, robust and individual. That's where the clinician comes in. This book lays out those sequences—what to observe, what to ask and what type of anticipatory guidance is appropriate at a specific time in development. There is no need to bore yourself or the child or waste time with "old hat" activities. Ask about newly acquired skills and follow with some carefully honed activities. Use what is known about developmental sequences to make focused inquiries and expand them up or down, depending on the parent's response. Alternatively, use parent questionnaires BEFORE the visit to get parental input and identify concerns.

   The targeted child assessment, along with a focused history, is completed in a few minutes. Trainees often ask how we get children to do specific things with blocks or with paper and pencil. They act as though it is a miracle when a child demonstrates exactly what they are supposed to do. Perhaps it is a miracle, but it is one that can be reliably repeated. A knowledge of child development allows us to be efficient and even downright lazy as we get the child and family to do all the work.

- **Interventions have to be built on strengths, not deficits.** A good intervention starts with an appraisal of positives, as well as concerns. Every visit offers the opportunity to better the lives of a child and family, so every visit is an intervention. If there is a specific concern, the process is one of building a program, an intervention or a change in the child's care or education. *Lining up assets and deficits is a place to begin, and communication with parents is fueled by the asset column.* The strengths will allow a child to get around barriers. It is also a way to put energy into a situation so that changes can be made by the child, the family or others who have an impact on the outcome. For example, a shy, physically awkward, but bright boy can be part of the basketball team as the keeper of statistics while having his own "personal trainer" (read adaptive physical education teacher) work with him separately. His abilities give him a meaningful social role while his deficits are addressed in another way. An artistic child with poor verbal skills can do her school project as an art presentation rather than as a long written report.

   Words used to describe children can be an intervention in themselves, and they can be both positive and accurate. With a positive perspective and optimistic tone, a family can hear what can be done to assist their own individual child.

- A talkative child can also be called sociable.
- An active child can be energetic.
- An irritable infant can be labeled sensitive.
- A hypotonic infant can be described as overly relaxed.
- A withdrawn child can be called shy.

The clinician can then proceed to describe what she thinks needs to be done to support that child so that he will be successful. This does not mean ignoring problems or glossing over concerns. It does mean reframing them so that there is respect for the child and family and motivation to face the issues together. This approach gets one farther down the road.

- **Child health care should be fun.** Although we all confront horrendous disease and miserable circumstances for children and families, our regular work should overall be fun. It stays in that realm if we continually marvel at the exciting development of children, the way they and their families overcome obstacles and the incredible adaptability of children and families. Watching these processes and seeing children grow and develop in individual ways should add delight to one's practice. Clinicians who get overwhelmed with the mounds of paperwork, the restrictions in practice we all experience these days and the continual pressure to do more for less need to change perspective. Through setting the agenda for each visit, setting up an office with a developmental focus and really connecting with families without hiding behind forms and checklists, the clinician can claim back some of the excitement of pediatric practice. This book teaches health care providers how to have fun as well as do a better job for their patients and families.

There is a real danger of child health care clinicians becoming technicians whose success is measured by their immunization records, complete review of systems and compliance with form completion and other non–patient care tasks. We think that the profession and patients are ill served by this technical approach. This book allows one to have a professional perspective on the overall well-being of the patients seen and the families met. We hope that those in training and in practice will take this opportunity to keep a broad perspective on the developmental forces that move children forward and require their families to change and adapt. This perspective should make practice not only more professional but also more intellectually satisfying. Being less bound by lists and guided more by an understanding of child development and family needs, one can have the freedom to determine the agenda of each encounter and set the stage to evaluate the really important issues affecting a child and family.

This book, then, is a guide for learning normal child development and a guide for clinical practice. It is meant to be useful for learning one of the vital basic sciences of pediatric health care and to be a guide for adding behavioral and developmental depth of knowledge to the practice of pediatric medicine. It provides the matrix onto which one guides developmental surveillance. It is a roadmap to allow one, from personal experience, to learn the principles of pediatric behavioral medicine, build a matrix of developmental expectation and understand the patients and families one encounters each day in child health care.

RECOMMENDED READINGS

Berk L: *Child Development*, 6th ed. Boston, Allyn & Bacon, 2003.
Cole M, Cole S: *The Development of the Child*, 4th ed. New York, Worth Publishers, 2001.
Shonkoff JP, Phillips D (eds): *From Neurons to Neighborhoods: The Science of Early Child Development*. Washington, DC, National Academy Press, 2000.

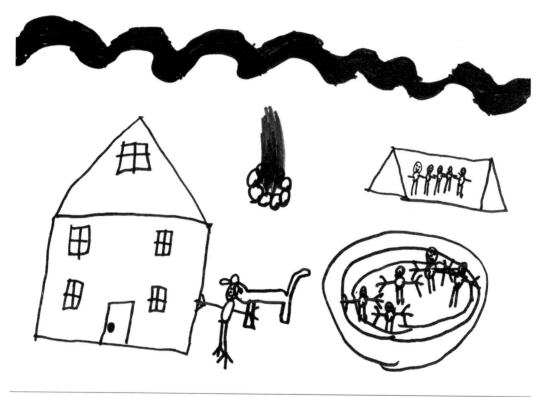

"My family outside." By David Betts, age 11.

CHAPTER 2

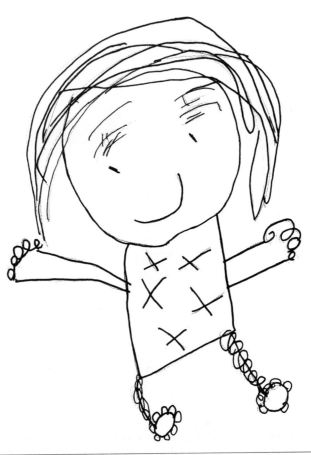

A girl shows her exuberant sense of self. By Dori Dedmom, age 6.

Understanding Children: Theories, Concepts and Insights

SUZANNE D. DIXON

This chapter presents the major theoretical perspectives on child development that contribute to our understanding of children. The major points of each theory, their enduring features and areas where each is most applicable are presented. The thinkers, experimenters and clinicians who have shaped our understanding are named within their own schools of thought. This chapter educates the health care provider on the basic lines of thinking that give us established and emerging insights into the development of children.

> *There is nothing as useful as a good theory.*
> KURT LEWIN

Systematic study of the behavior and development of children began its period of tremendous growth in the 19th century and is flourishing today as an area of rich scientific inquiry and research. Although all cultural and even religious traditions have harbored a distinct view of children and how to raise them, these folk theories are currently augmented by observations in natural settings and the laboratory and by the thoughtful reasoning of a now large gallery of eminent thinkers. We know more about children than ever before and the wealth of information is growing exponentially. Moreover, like the child himself, this theoretical bedrock of our understanding of our work with children is always changing and developing. This chapter presents the major, enduring theoretical perspectives that have shaped our views of the child. These perspectives provide insights for our everyday encounters with them. You can expect that these perspectives will evolve, will be modified or even debunked. So why bother with this theoretical stuff at all?

First, the science of child development is a core science that touches our professional lives. It is imperative that we have a professional level of knowledge of this science, just as we do in genetics or pathophysiology. The major theoretical perspectives add a high level of understanding of those we work with every day. It is amazing to me that as the discipline of child development has marched on, the training of most child health care professionals in this area remains elementary. We should know more and we should be familiar with these perspectives, both the classic and the new. **Theories allow us to think about behavior, family interactions and new achievements and to then make sense of them.**

13

Second, the theoretical insights do for us what they are generally designed to do: **organize observations**. With theoretical perspectives on a child, we are helped to organize the seemingly random or chance behavior of a child into recognizable patterns. When we have a view of what a child is up to broadly from a developmental perspective, small behaviors, incidental observations and expected and unexpected responses all become recognizable units of data that help us broadly in our understanding of a child and his family. Rather than be over-whelmed by the behavior and development of children, a theoretical framework will add some explanatory foundation, as well as some interest and delight to our work lives. With a strong theoretical framework, a clinician can make use of every behavior, every action and every inter-action with a child to gather and use data.

Anticipatory guidance becomes easy when we really understand what will come next and why. Developmental surveillance becomes a professional matter of monitoring the progression of expected events rather than the technical job of just checking off items on a list. These days, our clinical encounters are foreshortened, often pressured and stuffed to the gills with required components and paperwork. By having a big picture of what development is all about, we can maintain a high level of awareness of the core issues of our patients. When we encounter an unusual or troublesome behavior, we can be intrigued by what it means rather than be derailed by what it does to our schedule. An understanding of theoretical frameworks allows us to explain and intervene for a child and family that need us. We cannot do efficient work with excellence if we do not have the mental structures to make use of every bit of data in front of us. **Theories make us better observers and better thinkers.**

However, thinkers need help to put ideas and observations together. Theories on the development of children support our thinking processes by grouping behavior into manage-able packages to remember and to guide further observations. Accordingly, if I observe a child having a tantrum, I see that as part of the greater process of acquiring independence, so it is logical that other behavior may reflect this process, such as food refusal and sleep resistance. I can ask the right questions, provide guidance that anticipates these bumps in parenting and frame it all as normative and not pathological. I can also generate additional observations based on what I see as the organizing theme of the child's behavior. We can tie up packages of observations about a child to give them meaning and cohesiveness for our own thinking and that of families.

Organization of the facts and observations along with the guidance that such organization provides for further inquiry is a basic function of a theory for scientists working in research on the development of children. **As professionals we should be informed consumers of that research** so that familiarity with its foundation will better prepare us for that job. We will see the understanding of children grow over our professional lives, so a sense of the theoretical foundations for these investigations will put the hypotheses, the methods, the language and the conclusions of research reports into some mental structure. The important words that have entered the lexicon of child development from each theoretical perspective are shown here in italics. It is imperative that as health professionals we not be left behind as new insights are made by the allied scientists who study children.

There are a few special points that the reader should know about theories. First, theories come out of cultures, a time in history and even the political milieu in which they were born; they reflect all these factors to some degree. They are also often put forward by individuals who have a personal history that comes to bear on their intellectual work. The lives of these personalities make fascinating reading and should be considered part of the evaluation of the theory. (The major names in developmental theory are printed in bold here.) Second, new theories evolve not so much by building on the past but by challenging the old through highlighting the discrepancies and deficiencies in current thought and then proposing alternatives. This is why we see big shifts in thinking over time, with most perspectives mellowing under the harsh light of scrutiny and with the forces of the antagonistic views challenging those perceptions. I have tried to distill the enduring aspects of each school of thought, even if orthodox adherence to that theory is no longer common. They all have left us a legacy of understanding some aspect or characteristic of the child. Finally, few theories claim to give us all the answers on all aspects of development or claim to explain all types of behavior. Typically, theories focus on one area and spend only passing reference to other areas. So some aspects of the child are more readily explained than others are. Generally, as consumers of this work we should look where the light is shining from each perspective and use it if makes some sense.

When reading through this chapter, evaluate how each school of thought addresses four prime questions as conceptualized by Patricia Miller:

- **What is the basic nature of the child?** Is the child a rational scientist or a very irrational package of reflexes or emotions? Is the child an individual evolving pretty much on his own or is he merely a part of the fabric of a culture, a family? Is he like a machine, a plant, a computer, a whirling spiral or a thread in a tapestry? Why is a child's behavior so different from that of adults?

- **Is development quantitative or qualitative?** Does the child grow by adding new skills, becoming just more of what he was? Or does he make substantial, fundamental shifts in his capabilities and become something different than he was before? Are there stages in development or is it linear or just lines with more connections as in a network?

- **What is the balance of nature versus nurture?** What is primary in the force of developmental change, the child internally or the environment externally? Although no one takes polarized positions on this issue anymore and even the nature/nurture question itself is outmoded, differing theories add weight to one side of this equation over the other.

- **What develops?** This has to do with the level of analysis and the type of observations used to develop and test these theories. Is it cells in the nervous system or systems of reinforcement in the environment? To use The Institute of Medicine report's phrase: "Is it the neurons or the neighborhoods that are the unit of change? Is it brain modules or the processes that connect them? Is it cognition or emotions? Thinking or behavior?"

Universals

If there are a few universals we know about children that are endorsed by most developmentalists, they can be summarized as follows:

- **Children are active participants in their own development, at some level and in some or many ways.** Children are not passive recipients of nurturance but take what they need from the environment and do what they need to do to move themselves ahead. There is an internal drive to master the world, the challenges of life and the barriers that come up.

- **Children are inherently self-regulating.** They respond to stress, change, upheaval, the demands of the environment and their own maturation by getting back in balance. They are seen as learning new skills, handling emotions and altering their course if required. They can be expected to work at resolving discrepancies and crises in their views of the world, minimizing emotional pain and getting what they need from the environment by drawing on internal and external resources.

These two themes, which should spark both respect and trust for the child, should be guiding ones for the clinician.

As clinicians, we don't have to (and shouldn't, in my view) subscribe wholly to any one theoretical perspective. We can pick and choose what seems to fit for a given child at a given time and in a given area. This eclectic approach, however, requires that we have a solid grounding in the science so that our application is neither random nor glib. Throughout this volume, we have tried to highlight the perspectives that seem salient to the age and event before us as examples of this flexible approach.

We can draw on all the rich insights available to us to give our work professionalism, perspective, focus, interest and amazement as children become at once predictable and totally surprising as individuals.

MATURATIONAL THEORY–NORMATIVE APPROACH

Proponents of the maturational theory regard development as the inevitable unfolding of events determined internally by the forces of genetics and the neuromaturational processes that the genes direct. Development comes from within. This perspective began in the 18th century but flowered under **G. Stanley Hall** and his student **Arnold Gesell** working at Yale University in the early to mid-20th century. This perspective is most familiar to child health care professionals because it runs parallel to our understanding of embryology, developmental physiology and physical growth. It is also the perspective that underlies much of the traditional, often rudimentary material on child development that was presented in school and training, where the focus was on milestones and norms being on time or delayed. In this model, development depends entirely on neurological and physical maturation, and it proceeds in fixed sequences. The child is seen as an immature or incomplete organism that moves in predictable patterns of behavior during the course of continuous maturation. It is a linear model, with development seen as quantitative gains in competencies. The concept of cephalocaudal progression of development originated here; for example, control of the head comes before control of the legs. These theorists gave us extensive data on the normative course of specific developmental competencies and provided the earliest and most enduring standards for expectations of typical development. Although these milestones and age norms have been modified slightly over time, the sequences still ring true. They form the core for most developmental tests currently in use. Classification of children as delayed, deviant or normal based on varying rates of emergence of specific skills follows from these observations. The child's place in the continuum in comparison with that of his age-mates is the basis for a diagnostic formulation.

From the maturational perspective, the child's environment is seen as having an impact in a subordinate way; it may have a detrimental impact and impede the developmental sequence. Temperament and individuality are acknowledged, but not specified. Gesell's concept of internal readiness for a task has endured in the child care advice that began with Gesell but has influenced **Benjamin Spock's**, **T. Berry Brazelton's** and others' perspectives to the present. Gesell saw babies as inherently self-regulating and self-righting, progressing from periods of imbalance and instability to new levels of organization as they acquired new abilities. Very little depended on parents; they were supposed to step back, marvel and follow the child's lead. Gesell's books guided much of child-rearing practice in the mid-20th century.

Today we retain the norms of expected development in children that were built on this theoretical framework, but no one now weighs in on the extreme view that nature alone determines development. The powerful role of the environment has been identified. We now know that learning and teaching affect behavior and experience and even shape brain architecture. Furthermore, the discontinuities in developmental processes, abrupt shifts in competencies and new abilities that seem to appear without an antecedent basis are all at odds with orthodox maturational models. Much of the complexity and variability in development is left unexplained by this model. Gesell's norms were based on upper–middle-class U.S. children and need modification when applied in other contexts. We now know that newborns are more competent than they are formulated to be in this perspective and that much of the richness of toddler cognitive development was not appreciated by this school. Affective and cognitive development is not adequately addressed in this model. The major contribution of maturational theory stems from the valuable norms that it has provided for the systematic observation of development in children. We still need and use these norms today. We will see this application most clearly in the chapters on motor development (Chapters 12 and 14). Gesell's own perspective that babies are inherently "wise," being the depository of millions of years of evolutionary adaptations, is an important perspective for the clinician and parent alike (Box 2–1).

BOX 2–1   KEY INSIGHTS–MATURATIONAL THEORIES

- Children develop along fixed sequences, a continuum of developmental gains.
- Development is determined primarily by internal factors controlled by genes.
- We can characterize children as following a typical, accelerated or slowed course of development when compared with large population norms.
- Rates of development vary by individual but the sequence does not.
- Behavioral change is linked to physical maturation.
- Children must have an inner readiness to perform a task for teaching to be effective.
- Children have inherent abilities to self-regulate in terms of sleeping, eating, activity and engagement.
- Children are "wise" because they carry thousands of years of evolutionary adaptiveness.
- Appropriate child rearing is responsive to the individual child, not as predetermined by adult care providers.

PSYCHOSEXUAL THEORY: FREUD AND FOLLOWERS

Sigmund Freud made a significant contribution to our understanding of personality development through his retrospective observations and thoughtful theoretical formulations. He drew our attention to the consequences in later life of early childhood experience and the centrality of emotional life in shaping personality. This model emphasizes the importance of both unconscious and conscious mental processes that shape development and influence behavior. A person's self-concept results from the interface of the child's inner needs (*biological drives and instincts*) with the demands of the external world around him (*social expectations*), which are viewed as conflicting.

The three parts of personality were described as the *id* (housing the basic drives and instincts), the *ego* (the aware and rational self), which develops in late infancy and toddlerhood, and the *superego* (the conscience), which emerges from ages 3 to 6. The way these components are integrated and function in concert in early childhood determines the individual's ability to function over the long term.

Each stage in life revolves around the resolution of a particular "*psychosexual tension or conflict*," with sexual meaning centered on one body area in any given stage. Infancy is the *oral stage* (when the sensations of sucking and feeding and then biting are central to the child), and toddlerhood is the *anal stage* (when the pleasures and pains of eliminating or withholding are experienced). The 4- to 6-year-old period is the *phallic or oedipal stage,* when interest in the genitals and the relationship with one's parents take on a sexualized tone. Grade-schoolers are in the *latency stage,* when sexual feelings are said to go quiet, and adolescents are in the *genital stage,* with renewed interest in sexual activity. Most importantly, all stages involve the changing relationship with one's parents. The ability to form relationships with others is determined in part by the nature of these primary interactions.

Successful *resolution of specific inner conflicts* at each stage leaves the child ready for a new level of emotional and social maturity. Freud was the first to introduce the concept of distinct stages in development. His model is like a staircase, not linear. He viewed the source of mental illness as an outgrowth of developmental failure, not moving along satisfactorily to the next stage. Disruptions or abnormalities at a specific stage (e.g., anal) are seen as the basis for psychological conflict (e.g., obsessive behavior) that continues into adult life, when it results in unresolved anxiety (*neuroses*) or major psychological disturbances (*psychoses*).

Psychoanalytic theory was built from adult memories and observations, a clinical approach; it has not been submitted to experimental testing. This perspective has been described as having an inherent cultural, historical and perhaps male bias. Few adhere to the original, strict formulations, but Freudian thinking (as well as his words) has profoundly influenced our views on development and behavior (Box 2–2). Analytic thinking provided the fundamental insight on the development of self-concept and sexuality (as discussed in Chapter 18) and on the struggles for independence in the toddler and teen years (Chapters 15, 22, 23 and 24).

NEO-FREUDIANS

Following Freud, other important thinkers emerged and provided additional insights. **Margaret Mahler** and her colleagues taught us that a child's mental and physical relationship with his mother gradually moves from one of total *symbiosis* (as in pregnancy) to independence through a series of stages in the first 3 years of life. These predictable landmarks of emotional development allow for the child's increasingly solid sense of self as an individual. These processes of *separation and individuation* become increasingly complex with time. Chapters 15 and 16 on the toddler years draw on this construct.

BOX 2–2   KEY INSIGHTS–PSYCHOSEXUAL THEORIES

- Development occurs in distinct stages that vary by the drives and interests to be mastered in the service of meeting social expectations.
- Emotional life has a powerful influence on behavior and development.
- Emotions, dreams, disappointment, feelings and frustrations matter.
- Unconscious processes shape behavior, concurrent and ongoing.
- Interactions between parent and child influence personality, resiliency, adjustment and behavior into adulthood.
- Children do have an active mental life even before the emergence of speech.
- This mental life contributes to the child's adjustment both during childhood and later in life.
- Unconscious wishes and thoughts influence both present and future behavior, thus making it imperative when assessing behavior to look at the child's history, particularly his emotional past.
- Psychological growth is prompted by a moderate degree of frustration.
- The child's interpersonal experience with loved ones, most often his parents, is central to his overall adjustment and functioning.

Freud's daughter, **Anna Freud**, extended psychoanalytic thinking to specific observations of young children. Using individual play therapy and studies of orphan children, she conceptualized *"lines of development"* based on psychosexual theory. Examples of developmental maturation in this context are maturation from dependency to adult relationships, from sucking to rational eating, from egocentricity to companionship and from play to work.

Erik Erikson broadened and extended Freudian theory to include the whole life cycle. He brought in the influence of society beyond the family in determining the outcome of each developmental stage. His *psychosocial stages* are shown in Table 2–1. Each stage is characterized by negotiation of one central issue that is necessary for emotional advancement to the next

TABLE 2–1   Erikson's Stages of Development

Stage	Age	Issue
1	Birth–18 mo	Trust vs. mistrust
2	18 mo–3 yr	Autonomy vs. shame and doubt
3	3–6 yr	Initiative vs. guilt
4	6–11 yr	Industry vs. inferiority
5	Adolescence	Identity vs. role confusion
6	Young adulthood	Intimacy vs. isolation
7	Adulthood	Generativity vs. stagnation
8	Old age	Ego integrity vs. despair

stage. Variation in these stage-locked tasks through the forces of culture, family, individual differences and the changing demands of society makes it widely applicable. Erikson's theory extends through adulthood and highlights some of the generic issues confronting parents as part of their own development. Erikson believed that "the child can be trusted to obey the inner laws of development." Under this umbrella, child rearing calls for child responsiveness rather than a prescriptive process. These Ericksonian broad themes can help us step back from specific issues or types of behavior that are brought to our attention clinically. If we see what the child's "big job" is at that stage, we can often find a way out of an immediate dilemma.

Kari, age 5, was always the object of her mother's annoyance. Everything in her room was a mess, and when she was given an order to clean it up, the task was overwhelming. She just left it and skipped out. Her mother asked advice about this, saying that she worried about what would happen in adolescence if obedience was such a problem now.

The clinician asked Kari why she didn't clean up her room. Kari said it was "too much." Through a system of baskets, breaking the task down to manageable units ("now pick up all the blocks") and a series of rewards for a job well done, Kari and her mom got along much better. Kari proudly brought in her star chart of successes at the next visit. Initiative replaced guilt when she was able to be successful. Initiative wins out without conflict.

In the Ericksonian formulation, life is a journey to establish a *personal identity* that is built over time. Inherent factors such as physical maturation pose a series of crises; how each is resolved is influenced by one's place in a culture, in history and even in the political dimensions that surround us.

Erikson gave us a broad synthesis on development by using Freud's ideas of stages, but he incorporated perspectives of these stages across the age span. He taught us that current behavior is influenced by a person's past history, his present situation, his culture's history and even the current sociopolitical milieu. When evaluating a behavioral concern, Erikson taught us to look broadly and intervene widely. His work highlights the processes of adult development that shape the families we serve. Although experimental work is sparse, these perspectives are still influential in the thinking about and support of development. He drew our attention to the influence of each person's unique life history in determining the self. Many psychotherapeutic approaches that incorporate Erikson's ideas have this aspect as a theoretical base. Erikson's language in labeling the core developmental task at any given time is helpful in organizing our own thoughts, especially those regarding atypical behavior, and in communicating issues with families (Box 2–3). The infancy chapters, particularly Chapters 11 and 13, use this framework to look at affective development, and the school-age years, as developed in Chapter 21, highlight this construct.

BEHAVIORISM AND SOCIAL LEARNING THEORY

This group of theorists, dominant in American thinking for most of the 20th century, shares the perspective that only behavior that is observable can be studied (i.e., not motives, beliefs, unconscious forces) and that the environment is the primary source of behavioral change. The

---

BOX 2–3 KEY INSIGHTS—ERIKSON AND FOLLOWERS

- Development continues across the life span. We all have a developmental dimension, young and old alike.

- The process of development is the building of a personal identity.

- Biological maturation creates a series of crises that have to be resolved by each person, dependent in part on the wider social milieu.

- Society as a whole and historical and sociopolitical factors, as well as cultural ones, have a powerful influence on how these developmental hurdles are negotiated. Explanations for variations in human behavior and development must take these factors into account.

- The social context of a person strongly influences behavior. Look at the context.

- Each person's unique life history shapes his individuality.

---

environment supplies *patterns of reinforcement* or rewards that shape the child's behavior. The child becomes "*conditioned*" to respond in a certain way based on the environment's shaping of his behavior. The child's association of certain stimuli with responses influences behavior in increasingly complex patterns over time. The *stimulus-response model* explains all behavior. These theorists sought to make the study of child behavior an objective science and applied their efforts in laboratory settings. Although biology sets limits on what, when and how quickly children learn particulars, these internal factors were minimized. Types of behavior that are rewarded stay; those ignored or punished disappear or are "*extinguished*" with predictable regularity. Children are seen as lumps of clay to be shaped through experiencing positive and negative consequences of their actions. Behavioral problems and solutions come from patterns of reinforcement in the environment. Child rearing was seen in the earliest days (1930s–1940s) as "*child engineering.*" Much of the early work was a transposition of animal studies to children. Indeed, the behaviorists were the first to apply a theory to rigorous laboratory studies. **Ivan Pavlov**, **J. B. Watson** and **B. F. Skinner** are names associated with the earliest behaviorist perspective.

Social learning theory, with **Albert Bandura** as a major figure in this school, evolved from behaviorism. It highlighted the importance of modeling in the processes of development. Children learn within a specific social context that provides feedback on behavior. This theory has now evolved to account for the child's internal processes of organizing, regrouping and drawing on memory to shape a behavior in a new environment or situation. Although a lot of learning is still derived from observation, other types of behavior emerge from a child's ability to combine patterns and learn from imaginings of his own and through processes of self-evaluation. Children become more selective in what and whom they use as models, in line with an increasing sense of self and self-efficacy in their own worlds. Bandura now sees children as very active mentally in constructing models and developing behavioral patterns on their own. They are like student artists who study the paintings around them to pick up ideas and techniques, but then paint an original themselves. Children increasingly monitor and adjust their own behavior so that their own self-efficacy is enhanced. This model presents development as a series of upward spirals, with forward progress fueled by the experience of successes or failures in the past. The model is one of a steady uphill progression, shaped by what you encounter on the journey.

Behavioral theories have prompted a great deal of applied research, as well as clinical intervention strategies, including conditioning children to consequences (*reinforcers*), positive and negative, associated with problem behavior. Programs targeted to get rid of undesirable behavior through withdrawal of privileges or through punishment rely on these *behavior modification* techniques. Therapies designed to foster learning to deal with fears and phobias are also based on these principles. Programs for discipline, for eliminating fears of medical treatments and for managing bedwetting are examples of interventions founded on this theoretical base. Many programs for children with mental retardation or autism depend heavily on these techniques to eliminate disruptive behavior, prompt communication and teach simple skills. Research on the learning of aggression from models in the child's environment is built on this perspective.

Strict behaviorism does not take into account a child's inner life, emotions, motivations and style in adapting to new circumstances and demands, and its influence is on the decline. Minimal weight is given to the child's own internal processes of maturation and the contribution that the child makes to his own development. In addition, many types of behavior emerge without environmental prompts, in spite of incredible environmental barriers and a complete lack of models for that behavior. Language development particularly highlights the deficits in a learning theory model. Finally, the environment in which children develop is much more complex than a series of reinforcers or even a series of models. The view of learning theorists on the environment itself may be too narrow.

Behaviorist techniques are attractive to clinicians because they can be prescribed for almost any condition or situation presented by a troubled parent. Moreover, in many circumstances the techniques work, provided that one has typical children and typical circumstances. Caution should be exercised, however, because these techniques are directed at changing behavior alone and not at addressing the basis for that behavior. Children's behavior has meaning, no matter how seemingly maladaptive or disruptive. The clinician should attend to what that behavior is revealing before prescribing a "cure" for it. Failure of these behavioral techniques to change behavior is seated in the complex interactions between a child and care provider, inappropriate environmental expectations or needs that go beyond the immediate. The clinician should probe these possibilities as part of a complete clinical intervention, not simply provide a "*behavior mod*" solution.

Social learning perspectives push the imperative to look broadly at a child's environment when disruptive behavior emerges, thus suggesting the possible roles of inappropriate models or atypical social situations. A therapeutic intervention to change the environment often changes the seemingly maladaptive behavior of the child. One should closely evaluate what forces the environment is providing before labeling the behavior deviant.

Marci, a 5-year-old girl, was placed in foster care after her mother, an alcoholic, was found to be neglectful. Her foster mom was troubled that Marci continued to take and hoard food months after the placement. "Food is always there and she was never starving. Even when she came to us, she was too fat."

Note: The erratic care and attention given by Marci's birth mom probably set up an anxiety in Marci about getting what she needed. Overeating and hoarding seem like sensible responses to that experience. (In my experience, hoarding may go on for years in even the best of care.) Merely punishing Marci's behavior was not appropriate until her anxiety was addressed and trust in the environment was established.

Behavioral techniques require close and consistent linkage between a behavior and a consequence. Inconsistency in response doesn't allow that linkage to be established and may even set that behavior in concrete because of intermittent reinforcement.

Mrs. Johnson wanted Jared to sleep in his own bed, not hers. She would put him back and tuck him in for several nights in a row and then give up for a week or two. Jared learned that if he kept coming in, his mom would just give up. "I'm so tired by then," she said. Note: This intermittent pattern of reinforcement is doomed to failure because it sets up Jared's behavior to

The younger the child developmentally, the closer the link must be between the behavior and the consequence for the child to learn. Delayed praise or punishment does not work for children younger than 6 chronologically or developmentally. For children younger than 2, the link has to be nearly immediate for the child to learn. Finally, positive reinforcers are much more powerful in shaping human behavior than negative ones are; rewards work better than punishments. Furthermore, social, interactive rewards are the best of all—hugs, smiles and praise (Box 2–4).

BOX 2–4 KEY INSIGHTS–LEARNING THEORIES

- The environment, especially the social environment, has a powerful influence on behavior. Look at the environment when you evaluate behavior.
- Behavior is shaped (at least in part) by reinforcers in the environment. This concept can be used to change specific behavior.
- Children learn from the models, adults and children, around them, particularly in such matters as aggression, gender roles, social consciousness and action and social norms of behavior. Evaluate the models when you evaluate behavior.
- Children learn from seeing and experiencing the consequences of their own behavior and adjust accordingly.
- Behavioral change is promoted by an ever-advancing sense of self-efficacy. Without a sense of efficacy and the experience of success, children will withdraw from the failure milieu, either physically or psychologically.
- Behavior modification programs do work to change behavior, but not to address the basis of that behavior.
- The closer the reinforcer to the action, the more likely one is to link the two.
- Positive reinforcers work better than negative ones.
- Social reinforcers work the best of all.

PIAGETIAN PERSPECTIVES

Jean Piaget revolutionized our "thinking about thinking" in children by proposing a new idea: children think differently than adults do. He posited that children learn through active interaction with the environment. Piaget developed his view of the active role of the child through detailed observations of children; he attended as much to their errors in problem solving and the patterns of exploration as to their successes. These "mistakes" told him how children reason about and understand their world. The funny things little kids say often reveal their beliefs about the world, beliefs that they have constructed through perceptions mulled over in a very active mental life.

His observations led to a *stage theory of development.* A child's way of acting on the world, physically and mentally, shifts radically between these stages. Table 2–2 shows these stages. This sequence is invariant, although the rate of progression may vary. The world is understood by

TABLE 2–2   **Piagetian Stages of Development**

Stage	Approximate Age	Ways of Understanding the World	Basic Concepts to Be Mastered
1. Sensorimotor	Birth–2 yr	Through direct sensations and motor actions	Object permanence; causality; spatial relationships; use of instruments; etc.
2. Preoperational	2–6 yr	Mental processes that are governed by the child's own perceptions and linkage of events; no separation of internal and external realities	Sense of animism; egocentrism; idiosyncratic associations; transductive reasoning
3. Concrete operational	6–11 yr	Can reason through real and mental actions on real objects; can reverse changes in the world mentally to gain understanding; can reason with a stable rule system; understands some patterns	Mass, number, volume, linear time Deductive reasoning Conservation tasks Objective causality De-centering—can see another's perspective
4. Formal operations	12 yr and older (variable)	Abstract thought; can reason about ideas, impossibilities and probabilities; broad abstract concepts	Mastery of abstract ideas and concepts; possibilities; inductive reasoning; complex deductive reasoning

the child with increasingly complicated mental structures. The model here, again, is a staircase, but one that a child actively climbs, dancing a bit on each step.

Piaget's insights dramatically changed the dominant behaviorist schools in America through his premise that the child is an active learner rather than a passive recipient or target of environmental forces. Such concepts as the importance of discovery and exploration to the child, now the foundation of early education, come from his work. Much work in developmental psychology today has Piagetian ideas as the explicit or implicit foundation.

Children develop, in this view, by a process of *assimilation* (taking in information through any and all the senses), *accommodation* (taking one's current abilities/understandings and modifying them to adjust to the new circumstance or challenge) and organization of this into a new mental structure or physical action, a *schema*. Such development creates a new level of mental *equilibrium* that lasts until there is something new experienced in the environment. Growth in cognition then begins with identifying an event that is surprising, discordant with previous perspectives or novel. Children do show most interest in novel events in their environment. The environment nourishes, stimulates and supports this active exploration. They learn alone, but in the context of an environment that challenges, prompts and interacts. The social as well as the physical environment is an important part of learning. The interaction with others prompts one to construct new schema, provided that one is ready to assimilate that information. Teaching logic to a 3-year-old or abstract math to a 7-year-old doesn't work because the new understanding is too far away from the existing mental structures.

Important ideas in infant cognition, in the *sensory motor period*, are that infants learn through their own senses and actions on objects. These baby "experiments" begin with reflexes and the infant's spontaneous actions. The infant observes the results of such behavior and repeats it. Then he modifies his actions slightly and observes this outcome. These are called "*circular reactions.*" Through increasingly complex interactions, the infant constructs his own world view. This world is eventually found to contain objects and people that exist even when you don't see them, a concept called *object permanence*. It also has consistent connections between actions and results (*causality*) and is mapped in three dimensional space (*spatial perception*). These core concepts and others are built in predictable sequences as the infant matures, plays and "experiments." An infant banging a rattle in more and more complex ways, a baby playing peek-a-boo and a young child winding up a toy or finding a hidden toy are examples of this infant scientist at work. More specifics of these observations are covered in the infancy chapters (Chapters 11 to 14).

The *preoperational period* (preschoolers) is cognitively egocentric. Youngsters at this age believe that the world is organized around them and their wishes; events depend on their actions. Objects are viewed as having a life (*animism*), such as stars shining for their benefit. They are impulsive generally, particularly in assigning causes for events around them and justifying actions of their own, and have difficulty classifying objects into groups or seeing broad characteristics. They reason *transductively*, assuming a causal link or a permanent association when two events are experienced in close proximity (e.g., I had a temper tantrum in the clinic, so now I get a shot; the nurse blows up my mom's arm every time she gets checked because she is having a baby—that's why her belly just keeps getting bigger). Their logic is faulty, although they are mentally active in creating linkages and associations. Fantasy, imagination and their own desires influence thinking at this age. The world is a magical place, and they see themselves pulling the strings. Chapter 17 in particular uses these themes.

The *concrete operational child* (grade-schooler) becomes more logical and can reason about objects in front of him. He can imagine that changing the shape of an object or the distribution of an array of objects does not change their essence such as mass or number. He can imagine changes in real objects in his head. This mind-set is called *conservation* and is the mental basis for much of school work, games and sports (mental aspects) and social interactions. Deductive reasoning becomes possible. He can understand causality beyond himself and his own perceptions. He can "*de-center*" enough to understand that others may have ideas, feelings and desires different from his. He can look for the order of things beyond his own idiosyncratic groupings. The tasks of school and learning call up these perspectives and are applied in Chapters 19, 20 and 21.

With the *formal operational* person, an adolescent or adult, abstract, theoretical, inductive thinking becomes possible. Hypothetical situations, multifaceted causality and consequence networks can be imagined. This is discussed in the adolescent chapters (Chapters 22 to 24).

The chapters on illness (Chapter 26) and on stress and loss (Chapter 27) use this framework to explain childhood thinking in these circumstances. Our clinical approach changes when we know children experience the world qualitatively different than we do.

Recent observations indicate that Piaget may have underestimated the capabilities of infants and toddlers. In addition, familiarity with the tasks used to test these cognitive structures, as well as past teaching and practice, seems to enhance performance more than previously thought. With support, a child can function at a higher level (optimal level) than his usual one (functional level). Redefinitions of these stages abound. Boundaries between the stages may be blurred because of teaching and experience and are different in different domains, with different objects or in different circumstances, a process of unevenness called *decollages*. Cross-cultural observations support Piaget's ideas about the universals of cognitive development in young children, but the mental structures of older children and adults seem to vary across the globe, seemingly in response to the particular cognitive demands placed by a specific environment. Finally, the Piagetian stage theory has been abandoned or modified by many in favor of a more continuous and heterogeneous view of mental development in children. Children roll along rather than bounce from one stage to another in these revisionist views. Other Piagetians fill in the missing explanations for the changes from one state to another by highlighting the new discoveries on anatomical and functional aspects of brain development that coincide with developmental shifts. These changes create more brain capacity for the child to remember, organize and combine ideas at new, more complex levels. The leading edge of research on cognition abuts the new sciences looking at information processing systems, complex neural networks and ever-evolving systems of thinking (see later). However, Piaget's work contains a rich legacy of important insights and probably inspires more current research in child development than any other view (Box 2–5).

Beyond Piaget: The Stages of Moral Development

Piaget applied his theories to moral development with the description of two stages, divided at about age 10. At the younger stage, children see rules as immutable, handed down by an authority and requiring obedience to the letter. The seriousness of a crime is judged by the damage done or the extent of the violation, not by motivation. After age 10, children appreciate that people have different perspectives on what the rules that guide conduct are or should be

---

BOX 2–5   KEY INSIGHTS–PIAGET AND FOLLOWERS

- Learning is an active process for children. They build their own mental constructs from environmental input.
- Children understand, reason about and act on their world in qualitatively different ways than adults do.
- Cognitive development proceeds in stages that are distinct and invariant in sequence.
- Perceived moderate novelty, surprise or disappointment prompts interest and a reorganization of mental structures, thereby resulting in enhanced mental or physical abilities.
- The child is self-regulating in what he takes in and how it is organized.
- Readiness to learn a specific task is necessary if it is to be achieved.
- Supports, prompts and interaction with objects and people can move a child up the next level but cannot advance him beyond his ability to assimilate that input.
- Shifts in cognitive development are associated with changes in social interaction and competence, moral judgments and emotional regulation.

---

and that these rules might be changed. **Lawrence Kohlberg's** work evolved from Piaget; he also used stages to describe the generic characteristics of children's moral problem solving, the way in which they reason about moral situations. Children and adults all over the world seem to solve moral dilemmas along this continuum, although the context and values may vary by context, culture, religion and even sociopolitical influences. Those in industrial societies and those exposed to higher education advance through the stages faster, and many go further along the continuum than do those in simpler societies, in which judgments remain at the lower level of the continuum.

Kohlberg's view of the progression of moral judgment has been challenged by several investigators, prominently **Carol Gilligan**, in whose view this schema is inherently male, Western and falsely hierarchical. Values placed on cooperation, caring and compassion are more characteristic of the way women and indigenous cultures make moral judgments, and these factors are not accounted for in Kohlberg's scheme. Experimental work supports these differences but still shows that young children see rules as rigid and absolute, that guilt depends on the damage done rather than motivation and that the likelihood of punishment has strong sway. Lecturing a preschooler on the broad social order, the perspectives of others or even empathy is unlikely to have much salience or effectiveness. In contrast, many adolescents will love to discuss the complexity of moral decision making and will broaden their own perspective when exposed to others who base judgments on the values of adherence to human rights, the dignity of man and other broad values.

Social learning theorists disavow this stage-related explanation in the maturation of moral judgment. As expected, they identify the models that a child has in his life to shape these judgments. The ability to take more factors into account allows children to have more complex judgments with time.

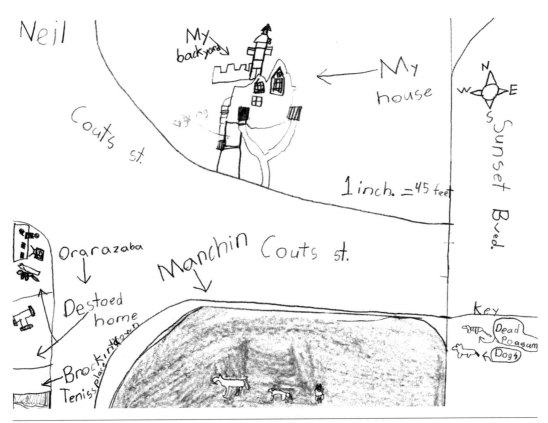

The child in context, in the neighborhood. Note the size and centrality of the child's house and the animals, including a dead possum, which are features most adult inhabitants would miss.

SOCIOCULTURAL THEORIES

The current era has seen a rediscovery of this school as initiated by the work of the Russian **L. S. Vygotsky**. With an eclectic background, an Eastern approach to life and living in a Marxist regime, Vygotsky provided an entirely new view of the child. He saw a child as embedded in the whole of the cultural, historical and social milieus; no behavior or developmental gain can be explained without taking these influences into account. The culture defines what skills are needed for functioning and then gives the child tools in the form of language, numbers, writing, technologies, ideas and patterns of behavior. With these they solve their own social problems, seen broadly as how to get along and succeed. The *child-in-context* is the only observable unit— a given child is inherently different in different contexts. A change in a child's routine, physical attributes and skills changes everything. Newer research in psychological anthropology, sociology and developmental psychology has incorporated these ideas with greater specification of the context of each child's behavior and evaluation of a child in an activity or within a specific surrounding. Cross-cultural work has changed significantly with this perspective. We no longer make head-to-head comparisons of populations (e.g., is this one smarter, faster, better than the child in another context), but rather look at variation within the context of cultural forces and the pressures of social change, with the concept of adaptability being the key observation. These perspectives are used in Chapter 3 to look at culture and child development.

Perhaps a greater contribution of the sociocultural model is the framework for learning that has influenced education. This construct is also helpful in considering children's functioning in the various learning milieus—with parents, in school, in early intervention, in sports, in the arts. Vygotsky proposed a "*zone of proximal development*," or the range of environmental influences (I will use the words stimulation or input) that prompt learning. A child on his own will function at the bottom of that zone, the *functional level*. However, with good teaching, parenting, coaching, motivation and modeling, the child will function at a much higher level, his *potential level*. This higher level is achieved through a process of "*scaffolding*," where the mentor assesses what the child can do and then builds on that, step by step, by guiding, modeling and suggesting strategies or approaches. This entails presenting activities just above the child's current level of functioning and helping him reach for that new level, to function "a head taller than himself." If the level of input is too low, the child gets bored and disengages or makes things more lively. (Envision the child throwing spitballs instead of doing his spelling words.) If it is too hard or presents unattainable tasks, the child simplifies the task, does part of it or disengages. (See the child daydreaming, doodling and asking to go to the restroom at math time.) The child will stay within his own zone of development as he regulates what he attends to and what he does with it. An environment that prompts healthy development is one that keeps the child at the top margins of his zone, with adjustments made for his advancing skills and backtracking if the child becomes overwhelmed. This process depends on the adult being attuned to the child, and as Vygotsky would say, all the better that they share a culture, a history together and a very strong relationship. All learning comes as part of a social relationship, a socially mediated process.

This theoretical model has applicability in education, parenting, early intervention programs and even the teaching of arts and sports. When a given child is failing, we need to look first at his abilities, but then develop a program or action that pushes him just beyond those. Close relationships and adjustments made from precise and sensitive observations are keys to success.

BOX 2–6   KEY INSIGHTS–SOCIOCULTURAL THEORIES

- The child's development is enmeshed in a social, cultural fabric from which he cannot be separated.
- Behavior can be understood only as a child-in-context.
- Children learn only in social contexts. They solve social problems presented by the real world in which they live. They learn the skills and acquire the tools that allow them to survive and thrive.
- Children learn within a certain range of environmental input, at the lowest level when left to their own devices, at the highest level when given appropriate support. If the environment is overwhelming, they will do something to lower the input or alter the task downward. If too low, they will add some spice to the situation.
- Development is better characterized by what children can accomplish with support and how they evolve over time in an environment of social support. Assessment should be interactive and dynamic over time.
- Teaching, coaching or parenting at its best teaches strategies to learn, not specific skills or information.

In clinical settings we are often looking at mismatches between the child and his milieu, but the source of that misalignment is not clear; that's where we need observations, assessments and identification of successes and the circumstances of failure. Static assessments of what a child does on his own are not as helpful as what he does with appropriate and individualized help. Moreover, the picture of the child's skills at any one point in time is not as helpful as the characterization of development over time, with support. These perspectives echo the Freudian notion of *moderate frustration* as a prompt for emotional growth and the centrality of relationships to developmental change. They also echo the Piagetian notion of *moderate novelty* prompting cognitive growth. Kohlberg described young people functioning at a higher moral level when they interact with others who have more advanced moral reasoning. Generally, this perspective calls on us to assess whether a child is "in his zone," be it in school, at home or on the playing field, and then asking what needs to be changed to allow him to function at a higher level without being overly taxed, physically, emotionally or cognitively (Box 2–6).

ECOLOGICAL SYSTEMS APPROACH

Closely allied with the sociocultural views are those with *ecological* perspectives as influences on child development. In this view, a broad and interlocking set of systems influence the developmental processes. Table 2–3 describes these systems. No longer is the child viewed as being influenced by the interface with family, peers and school alone. Rather, the whole sociopolitical and cultural environment has a profound impact on the one hand and incredible potential for intervention on the other. Beginning in infancy and increasing dramatically as they age, children shape these environments and make critical choices about even which environments will touch their lives (e.g., Will it be the soccer team or basketball? Will I do drama or be on the debate team?). **Uri Bronfenbrenner** is a key proponent of this perspective, which was inspired by his work on daycare. In related work, **Michael Rutter** and colleagues

TABLE 2–3 **Ecological Systems That Influence and Determine Child Development**

System	Description	Examples
Microsystem	Direct, reciprocal interactions between adults and children; also includes others who influence those directly acting on the child	Parents, siblings, care providers, teachers
Mesosystem	Environments that serve as connections between individuals in the microsystem	Home, school, daycare
Exosystem	Social settings that affect children, but do not contain them; community-based organizations, services and forces that influence the child-family microsystem; and informal community support systems for families	Health and welfare services, workplace policies and programs, social networks, financial aid, jobs, recreational opportunities for families
Macrosystem	Cultural values, laws, customs, resources and the priorities that children and children's issues have in the community	Daycare standards, educational standards and expectations, laws

have called attention to the tremendous impact of the school milieu on children. Such forces as the media, violence, cultural diversity and the prevalence of computers and the Internet shape development in many ways, for good and ill.

The essence of this theory is that all the outer systems mediate their effects through alteration of the microsystem that surrounds the child, the interaction and care within the family. The child is nested in these concentric circles. For example, homelessness, isolation, job stress and lack of health care all influence the interaction between parent and child through depression, lack of focus, tension, lack of time for the child and physical hardship. Perturbations at one level rattle the whole system and make profound changes in the child's world. For example, the events of 9/11/2001 have profoundly shaken American life. Children even at a distance were deeply affected by the media presentation of destruction, the change in family vigilance and the economic fallout that ensued. In another example, the structural components of a health care system will change when, how and where a child gets care and even what elements will be included in that care. Religious beliefs may determine how many children are in a family or what kind of discipline is used. These, in turn, will act through alterations in the parent-child interface. The impact of each factor will vary, depending on the developmental status of the child and all the other factors in this system. The child is enveloped by the family; however, this is not an impervious cocoon, but an ever-changing environment. It's also a two way street—the child's own needs, personality and developmental level prompt change in the interface between him and his family, which in turn prompts changes in the family's interface with society.

To the child health care clinician, this is no surprise. Many issues in behavior and development have their genesis in the child's surroundings in the broadest sense. An ecological systems approach mandates a broad perspective on pediatric care. Sometimes we can act at

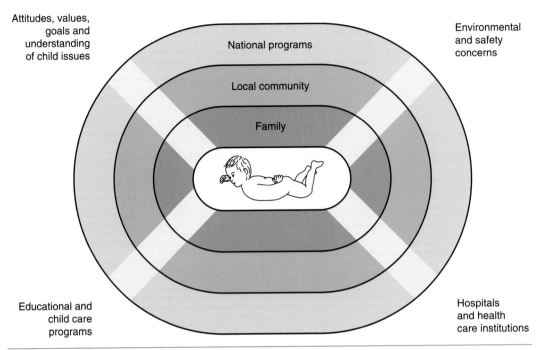

Attitudes, values, goals and understanding of child issues

Environmental and safety concerns

National programs

Local community

Family

Educational and child care programs

Hospitals and health care institutions

Figure 2–1   Spheres of advocacy in pediatric practice.

BOX 2–7   KEY INSIGHTS–ECOLOGICAL SYSTEMS

- Development is determined by a child's interaction with his family.
- The interface between the child and the family is in a state of constant change in response to intrafamilial and extrafamilial forces.
- Societal forces have a powerful influence on the child, primarily through the medium of alterations in the interactions in the family.
- The child's own behavior alters the caretaking milieu.
- To solve a child's issues, one may need a family systems approach or community advocacy.
- The caretaking system is the patient or the target for intervention.

---

one level and sometimes at another in the course of taking care of our patients. These spheres of advocacy are seen in Figure 2–1. One cannot care for children without taking these systems into account. At one level, these systems become the patient, the target for intervention (Box 2–7).

MONTESSORI APPROACHES TO CHILDHOOD EDUCATION

Maria Montessori's perspectives on the learning of young children have had an influence on preschool education and our thinking about early childhood beyond the confines of any Montessori school. Her view of children was that

- Children learn on their own if they are set in the right milieu.
- Children think and learn quite differently than adults do; they need to discover concepts and ideas on their own.
- Children have "*sensitive periods*" when they are naturally inclined to learn certain tasks.

Working with children in some of the poorest communities in Italy in the mid-20th century, her goal was to set up experiences for children at home and in her "*children's houses*" schools so that children work on their own with only infrequent adult prompts and simple opportunities to learn by building on their own areas of interest. Tasks of ordinary life, such as cutting vegetables, setting a table or pouring tea, have much interest for the child and should be presented to him. Children have an inherent sense of the need to put things in order in the first 3 years (e.g., lining up blocks, counting cars) and focus on small details of their world in the first 2 years (e.g., watching a fly on the wall, picking up a small rock on a hike). The complex use of hands is the work of 18 to 36 months. She saw walking as a "second birth" and highlighted the need to support, not inhibit, the exuberance that accompanies motor achievement. There was a strong belief in the importance of nature settings in the learning of young children. Because a classic children's house has a mix of ages from 2 to 6, children learn from older children and provide care and direction for younger children. Uneven development becomes hidden by the wide range of abilities seen in these mixed age environments.

Strict adherence to Montessori methods downplays free, imaginative play, drawing or cooperative role-playing. Fairy tales are discouraged. The classroom is filled with children working independently with specific apparatus (e.g., red and blue rods, gold beads) designed to teach basic concepts such as number and size comparisons. Teachers are more like personal trainers for each child. The classroom often has a quiet formality about it as children work independently in their own spaces with one specific activity at a time. Rituals of greeting and interaction constitute important parts of the day. However, Montessori schools vary widely from this orthodoxy, so each must be evaluated; how the theory is applied varies broadly. Many non-Montessori preschools have incorporated parts of the Montessori program without the label and often not even knowing where the notions that guide the program came from. Many studies suggest enhanced concentration, confidence, independence and enthusiasm, and performance are at least on a par with those of children in other early childhood educational programs. Maria Montessori would have liked that (Box 2–8).

MINI-THEORIES AND EMERGENT IDEAS

Other theoretical models have some valuable insights without presenting a broad structure of development. Others are in their own infancy but promise to give us new understanding. Some of the newer concepts are presented here.

BOX 2-8   KEY INSIGHTS—MONTESSORI

- Children are naturally curious about their world and will learn new things without prompting if given the opportunity.
- Early childhood is the time to allow a child to discover and explore by using his innate sense of order, attention to details and exuberance with physical movement.
- There are critical periods in early childhood to build key concepts and mental structures.
- Free play is not frivolous.
- Children learn at different speeds, in different ways, and have varying interests that guide learning.
- If we follow a child's own enthusiasm, learning is more likely.
- Education means creating opportunities to learn.
- Nature is good for children. Send them outside often.
- Grace, courtesy and respect for the rights and properties of others are important to instill in early childhood.

Dynamic Systems Theory

This theory is an application of physics and mathematics principles to the development of humans. It proposes that children develop with patterns of behavior that change in complex ways over time and space like a calculus function with endless feedback loops. Behavior isn't seen as just one action, but as a whole pattern that changes under changing circumstances and through feedback both from the environment and from within the child. This can be seen in the motor behavior of the human infant, where no reach is the same as the last one because it is changed by the child's last experience with reaching and is being done under necessarily new conditions. So the infant doesn't just reach but develops a modifiable pattern of behavior that is applied as needed in changing circumstances. The developing human is *inherently self-organizing*, predisposed to adapt to an ever-evolving environment, including the internal environment of the child himself. Any given behavior is the result of multiple, continuous interactions within and without. The cause of developmental change is multiple and continuous. A change in one area of competency will have widespread change in all systems of behavior. Although this kind of thinking has been applied to all areas of development, it is most studied in application to motor development. We will discuss it again in Chapters 12 and 14. Certainly, motor development has never been quite as interesting or as complex as this approach has made it.

Modularity Nativism

In this view, the child's mind contains a set of loosely connected, *preset modules* or structures that are uniquely primed to respond to a specific kind of input at a specific point in the child's life. Each unit is pre-established to allow development in a particular domain. Knowledge, skills and understanding are domain specific in this view. There needs to be very little in the way of developmental prompts to begin these processes. This view attributes the source of developmental change nearly entirely to innate processes. These processes are in turn determined by a long evolutionary history that makes those modules in the human uniquely adapted to the human condition. If a critical time period is missed, learning in that area may be compromised over the long term. The most famous proponent of this view is **Noam Chomsky**, who proposed a "*language acquisition device, or LAD,*" that is critical to the learning of language. We discuss this concept in the chapter devoted to language (Chapter 16). More recent applications have been to cognition. This view is in direct opposition to the connectionist perspectives described later.

Multiple Intelligences

Howard Gardner's ideas are allied to some degree with the modularity ideas just described. In his view, some individuals are particularly primed to be responsive to certain kinds of information and skill acquisition. They are innately set up to process information in specific ways, to learn in specific ways more easily than in others. Called "*multiple intelligences,*" these clearly varying differences in a child's "hard wiring" identify strengths and vulnerabilities that influence how a person functions. Each type is neurologically based with its own developmental course (Table 2–4). Gardner dismisses the notion of general intelligence entirely. Schools base their teaching and assessment on linguistic intelligence, but a child with strengths in other areas may not be successful in that particular milieu. Gardner's theories allow the framing of many difficulties with learning as "*learning differences*" rather than learning "disorders." His view is that we miss a lot of human potential when we fail to allow these other mental abilities to blossom.

Little research exists to substantiate this theory, and some observations indicate that these specific abilities may not be so distinct. However, these insights focus us on the individuality of

TABLE 2–4   **Multiple Intelligences**

Intelligence	Description
Linguistic	Sensitivity to language; language-based functions
Logicomathematical	Abstract reasoning, manipulation of symbols, detection of patterns, logical reasoning
Musical	Detection and production of musical structures and patterns; appreciation of pitch, rhythm, musical expressiveness
Spatial	Visual memory, visual-spatial skills, visualization
Body—kinesthetic	Representation of ideas, feelings in movement; use of body, coordination, goal-directed activities
Naturalistic	Classification and recognition of animals, plants
Social	Sensitivity and responsiveness to moods, motives, intentions and feelings of others
Personal	Sensitivity to self, feelings, strengths, desires, weaknesses and understanding of intention and motivation of others

each child. Children failing in one domain should be encouraged to develop other areas in which their unique ways of learning may be successful. Identifying these varying competencies to parents allows them to see strengths and virtues in their child, abilities that may flower later than others because of the differential rate of development of these multiple areas. Parents who have children with atypical development will benefit from reading this perspective.

Neural Networks and Connectionism

Rather than advocating a comprehensive or even a unified theoretical approach to development, diverse groups of scientists are using the computer as a model to look at human learning. These approaches vary from using the information processing capacities of computers as a metaphor to explain how children and adults learn, to actual construction of computer models that replicate those processes and/or predict learning behavior. The latter type of approach is particularly exciting in that it gives us insight into the basic processes of development and accounts for both internal capacities and the role of input from the environment. These approaches have further appeal in that they present the most coherence with what we know about the structure and function of the brain down to the cellular level. The process of developmental change is seen as taking information into the nervous system by means of a variety of neural structures designed to respond to varying kinds of input, including internal stimuli. This is the *input layer*. These cells then act on another layer of cells, the *hidden layer*, that form a network of activation dependent in some part on previous experience. These in turn activate another unique network of cells, the *output layer*, that produce action, including backward feedback. The process of learning, then, is the construction of networks of activation that become both more complex and more specific with time. These layers are not domain specific, so networks may be used for a variety of functions. A very small difference in activation can produce very different patterns down the line, both in the immediate sense and later in life through the construction of very different networks. Late-appearing problems may have their origin early in development through this cascading of effects across networks and over time. Small differences in neural network activation can lead to large differences at the behavioral level.

These perspectives see the human brain as a highly interactive, dynamic system with always emergent patterns of network activation. Knowledge is seen as a distributed pattern of activation that involves connections with various weights or strengths. Maturation provides for more capacity to refine such networks and improve processing speed through enhanced efficiency.

The models created laboriously in the laboratory do replicate human learning very tightly in these types of experiments. These approaches have the potential to explain individual variability in development, as well as patterns of atypical development, particularly those linked to specific genetic conditions such as Williams' syndrome or fragile X syndrome. In such circumstances, a small change in neural structure evolves into a distinct pattern of behavior and development. These approaches appear to be getting us closer to understanding the brain/behavior linkages.

Application to education has been swift, though limited. Whole curricula have been designed to teach the development of learning strategies and approaches rather than specific information or skills. The characterization of learning disabilities as malfunctions at very specific parts of the process of information handling by an individual has led to some rethinking of the approach to remediation for an individual child.

Weaknesses include the limitations of behaviors modeled by these approaches, now primarily language, cognition and social development. Most work has been done on adults and older children and very little on infancy. No computer model has been able to replicate the phenomenon of rapid insight that humans can exhibit: putting together bits of information in an explosion of consolidated thinking. The idea of stage shifts is not explained at all by such modeling, given that development is seen as largely quantitative in nature. Finally, the human context of development and emotional states that influence all types of development is not addressed in these approaches. This group of approaches, network models and connectionism, is in direct opposition to the modularity approaches described earlier. Nevertheless, neural network studies are some of the most exciting new ways to look at development.

TEMPERAMENT

The way a child behaves and develops, not just how, is an important perspective on a child and the foundation of much research in child development. This is called temperament. *Temperament can be defined as stable, individual modes of responding to the environment based on differences in emotional reactivity, activity level, attention and self-regulation that appear consistently across situations and are relatively stable over time.* The concept of temperament as an important characteristic of a child and a strong predictor of behavioral concerns and problems began in earnest with the seminal work of **Stella Chess** and **Alexander Thomas**. Their longitudinal studies clearly showed remarkable stability of the characteristics of temperament and their relevance in understanding the responses children generate in the caretaking environment. Temperament influences all aspects of development and is often the source of many behavioral concerns.

The dimensions of child temperament often used in clinical practice and some research are shown in Table 2–5. Clinical appraisal of these dimensions can be done informally in a primary care setting over time, but it has been standardized by **William Carey** and **Sean McDevitt** (see

TABLE 2–5 **Temperament Dimensions**

Dimension	Description
Activity level	Amount of physical movement during sleep and awake periods
Rhythmicity	Regularity of physiological functions, such as sleep, hunger, elimination
Approach-withdrawal	Nature of the initial response to new stimuli
Adaptability	Ease or difficulty with which reactions can be modified
Persistence–attention span	Length of time that an activity is pursued
Intensity of reaction	Energy level of the responses regardless of quality or direction
Distractibility	Effectiveness of extraneous environmental stimuli in interfering with ongoing behavior
Threshold of responsiveness	Amount of stimulation (e.g., light, sound, touch) necessary to draw a discernible response from the child
Quality of mood	General emotional tone of the child's response and interactions

Appendix) with the use of questionnaires. A child is characterized in these dimensions in comparison with other children his age. Though standardized on typically developing children, these same dimensions can be applied, with care, to those with atypical development. Adjusting for developmental rather than chronological age is one consideration. Other researchers such as **Mary Rothbart** use slightly different language and clustering, but there is considerable overlap in all schemas.

Substantial evidence indicates that these characteristics are "hard-wired" in any individual and, indeed, in the family and in cultural clusters. Twin studies show that identical twins are more alike temperamentally than fraternal twins are, even when raised apart. Some characteristics group in families, such as shyness, poor adaptability and irregularity in biological functions. Additional evidence shows that resting heart rates, cortisol levels and even frontal lobe electro-encephalographic activity vary by temperament in infancy and beyond. A subdivision of research is evaluation of the temperamental phenotypes of children with these characteristics as a result of specific genetic conditions (e.g., Williams' syndrome, Lesch-Nyhan syndrome, Angelman's syndrome).

The way in which these characteristics cluster strongly influences the perception and reality of difficulty in child rearing. In western societies (i.e., where this subject has been studied in large groups), the population of infants is divided into three groups:

- Easy (40%). Regular routines, cheerful and adaptable
- Difficult (10%). Irregular, slow to accept change and tending to respond negatively
- Slow to warm up (15%). Inactive, mild, low-key responsiveness, negative or neutral mood and slow adjustment
- Mix of characteristics (35%)

Behavioral concerns are predicted by temperament. Difficult babies are four times as likely as easy infants to have preschool and school difficulties. Children who are slow to warm up are likely to have adjustment difficulties in middle childhood and beyond. Shyness, anxiety and social withdrawal are all problems with which they may have to cope in greater frequency than children with easy profiles do. These links are particularly strong for children who are at the extremes, such as a very fearful infant or a very active toddler. If temperament is measured in infancy, stability over time is at the modest level; if evaluated after the first year, the continuities are very strong, into adulthood.

There is cultural variability in temperament, with infants in different groups clustering in one direction or another. For example, Chinese infants were found to have less intensity of responsiveness and less activity and to be less easily irritated than western infants. Other examples are presented in Chapter 3.

Being difficult is not always bad: in some emerging cultural societies, having a difficult temperament as an infant was more predictive of survival under harsh environmental conditions; in others studies, an active demanding and irritable child elicited more parental attention and, over time, a better adjustment. Some preliminary work suggests that more irritable, demanding and not easily consoled preemies are more likely to survive their lung immaturity than similar infants with a more placid approach to the challenges of life. Finally, certain difficult temperaments in infancy have some advantage in adult life when people choose environments where their personality traits work to their advantage. Active, gregarious, talkative school-age children may spend a lot of time in the principal's office but be very successful salespeople, entrepreneurs and activists. Children labeled slow to warm up may find a niche in a profession that requires precision and caution.

Developmental tasks themselves will be approached differently based on temperament. A quiet child who is slow to warm up may try his first steps hesitantly, even late, but demonstrate a relatively well coordinated gait once he makes the leap to independent walking. Clinical assessment of developmental tasks should take a child's temperamental characteristics into account.

Characterizing a child's individuality on dimensions of temperament allows the clinician to assist parents in seeing the child's unique needs and in developing behavior management strategies that are likely to be successful. For example, a child with low adaptability will need help in anticipating and coping with change. A high-activity child will need to wind down before bed. Good advice follows from a clear understanding of these individual characteristics. The concept of temperamental match or *"goodness of fit"* between parent and child predicts adaptability and resilience in the face of stress; poor alignment is often the source of interactional difficulties and behavioral complaints. For example, a quiet, low-intensity boy who withdraws initially in new situations may be regarded by his dad as a "sissy." A high-intensity girl with a negative mood who is also highly persistent may have trouble making friends. She may be regarded by her parents as antisocial, ungrateful and generally difficult, particularly if the parents are gregarious, flexible and generally low key. In these circumstances, the clinician must help families see these differences as hard-wired and part of the individuality of the child. If they respond with altered expectations and a child-rearing style that is supportive and not destructive, the child is likely to do well, with some shift in personality to more adaptive functioning. A child with a negative mood, poor adaptability, irregularity in habits and a highly intense reaction presents a challenge to any parent and calls forth a punitive, negative, angry parenting style unless such behavior is seen in the context of an individual style and responded to positively and consistently. *Temperamental mismatch* is often the underlying diagnosis for troubles at home, in school and in the social milieu. Temperament will enter into many chapters because it is an important concept.

Other longitudinal work done in Hawaii by **Emmy Elizabeth Werner** and colleagues, though not strictly of temperament, shows the role of these individual factors in development. The concept of the effect of *resiliency* in the face of overwhelming stress on the processes of development was evaluated over the life span. This work showed that children with a positive demeanor, a ready approach to what life brought and an ability to inspire passionate devotion in at least one adult care provider were more likely to succeed in all aspects of their lives despite a myriad of risk factors. These individual features were more predictive than other biomedical (except direct insults to the central nervous system such as meningitis) or even sociological variables when examining the outcomes of children monitored into adult life. Such is the power of temperament to influence development. Without a strong understanding of how temperament influences behavioral and developmental issues, the clinician will have a hard time evaluating behavior, behavior problems and difficulties that children and families face in all the systems that change their lives.

LONG-TERM STUDIES

Although there are weaknesses in longitudinal research, these efforts do give us perspectives on the development of children. Students of child development should be aware of some of

TABLE 2–6 **Perspectives of Human Behavior**

	Theories of Development			Skill Areas		Possible
Age	Freud	Erikson	Piaget	Language	Motor	Psychopathology
Birth–18 mo	Oral	Basic trust vs. mistrust	Sensorimotor	Body actions; crying; naming; pointing; shared social communication	Reflex; sitting; reaching; grasping; walking; mouthing	Autism; anaclitic depression; colic; disorders of attachment; feeding and sleeping problems
18 mo–3 yr	Anal	Autonomy vs shame, doubt	Symbolic pre-operational	Sentences; telegraph; unique utterances; sharing of events	Climbing; running; jumping; use of tools; using toilet; early self-care	Separation issues; negativism; fearfulness; constipation; shyness; withdrawal; aggressiveness
3–6 yr	Oedipal	Initiative vs. guilt	Intuition, pre-operational	Connective words; can be readily understood; tells and follows stories, questions	Increased coordination; tricycle; jumping; writing	Enuresis; encopresis; anxiety; aggressive acting out; phobias
6–12 yr	Latency	Industry vs. inferiority	Concrete operational	Subordinate sentences; reading and writing; language reasoning	Increased skills; sports; recreational cooperative games	School phobias; obsessive reactions; conversion reactions; depressive equivalents; anxiety; attention deficit/hyperactivity disorder
12–17 yr	Adolescence (genital)	Identity vs. role confusion	Formal operational	Reason abstract; using language; abstract mental manipulation	Refinement of skills	Delinquency; promiscuity; schizophrenia; anorexia nervosa; suicide
17–30 yr	Young adulthood	Intimacy vs. isolation	Formal operational	Reason abstract; using language; abstract mental manipulation	Refinement of specialized skills; sports skills peak	Schizophrenia; borderline personality disorder; adjustment disorders; development of intimate relationships; difficulties with relationships
30–60 yr	Adulthood	Generativity vs. stagnation	Formal operational	Reason abstract; using language; abstract mental manipulation	Refinement of skills	Depression; self-doubts; career development issues; family; social network; neuroses
>60 yr	Old age	Ego integration vs. despair	Formal operational	Some loss of skills; decreased memory, focus	Loss of functions	Involutional depression; anxiety; anger; increased dependency

these famous studies because they are still invoked today to explain the continuities, consistencies or lack thereof in the development of children. The studies from Hawaii (The Children of Kauai, Kauai Revisited, etc.) are examples of some of the large longitudinal studies of children that give us long-term perspectives and some ideas of linkages. Other studies performed on the stable population of the Isle of Wight gave us new insight into several aspects of development. The Guidance Study out of Berkeley (also know as the Berkeley Growth Study) began in the 1920s and has yielded much important data about a U.S. population. Jerome Kagan's long-term study of personality and outcome traced children from birth into adolescence.

SUMMARY

There is a wealth of information on the development and behavior of children that is waiting to be applied to the clinical encounters we have every day. A comparison of the major theories is presented in Table 2–6. These perspectives help us organize our observations and our thinking, they assist us in becoming efficient in data collection, and they give us insight into many behavioral tools at our disposal to assist families in supporting their own child's development. These disciplines are the foundation for care. A knowledge of these core sciences will help us function at a professional level in our work and will make us good consumers of the research that expands our knowledge every day. No one perspective tells us all we need; we have the luxury of an eclectic and evolving approach in our views of our young patients and the forces that shape their development.

RECOMMENDED READINGS

Crain W: *Theories of Development: Concepts and Applications*, 4th ed. Upper Saddle River, NJ, Prentice-Hall, 2000.
Kagan J: *The Nature of the Child.* New York, Basic Books, 1984.
Miller PH: *Theories of Developmental Psychology*, 4th ed. New York, Worth Publishers, 2002.
Thomas RM: *Comparing Theories of Child Development*, 5th ed. Belmont, CA, Wadsworth/Thompson Learning, 2000.

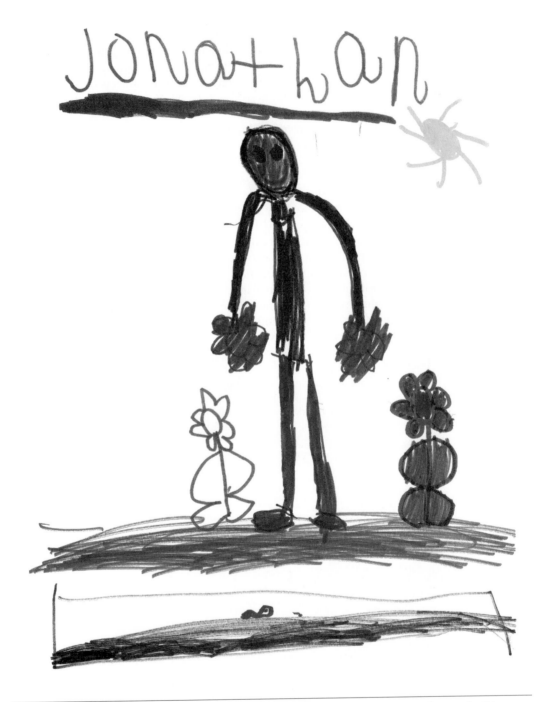

Developmental Parallels. "Jonathan," a 6-year-old sets himself amidst the growing flowers. By JM.

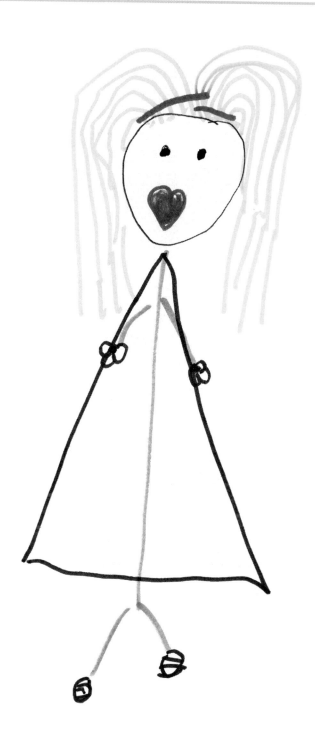

CHAPTER 3

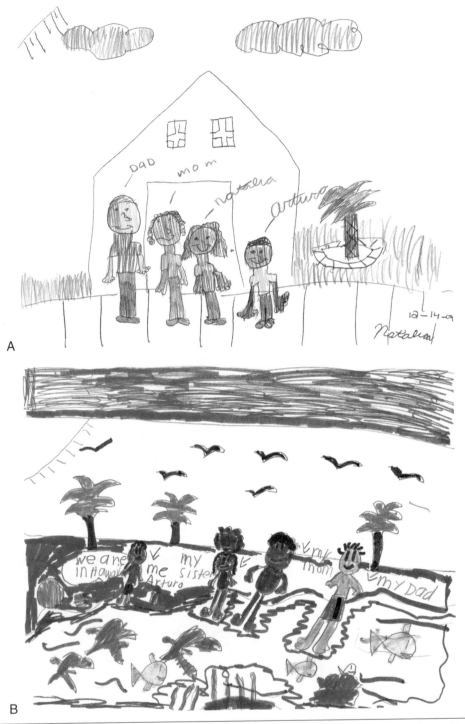

A bicultural/biracial family as seen by two siblings. **A**, An 8-year-old girl draws her family in front of her home. Dad is Latino. Mom is African American. By Natalia Jacobo. **B**, A 6-year-old boy draws his family at the beach. He pointed out that he was doing his best to get the skin tones "just right."

Cultural Dimensions in Child Care

LORI TAYLOR, LINDIA WILLIES-JACOBO and SUZANNE D. DIXON

This chapter describes the cultural variation that alters a family's view of the child, the role of parenting and the understanding of health, disease and healing. This variation will influence all encounters between the health care provider and the child and family. The specific issues related to the most commonly encountered cultural groups in the United States are presented. These insights should enable the practitioner to become increasingly culturally competent in provision of care. It will also enrich all practice experiences through this broadening of perspective.

The impact of a child's cultural background during any pediatric encounter is pervasive. Culture influences parenting practices, developmental expectations and perceptions of the child's behavior as well as the behavior itself. It also affects the way in which families seek medical care and interact with health care providers and the western medical system. Even if a family speaks without an accent, lives a very westernized life and appears to fully embrace the majority culture, the deep psychological dimensions that culture imparts will still influence all aspects of child rearing and care. These differences may also be a source of misunderstanding between the family and health care provider and may explain many cases of poor compliance and lack of follow-up. An enhanced understanding of the cultural dimensions of care will help avoid this source of miscommunication and disappointment on both sides of the care partnership.

WHAT IS CULTURE?

Our knowledge about the importance of culture in medicine begins with an understanding of the differences between "race," "ethnicity" and "culture." In its most common usage, the term *race* implies shared attributes that are purely genetic and/or physical, the color of one's skin, body shape and hair texture and distribution, for example. The word *ethnicity* implies a sharing of heritage, customs, foods and other aspects—the outward practices of a group of related peoples. *Culture* is the most complex of these terms and has the broadest definition. The word is derived from the Latin root "*colere*," which means to cultivate or nurture like a plant.

Culture consists of traditional or learned patterns of thinking, feeling and acting that become established within a social group and are transmitted from one generation to another. Culture encompasses shared beliefs, customs, traditions, values and one's sense of self and place in the universe.

It is the similarity in psychological makeup that is important here. Culture also implies an ongoing transmission of these mental structures to the next generation, often through implicit rather than explicit means. Members of a cultural group often, but not always have ethnicity and race in common. As an example of incongruity in these aspects of self, consider the deaf culture. Members are heterogeneous in race and ethnicity but nonetheless share many beliefs, values, world views and practices—they share a culture.

SEEING YOUR OWN CULTURE

The first step in understanding culture is to be aware of one's own. Many Americans, including educated western professionals, may counter with, "But I don't really belong to any particular cultural group." Lack of perspective on one's own culture is a sign of ethnocentrism, the belief that one's own values, beliefs and perspectives are the norm or gold standards and everyone else is defined by comparison with it (Box 3–1). This view makes one blind to the richness and value of other cultures and thus impoverishes oneself and makes one less able to work with others. It should be avoided.

Those who consider themselves to be "cultureless" might consider the following eight values and beliefs that have been identified as characteristic of dominant American culture:

1. Importance of individualism and privacy
2. Belief in the equality of all individuals
3. Informality in interactions with others
4. Emphasis on the future, change and progress
5. Belief in the general goodness of humanity
6. Emphasis on the importance of time and punctuality
7. High regard for achievement, action, work and materialism
8. Pride in interactional styles that are direct and assertive

Most of the world does not share these values. Clinicians in the mainstream American culture may not appreciate the extent to which their own cultural values, such as those just described, affect

---

BOX 3–1   AVOIDING ETHNOCENTRISM

Ethnocentrism is the belief that one's own way of living and doing things is the best way, simply because it is one's own. Cultural practices that appear different are dismissed as "wrong" or "inferior" on the basis of unfamiliarity. An ethnocentric viewpoint is clearly detrimental to anyone working with families from diverse cultures. Consider the following description of a daily ritual of a certain cultural group:

The daily body ritual performed by everyone includes a mouth-rite. . . . It was reported to me that the ritual consists of inserting a small bundle of hog hairs into the mouth, along with certain magical powders, and then moving the bundle in a highly formalized series of gestures.

This is a description of tooth brushing in the fictitious culture of Nacirema (American spelled backwards) created by an anthropology professor in a humorous attempt to illustrate how something that is perfectly natural in one culture can be seen as strange when viewed from the outside.

their practices. For example, clinicians who value punctuality may become frustrated with families from other cultures in which the concept of time is less meaningful. Other clinicians who value a direct interactional style may doubt the sincerity or attentiveness of a patient whose culture discourages eye contact. Those who value privacy may have difficulty understanding why a preschool-age child is still sleeping in her parents' bed. To support all these families, one must be able to enter into their own cultural system.

CULTURE AND CHILD REARING: CULTURE IS BOTH INHERITED AND ACQUIRED

Culture and the ways in which children are raised interact in a bidirectional way. The child's individual characteristics influence how he is raised, and the culture's view of the child, his role and societal requirements act to shape child-rearing practices. The varying behavioral profiles of neonates born into different cultures provide examples of how the infant contributes to his own rearing. Japanese and Chinese infants are less active, less irritable and less vocal than comparable neonates from a western European heritage. This prompts a toned-down interactional style with their moms, but also with a western adult—the baby's temperament influences the adult. African infants have higher motor tone at birth and have some acceleration in motor development. Vigorous handling of them by care providers and investment in motor development follows from these infant characteristics.

Culture influences the behavior of adults with children as they consciously and unconsciously reflect the culture's values. For example, Japanese moms see their role as bringing a child into compliance with the rules and required behavior of the family. The Confucian values of strict obedience and responsibility to others are acting here. The infant is swaddled tightly, fed at the first whimper and kept quiet much of the time. Independence and individualism are not valued—control of the child is fostered instead. Similarly, when Chinese moms are asked, in an experimental setting, to narrate a past family event with a child, they often mention the child's misdeeds and the embarrassment such behavior brings to the family. Irish American moms with the same direction gloss over any misdeeds and emphasize the individual joy and achievement of the event. In face-to-face interactions, American parents engage their young infants with eye-to-eye contact and aim to get big smiles and exuberant movement from them. In African cultures, where restraint in emotional expression is an important underlying norm, moms will damper that same face-to-face interaction to keep the infant's emotional expression in a narrow range. The rules of affective expression and appropriate behavior are being transmitted very early in Asia, in Africa and in America.

The western institution of preschool provides a useful example of how differing cultural values influence a parent's perspective. The concept of 3-year-old children in a classroom with same-age peers and a teacher as authority figure is foreign to many, if not most of the world's parents. In fact, the idea of an adult who is unrelated to a child spending significant time guiding and nurturing that child would be unacceptable in many cultures. Western parents, on the other hand, are thrilled that their children can separate from them and spend time meeting new people, cooperating with peers, mastering new skills and learning to be independent and self-reliant. These early achievements are seen as a step toward becoming successful members of the dominant American culture.

WHAT IS "NORMAL" IN THE BEHAVIOR AND DEVELOPMENT OF CHILDREN?

Much of our understanding of child development comes from studies of western, often affluent western populations. Although there is an ever-growing body of cross-cultural comparative research, much of what we assume to be normal has a cultural and frequently socioeconomic bias. This narrow perspective of child development may not be applicable to the majority of the world's children.

Systematic studies of behavior and developmental expectations initially characterized populations as either accelerated or lagging behind the dominant American culture in one or more areas. Contemporary research on behavior and development focuses on the connections between child-rearing patterns and the cultural forces that both promote and shape these patterns, at least in the environments in which such practices evolved. Child-rearing practices that are long established in a cultural tradition were adaptive in that culture's setting even if they appear poorly adaptive to the current circumstances. Studies on cultural adaptations prompted by the environment describe universal themes of human development, as well as the limits of adaptability. What is normal should be evaluated within its evolutionary cultural milieu. With this perspective, practices are neither good nor bad, although they may be poorly adaptive to the current situation.

OUR MULTICULTURAL PATIENTS

All child health care practices contain a bright array of cultural traditions, and that trend is here to stay. The United States is continuing its historical legacy of cultural diversity. People born in another country now represent a larger segment of the U.S. population than at any other time in the past 5 decades, and the trend is anticipated to continue. By 2010, the number of Latino children in the United States is expected to rise by 5.5 million, the number of African American children by 2.6 million and the number of children of other nonwhite races by 1.5 million. In this same period, the number of white children will fall by 6.2 million. By the year 2020, an estimated 40% of school-age children in the United States will be a member of a minority group.

All health care providers need to develop tools that allow them to adequately address the needs of children and families from these many cultures to become "culturally competent." Knowledge begins this process. The following sections are devoted to a discussion of several major cultural groups within the United States, with specific attention paid to aspects that may affect child development, child-raising practices and interaction between families and the western medical system.

Each cultural group is quite large and heterogeneous and contains many subgroups that differ in language, customs and values. For example, the cultural group "Asian" encompasses the Far East (Japan, China), Southeast Asia (Vietnam, Laos, Cambodia) and, in some discussions, the Near East (India, Pakistan), Indonesia and the Philippines. Clearly, this is an incredibly rich mixture of people, with many different languages, religions and traditions. However, there are specific themes shared across many of the subgroups, and it is these themes that justify this brief presentation of the larger group as a whole. A list of resources for further information on individual cultures can be found in the reference section.

A word of caution: Specific beliefs and practices regarding child rearing, health and illness are often, but not always shared by members of a cultural group. A person's identification with a particular culture is not a guarantee that the individual subscribes to all the beliefs of the group. Many factors contribute to interculture variability, including age, place of birth, socioeconomic status, education level and degree of acculturation into the "American culture." Clinicians should regard the information on different cultural groups as background data to open dialogue with children, adolescents and their families rather than a substitute for the discussion itself. Exploring the cultural dimensions of a patient/family is a process of individual discovery.

Latinos

An 18-month-old Latino boy is brought to the clinic for a health supervision visit. During the developmental assessment, his mother states that the child says two words ("mama" and "papa") and is able to follow simple commands. English and Spanish are both spoken in the home. You express your concerns to the mother regarding the child's paucity of expressive language; however, she does not appear concerned. You ask her if someone reads to the child at home on a regular basis, and she responds with a smile, "He's only 18 months old." Note: This case illustrates the differences in expectations for behavior and development and in the role of parents in Hispanic culture. It also illustrates the issues of language assessment in a bilingual setting.

Latinos are defined as people living in the United States with the background of Spanish-speaking peoples of Latin America. This diverse group comprises approximately 13% of the U.S. population and is increasing.

The View of the Child Children are highly valued in the Latino culture, and higher rates of fertility and birth in Latinos are well documented. Both men and women spend much time with children and have a nurturing role in their lives, although most direct care is the responsibility of the women in the family. Babies are to be cuddled, protected and fed, not talked to excessively. Chubby children reflect well on parents; feeding difficulties and poor growth are a serious ego blow to mothers in these cultures because physical nurturance is central to the definition of a good mother.

In interviews of immigrant Latino families, verbal communication with babies was viewed by the parents as "silly" because they believed that children could not understand them until later ("after they began to talk"). Spanish-speaking mothers of Mexican origin talk less at 1 and 8 months to their infants and hold their premature babies more at 1 month of age than do English-speaking mothers of various ethnic backgrounds. Early interactions of Mexican American mothers are predominantly nonverbal. Other comparative studies of maternal teaching behavior found that Latina mothers viewed themselves strictly as "mothers," not teachers. They believe that the education of their children is the responsibility of schools, not the role of the parents.

In contrast, parents of children in the dominant U.S. culture are often very concerned if expressive language does not emerge early. This worry comes out of a broader view of what is

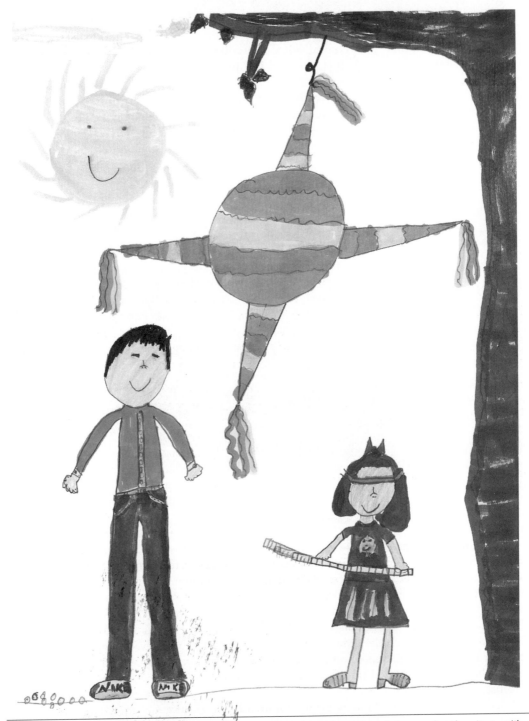

Cross-cultural perspectives. A Mexican American girl, age 11, shows herself ready to go after the piñata with a smiling dad nearby. Cultural traditions anchor childhood memories.

appropriate for children. These westernized families tend to encourage and reward individuality and assertiveness and place significant value on children participating in adult conversation. Latino families may see this behavior pattern as socially unacceptable, disrespectful or disruptive. The apparent "lack of concern" of a Latino parent whose child is language delayed (see the opening case) may be due to different expectations about what is normal and abnormal.

Although children in Latino families are highly valued, they are expected to behave. Parents may have authoritarian parenting styles and use threats, shame and embarrassment to change behavior. Strict disciplinary practices in the Latino culture may be counterbalanced with a permissive attitude toward children in other ways. Alternating authoritarian and permissive child-rearing practices may at times lead to confusion, both in the family and in an individual child.

Respect for elders, especially the father, is a highly valued trait. The expectations of boys and girls tend to be different; boys are more indulged, whereas girls are protected. Disciplinary roles may be different among parents in a Latino family; the mother is often the primary care-taker, and disciplinary issues are typically left to the father.

Family Values Families and society as a whole emphasize interpersonal harmony; cooperation is encouraged. The competitive edge that characterizes mainstream American families is typically absent in Latinos. It has its roots in the peasant organization that was the original societal structure from which these groups came. Cooperation within and between groups is key to survival in such settings. In the current era, the poverty and discrimination that families experience may make getting along with one's group as vital to survival as it was when these traits evolved.

Clinicians who provide health care for children in Latino families must be aware of the importance of the extended family, known as "familismo," or collective loyalty to the extended family. This is especially important when discussing sensitive medical issues that require decision making and consent.

One application of "familismo" is that parents may delay an important decision until they consult with an extended family member, such as a grandparent. Or they may decide to defer some intervention because of the competing needs of another family member, judged to be more urgent at the time. When decisions are not urgent, families should be allowed appropriate time to make a clinical decision, including all who have a part to play in the process.

Illness and Healing Illness in the Latino culture is believed to result from hot-cold imbalances, drafts or winds and decomposed foods. In a study of 100 Latina mothers who were asked about the cause of their children's illness, 80% believed that cough resulted from an imbalance between hot and cold forces, 36% believed that their child's diarrhea resulted from "something they ate," and 53% believed that conjunctivitis was caused by an "air." What is notable about this particular study is the disregard for the "germ theory" as a causative role in illness. Many home remedies used by Latino families are perceived to restore the balance between hot and cold forces. Such remedies include teas, baths and some special foods.

Folk illnesses are distinctive ailments that belong to a particular cultural group. A large percentage of Latino primary caretakers acknowledge a belief in folk illnesses. Common folk illnesses in the Latino population that clinicians will encounter include "mal de ojo," "empacho," "susto," and "mollera caida" (Box 3–2).

BOX 3–2   LATINO ILLNESS TERMS

- Mal de ojo—Evil eye
- Azabache—Seed charm
- Curanderos—Traditional healers
- Empacho—Blocked intestine
- Greta—Medications containing lead
- Azarcon—Medications containing lead
- Botanicas—Drugstores selling traditional medicines
- Susto—Fright
- Mollara caida—Fallen fontanel

"Mal de ojo," also known as the evil eye, occurs when a person with "strong eyes" looks at a child. The strength of the eyes is believed to heat up the child's blood, which leads to inconsolable crying, fever, diarrhea and gassiness. Wearing an "azabache," or seed charm, on a necklace or bracelet is believed to protect against this illness. Many children may come to their medical visits wearing these charms, and a clinician's knowledge about its meaning may be extraordinarily useful. Folk healers, or "curanderos," are often called on for assistance to cure this illness. Mal de ojo is said to be cured by rubbing the child's body with an egg, breaking the egg into a glass of water and placing it under the head of the child's bed overnight. If the egg appears solidified and milky white when it is examined in the morning, the child is said to be cured.

"Empacho," or blocked intestine, results from food sticking to the walls of the intestines and causing an obstruction. Symptoms include abdominal pain, vomiting and diarrhea. There are a variety of folk remedies for empacho, including the use of herbal teas and abdominal massage with oils. The goal of therapy is to dislodge the offending agent from the intestines. The most problematic treatments of empacho are "greta" and "azarcon." They contain lead oxide, which can cause lead toxicity. These substances are readily available to Latino families at "botanicas," or drugstores, in Mexican cities along the U.S. border.

"Susto," or fright, occurs after a frightening experience. The symptoms are usually insomnia, nightmares, fever and diarrhea. A variety of rituals, including prayer and other religious practices, are often performed to cure susto. The goal of treatment is to eliminate "fright" from the child's body.

"Mollera caida," or fallen fontanel, occurs if an infant is pulled too rapidly from the breast or if a bottle is pulled away from the infant too quickly. The soft palate is believed to sink in, thereby leading to difficulties feeding and swallowing, as well as fussiness, fever and diarrhea. Some of the folk remedies for mollera caida include sucking on the fontanel or pushing up against the soft palate. Therapy is aimed at "realigning" the fontanel. The most dangerous remedy involves hanging the infant over a basin of hot water and tapping the feet. There is one report of a Latino infant's death resulting from subdural hematomas that occurred after his grandmother held him by the ankles and partially submerged his head in boiling water while shaking and tapping his feet.

"Fatalismo," or fatalism, is expressed in the Latino culture when a parent accepts adversity with the phrase "lo que Dios quiera" ("whatever God wills"). Pediatricians may experience fatalismo when a parent seems less concerned than expected when faced with a difficult diagnosis or treatment. This attitude may be interpreted as lassitude, laziness or lack of understanding.

Asian Americans

At the 9-month visit, Dr. Smyth asks Mrs. Nguyen how her daughter is sleeping. Mrs. Nguyen reports that her daughter is sleeping very well; in fact, she sleeps in bed with the parents all night and wakes to nurse several times. As part of his anticipatory guidance, Dr. Smyth recommends to Mrs. Nguyen that her daughter sleep in her own crib and suggests that she let her "cry it out" for increasing periods to learn to sleep alone. His suggestion is met with a "Yes, doctor," and a puzzled look on Mrs. Nguyen's face. Note: This example illustrates differing perspectives on the goals of child rearing and a common misconception that one is communicating when just the opposite is true.

Asian Americans are a heterogeneous group consisting of people from Japan, China, Taiwan, Southeast Asia, Indonesia and the Philippines. In some ways, many of these subgroups are more different than alike, but they share many common values and beliefs.

A Different Sense of Self Asians generally see themselves and define themselves by their placement in a family, in a community and in a history. Individual traits are less important than one's place and the role that is demanded of that position. This attitude evolved from the hierarchical cultures that are the traditional norm in most of these regions, where one's role and place in life are strictly determined. Confucianism tradition adds to one's sense of duty, the importance of obedience and restraint of personal desires and goals. Asian culture does not stress independence and autonomy; conformity and obedience are valued. The individual is viewed as secondary in importance to the family and community. In a study from Great Britain, Asian and white parents were asked to rate the importance of various child qualities. Whereas white parents rated traits highly that promoted self-direction in children (having good judgment, self-control, being responsible, being interested), Asian parents tended to rate traits highly that promoted conformity in children (good manners, honesty, being clean, obedience). Emphases are placed on harmony and maintaining good relationships in the home, workplace and community, all in line with the broader cultural values.

Child Rearing When the desired outcomes are obedience and conformity, Asian parents might be expected to rule with a strict, iron hand style, but such is not usually the case. In general, Asian parents use a disciplinary style that may seem superficially indulgent from a Western perspective, one that is guided by the principle of mutual cooperation. There are subtle forms of behavioral shaping to mold this cooperation and obedience over the long term. A traditional Japanese belief is that it is not appropriate to use "controlling" types of behavior, such as anger or impatience, to influence the child because it is feared that resentment and disobedience will result. Young children are raised without strict discipline or limit setting during infancy and toddlerhood, but there is close hovering over the child so that any unacceptable behavior is clearly, but gently shaped in another direction.

With age, there is a growing emphasis on conformity and mutual respect with explicit teaching of the rules of conduct. Identifying the effect that one's behavior has on the reputation and well-being of the family becomes increasingly important. Asian parents use shame, embarrassment and guilt because these are well-regarded, well-accepted disciplinary methods used by Asian parents. It is not unusual for parents to poke fun at children or to recount stories of misbehavior to emphasize the importance of not embarrassing or shaming the family in the future. Proper form and decorum are valued in social practice, and this formal style of interaction is modeled for children at an early age. Love and affection are openly and visibly expressed primarily with infants; thereafter, parents demonstrate love for their children by providing and caring for them rather than by openly displayed physical affection. Lack of restraint in any emotional valence is humiliating to families. Western clinicians may think that such responses are cold or unfeeling or wonder whether they have gotten through at all.

> Dr. Garrity just finished making a tough disclosure to the Chin family that their 3-year-old, Alex, has leukemia. The family was stone-faced, asked few questions and agreed to all that was suggested. She wasn't sure the family understood what she had tried hard to explain and was particularly concerned whether they understood the seriousness of the diagnosis and required treatment. Note: There is a difference in the norms of emotional expression here, not in commitment to the child.

Kagan studied early interactional patterns of Chinese American and European American infants and found that Chinese American infants vocalized less, were less likely to smile at external stimuli and demonstrated more social restraint and inhibition than European American infants did. These neonates were quieter, less irritable and easier to calm when upset. Chinese American parents may be less likely to reinforce verbal and affective displays by their children, consistent with the Asian value of social restraint. In contrast to Western families, some Asian families may not value or encourage early language skills. A child who talks excessively may be considered rude and obnoxious. His behavior may reflect poorly on the mother, whose job is to anticipate her child's every need so that there is no need for the child to use words for requests. Clinicians who evaluate the language development of children from Asian families may face challenges that go beyond language barriers. For example, a pediatrician who recommends that a child be engaged as a conversational partner to prompt language development may be met with a blank stare by an Asian parent to whom this concept is completely foreign.

Cosleeping is practiced in most Asian cultures, at least partly as a reflection of the early promotion of interdependence. This custom stands in contrast to most Western parents, who value self-sufficiency and independence in their children and therefore expect their offspring to learn quickly to sleep by themselves. In fact, the first night of uninterrupted solo sleep is often a cause for celebration in mainstream American households, a concept that would baffle traditional Asian parents.

Avoiding Confusion in Communication Many Asian parents will answer "yes" or nod out of respect for the clinician, regardless of whether they agree with or understand what is being said.

Dr. Thomas: "Your son has an ear infection that is not severe. I think he will get better on his own in a short while. You can use ibuprofen to treat his pain. It is very important that you bring him back in 2 days so that I can recheck his ears, okay?"

Mrs. Vo: "Yes, doctor."

Dr. Thomas: "I know that this can be a lot to remember, so just to be sure that everything is clear, can you tell me your understanding of his illness?"

Mrs. Vo: "Doctor, I'm sorry but I didn't really understand …"

Dr. Thompson recognized that "yes" does not always mean "I understand" and pursued the topic further. Had she not done so, Mrs. Vo would have left the office with a poor understanding of her son's condition and may not have returned for necessary follow-up.

Health, Illness and Interactions with the Health Care System Many Asian health-related belief systems center around balance and harmony to ensure spiritual and physical health. There are three basic causes of disease in traditional Asian medicine:

- Metaphysical
- Naturalistic
- Spiritual

Most traditional Asian cultures ascribe importance to *metaphysical balance between "hot" and "cold" forces.* Certain foods, parts of the body or experiences are designated as having either "hot" (energizing) or "cold" (calming) properties. Treatment of illnesses caused by a hot or cold imbalance relies on the principle of opposition. For example, childbirth is termed a "cold" experience because of the loss of blood and vital fluids, which are "hot" substances. To restore balance, in the postpartum period women consume "hot" foods such as meat and spices. In Cambodia, the balance is also restored by a tradition known as "mother roasting," in which the new mother spends her first postpartum weeks lying in a bed with a fire continuously lit beneath it.

Naturalistic causes of disease refer to the belief that an individual can become ill because natural forces known as "winds" can enter the body. At times the "winds" refer to actual weather changes; however, more often they refer to changes in environmental "energy flow." Newborn infants are often swaddled extensively, despite the temperature, to protect them from the "winds" during the vulnerable neonatal period. Physical treatments such as rubbing the skin with eggs or coins (in Vietnamese called "cao gio," or "coining"), applying warm cups to the skin or acupuncture are often used to alter energy flow and/or draw bad "winds" to the surface so that they may be eliminated from the body. Many clinicians are familiar with the Southeast Asian practices of coining and cupping, which leave marks on the skin from friction (coining) or suction (cupping). Without knowledge of this practice, the ecchymosis and petechiae produced by coining and cupping may inappropriately suggest child maltreatment or a bleeding disorder.

Spiritual beliefs about health and illness are found among many in the Southeast Asian culture, especially the Hmong of Laos. This Asian culture is a past-oriented culture, in contrast to traditional Western future orientation. Honoring tradition and the worship of ancestors is emphasized. Ancestors are often believed to play a role in a person's current physical and spiritual well-being. Failure to honor ancestors is a potential reason for an individual to fall ill. Spiritual harmony may also be disrupted if a person experiences fright or grief or is the recipient of unkind words. In Taiwanese folk medicine, for example, if a child has colic and is irritable but has no fever, he has "ching" (fright), which is a condition of soul loss. Prevention of such illnesses takes the form of charms, strings and other jewelry that is believed to "lock" the soul and prevent it from leaving the body. Clinicians should be aware that what seems to be adornment on children may actually have greater significance to the family. Spiritual illnesses are often treated with soul-calling ceremonies performed by spiritual healers, or shamans.

Herbs and natural remedies are also widely used in many Asian communities. Most are harmless and some, such as ginger, may be helpful. A dangerous home remedy is "pay-loo-ah," a lead compound sold by traditional healers and traditional Chinese medicine practitioners. Parents give this reddish orange powder to their children for fever and rash. Many Asian Americans consider home remedies, herbal therapies or traditional Chinese medicine as their primary resource when ill and will turn to Western medicine as a "last resort."

Clinical Encounters Clinicians should be aware of other cultural norms when interacting with Asian patients. Conflict is to be avoided in Asian cultures, consistent with the emphasis on harmony. Many Asians will avoid saying "no" to prevent any offense or hurt feelings, especially to a figure of authority such as a health care provider. Clinicians should be aware that a "yes" answer may not mean "I agree," but rather "I respect you" or "I have heard you." Open-ended questions that allow the patient to elaborate or repeat instructions will help avoid confusion.

Asian patients may also demonstrate respect for authority by avoiding eye contact, which to the uninformed clinician may seem suggestive of disinterest, insincerity or dishonesty. Formal introductions and terms of address are generally better accepted than a more typically western casual style, at least when first meeting a family.

In many Asian cultures, especially Southeast Asian, it is considered offensive to touch another person on the head because that is where the soul is believed to reside. Clinicians should proceed slowly with a head examination and explain what they are doing. Avoid casually patting infants on the head. Conversely, the foot is believed to be the "lowliest" part of the body, and to point it at another, such as occurs with certain body postures, or to expose the sole of one's foot to another is considered insulting. Explaining what one needs to do and why will help alleviate some discomfort.

Personal and family problems, including most mental health conditions, are often a source of shame for Asian families. Many patients will discuss these issues in an indirect manner, with veiled references to the problem. The same process may occur with serious pediatric developmental concerns, for which Asian parents often feel a sense of blame. When there is a need to ask direct and focused questions, a careful explanation about why such questions are necessary demonstrates cultural sensitivity to how disquieting and uncomfortable this approach is for a family. Mental health issues are frequently somaticized because it is much more acceptable to have a physical ailment than a "mental problem." Complaints of headaches, digestive problems and other seemingly nonspecific illnesses may be the family's way of bringing forward behavioral and developmental complaints. A wise clinician will sensitively probe the matter beyond the initial complaint.

African Americans

A 20-month-old African American boy is brought to the clinic by his mother for an uncomplicated acute illness. At the end of the encounter, she states that she is very worried that her son is not yet potty trained. She further expresses concern and frustration that he "doesn't even try." By the time her daughter was 20 months old, she was already "fully" potty trained. The child's grandmother believes that he is simply "lazy."

African Americans are a diverse group of people with ancestry primarily from Africa and the Caribbean. The greatest concentration of this group is in the Southeast and mid-Atlantic regions. African Americans constitute approximately 12% of the U.S. population, with a projected growth to 14.3% by the year 2035.

Family Foundations Family and church shape the beliefs, value systems and health-related behavior of African Americans. Adults in addition to the parents are often part of these families—grandparents, godparents and other relatives or friends with only a very distant connection. This family-like relationship with friends and neighbors—classificatory aunts, uncles and cousins in anthropology terms—means that the network of care and influence may be very wide for African American children. They see more relatives per week than children in other groups do, and this extended kinship system may have a more important role in children's lives. African Americans tend to do more explicit teaching about their social and religious traditions than other groups do. The central role of senior women comes from matriarchal traditions that still exist in West Africa. One way to demonstrate understanding of this value of respect for elders by children is to use appropriate titles such as "Mr.," "Miss," or "Mrs.," unless invited to do otherwise. A wise clinician will follow suit unless given explicit permission to do otherwise.

Churches have been the cornerstone of stability for African American families. During and after slavery, the church was a major support system to the African American community. Religion plays a major role in the health beliefs, practices and behavior of African Americans. Church ministers often have powerful influence in the community. Public health programs, advocacy campaigns and establishment of new health programs and initiatives will benefit from consulting and including the religious leaders in the African American community.

Child-Rearing Values African American children are taught to be devoted, respectful and loyal to their relatives. However, the values of assertiveness and independence are also encouraged. Both self-reliance and self-control are values to be encouraged. Children are often responsible for the care of their younger siblings or other young children, a practice that has very long roots in African tradition. Child health care providers should be aware of these care arrangements when providing health and safety counsel.

The firm, authoritarian mode of discipline practiced by many African American families is often in contrast to the "democratic" manner in which mainstream American families discipline their children. Immediate obedience is often demanded by parents. During a clinical encounter, it is not unusual for a parent to share with a clinician that the child gets "a good whipping" if he is not behaving. There is typically little room for discussion or negotiation between the parent and child. The biblical adage "Spare the rod, spoil the child" is a part of child-rearing beliefs in many African American families.

The way in which various cultures approach toilet training and how they traditionally go about it tell us a lot about the differing views on raising a child. In a comparative study of African American, Latino and white parents, African American and Latino parents indicated that they expected their children to overcome the "dependency" of infancy as soon as possible.

In another study of the developmental expectations of four cultural groups (African Americans, Puerto Ricans, European Americans and West Indian/Caribbeans), Pachter and Dworkin inquired about the age at which children should be toilet trainable. African American mothers' response was 20 months, as compared with a response of 28 months by European American mothers. The response by Puerto Rican and West Indian/Caribbean mothers was intermediate at about 22 months. Many African American families expect toilet training to occur at an early age, and there may be limited tolerance when it occurs later than expected.

An extreme of this expectation is seen in an East African culture. The Digos believe that infants are toilet trainable soon after birth and, in fact, are successfully toilet trained by 5 or 6 months of age. The model for toilet training used by this tribal group is considerably different from that used in Western culture; it relies on the mother recognizing the child's signals of the need to eliminate. The U.S. approach is that this is a child-initiated activity.

The communication style of African Americans has been viewed as aberrant by some in mainstream American culture. Many African Americans speak with a culturally distinctive, nonstandard dialect of English often referred to as "black English." It is typically characterized by omitting the verb "is" in the present tense, using singular nouns for plural objects and dropping final consonants. These forms have their roots in traditional African languages. Some health care providers view this particular dialect as substandard English. African American children may even be identified as having speech or language problems. The use of these dialects by African American children should be viewed as a language "difference" more than as a disorder. The recommendation by many linguists is that children be taught to use the "nonstandard dialect" when in a home environment and reserve the "standard dialect" for formal speeches, as well as classroom conversations with teachers.

Illness and the Health Care System Illness in the African American community is described as *natural* or *unnatural*. *Natural illnesses* result when an individual fails to maintain harmony in the physical or natural world. Examples of *natural illnesses* are "high blood" (hypertension) and "low blood" (anemia), conditions perceived to be caused by lifestyle excesses and as a punishment from God. An herbalist often treats these conditions, whereas a Western-oriented clinician is sometimes a last resort. Knowledge about the specific names for *natural illnesses* and conditions used by African American families is useful to clinicians who care for African American children (Box 3–3).

Unnatural illnesses occur when the individual is the victim of a hex, curse or spell. When the "plan of God" is disrupted, the illness is perceived as "unnatural." These illnesses are often behavioral (e.g., autism) or gastrointestinal in nature, and blame is assigned to a patient if there is no specific diagnosis or the treatment has failed. Treatment may involve the recruitment of a "conjurer," one with specific "powers" to cure someone who has been "hexed." Prayer and incantations are used.

> ## BOX 3–3   PHRASES AND TERMS USED BY AFRICAN AMERICANS TO DESCRIBE ILLNESS
>
> - Falling out—Fainting or loss of consciousness
> - Falling off—Weight loss
> - Sugar—Diabetes
> - Low blood—Anemia
> - High blood—Hypertension and/or polycythemia

Many African Americans perceive themselves not as equals to the white majority. There is often a distrust of mainstream institutions and health care providers who are members of the dominant culture. This distrust is based not only on memories of slavery but also on more recent historical experiences, such as the abuses of the 40-year Tuskegee syphilis study, in which African American men recruited for the study were promised, but never given treatment. This type of experience often makes it difficult to recruit African American families into any form of experimental research because it is often met with suspicion. Even health advisories come under suspicion. The directive to put infants on their backs to sleep to prevent sudden infant death syndrome has been poorly accepted among African Americans. Suspicion about this change in "traditional" baby care seems to explain most of the failure to adopt this practice.

Native Americans

Mr. and Mrs. Running Bear called to say that they were canceling knee surgery for their son John. When they arrived at the hospital, John said he wanted to go home. The parents said that it was his choice. Note: This case illustrates the individual locus of control and decision that is typical of Native American groups but often seems inexplicable to western health care providers.

The term Native American refers to a large and heterogeneous population of more than 500 different tribal groups. These tribes differ widely, and a wise clinician should seek specific information on groups in his area.

Stereotyped and homogenized images of Native Americans in books, television, movies and toys shape our ideas of their culture, which is really quite varied and complex. These images depict Native Americans as either fierce savages or dreamy "nature people" who talk to plants and animals. Such portrayal of Native Americans is culturally and historically incorrect. Native American children who encounter such stereotypical images may be hindered in the development of pride in their heritage, self-image and cultural identity. To correct these errors, school curricula now include accurate information about Native American history and the culture of contemporary Native Americans (see *www.nativechild.com*).

Without yielding to the blender error of overgeneralization, some common themes are relevant to many of America's native peoples. These cultures value conformity to specific

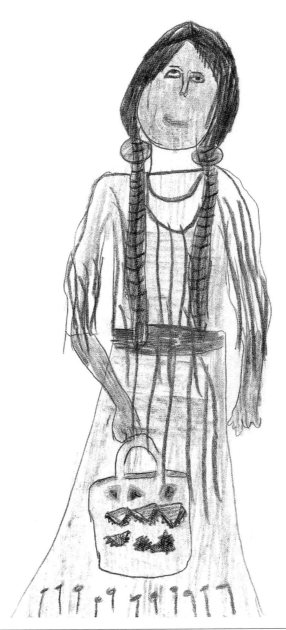

A Native American girl is shown in all her finery, her traditional dress (original in colored pencils). By M. D., a girl aged 11.

behavioral standards and group solidarity. Patience and honesty are important. Harmony within the family and community is connected to harmony with nature; both are sought as key goals in life.

Central to the Native American value system is a belief in the inviolability of the individual, or the idea that persons of any age have the right to make their own decisions with respect to personal action. It is seen as rude or improper to directly order or force anyone to do something against his will. Individual freedom is accorded to all members of the tribe, regardless of age. As one example, in Sioux tradition, a deep respect for individual autonomy is granted to even the youngest children. They are permitted to participate in decisions that may affect their risk for injury, health and illness and career path. In medicine, this belief may translate into children deciding whether they want to participate in certain therapies (e.g., a surgical procedure as in the case study presented earlier, chemotherapy, counseling or speech therapy). Parents who are noncompliant with a prescribed medicine or treatment may simply state, "He didn't want to do it." Western medical providers may incorrectly interpret this response as laziness or lack of responsible parenting skills when in fact, it is consistent with the cultural value of individual freedom of choice.

Child Rearing The emphasis in the rearing of children is placed on respecting the child's own freedom of choice, with the expectation that the child will likewise respect the individual choices of others. Children are responsible for knowing and choosing the proper path. Knowing comes from one's own inner reality, as well as from the implicit and explicitly taught norms of the tribe. Discipline techniques that attempt to constrain or control the child are used rarely. Physical punishment goes against traditional approaches.

Interactions between people of Native American cultures are rich in nonverbal communication. Parents often use "silent language," such as gestures, body language, touch and facial expression, to communicate with their children. In a study of parenting practices among mothers from different cultural groups, it was found that Navajo mothers had a more passive and silent interactional style with their infants than African American or white mothers did. Clinicians who assess language development in Native American children should consider the child's total language environment. A suggestion to "narrate the day" with a toddler or preschool child to stimulate language development may seem absurd to Navajo and other Native American parents. Moreover, it is likely to be foreign to the child as well because verbal interaction with an adult is not usually expected of them.

Raising children is seen as a tribal responsibility, with active participation of extended family members. Tribal elders perform the vital task of passing on the tribe's history and the culture to children through a rich inheritance of folklore and storytelling. Many tribes have a matrilineal heritage structure, so a child's maternal uncles may have a very important role to play in the child's life (Box 3–4).

Concepts of Health, Illness and Healing In traditional Native American folk medicine, the health of an individual is linked to the people and objects in that individual's environment. Illness occurs because of an imbalance between the individual and that universe. This imbalance can take on many forms or have several components. There are spiritual, mental and physical elements of a person's state of health, and healing must address all these elements. Native American medicine uses a holistic approach that emphasizes the treatment of mind, body and spirit together. Treatment of an individual may involve the participation of family

BOX 3–4

Early in the 20th century, developmental psychologists and anthropologists believed that Hopi infants were delayed in onset of walking because of the use of cradleboards. It was assumed that the constrictive nature of the cradleboard and the long periods of constraint did not allow them to practice the skills needed for ambulation. In 1940, Dennis found that Hopi infants were slower in onset of walking than their mainstream American peers were, with a mean age at onset of approximately 15 months, regardless of whether a cradleboard was used. A 1982 study, however, demonstrated an average age of walking of 12.5 months for Hopi infants; infants reared on the cradleboard walked as early as unrestrained infants. The authors evaluated possible reasons for the difference in findings between their study and Dennis' study and concluded that an inadequate diet of the infants evaluated in the earlier study was the most significant contributor. They hypothesized that the accelerated rate of walking reflected the enhanced quality of Hopi infant nutrition from programs such as the Indian Women, Infants and Children's Program. This series of events illustrates the potential pitfalls of making assumptions about child-rearing practices without supportive data (e.g., the incorrect assumption that cradleboard use leads to a delay in walking). It also highlights the importance of considering potential contributing environmental factors (e.g., nutritional status) when evaluating the development of an individual or a population.

members, friends or the entire community. The spiritual world is inseparable from the material one, and this belief may affect the way in which "health" is perceived. For example, an American pediatrician may consider attention deficit/hyperactivity disorder (ADHD) to be a physical/psychological disorder, whereas a Native American parent may describe her child's ADHD symptoms as "spiritual gifts."

Although the specific details of treatment methods vary from tribe to tribe, most forms of traditional Native American medicine incorporate the following four practices in some way.

First is the involvement of *traditional healers,* sometimes referred to as "medicine men/ women." These healers are considered to be links to the spiritual world. The relationship between the patient and the healer is of considerable importance and provides the energy needed to begin the healing process. The healer may go into a trance-like state to seek help from "spirit guides" in order to address the spiritual part of a patient's illness.

The second practice is the use of *herbal remedies.* Herbs are either ingested or burned ceremoniously and wafted over the patient.

The third practice is that of *purification or purging rituals.* The most familiar of these practices is the use of sweat lodges, in which the patient and healer sit inside a small covered structure and engage in healing ceremonies in an environment of steam made by water and hot stones. These rituals allow for the patient's intentions and beliefs to work together for healing. They often involve the idea of passage from one state to another, one place to another. The ceremonies vary between tribes but usually consist of a combination of dancing, painting, chanting and drumming in combination with feathers, rattles, sacred stones and other sacred objects.

Interactions with the Health Care System Interactions between Native Americans and the western medical system are shadowed by a history of oppression and mistrust. For 300 years before the 20th century, many tribes were decimated by westward-moving white soldiers and settlers. These historical memories are often associated with significant discomfort among Native Americans when interacting with "authority." They may view the medical system with suspicion and distrust because it is perceived as being an extension of the government and colonialism. Clinicians may find Native American patients reluctant to disclose personal information. A patient's trust must be gained over the course of several visits before attempting to discuss sensitive matters. Medical information about birth control and family planning may be met with suspicion because it may be seen as an attempt to reduce the tribal population. It is not in keeping with traditional Native American values to try to control birth rates and fertility because interference in these natural processes is not embraced. Additionally, most tribes desire increases in their populations.

As in other cultures, Native Americans may avert their gaze to demonstrate respect; prolonged direct eye contact is considered rude. To the Navajo, in particular, direct eye contact is believed to create a conduit by which the evil spirits of one person may travel toward and enter another. Eye contact is not a reliable indicator of attentiveness or sincerity. The preferred social communication style is quiet, reserved and respectful. Native peoples expect long pauses to allow the participants to process information and carefully craft a response. Loud, enthusiastic or boisterous conversation is usually offensive. Pressure to respond is regarded as rude.

Many tribes, such as the Sioux and the Navajo, traditionally have no concept of time; "waiting" and "being late" may be unfamiliar ideas. A traditional Native American belief is that the time when an event should take place is when things are in order for the event, which may or may not correspond with a set appointment time. This outlook has obvious implications for interactions between Native Americans and the western medical system.

The Arab Culture

Dr. Lake is concerned with the frequency of asthma exacerbations being experienced by her 5-year-old patient Nadir. On numerous occasions she has discussed with Nadir's parents the need for inhaled corticosteroids to prevent further episodes. The family refuses such therapy, which has left Dr. Lake frustrated with her apparent inability to convince the parents of the seriousness of Nadir's disease. Note: This case illustrates the cultural basis as a source of poor compliance with a prescribed medical intervention. Preventive care doesn't make sense to this family, and it may even be seen in their attitude toward treatment.

Arabs have cultural origins from over 20 countries in the Middle East and North Africa. Though a rich and varied group, Arabs share a common ancestry, history and language, which gives them a common cultural identity. Although a significant proportion of Arab emigrants to the United States are Christian, many Arab Americans endorse the beliefs of Islam.

The Role of the Child within the Family In Arab culture, the extended family is the strongest social unit. Elders are often given the major decision-making roles. The needs of the individual always come second to the needs of the family. Core cultural values include commitment to family, honoring of obligations, loyalty, responsibility and unity. Gender and age define strict roles. The father's role is to provide for his family and protect them. The role of the mother is to nurture her spouse and children and ensure good social standing of the family within society. As such, she is also expected to raise her children according to Arab culture and tradition.

Children are highly valued for many reasons. They provide their parents with continuation of the family name, with greater connectedness to society and with higher social standing. As an example of this greater social standing, consider the renaming of parents that occurs after the birth of a male child. If the son's name is Raja, the father's name will become Abu Raja (father of Raja) and the mother's name will become Um Raja (mother of Raja). These highly valued children are not without their own roles and expectations within the family, however. Children are expected to obey and honor elders and parents and to put the family's needs before their own. A "good child" is one who is obedient, polite and disciplined and conforms to the values of the group. A child's behavior reflects on the family; a misbehaving child or rebellious teenager can be a source of shame and embarrassment. Parents are blamed for the misbehavior of children, especially that of adolescents. Children are expected to care for elderly parents.

Arab families who immigrate to the United States may struggle with the individualistic values that are omnipresent in American society and are often reinforced in American schools. The concepts of "independence" and "looking out for oneself" fly in the face of the traditional Arab values of group unity and placing one's own needs second. Parents may fear losing control over their children and thus over their own values and traditions.

Children are often indulged as infants; they are frequently held, caressed and talked to lovingly by all members of the extended family. Breastfeeding and cosleeping are common into the third year. As children enter toddlerhood and middle childhood, responsibility increases, as does the mandate for parents to teach them. This includes formal education and the inculcation of social customs. Parents are to treat children with respect and without violence. They are to provide guidance to the teen but show increasing respect for the young person with consideration of his opinions.

The concepts of "maturity" and "adulthood" may pose problems for Muslims among the Arab community and others from the Arab world as they interact with the western medical system. In American society, by secular law, an adolescent is an adult, free to make medical and legal decisions at the age of 18 or even younger in some circumstances. In Islamic teachings, however, an adolescent is considered to have reached adulthood when he or she is "intellectually mature." This is determined by the family's assessment of the adolescent's ability to live and function independently. An adolescent who is *legally* able to make health-related decisions may not be considered by his parents to be mature enough to do so.

Nineteen-year-old Muhammad suffers from supraventricular tachycardia. Dr. Blake discusses several options with him, including an ablation procedure. Muhammad elects to go ahead with the procedure, and it is scheduled for the following month. The next day, Dr. Blake takes a telephone call from Muhammad's parents, who do not feel that he is mature enough to make such decisions. They state angrily that their rights as parents have been violated.

Health-Related Beliefs and Practices The Arab culture is present oriented; a preoccupation with the future can be seen as unnatural and unhealthy. The future is thought to be in God's hands, and any attempt to predict or control it may be perceived as defiance of God's will. This belief has obvious implications for the delivery of health care because Western clinicians place a high value on the anticipation and prevention of future problems. For example, a parent of a child with a developmental disability may refuse to plan for declines in the child's functioning. Clinicians unfamiliar with the culture might incorrectly interpret such refusal as lack of understanding, denial or indifference. Disease prevention defies this perspective on illness causality, as illustrated by the case of Nadir with asthma described earlier.

Some Arabs believe that even speaking about something bad may bring it about or that thinking about accidents or diseases may actually cause them to occur. Illness may be treated once it appears, but to plan for such an occurrence is believed to possibly affect the future adversely.

Arab cultures share with others belief in the evil eye and in hot/cold imbalance as a cause of illness. "Evil eye" is thought to occur when a child is admired in a boastful way without mentioning the name of God. It may also occur when an individual or family has some good fortune that evokes jealousy in others. Arab parents may protect their children from the evil eye by having them wear amulets or by burning incense nearby. Traditional healers may be used to cure the evil eye through the use of herbs, incense and prayer. Exuberant praise of a child is believed to be dangerous under this belief system.

Cold is often seen as causing illness, and a hot remedy is required. The offending agent is usually a cold current or draft causing gastrointestinal, respiratory and muscular symptoms. Treatment is aimed at restoring balance through hot foods and heavy blankets.

Many Arabs use home remedies before seeking care from the western medical system. Such remedies include "sweating out a fever," herbal teas such as chamomile and mint and concoctions of sugar, fruit and honey. Although most of these interventions are safe, clinicians would be wise to ask parents about any home remedies used so that appropriate counseling can be initiated (i.e., regarding the inadvisability of giving honey to infants or of overbundling an infant who is already febrile). Although Arabs may use these home remedies, most place high value on the western medical system and have confidence in the healing abilities of doctors. They do not usually delay long in seeking care when ill.

Another time-honored healing tradition is that of prayer. Many Arabs will read verses from the Quran or the Bible to give comfort and enhance recovery of the patient.

Communication and Expectations An ill person, whether child or adult, is expected to take on the "sick role." This person is neither to perform self-care nor to participate greatly in discussions or decision making. Decision making is left to the patient's family. It is expected that the clinician will tell the patient only the good news about his condition. In fact, the entire family may prefer a positive outlook with negative details played down. Talking about a bad thing is believed to cause or expedite its occurrence; talking about death hastens it. Hope is critical both for the patient and for the family. These expectations surrounding health communication can clearly pose problems for clinicians. Western medicine operates under the principle that patients should be fully informed of their condition, as well as treatment options. A wise clinician will proceed with caution when a child is severely ill. Under such serious circumstances, it may be prudent to consult the eldest family member and enlist the support and negotiation skills of a hospital ethics team, religious leaders or community leaders.

Privacy is highly valued in the Arab culture. Patients or parents being interviewed may prefer to give as little information as possible. They may feel that a clinician should be able to diagnose and treat a problem simply by seeing the patient and may grow frustrated with in-depth questioning. Medical histories are often viewed as quite intrusive. Psychological and emotional information is guarded especially closely, and many Arab patients resent discussing problems in such areas. For example, a study of parents in the United Arab Emirates found that only 38% of parents would seek help from a mental health specialist in the event of psychiatric problems in their child. As in many cultures, there remains a stigma attached to mental illness. Emotional or psychological problems may be brought to a clinician's attention in the form of vague somatic complaints. If the situation is not an emergency one, it is advisable to try to divide sensitive questions among multiple visits so that a patient or parent is not overwhelmed by too much in-depth questioning.

FROM PRINCIPLES TO PRACTICE

Once we understand and acknowledge the impact that culture has on a patient's health beliefs, practices and behavior, how do we incorporate these concepts into daily practice? How can we apply this cultural information to each clinical encounter, regardless of the patient's specific cultural background?

Lee Pachter proposed a model for cultural competency known as "*awareness-assessment-negotiation.*" This model can be applied in visits with patients from any cultural traditions, regardless of whether the clinician is familiar with that specific tradition. It is especially helpful when working with children, adolescents and families whose beliefs about health and illness do not fit into a standard Western biomedical model.

Awareness Comes First

The clinician must learn the commonly held beliefs, practices and values specific to the patient population that is being served. Knowledge is part of this step, but cultural awareness extends to how we present ourselves as health care providers as well. Realizing that our own perspectives shape our interaction with patients sets the stage for us to consciously modify our approach in line with the family's expectation. The concept of "professionalism," for example, is embedded in our Western style of communication. We tend to hold a strong belief that our professional self is significantly different from our personal self. We place a significant value on "directness" and "getting to the point." Some cultural groups find this approach offensive. Many Latino families, for example, place a greater value on the concept of "personalismo," or formal friendliness. The expectation is that the clinician will show considerable warmth toward the patient and develop a more personal relationship with the family. Awareness of this difference allows for modification of our behavior in a clinical encounter. One way to demonstrate this might be by sitting closer to the family during the visit or by ending the visit with a tap on the caregiver's shoulder in addition to a handshake. Awareness of this particular value leads to better communication with this specific cultural group, a more rewarding interaction and better outcomes.

Assessment Is Next

The second part of the model asks for *assessment* of whether the family with whom we are interacting embraces a particular belief system and under what circumstances. There is always the risk of stereotyping when dealing with people from other cultures. One cannot assume that everyone who is African American is a proponent of corporal punishment, for example, nor can we assume that all Asian Americans practice coining.

One way to obtain information about the level to which a patient or family subscribes to some of these beliefs is to first share with them what you know specifically about their culture. Follow this with a direct inquiry, preferably with an open-ended approach. This assessment will need to be done for each specific issue. Families vary in the level of acculturation or inclusion in the mainstream culture. Practitioners who wish to explore health-related belief systems may use the questions from Figure 3–1.

The Kleinman Cultural History

1. What do you think has caused your problem?

2. Why do you think it started when it did?

3. What do you think your sickness does to you and your body? How does it work?

4. What are the chief problems your sickness has caused for you?

5. How severe do you think your sickness is? Do you think it will have a long or short course?

6. What do you fear most about your sickness?

7. What have you done to treat your sickness so far?

8. What kind of treatment do you think you should receive?

9. What are the most important outcomes you want to receive from this treatment?

(From Kleinman A, Eisenberg L, Good B: Culture, illness and care: Clinical lessons from anthropologic and cross-cultural research. *Ann Intern Med* 88:251-258, 1978.)

Figure 3–1 The Kleinman Cultural History

Now the Balancing Act

The third part of the model calls for *negotiation*. The health care provider must find ways of compromising with families if there is an area of conflict resulting from cultural differences that has significant consequences for the child. It is at this point that a clinician's cultural awareness and sensitive assessment are put to the test. If a parent has inappropriate expectations and a punitive approach to toilet training, for example, the health care provider may encourage the parent to delay toilet training until the child demonstrates signs of readiness for bowel or bladder control and to use positive rewards. The parent may continue to feel empowered, and at the same time the child will no longer be subjected to punitive consequences. The clinician can explain his own view, starting with the word "I" ("I think that force feeding a child ..."). Always supply an explanation for the view or the belief, perhaps with a statement about the evolution of that view ("We used to have no treatment for this condition, but now we ..."). Clearly state your recommendation and your view of the consequences. Reflect the parent's perspective as a positive one, but clearly state the consequences of that approach as you see them. Start with "I" ("I think that failing to give the medication will ..."). Then solicit a response, and wait for as long as it takes. The dialogue can then begin.

Although we cannot become experts on every cultural group, awareness coupled with knowledge of the health beliefs, practices and expectations of families from the cultures that we serve promises to be beneficial to each clinical encounter. Cultural competency adds effectiveness, flexibility and sparkle to our clinical lives.

For some practices that are not harmful but are just different, a wise clinician may wish to point out the differences, provide information as the parent requests and leave the matter alone. Interest in cultural traditions, respect for practices that are not harmful, and willingness to hear about these matters will set the stage for further positive interactions with a family involving both small and large concerns.

For seriously harmful practices, the health care provider may want to bring in key decision makers in the cultural group. These participants should have the issues laid out clearly, the recommendations made explicitly, and the clinician's view of the time frame for action. Areas of disagreement should be explored with patience and respect. For serious matters, the clinician may need to bring in key influencers such as elders, clergymen and grandparents. The foundation for these discussions should be that everyone, no matter their tradition, wants the best for their own child and that traditions different from our own have evolved because they were successful over the longer term in rearing children to survive and thrive in the culture in which they evolved.

HEADS UP–CULTURAL DIMENSIONS

Key Points in the Road to Cultural Competency
- The more we understand our own cultural biases, the more effective we are at caring for children and families from other cultures.
- Nobody is truly "cultureless"; the dominant American culture has its own characteristic set of values and beliefs.
- Culturally dependent variations in child-rearing practices often reflect different expectations from children that are culturally based.
- A person's identification with a particular culture is not a guarantee that the individual subscribes to all the beliefs of the group.
- Most cultural groups have explanatory models about health and illness that are divergent from Western medical theory.
- Many families will use traditional physical, herbal or spiritual healing remedies in addition to seeking Western medical care.

Cultural "Musts"
- Know who your patients are: Where do they live? What language do they speak? What is their background?
- Become familiar with the health-related beliefs and practices of the predominant cultural groups in your practice.
- Determine at each clinical encounter what, if any, cultural forces are at play.
- Assess whether individual patients subscribe to commonly held beliefs of their cultural groups; do not make assumptions.
- Negotiate a compromise between traditional remedies and Western medical therapies when possible.

INTERNET RESOURCES

Diversity Rx: http://www.diversityrx.org. Provides information for policymakers, health care providers and consumers on language and cultural competence in health care and program and policy design; also offers networking opportunities.

National Center for Cultural Competence: http://www.gudcd.georgetown.edu/nccc/. Provides information on cultural competence at a systems level; also gives links to other related web-based resources.

The Cross-Cultural Health Care Program: http://www.xculture.org. Has resources to help health care institutions provide accessible quality cross-cultural health care; also has very practical information "synopses" on a variety of different cultural groups.

RECOMMENDED READINGS

For Professionals

Fadiman A: *The Spirit Catches You and You Fall Down.* New York, Farrar, Straus and Giroux, 1997.

Johnson-Powell G, Yamamoto J (eds): *Transcultural Child Development.* New York, John Wiley & Sons, 1997.

Slonim MB: *Children, Culture, and Ethnicity: Evaluating and Understanding the Impact.* New York, Garland Publishing, 1991.

Small MF: *Kids: How Biology and Culture Shape the Way We Raise Our Children.* New York, Doubleday, 2001.

West C: *Race Matters.* New York, Vintage Books, 1994.

For Children

Ajmera M, Ivanko JD: *To Be a Kid*. Watertown, MA, Charlesbridge Publishing, 1998 (also available in Spanish).

Ajmera M, Ivanko JD: *Be My Neighbor*. Watertown, MA, Charlesbridge Publishing, 2004.

Ajmera M, Versola AR: *Children from Australia to Zimbabwe*. Watertown, MA, Charlesbridge Publishing, 1997.

Bernard E: *A Ride on Mother's Back*. New York, Harcourt Brace, 1996.

Pinckney S: *Shades of Black; a Celebration of Our Children*. Scholastic, 2000.

Shetterly SH: *The Dwarf-Wizard of Uxmal*. New York, Atheneum Publishers, 1990.

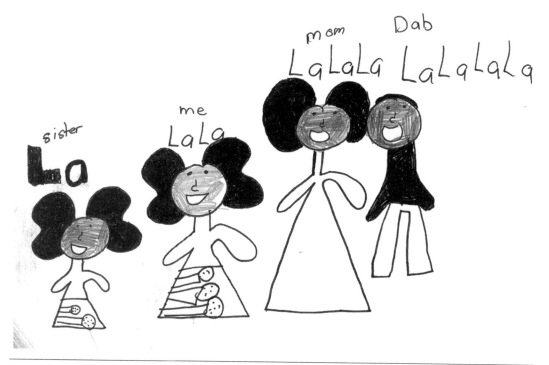

"My Family Singing." This child's ethnicity as an African American rings out in this family drawing. By Shaiete K. Brown, age 8.

CHAPTER 4

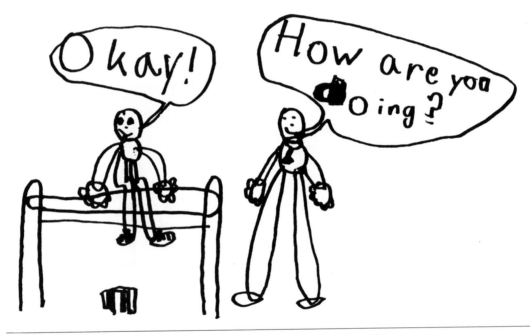

"Talking to my doctor." By Ryan Hennessy, age 7½.

Developmentally Based Office: Setting the Stage for Enhanced Practice

MARTIN T. STEIN

This chapter describes a developmental focus that can make clinical encounters with children and parents more efficient and productive. Specific components and methods of interviewing are illustrated to show how clinical tools can be used to make the most of each encounter. The physical layout of the office and the structural elements of the practice can enhance the quality and efficiency of care for the child and the whole family.

Key Words

- Interview
- Transactional-Educational Model
- Dual Patient
- Verbal and Nonverbal Communication
- Process and Content
- Explanatory Model
- Active Listening
- Transference
- Reflection and Self-awareness

Families are the primary context in which life is experienced, especially for children. Pediatricians tend to focus on the child's symptoms, developmental skills and behavior and spend less time assessing family strengths, stresses and life event changes. By incorporating the parents and the child as equal partners during the clinical **interview**, the clinician discovers important information about a family's strengths and potential stressors, such as marital discord, depression and economic and social uncertainties, along with specific data about the child's place in the family and community. The family-directed interview model supports the notion, confirmed by research and clinical experience, that the developmental potential of children is affected by the environment in which they live. Family-directed interviewing also encourages the generation of data about the child's home environment, which has been shown to have an important impact on a child's development.

THE ENCOUNTER AS A PLANNED EVENT

The clinical practice of preventive pediatric care is built on a **transactional-educational model**. When the clinical encounter is orchestrated in a manner that provides an educational experience for the parents, child and clinician, expanded gains emerge from the encounter. By *planned orchestration* of the style and content of the interview, a new dimension is added to the practice of pediatrics that makes it both more effective and more rewarding. The manner in which questions are asked, the types of questions asked, the direction of the questioning (to the parent and to the child) and the actual interaction with the child are critical components of the interview. They control not only the informational data base but also what parents and children learn about growth and development during times of illness and health.

THE PHYSICAL LAYOUT

The potential for an "educational experience" during a pediatric office visit begins before the actual visit. The physical and social ecology of a medical office that serves the needs of children requires forethought in planning and continuous modification. An appreciation that personnel, space, color and design can interact to create a positive, health-promoting atmosphere may generate interesting ideas that allow the office environment to enhance child development, parent-child-clinician interactions and assessments of health and development. The pictures or children's drawings selected for the walls, the availability of crawl and walk spaces, the toys in the reception area and the educational material made available to parents and children are at first seemingly unrelated decisions, but they create a unique theme in each office. A special message will be given to families even as they enter the clinic or office that this is a place for children and families, that children are expected to explore and that developmental concerns are front and center at this practice.

Whether a new office or clinic facility is being planned or modification to an established office seems possible, two questions should be asked:

"How can we plan to use the available space in a manner that is consistent with the developmental needs of the children and parents who will come to the facility?"

"Can the design promote comfort, relieve anxiety, nurture the parent-child relationship and maintain a learning and educational milieu?" Priorities, budgets and available space will vary among settings, but a core group of developmental principles are applicable to most pediatric offices, including the following:

- *A busy waiting room is like a neighborhood park.* Parents can observe their children learning to play and interact with other children. Toys, books or a wall board equipped for drawing will make these interactions more interesting for parents and children. The waiting room might also serve as an after-hours meeting place or informal classroom. It can be used for educational events, group care visits or places for families of children with special needs.

- *The waiting area should allow for movement and play of children.* The choices of flooring, wall covering and furniture should take into account the developmental requirements of children at various age groups. Safety, clean lines and cheerfulness are key elements. Avoid overstimulating, noisy or trendy decor. Doors should shut off main traffic areas.

- *Furniture and play objects can be safe, but still engaging and instructive.* A concern for a safe environment should not create a sterile office. Providing a space for containment of busy toddlers and a separate area for teens is ideal. Smaller, semicontained areas set a quieter and more contained tone for families.

- *Pictures of children and their families or drawings created by children* in the practice invite children to feel comfortable in the office and encourage conversation about the pictures' content among parents and other children.

- *A fish tank in the waiting room* may help alleviate the anxiety and fears that many children experience when visiting a physician's office.

- *Tables and chairs designed for toddlers and young children* and placed in the reception area may encourage a child to separate from the parent and independently open a book or play with a puzzle. Anxiety may be momentarily decreased as the child learns to manage a fear independent of the parent.

- *The availability of paper and marking pens or a chalkboard* will encourage children to draw pictures that may help them redirect fears about their symptoms, an illness or the concern observed in a parent. These drawings can be shown later to the clinician; they may provide valuable insight into the child, family or illness (see Chapter 5).

- *Observation of children and parents together by office personnel* allows data to be collected about developmental and interactional issues. Mechanisms in place to periodically assess these important "naturalistic" observations by an experienced office staff can be invaluable to a busy clinician. It also creates a sense of teamwork in the holistic care of a child and family.

Televisions in the waiting room may give an unintended message to a parent that TV viewing should fill in life's empty spaces. Monitoring appropriate content is an added burden for staff. Consider getting rid of the TV *or* be very vigilant about what's showing—it's a reflection of your values and may or may not help your patients.

AN INTERACTIVE MODEL

As the clinician acquires information from the parent and child, a broad social and medical data base is generated. The parent and older child receive information from the clinician that focuses on diagnosis, treatment and education. During the interview, parent-child interactions provide the clinician an opportunity to assess developmental skills of the child, as well as parenting skills and the dynamics of family interaction The interview is an opportunity to observe the interaction between child and parent—how the baby is undressed/dressed, fed, spoken to, spoken for and disciplined and how the child looks for comfort and receives it. The rewards of the clinical interview can be a shared learning experience. Careful engineering of this process can provide long-term gains in understanding the family and a clearer focus for care and guidance.

THE DUAL PATIENT

The pediatric interview encompasses the notion of the **dual patient**. The parent and child are the patient, both as individuals and as an interactional unit. We do not see any of them as "clients."

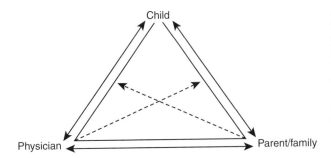

Figure 4–1 The therapeutic triangle in pediatrics. The educational model for the clinical pediatric interview should follow a pattern in which information exchange is dynamic for the three participants. (Adapted from Doherty WJ, Baird MA: *Family Therapy and Medicine: Toward the Primary Care of Families.* New York, Guilford Press, 1983, p 13.)

Although most of the historical facts during an interview will come from the parent, the child often provides important clues through verbal and nonverbal interactions. A frequent shortcoming of the pediatric interview is that the clinician, rather than actively involving the child, communicates exclusively with the parent. In a 3-year-old, expressive and receptive language skills provide the child with the ability to communicate symptoms and concerns to the clinician. If you find yourself talking more than half the time, it usually means that you aren't getting what *you* need from the interview. As a rule, patients should talk more than the clinician.

The interview should provide information and supportive care of the "third patient," the interaction between the child and the family unit, through direct questioning of the participants and sensitive observations of their interactions. It is useful to think about the process as involving a story or stories from the family members, and the work of the clinician is to hear the story and its personal meaning for each participant. The "therapeutic triangle" (Fig. 4–1) illustrates the influence of parents (and the extended family) on the relationship between the clinician and child; simultaneously, the child's clinician supports the relationship between the child and family because this is the vehicle of intervention, care and support for the child.

Questions should be directed to children with age-appropriate words and eye contact that will encourage the child's participation. Direct interaction with a child of any age acknowledges the important contribution that any individual child has on his own rearing, health and development. An appreciation of the dual patient directs the clinician's attention to concerns of both the parent and the child and to the important role that the interaction between them really plays. This approach enhances traditional pediatric advocacy for the needs of the child. (See Chapter 18, the 4-year-old health supervision visit, and subsequent chapters for examples of a coordinated parent-child interview.) One way of emphasizing the child's importance is to ask a child familiar to the office to state his reason for the visit first and to give him the last word as well.

LISTENING WITH YOUR EYES

Information from the clinical interview is derived from two major sources: **verbal and nonverbal communication** (Box 4–1). Interactional behavior—how the baby is held, fed, stroked, spoken to, looked at and so on—is also part of the nonverbal data base. Similarly, the relationship between an older child and parent should be observed and assessed during the

---

BOX 4–1 VERBAL AND NONVERBAL COMMUNICATION: MAJOR INFORMATION SOURCES

- **Verbal information** refers to the data that patients tell us about themselves, the core of the traditional medical history.
- **Nonverbal information** refers to observations we make about the style, timing, emotive ambience, flow of the interview and even what's *not* said. Facial expressions, posture, movements of the extremities and the quality and tone of speech are examples of important observations that frequently provide clues to critical aspects of a child's life and family environment. Clinicians often neglect this source of important information, and as a result their data gathering is less efficient and less accurate.

---

interview. Observations about communication style and content regarding discipline and self-help skills (e.g., undressing and getting on the examination table) can provide important clues about parent-child relationships, as well as developmental capacities. Children who are delayed or whom the parents perceive to need care appropriate for a younger age will show this behavior during the interaction. In fact, motor, social, adaptive and individual temperament skills can be assessed in a young child by observing the child's activity while the parent is providing the medical history, provided that the room and your focus are set in that direction.

Nonverbal data are as real as verbal statements and should therefore be incorporated into the medical evaluation. Often they give clearer and added information—information that may *not* be available verbally, no matter how exhaustive the interview may be.

Because pictures are worth a thousand words, these observations add to the efficiency and accuracy of the data set assembled by the clinician. In these days of rushed visits, one cannot afford to miss anything from the clinical encounter.

These observations should be written in the medical record and be given diagnostic status when appropriate (e.g., a sad child—rule out depression; a parent with multiple tics and a halting voice—consider parental anxiety; an active and difficult-to-comfort infant—keep in mind an active infant temperament). They should be incorporated into the problem list to ensure appropriate attention during follow-up care. In practices that use a child behavior checklist or a parent-family psychosocial screening instrument completed before the office visit (see Appendix), nonverbal observations can be compared with the parent's written observations. Confirmations and discrepancies may provide useful clinical information.

Nonverbal cues given by parents and children are a component of the **process** portion of the interview as opposed to the **content** portion. Although the process of an interview is interwoven with the content, it is helpful for the clinician to be aware of the two components as separate. In that way, verbal data can be understood within the context of the nonverbal information that was generated simultaneously by the parent or the child and monitored by a sensitive clinician. For example, a mother of a 2-month-old infant who demonstrates her anxiety as she states her concern about multiple minor somatic symptoms is understood more clearly when observation of nonverbal clues suggests maternal sleep deprivation or depression after birth of the child.

POSITIONING THE PARTICIPANTS

Certain aspects of the interview environment controlled by the clinician determine the quality and quantity of data that will be obtained. Planning the clinical space in an examination room may be guided by knowledge that the word *interview* is derived from *between* and *seeing*. By implication, the process of interviewing is a mutual communication of thoughts that can be influenced by the nature of the space between the clinician and patient. The clinician can and should actively determine that spacing. The following are issues to consider to create the best interview environment possible:

- The clinician and parent should be positioned at the same level to ensure eye contact and to prevent a subservient positioning effect. Both sit down or both stand up.
- The decision to conduct the interview in a sitting or standing position will change with the type of visit.
- For a new patient or a new problem that requires an extensive history, sitting down with the parent and child may encourage greater information exchange, as well as allow the clinician to pay more attention to nonverbal cues.
- For an established patient with an acute illness, the history may be taken while the parent and clinician are standing.
- A young child who is ill may remain in the arms of the parent or in close physical contact.
- The placement of chairs in an examination room and the proximity of the clinician and patient influence the style and content of the interview.
- A desk between a practitioner and the parent and child can be a barrier to optimal communication.
- Picking up a chair and moving it closer to a parent may facilitate the exchange of information; the act itself may enhance a therapeutic relationship.
- When interviewing a child or a teen, apply the same principles of spacing and eye contact.
- A cautionary note on use of an electronic medical record during an interview: remember that you are interviewing the parent and child, not the computer screen. Frequently turn to the parent and child, make effective eye contact and send a visual message that they are important. Alternatively, take notes and convert them to the electronic record later.

To maximize the quality of the interview of a child at any age, the clinician should be at the same level as the child. For a tall clinician, positioning is especially important when interviewing young children and parents. A younger child should be allowed to scan the physician at a distance first and become familiar with her. Eye-to-eye contact is an intense, invasive interpersonal maneuver and may be very threatening to a child younger than 2 years or to a child of any age if the contact is initiated early in an interview. A friendly interchange with the parents first allows the child to size the clinician up before the interaction.

TALKING WITH CHILDREN: WORDS AND FEELINGS GO BACK AND FORTH

When interviewing a child who has achieved interactive language skills at about 3 to 4 years of age, the clinician can speak directly to the child, ask questions and listen carefully to responses.

It is helpful to remember that receptive language development is often ahead of expressive language. A 2-year-old may understand as many as 300 words, but expression may be limited to 50 to 100 words, for example. Children may reveal information of which the parent is either unaware or has suppressed. In addition, allowing the child to participate in the interview provides an opportunity to assess language development and auditory functioning. Furthermore, it provides the child with an experience of actively participating in the visit to the physician, which may encourage a sense of responsibility and participation in personal health and medical care. It may also provide a model for parents in listening to and respecting the opinions of the child. Beginning with the health supervision visit for a 4-year-old (see Chapter 18), the clinician has the opportunity to conduct the interview with the child and parent in a parallel fashion. This rich clinical experience requires a knowledge of age-appropriate developmental skills and a comfort level in communicating simultaneously with an adult and child. The rewards are tremendous. This approach adds minimal time and a much-expanded clinical data base. This book describes what to observe at each encounter and say at that age. The more targeted the questions and comments, the more efficient the visit. A prepared mind sees and hears the relevant material, usually in quick order.

EVERY VISIT AS AN INTERACTION

The clinician's interactions with the child during the interview and physical examination provide an opportunity to model certain types of behavior for the parent. For example, a physician holding, rocking and stroking the infant while talking to the parent can give a young, uncertain mother a chance to observe effective soothing techniques. Providing firm discipline to an uncontrolled toddler with a concise and authoritative statement may help the parent experience the effect of appropriate limit setting and discipline. A note of caution—there can be a fine line between supportive modeling of discipline and implied criticism of the parent for not doing it herself. When an older preschool or early school-age child misbehaves in the office, there is an opportunity to ask the parent to assert control over the child and, if she is unable to do so, to capture the moment by asking whether the child's behavior has been a problem. These chance events, when a behavioral or developmental issue naturally comes up, open up "teachable moments" that become part of the real output or gain of the encounter itself.

Giving a 5-year-old the choice of using the left or right arm for an immunization or a tuberculin skin test may illustrate to the parent the value of providing some kind of option for a child facing something that is really non-negotiable. In addition, the clinician may demonstrate to the parent the powerful effect of reflecting on a child's feelings when an emotional response is intense. For example, to a tearful youngster about to undergo a painful procedure, the physician might say, "You're worried that the stick is going to hurt, aren't you?" The child's altered emotional response to these "feedback" statements is often dramatic and encourages further communication about the child's feelings. In general, clinicians should be sensitive to the effect that their behavior vis-à-vis the child has on the parent's behavior and style of child rearing. These modeling experiences are more effective than any amount of formal instruction or critiques of the parents' own behavior.

Sensitivity to verbal cues and emotional experiences during a clinical encounter may introduce unexpected opportunities that lead to an understanding of the parent-child relationship. In addition, it may provide insight into the important relationship between the child, parent and clinician. These events, characterized as "critical incidents," require clinical vigilance. They may be fleeting and awkward, as seen in the following case study, "Jake: A Teachable Moment."

Jake has been a healthy child before his health supervision visit at 18 months old. As you enter the examination room, you observe Jake playing on the floor with a plastic toy that has several movable parts. He appears engaged and intent on mastering the toy. You also notice that his fine motor skills are mature for his age when you observe Jake drawing and scribbling on paper with a fisted grasp. Jake appears not to notice you when you enter. Shortly after you begin to gather information from his mother, Jake's activity level and focus change dramatically. He starts hitting the toy, screams "bad … bad," and throws the toy into a wall. He starts to cry, resists his mother's attempt to hold him while she provides reassuring words and hits her with his hand several times. His mother begins to cry and says, "He was such a good baby. In the last few months he's a different child— selfish, angry and always throwing a tantrum." You are faced with several options at this point:

1. Quickly perform a physical examination, check the growth chart and order immunizations (and a blood lead level and hematocrit if appropriate).
2. Talk to Jake's mother about tantrums and the need for discipline and provide a handout on toddler development and discipline.
3. Attempt to engage Jake with words and a toy (e.g., sit down on the floor, play with the toy and say something such as "Gee, this is a great toy. I can make the door open so the boy can go inside."). Alternatively, address Jake and say, "It's real hard to come to the doctor!" or "You are real upset at the doctor's office." Follow these words with silence and wait patiently for Jake's response.

The first option brings closure to the office visit but does not address Jake's behavior. The second option demonstrates recognition of a problem and expands the mother's knowledge about toddler behavior and approaches to discipline, but it is not personalized to this family and does nothing to build your own relationship with them. The third option illustrates immediate recognition of a "teachable moment." The pediatric clinician chooses to model an age-appropriate response to a tantrum through action and language. Engaging the child alters the scene in response to the child's reality. The pediatrician's language is direct and brief; she tries to mirror the child's feelings with a few words and waits for a response. This technique, known as "active listening," encourages Jake's mother to learn that she can interact with her son at these difficult moments by feeding back to him the feelings he is experiencing. The clinician's modeling of the behavior can be followed by the information exchange illustrated in the second option.

STRUCTURING THE INTERVIEW

The clinician sets up an effective and efficient practice by structuring the well-child medical interview. Such orchestration of these visits is helpful in ensuring complete data collection, as well as providing a framework for controlled digressions. An opening statement should include an introduction by name if this is the first visit. A concerned, friendly and empathetic demeanor has been shown to be the approach that is most effective in child health care practice. It can be established by a warm introduction and immediate eye contact with the parent. The intensity and duration of eye contact may need to be modified according to the cultural context (see Chapter 3). Some clinicians find that an extended hand assists in the development of a medical relationship. A brief statement about the goals for the visit may be helpful at the beginning of the interview. This can be followed by asking, "What concerns about your child's health would you like to discuss during this visit?" A similar question might be directed to an older child. This approach, early in the visit, ensures that the parent or adolescent has an opportunity to state the agenda for the visit; it allows the clinician an opportunity to structure and address that agenda.

The content of an interview depends on the child's age and significant developmental themes. Specific chapters in this book provide directions for each age so that the themes or issues most likely to emerge can be targeted at that time. To encourage a developmental perspective for the well-child visit, questions and educational information should be organized around the major issues at a particular age. In this manner, specific goals can be established for each visit. For example, at the visit when the infant is 6 months of age, the encounter highlights the emerging motor skills of grasping and reaching out. Advice about solids (especially finger foods), toys and poison prevention should be provided to parents in the context of specific current and anticipated developmental skills. Knowing this theme means that the clinician will put a block in her pocket and extend the block or a pen or a stethoscope to the child as she enters the room. The key observation is made in 3 seconds, and conversation, advice and teaching follow easily. *Choosing a central concern or theme gives the visit more cohesiveness* and less of a feeling of an assembly line or check-off list, both for the clinician and the parent. The chapters in this book on each health supervision visit prepare clinicians for this task. The contents of the clinical interview, both data gathering and instruction, for each age will be outlined in subsequent chapters.

WRAPPING IT UP

Parents appreciate a summary statement after the history and physical examination. When the child's health and development are satisfactory, the clinician should report that finding positively, emphatically and with enthusiasm. The parent should be congratulated on the care and health of the child. These supportive statements encourage a high level of self-esteem with regard to parenting skills and strengthen the relationship between the parent and clinician. Parents often feel that the visit is a checkup of them as parents. They hunger for affirmation of their parenting and their child's well-being. Give it honestly and enthusiastically.

When a problem has been uncovered and discussed during the visit, review the problem briefly during the summary statement. This should include an assessment of how serious the clinician judges the problem to be and the plan he advises. Provide a time frame for decisions, assessments or future reevaluations. Options for the parents and child should be clearly stated. The parents may raise an important question or concern when their options are reflected back to them and after they have digested the information presented to them. Don't be surprised if this summary prompts a whole set of questions, a new level of awareness and raw emotions. That's what such a summary is designed to do.

Each well-child visit should terminate with a *closing statement* that allows the parent and older child to express an uncovered problem or concern. "Was there anything else you wanted to bring up?" may encourage the parent or child to mention an emotion-laden problem that they are able to express only after a sense of trust has been established by the end of a visit. These *out-the-door questions* as the visit is about to end may be frustrating in a busy clinical setting. However, they frequently reflect significant issues that have previously been hidden.

After completing a health supervision visit for a 2-week-old, the pediatrician, with one hand on the doorknob, was told, "Oh, by the way, my 3-year-old has trouble with her bowel movements." A quick screening history revealed significant constipation for a year and a paucity of language development associated with apathy and social withdrawal during that time. She had not grown during the year. As the father described the history, the pediatrician saw a midline anterior neck scar on the child. When it was revealed that a cyst had been removed before the onset of constipation, the diagnosis was apparent. An iatrogenic thyroidectomy was the result of excision of a thyroglossal duct cyst in which most of the child's thyroid tissue was embedded in the lining of the cyst. A diagnosis of severe hypothyroidism (thyroid-stimulating hormone, 950; thyroxin, <1) was the result of an "out-the-door" question by a concerned parent and an attentive pediatrician.

If time for an adequate response is not available, a statement such as "It sounds like something we should talk about when we both have more time together" may be followed by arranging the next available appointment if the concern is of a nonemergency nature. Although the clinician should not feel obligated to answer all out-the-door questions, interest and concern can be expressed by making an immediate, appropriate follow-up arrangement as part of a new contractual agreement, thereby acknowledging that the concern was heard.

The same response can be made to families who are late for their appointments or who bring up big issues on visits for acute illnesses. The clinician can say, for example, "I just don't have the time today to really help you with that issue—it's too important for the very little time we have together today. Let's get a time when we can really work on this together." Then get specific and have the scheduling clerk, the nurse or whoever is responsible set up a time. Don't let the family leave without a specific appointment to address the issue. This practice helps clinicians feel as though they are in better control and able to do better work. Obviously, emergency concerns have to be fit in, but others can usually wait. Most families appreciate a little longer time slot when the clinician can sit down and really listen. Wise clinicians don't let out-the-door comments derail their day, but they do recognize them as entrees to important information.

Each clinician develops a personal style for interviewing that optimally encourages the establishment of a helpful and healthy therapeutic relationship with children and parents. If education, guidance and developmental monitoring are the objectives of a visit, a flexible, empathetic and compassionate approach is helpful to ensure optimal communication between the clinician and the family. Awareness of the tools available to the clinician in constructing the interview will create a form and foundation for the art of medicine.

"I think you should ask the patient what's wrong with him or her, not the parent. The parent is not sick. The kid is sick. He knows more of himself than anyone else understands. A patient. Thanks. Karen." A child reminds the doctor about the importance of talking to children. (This statement was discovered on a bench in a teaching clinic after all the patients had been seen. It was wrinkled and rolled in a ball. Courtesy of Dr. John Kennell.)

FINE-TUNING THE INTERVIEW

Open and Closed Questions

The interview should start with open-ended questions, such as "How is your baby doing?"; "What's new with the baby's development?"; or "What do you like about your baby?" Such questions generate more spontaneous, less structured responses. They allow the parents to bring up problems of greatest concern to them and acknowledge the parents' responsibility in establishing priorities in the interview. The interview should start with these types of questions. Open-ended questions allow the child's or the parents' **"explanatory model"** of the illness or problem to come out. The explanatory model is the culturally dependent perspective of an illness that the family brings to the medical encounter. This is the first step in meeting the family's needs for addressing an issue.

When open-ended questions lead to confusing or rambling answers, the clinician may want to get some clarity and focus. This should be done carefully and should always start with "I"— "I'm getting a little confused about what your main concern is" or "I'm not clear about when this problem started; help me understand that part better."

Open-ended questions can be followed by closed-ended questions that are focused, specific and more concrete (e.g., "Is the baby sitting up without support?" "How is breastfeeding going?" "Are you getting any help with child care?"). Such questions provide important concrete data and shift control of the interview to the interviewer. The clinician's explanatory model and agenda for the interview can be brought out by the careful use of these questions. Some cultural groups may have an initial negative response to an open-ended question at the beginning of the interview because they may be accustomed to a more formal health care encounter, with the physician being more directive. Putting the open-ended question into context can help, such as saying, "I like to hear a parent's concerns first" or "I always ask children why they think they came here today." Planned, thoughtful use of these types of questions allows the clinician to get the information needed and build a relationship.

Pauses and Silent Periods

When emotionally difficult issues are discussed, the use of silent periods is extremely beneficial. It allows the patient time to collect thoughts and express feelings. It carries with it the message that you care enough about the patient to take the time to listen to her deepest concerns about the child and family. This is not wasted time, but it is hard to do.

Repetition of Important Phrases

When a patient makes a statement that appears significant from either verbal or nonverbal cues but stops the communication abruptly, the clinician may choose to repeat or interpret an important phrase that was just mentioned. This approach encourages further exploration, clarification or modification by the patient.

The mother of a 6–month-old infant was told that her child, who had previously exhibited normal development, demonstrated early signs of spasticity. When the meaning of this finding was discussed with her, she said that she had worried about her son's breathing problems at birth. A period of silence was followed by a statement from the clinician: "You worried about the baby's breathing at birth?" The mother was then able to express her concern about the need for ventilation and oxygen supplementation during the perinatal period and her ongoing fear that it would affect her child's brain development.

Dealing with Surprise

When parents say outrageous or alarming things, the clinician should just repeat their comment back in an even voice without comment. For example, "You give him Coca-cola every night at bedtime." The ball is then passed to the parent to explain, clarify or expand the startling comment. The clinician can then gather the wit to respond appropriately. With some statements, we can make a supportive connection with a parent by acknowledging their intent (e.g., saying that corporal punishment has as its intent to help the child in some particular way and then listening to the parent's response before offering alternative forms of discipline). At other times, the use of an "I" phrase is usually the best way to begin a response to an alarming statement (e.g., "I'm really concerned about what you've just said" or "I think that's a pretty powerful statement"). To maintain a position of active listening in these situations, experienced clinicians remind themselves, "better curious than furious." Keep the tone even and your face and body silent.

Active Listening

Active listening refers to the process of giving undivided attention to what a person is saying through words and body language. It requires, above all, the ability to concentrate. The assumption underlying active listening is that the patient will provide most of the important information spontaneously, verbally or nonverbally, if given an opportunity and the encounter is set up correctly. A clinician who listens actively uses open-ended questions, pauses, silences and repetition of important phrases. Such an empathetic listener can discover, through a unique, interpersonal style, a way that brings about a succinct and accurate acceptance of the patient's feelings, concerns and perceptions. This understanding of the patient is communicated through facial expressions, posture, hand movements and head nodding. Active and empathetic listening can decrease a patient's anxiety, increase trust in the clinician, encourage greater patient participation in the interview process, yield more information and increase the clinician's satisfaction in the relationship. It is a skill that can be learned and is one of the most effective and efficient ways to build a complete data base. Henry Louis Gates, Jr., has observed that "the art of the interview … paradoxically depends at once upon the presence of the interviewer *and his or her absence, silence or invisibility*. The role of an interviewer is somewhat that of a catalyst in a chemical equation: elemental and essential, yet destined to disappear." Most mistakes have to do with too much talking. If one finds that one is doing more talking than listening, a great deal of needed information will probably be missed.

Transference

Primary pediatric care is based on the development of a long-term relationship with families. When continuity of health care is provided in this framework, a special relationship develops between the caregiver and the patient and family. In pediatric practice, parents usually have significant respect and admiration for their child's physician; it is the foundation for a trusting, long-term relationship. This relationship is the single most powerful tool in effecting change for the child. It is also one of the rewards of primary care. At the same time and to a variable degree as a result of this close and special relationship, a parent may respond to the pediatrician as someone who is symbolically and psychologically identified with another important person in her own life, past or present. For some mothers, the symbolic attachment may be a father or a mother and, for others, an uncle or other important person in their lives. This "**transference**" phenomenon may surface only at times of deep emotional expression, such as overwhelming joy, relief and admiration for the clinician after a successful therapeutic intervention. It may also be the unconscious source of hostility directed toward the clinician by the parent of a child with a chronic, functionally disabling illness. In some cases, transference is the source of some underlying sexual tension on the part of both the clinician and the parent. This relationship should be looked at honestly. The clinician may need to distance himself or provide some additional protection, perhaps by enlisting the help of a colleague to sort through the situation. An appreciation of parental reactions mediated by transference may assist the clinician in providing more appropriate and helpful responses during medical interviews and in understanding some aspects of the interaction.

In addition, it may sometimes allow for an understanding of strong personal feelings experienced by the clinician. This insight does not get rid of transference in an interaction, but acknowledges it, uses it for the healthy energy it provides and keeps in check the less helpful aspects of its presence. Monitoring of your own emotional response allows awareness of this phenomenon and use of it to advantage.

Reflection and Self-awareness

Effective clinicians monitor their work with patients through reflection and self-awareness to examine their own belief systems and values, manage strong feelings about patients and make difficult decisions. Dr. Ronald Epstein has described a clinician who practices in a reflective and self-aware manner as a "mindful practitioner" who "attends in a nonjudgmental way to their own physical and mental process during ordinary everyday tasks. This critical self-reflection enables physicians to listen attentively to patients' distress, recognize their own errors, refine their technical skills, make evidence-based decisions and clarify their values so that they can act with compassion, technical competence, presence and insight." Reflection and self-awareness during an interview can be achieved by conscious use of your own response to a child, parent and other family members as a therapeutic tool. *A clinician's emotional responses can serve as a barometer to enhance understanding and suggest new directions of inquiry.* Dr. Benjamin Spock's encouragement to parents, "Trust yourself—you know more than you think you do," is as salient advice to clinicians as it has been to parents.

Pay attention to your own feelings in an encounter, your own responses to a child. If you feel your shoulders slumped, your face dropped and your movement slowed, you may just have had a visit with a depressed parent and have soaked up some of the gloom in the room. If you find a child particularly irritating, demanding or obstructive, reflect on what such behavior is like at home and at school. If you find yourself handling a baby overcautiously or lowering your voice, look at what the source of that fragility is. Based on your own feelings, you need to change the agenda of the visit or make a plan to see the child and family again to investigate matters further.

Set for Success

Analyses of pediatric interviews through videotape records have documented the clinical skills to which parents are most responsive. Process and outcome measures, such as parental understanding of a diagnostic label and compliance with a medical regimen, have been evaluated and correlated with specific traits of clinicians that yield optimal results. Effective interviewing skills go a long way toward optimal results. Dr. Barbara Korsch, a pioneer in pediatric interview research, suggests that the following traits produce the most effective medical encounters:

- Pay attention to the *concerns of patients*. Three open-ended questions will elicit *most* parental concerns for a child with a problem:
  1. Why did you bring Jason to the clinic today?
  2. What worried you most about him?
  3. Why did that worry you?

- *Acknowledge the parent's expectation* for the medical visit and the parent's explanation of the child's problem, or the explanatory model. Parents may bring to the visit their own explanatory models of illness and health. It is important to bring those models to the surface and show the parents that you understand their perception, whether it is similar to or different from your own.

- Parents need an *explanation of the diagnosis and cause*. If the medical explanation is inconsistent with the parents' own understanding, the clinician should try to reconcile the difference. For example, a parent who believes that the child acquired a cold from rain exposure may be assisted by the statement, "The cold was caused by a virus he acquired rather than by your taking him out into the rain."

- Nurture the *doctor-patient relationship*. Be relaxed, friendly, positive and warm in manner.

- *Limit medical jargon*. This is often a protective barrier for yourself. Jargon can be used to establish power over another or to hide ignorance when you feel threatened. Rather than hide behind words, try to deal with the situation directly.

- Most parents prefer a *friendly, professional attitude* rather than an authoritative, business-like stature or an overly casual or familiar manner.

- *Attend to parental anxieties* as manifested by nervousness and tension during the interview. Examples of responses are the following: "You look nervous to me today . . . is there something you want to bring up?" or "You don't seem to accept my explanation of his sore throat."

These skills can be acquired during medical training or in pediatric practice. As with most aspects of learning, supervision is extremely helpful in gaining insight into interviewing techniques. A one-way mirror provides an opportunity for observing interviews. A videotape of a patient encounter can be played back in front of the student and teacher. Videotaping has the advantage of allowing comments periodically when the tape is stopped and replayed. Medical centers with teaching programs usually have video facilities that can be used by pediatricians in practice as a form of continuing education.

Communication is the high technology of the 21st century. However, without computers, satellites or forms of artificial intelligence, the primitive art of communication during the medical interview remains a powerful and effective way to gather data, teach and develop the specifically human way of connecting with another human being empathetically and therapeutically. It is still at the core of medical practice. We owe it to ourselves and to our patients to develop these skills optimally.

Recognizing Hidden Agendas

Parents who bring children to a physician for an illness visit are frequently motivated to come to the office because of a concern that is not immediately apparent. The "secondary diagnosis" often originates from a behavioral, psychosocial or developmental uncertainty that the parent may be unaware of at the time of the visit or one that seems inappropriate to bring to the attention of the child's clinician. The real concern must be uncovered or it will prompt additional, unnecessary office or emergency room visits.

Bass and Cohen investigated ostensible and actual reasons for seeking care in a pediatric office practice. Over a 3-month period they asked parents involved in 370 sick visits, "What are you concerned about?" When the parent responded with a physical symptom, the next question was, "Is there anything special about the (fever, cold or infection) that causes your concern?" In the 370 office visits, 34% of the parents expressed a fear not verbalized initially that appeared to worry them about a more serious condition than could be anticipated from the ostensible reason for the visit (Table 4–1).

TABLE 4–1   **Actual* Reasons for Visits to Pediatric Providers**

Reason	Patients (370 Visits)
Vulnerable child syndrome	39
Parent thought the worst	30
Parents' fear of cancer or leukemia	10
Authority figures raised concerns	10
Illness lasted "too long"	9
Death of relative or friend	8
Travel or moving	7
Symptoms of "vital organs"	7
Absent parent	5
	125 (34%)

*Actual reasons as opposed to ostensible reasons for the visits.

These parental concerns reflect fears and anxieties about the child's health and provide insight into family functioning and parental perceptions that are critical to growth and development of the child. Parents in 10% of the visits saw the child as "vulnerable" because of a previous illness or event in the life of the child, a family member or a close friend. Providing the parent with a brief opportunity to express any hidden agenda may be therapeutic in itself. The clinician then has a window of opportunity to place the symptom in perspective and, when appropriate, reassure the parent about the health of the child and the limited duration of the current illness. When these fears have created significant or chronic parental anxiety, a future visit may be necessary. If the agenda is not addressed, future visits to the office and emergency department or calls in the middle of the night for minor problems will continue to plague the clinician. Parents may not even be aware of these underlying concerns themselves. Like a hidden infection, they need to be identified or they will continue to fester.

These explorations in causality are the rewards of sensitive interviewing. For the child and family, the therapeutic value may be as important as discovery of the pathophysiology of a cardiac murmur. The long-term benefit comes from the relationship that begins to be built when clinicians give parents the message that their concerns are important and worthy of the physician's time. Dr. Leon Eisenberg captured this idea when he said, "**Time with the patient will remain the currency of medical care**" (personal communication).

Culturally Sensitive Interviews

In developed countries, cultural diversity is the rule rather than the exception. Although most of the general principles of effective medical interviewing reviewed in this chapter are applicable when there are cultural differences between a clinician and patient, such differences may pervade the encounter at many levels. Patcher has defined culturally sensitive pediatrics as "care [that] *respects the beliefs, attitudes and cultural life-styles of patients.* It acknowledges that concepts of health and illness are influenced by patients' ethnic values, religious beliefs, linguistic considerations and cultural orientations." A culturally sensitive pediatric clinician discovers ways to blend ethnomedical interpretations of a child's developmental skills and behavior with a biomedical understanding. Culture, however, does not dictate the beliefs and behavior of a child or parent in a specific way, but rather acts implicitly to guide a patient's decisions (see Chapter 3).

Some clinicians may be frustrated by a false impression that to accomplish an effective medical interview that also nurtures a therapeutic relationship, a clinician must possess specific information about a family's cultural beliefs and practices. Certainly, knowledge about some customs is useful, such as the reason for limiting direct and sustained eye contact in some Asian cultures; an appreciation of "mal de ojo," the evil eye belief found in many Hispanic cultures in which symptoms are perceived as arising from feelings of malevolence or jealousy; and the use of physical punishment for misbehaving children practiced by many parents in disparate cultures. However, two clinically useful techniques will guide and assist medical encounters across cultures without an extensive knowledge of specific customs and beliefs.

Explanatory Model for Symptoms All patients have a culturally based model for understanding health status at times of health and disease. Their interpretation and explanation of symptoms may be different from the assumptions of the clinician. Through a

---

BOX 4–2   QUESTIONS FOR A HEALTH BELIEFS HISTORY

- What would you call this problem?
- Why do you think your child has developed it?
- What do you think caused it?
- Why do you think it started when it did?
- What do you think is happening inside the body?
- What are the symptoms that make you know you know your child has this illness?
- What are you most worried about with this illness?
- What problems does this illness cause your child?
- How do you treat it?
- Is the treatment helpful?
- What will happen if this problem is not treated?
- What do you expect from the treatments?

Modified from Patcher LM: Practicing culturally sensitive pediatrics. *Contemp Pediatr* 14:139, 1997; and Kleinman A: *Patients and Healers in the Context of Culture.* Berkeley, CA, University of California Press, 1980, p 106.

---

process of specific questions, the family's explanatory model of health and illness will emerge (Box 4–2).

Mini-ethnography In the process of an empathetic, respectful interview with the parents and a child, the pediatric clinician should strive to understand cultural and personal meanings and interpretations of the child's development and behavior. When the patient is seen in the context of continuity of care, defining a mini-ethnography for a child and family over time is a clinically and personally rewarding exercise. Other family members and interpreters may be essential in the development of a meaningful history. Box 4–3 gives guidelines for a bilingual medical interview.

Eliciting Information

At its best, the clinical interview yields information that will elaborate on a particular diagnosis or parental concern. The priorities set by the clinician, nurse or telephone receptionist can enhance or suppress important information. After an appointment is made for a health supervision visit, a receptionist might routinely offer the following suggestion: "You might think about your concerns before the appointment. The doctor is interested in your child's development and behavior. Some parents find it helpful to make a short list of concerns before the visit." In the office, a medical assistant or nurse should inquire about specific concerns while preparing the child for the visit. Parent and child questionnaires for health supervision visits can also be used to enhance each visit (see Appendix).

Two studies suggest strategies for more effective acquisition of data and strengthening of the relationship between the child's clinician and parents by inquiring about specific behavioral concerns. The Pediatric Symptom Checklist (PSC) (see Appendix) was developed as a screening test for psychosocial dysfunction among school-age children seen in general pediatric practice.

BOX 4–3   GUIDELINES FOR A BILINGUAL MEDICAL INTERVIEW

- Always use an interpreter (ideally a trained professional rather than an ad hoc interpreter), unless you are fluent in the family's language.
- Try to match the individual interpreter to the individual patient and clinical setting.
- Reassure the parent or child regarding confidentiality.
- Avoid technical terms, jargon, lengthy explanations without breaks, ambiguity, idiom, abstraction, figures of speech and indefinite phrases.
- Use clear statements planned in advance with language appropriate for the interpreter, and expect to spend twice the usual time.
- Be prepared to obtain information via narrative or conversational modes.
- Ask the interpreter to comment on nonverbal elements, the fullness of the parent's or child's understanding and any culturally sensitive issues.
- Learn the basic language and common health-related beliefs and practices of patient groups regularly encountered.

Modified with permission from Putsch RW III: Cross-cultural contamination: The special case of interpreters in health care. *JAMA* 254:3334-3338, 1985.

While in the waiting room, the parent is asked to complete a 35-item list of symptoms by approximating their occurrence as never, sometimes or often, scored 0, 1 and 2, respectively. A total of 28 points or more constitutes a positive screen. Comparison studies of the established Children's Global Assessment Scale given blindly to the same sample of children revealed that about 15% of middle-class school-age children would screen positive versus 24% of economically disadvantaged children. Using 28 points as a positive screen, the sensitivity of the test is 95% (5% false negatives), and its specificity is 68% (32% false positives). A short form of the PSC is now available.

Although screening checklists in clinical practice are limited by their tendencies to over-simplify complex developmental and behavioral issues, they have the advantage of bringing clues to the child's behavior into the pediatric encounter for exploration. They also sensitize the parents to issues or concerns that they may not have fully formulated. In addition to the PSC, investigators have developed other parent-generated checklists for preschool behavior problems and school-age behavior. The Eyberg Child Behavior Inventory asks a parent 36 questions on behavioral problems common among children from $2\frac{1}{2}$ to 11 years old; the test has excellent sensitivity and specificity. The Family Psychosocial Screening Test was designed for use by pediatric primary care clinicians to assess family function with regard to specific types of behavior, including depression, substance abuse, parent abuse as a child and other risk factors for developmental and behavioral problems in children (see Appendix).

Epidemiological studies indicate that up to 15% of school-age children have a disorder in psychosocial dysfunction and that pediatricians identify only a small percentage of these disorders during most office visits. Some clinicians may find the PSC and other behavior screening instruments helpful in setting the agenda for health supervision by giving the parent (and child) the message that behavioral concerns are appropriate and that discussion is

TABLE 4–2   **Community Resources for Prevention, Evaluation and Treatment of Children and Their Families with Problems in Development and Behavior**

Early intervention services (0–3 years old)
Public school services for children with special needs
Home visiting networks
Mental health services
Recreation services
Nutrition services
Speech and hearing
Occupational and physical therapy
Programs for students with learning disabilities
Preschools/daycare—child care resource and referral agency
Early Head Start and Head Start programs
Parent support/respite care

encouraged during the visit. A behavioral screening test can be used as a springboard to initiate the dialogue and therapeutic alliance necessary to explore behavioral concerns.

COMMUNITY RESOURCES

Developmentally based pediatric practice means that a clinician has a comprehensive knowledge about resources in the community that enhance preventive and therapeutic goals for his patients. Community resources serve as an extension of the pediatric clinician for consultation, referral and intervention. An effective "medical home" means that the primary care staff can direct children and families to preventive and therapeutic services in the community. Knowing who your allies are in the community and in what situations they can be accessed is a critical element of effective primary care.

Community resources go beyond knowing about medical subspecialty referrals (Table 4–2). They include early intervention programs, effective ways to access school programs for children with special needs, services for children with language delays (including instances when the pediatrician has a concern about autistic spectrum disorder) and mental health professionals. Knowledge about community resources not typically considered to be medical is also useful—for example, after-school programs, recreation programs (including supervised sports activities) and summer programs for obese children or for shy children who may benefit from social skills training. In some communities, a social service agency may accumulate this information; in other communities, pediatricians have the responsibility to organize the resources available for their practice. Assigning the organizing role to an individual office staff person who maintains an up-to-date binder on a broad range of community resources is an effective strategy.

Innovations in Primary Care Pediatric Offices

GROUP WELL-CHILD CARE. In this practice model, children are seen for health supervision visits in the first 2 to 3 years of life in small groups of parents and infants. Beginning with the first well-child visit after birth, a group of five to six infants and parents meet (usually 45 minutes) to discuss the contents included in the *Guidelines for Health Supervision III* or *Bright Futures*. Parent concerns guide the discussion. The clinician is in the roles of both an educator and facilitator. With children of similar age, parents often have shared concerns. They learn from each other, as well as from the clinician-facilitator. After the group discussion, each child is examined; the physical and developmental assessments can occur within the group or individually. Group well-child care is cost-effective, efficient and satisfying to parents and includes all the content found in traditional individual care. It has the added advantage of creating a supporting group of parents who can share their parenting experiences while observing a range of developmental and behavioral characteristics.

PARENT GROUP DISCUSSIONS. Parents are invited to hear a presentation by a clinician in the practice, followed by a group discussion. The focus can be on a developmental stage (e.g., toddlers, school-age children, adolescents), a particular topic (e.g., nutrition, tantrums and discipline, home safety, school underachievement, substance abuse) or a condition (e.g., asthma/allergies, recurrent ear infections, attention deficit/hyperactivity disorder, eating disorders). Parent group discussions focused on a specific age group may also be organized before selected health supervision visits in the first 3 to 5 years of life, with the discussion being followed by an examination.

TEACHABLE MOMENTS. Teachable moments are opportunities when a clinician recognizes an occasion to comment about or demonstrate a response to a child's behavior or to communicate information during the physical or developmental/behavioral examination. They are unplanned opportunities to provide information, promote discussion and support parents. Observation of a difficult temperament, refusal to cooperate during a physical examination and concern about maternal depression are examples of teachable moments.

HEALTHY STEPS. Healthy Steps is an organized approach to primary care for children from birth to 3 years of age. The goal is to increase a clinician's ability to address behavioral, emotional and cognitive development. To achieve this goal and create a strong bond between clinicians and parents, a Healthy Steps specialist (trained in pediatric nursing, early childhood education or social work) is available to the practice to ensure enhanced well-child care, home visits, child development/family health checkups, availability of written materials, access to a child development telephone information line, links to community resources and parent groups. The Healthy Steps specialist performs a standardized developmental screening test at targeted times and meets with parents during well-child visits to discuss behavioral and developmental issues. Teachable moments in the office encounter are emphasized. Research has demonstrated that parents in the program acquire more knowledge about child development/behavior and are better able to use community recourses than parents exposed to traditional pediatric care.

REACH OUT AND READ. Developed to promote literacy, language skills and a close parent-child attachment through reading to children at an early age, the Reach Out and Read program offers a developmentally appropriate book to a family at each health supervision visit in the first 5 years beginning at the 6-month visit. The books may be taken home, and office clinicians and staff emphasize the importance of reading aloud to young children. In the waiting room, volunteers read to children, thereby modeling techniques for parents. Reach Out and Read has been shown to increase parental attitudes and activities that encourage early literacy and to improve language scores on standardized tests at 2 years.

SUMMARY

- The child and the parent are the patient.
- The "therapeutic triangle" illustrates the influence of parents (and the extended family) on the relationship between the clinician and the child.
- Between 6 months and 2 to 3 years of age, stranger anxiety often guides the examination, and the child may be more secure in the lap of a parent.
- By 3 years old, a child begins to contribute to the oral history; by 4 years, she is a major player.
- Adolescents should be interviewed separate from the parent to encourage autonomy and promote communication.
- Methods to enhance the clinical interview include the following:
  Open-ended and closed-ended/focused questions
  Pauses and silent periods
  Repetition of important phrases
  Active listening
  Transference and countertransference
- The processes of "reflection" and "self-awareness" by clinicians are associated with improved listening to patients in a nonjudgmental way, recognition of clinician errors and refinement of technical interviewing skills.
- Knowledge about and respect for the beliefs, attitudes and cultural lifestyle of children and their families yield important clinical information and enhance the therapeutic alliance.

! HEADS UP–DEVELOPMENTALLY BASED OFFICE

- Periodically review the content and quality of information in your waiting room about development and behavior for parents and children.
- Clinical data are generated from verbal and nonverbal clues. Both are important.
- When entering the exam room, address the child with a comment before opening communication with a parent.
- Look for "teachable moments" and the opportunity to model a behavior response and/or provide verbal/written information.
- Don't neglect an "out-the-door" question from a parent. It may be the main concern for the visit.
- Have paper and a marker (or crayon) available for drawing while waiting to be seen.
- The "explanatory model" of a parent or child for either health or illness may be different from the assumptions of a Western-trained clinician.
- A parent may have a "hidden agenda" that reveals a behavior or developmental uncertainty. Through active listening and focused questions, the hidden agenda often comes to the surface.
- Have an up-to-date, comprehensive list of community resources available for referrals.

RECOMMENDED READINGS

Allmond BW Jr, Tanner JL, Gofman HF: *The Family Is the Patient*, 2nd ed. Baltimore, Williams & Wilkins, 1999.

American Academy of Pediatrics: *Guidelines for Health Supervision III*. Elk Grove Village, IL, American Academy of Pediatrics, 2002.

American Academy of Pediatrics: Family pediatrics. *Pediatrics* 111(Suppl):1539, 2003.

Epstein RM: Mindful practice. *JAMA* 282:833-839, 1999.

Green M (ed): *Bright Futures: Guidelines for Health Supervision of Infants, Children, and Adolescents*, 2nd ed. Arlington, VA, National Center for Education in Maternal and Child Health, 2002.

Liu YH, Stein MT: Talking with children. In Parker S, Zuckerman B (eds): *Developmental and Behavioral Pediatrics: A Handbook for Primary Care*, 2nd ed. Boston, Little, Brown, 2004.

Stein MT, Jellinek M, Wells RD: The difficult parent: A reflective pediatrician's response. *J Dev Behav Pediatr* 24: 2003.

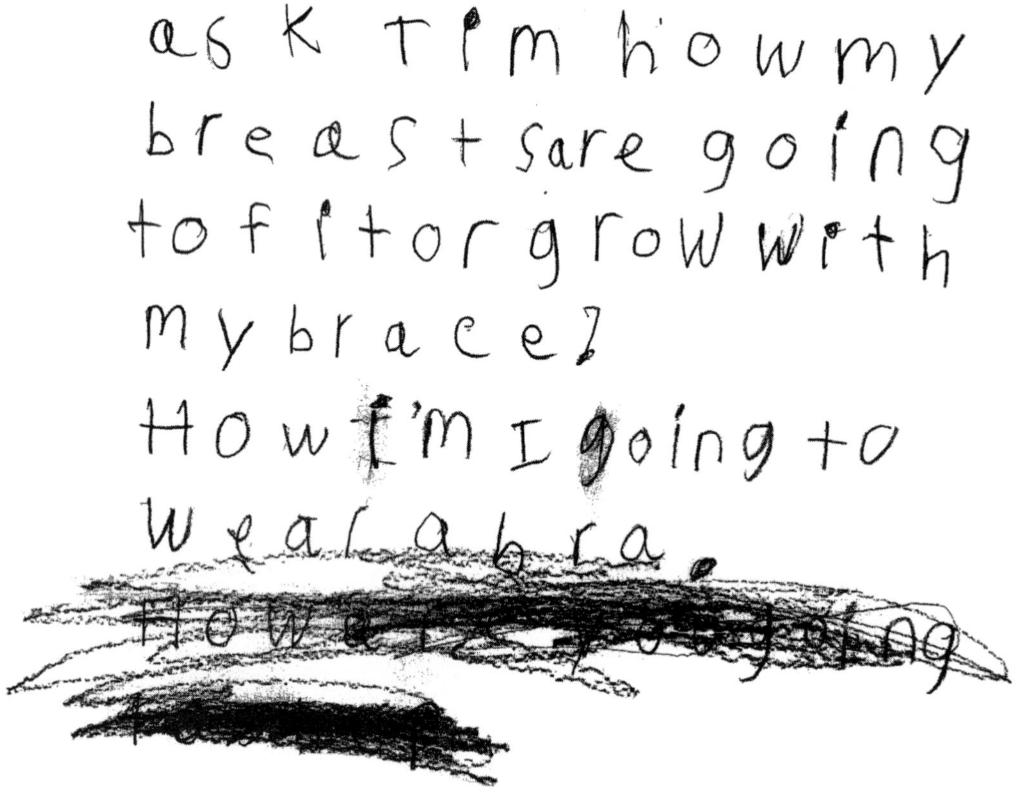

ask Tim howmy
breastsare going
tofitorgrow with
my brace?
HowI'mIgoing to
wearabra.

"Ask him how my breasts are going to fit or grow with my brace? How am I going to wear a bra. How are you going to … ?" A 9-year-old writes a note to her orthopedic surgeon rather than ask him directly a very concerning question. When the brace is to be worn by her to treat scoliosis, how will her maturation continue? By Kandace Faller, aged 9.

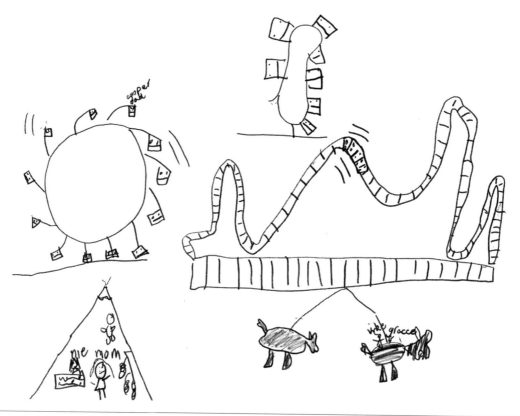

Some days in the office seem as busy and frenetic as a day at an amusement park, depicted here by a girl on an excursion with her family. The movement lines make it all seem to be whirling around. By, EB, aged 9.

CHAPTER 5

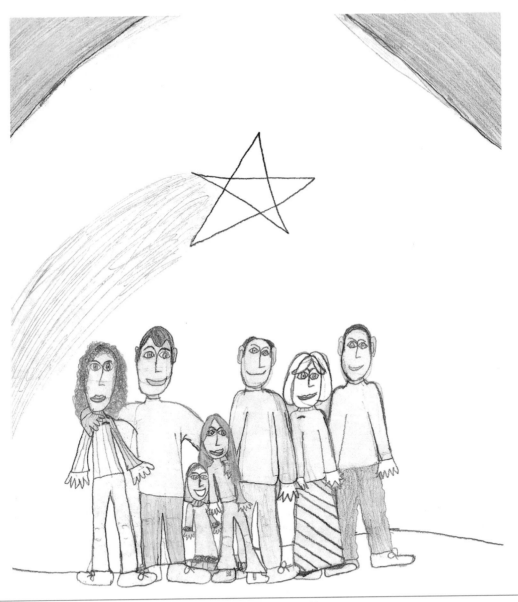

"My Family." By Robin Auerswald, age 8.

Use of Drawings by Children at Health Encounters

JOHN B. WELSH, SUSAN L. INSTONE and MARTIN T. STEIN

This chapter describes the use of children's drawings in clinical settings as probes into cognitive and emotional development. Scoring of figure, person and family drawings is featured. Ways to look at drawings as revealing of a child's inner life and social circumstances are described. Examples of typical and atypical drawings illustrate this presentation. Models for using these techniques in practice are presented.

Children can be asked routinely to "draw a picture of your family" at all health supervision visits beginning at 4 or 5 years of age. Drawing a picture may lessen the stress of the visit to the pediatric office, assess fine motor and visual-perceptual abilities and provide useful information about the child's sense of self, developmental status, family relationships and adaptation to stress. Talking about the drawing often opens up a resourceful and therapeutic discussion among parents, child and clinician. This chapter explains how to use, understand and enjoy children's drawings.

WHY DRAWINGS?

Children naturally like to draw. The regular use of drawings can make a number of contributions to a child's visit to the health care office or clinic. During these encounters, an invitation to draw creates a nonthreatening, relaxed ambience that allows clinicians to give recognition and encouragement and make meaningful observations of the child at the same time. Sequential drawings should be part of the medical record to mark the child's development, monitor both ordinary and extraordinary adaptive stress and serve as a developmental screen.

The manner in which the pencil is held and manipulated by the child to copy geometric shapes or draw pictures can be observed to assess fine motor skills, visual perception and visual-motor integration beginning at 18 months and continuing through adolescence. A child's drawing is often an opportunity to engage parents and children in discussion of an important event or concern that does not surface during the clinical interview. Making the child's drawing a regular part of the medical record gives it an individual identification that extends over time. Children are interested in their previous drawings; adolescents, in particular, are impressed with what they have done in the past, and this thread of continuity helps them in seeking a personal identity. A sense of control and ownership in the primary care visit builds a foundation for involvement in and responsibility for health and health care.

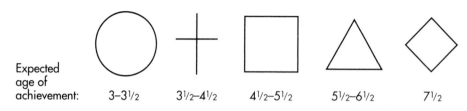

Expected age of achievement:

3–3½   3½–4½   4½–5½   5½–6½   7½

Figure 5–1   Screening test for visual-motor integration and fine motor coordination and the expected developmental sequence for copying geometric forms.

DEVELOPMENTAL ASPECTS

A definite sequence, beginning with basic scribbles that progress to more complex diagrams and designs, is seen early in the drawings of toddlers and young preschool children. The human figure emerges by the time the child is 3½ to 4 years of age. These drawings seem to be universal and cross-cultural in their progression toward meaningful, symbolic representation of the human figure. Drawing and symbolic representation lead naturally to writing and reading and may be useful precursors to the latter.

The emergence of visual-motor integration skills can be monitored by pediatric clinicians in formats suitable for primary care practice. Well-established norms have been documented for the sequence of copying simple geometric forms (Fig. 5–1). This sequence allows for a quick cognitive screen as children mature.

The Draw-a-Person test (described later) extends the information gained from geometric figures and correlates with mental age. It is used for children older than 3 years and has proved to be reliable for nearly 70 years as a general screening test for well children.

The evolution from subjective to objective realism marks cognitive maturation as the figures drawn progress from depicting the world as it seems to the child to the objective reality of the world as it really exists. These changes correlate with the child's evolving cognitive structures from *intuitive* or *egocentric* to those of a logical, *concrete* thinker (see Chapter 2). The "distortions" seen in the drawings of young children reveal the child's view of the world, often enlightening parents and clinicians alike. More accurate, realistic drawings come from grade-schoolers. Abstractions, or conscious distortions used to convey concepts, coincide with the emergence of abstract thought in adolescence.

The development of a third dimension, depth perception and visual occlusion (not seeing the parts of a figure through another object, so-called x-ray visibility) are marks of an intellectual maturity that gradually develops between the ages of 7 and 8 years through 10 to 12 years. Developmental psychologists acquire insight from observation of the changes as seen in this progression toward photographic reality. Although the emergence of these elements is quite standard, their use by any given child remains the unique product of that individual. Health status, temperament, family and sociocultural influences shape how these emerging skills are used.

PROJECTIVE ELEMENTS

The use of drawings as a projective technique, in which the child reveals inner feelings about himself and his world, significantly strengthens their usefulness. There is a large body of investigation of children's drawings in the psychological literature. The use of children's drawings in clinical practice builds on this foundation but involves a less formal use of drawings. This technique necessitates a wide range of symbolic interpretations of the drawings, and its effectiveness varies with the skill and experience of the viewer. Certain literature supports this approach to children's drawings. Of particular importance are family drawings, especially kinetic family drawings, or drawings of families doing something. The child is directed to draw a picture "with everyone in your family, all doing something." Considerable sophistication and objective verification of the family drawings have established this technique in child development. Several components of these drawings call for attention because they reveal a great deal about family dynamics:

- Where individual members of the family are placed in the picture
- Relative size and position of individuals on the paper
- Distortion of an individual or parts of an individual
- Omission of a member of the family
- Force lines (barriers) between members
- Relative amount of detail of a specific member

Studies using grid analysis and computer evaluation add considerable sophistication to the analysis of these components, but that isn't usually needed. Clinically, *the child lays out his internal perception of his family through these drawings.* Such information can be enormously helpful to the child's clinician in the process of assessing the child's self-image, patterns of communication and relationships with others in the family.

Psychological insights may be especially helpful in interpreting the drawings of children who are younger than 7 or 8 years. These drawings extend the child's language ability and allow access to his subjective reality. The threatening parent of the opposite sex, exaggeration of size, siblings missing, the magnified, nurturing mother or the threatening, menacing father occur with such regularity as children go through important social and emotional stages that these elements are seen readily in drawings (Fig. 5–2). Occasionally, parents can gain insight from such drawings into these special stages of development in ways that may not be apparent from the child's behavior. Drawings can also make parents aware of stressful experiences that have not previously been disclosed by the child. The drawing tells more about deep-seated emotional issues than the child can convey in words or the parent can see in behavior or speech (Figs. 5–3 and 5–4). When the child is able to describe his drawings, his verbal explanations can assist in the interpretation and should be encouraged.

Parents are often interested in interpretation of these drawings. Caution must be used to not overextend their meanings. At times, however, they can shed illumination on situations that would otherwise be obscure. The drawing, like a urinalysis or electrocardiogram, is only one piece of data at one point in time and must not be overinterpreted. However, the appearance of recurring themes in drawings collected over time can contribute to the validity of their meaning. At the very least, they can open up topics for discussion with the child and with the family.

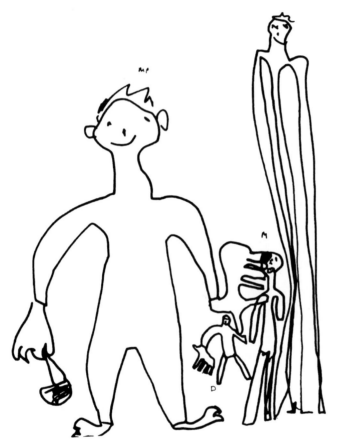

Figure 5–2 Kinetic family drawing by a 6-year-old boy who had a particularly close relationship with his mother. The mother is attached to a magnified left hand of the child, whereas the father (described as emotionally distant) is placed below the powerful hand and drawn as a smaller figure. An older brother is at the right side of the picture.

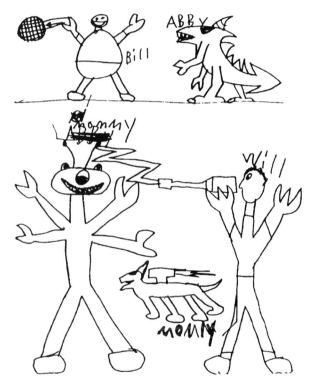

Figure 5–3 This drawing was done by a 9-year-old boy who had been admitted to the hospital on three occasions for severe abdominal pain and vomiting without a detectable organic cause. His parents had separated. In this kinetic family drawing the child demonstrates aggression toward his mother and separates his idealized father ("Bill") and a symbolized monster-sister ("Abby"). The child appeared depressed in the office, and his mother was concerned that "he wants to sleep all the time."

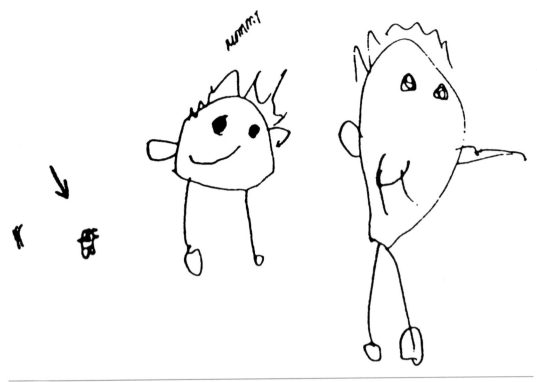

Figure 5–4   A 7-year-old boy, depicted by the *arrow*, drew this picture during an office visit initiated as a result of disruptive behavior and diminished school performance after his parents' emotionally conflictual divorce. (See details of the case in the text.)

DRAWINGS AND MEDICAL CONCERNS

Of specific importance to pediatric practice are certain drawing configurations of children with psychosomatic complaints such as recurrent abdominal pain and headache syndromes. The regularity with which these children produce characteristic pictures can be of considerable diagnostic aid in these clinical situations. The following are such characteristics:

- Rigid, stiff body images
- Fixed, uniform smiles
- Perfect symmetry
- Short stubby fingers
- "Cookie cutter" figures

These features often correlate with perfectionist, achieving children who have a significant need for approval and limited ability to ventilate feelings (Fig. 5–5). These styles represent a predisposition to the internalization of stress and pressure, which may result in recurrent somatic complaints. Reviewing these drawings with the child or family often serves to open up discussion of the background and dynamics of symptoms without an organic cause.

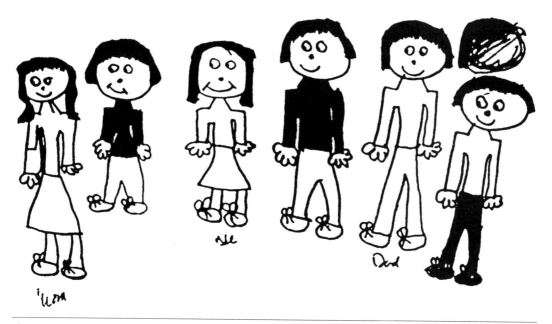

Figure 5–5 A 9-year-old girl with several months of nonorganic, recurrent abdominal pain drew herself, her parents and three siblings with a uniformity that lacked individuality. These "cookie cutter" drawings are seen in school-age children with limited ability to express their feelings associated with perfectionistic achieving patterns.

Assessing school readiness and neurodevelopmental status is an important part of pediatric practice. A child's drawing adds a dimension to this evaluation (Fig. 5–6). Studies of drawings of preschool children have identified particular characteristics that correlate with subsequent school dysfunction. Examples at this age are poor integration of the torso, absence of eyes or ears, unusual placement or size distortion, wobbly lines with overconnections or underconnections, reversals and difficulty sustaining effort such that the early part of the drawing comes out significantly better than the last part. Age-appropriate visual-motor integration in association with distortion of body image or other atypical features may point to psychosocial or emotional problems rather than difficulty with visual-motor integration. Figure copying may be aberrant at this age in high-risk populations who may otherwise appear developmentally normal in gross motor, expressive, language and social skills. Difficulties seen at this time call for early and specific assessment before school entry.

Many studies of the drawings of children with a chronic illness and abused children in hospital and community settings have been performed. Interpretation of these drawings may be therapeutic for the children and can give useful clues to the child's developmental stage and perception of the severity of the illness. Ill children or those undergoing procedures often show cognitive regression, emotional disintegration and signs of stress. The drawings of children with a serious chronic condition can illuminate the child's understanding of the illness, perceptions of being sick or injured and feelings of isolation. Specific indicators in the drawings can help the clinician evaluate the child's degree of psychosocial adjustment. For

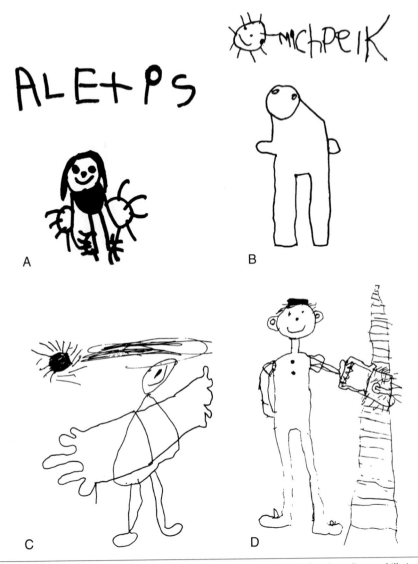

Figure 5–6 **A**, Drawing by a girl, 3 years, 10 months old, with advanced school readiness skills in language and in social and motor areas. This drawing indicates a mental age of 5 years, 6 months. **B**, Drawing by a 6-year-old boy who was small for gestational age and whose perinatal period was associated with distress and tremulousness in the nursery. Discipline problems characterized his early development. His drawing is atypical at school entry; it demonstrates a constricted sense of self with limited body parts, especially a paucity of facial features. The mental age assigned to the drawing is 4 years, 9 months. **C**, Drawing by a 6-year-old boy with attention deficit disorder associated with aggressive behavior and hyperactivity. At 4 years old he had viral encephalitis with a residual abnormal electroencephalogram. The mental age assigned to the drawing is 6 years. **D**, Drawing by a boy 6 years, 4 months old, which he described as "an engineer that signals to the train." He demonstrates advanced school readiness skills in the areas of fine motor, spatial and conceptual skills. The mental age assigned to the drawing is 7 years, 6 months. (A follow-up visit 20 years later revealed that he had completed a degree in architecture and was studying to become a stage designer.)

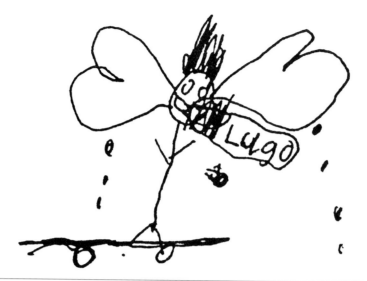

Figure 5–7   In some cases, a parent's wish to protect a child from the prognosis of a terminal diagnosis can have unintended results. This picture by a bright 9-year-old hemophiliac boy with asymptomatic human immunodeficiency virus (HIV) infection was drawn during a routine visit to the HIV clinic. His mother had not told him about his HIV diagnosis and prohibited everyone else from discussing it with him. The figure on a skateboard is spitting and has exaggerated ears that appear to be crying, thus suggesting feelings of distress and a need for reassurance about his diagnosis.

example, unusual treatment of certain parts of the body in drawings may suggest feelings of anxiety or worry (Fig. 5–7). Themes of threatening weather may suggest feelings of distress about the illness that the child may be unable or unwilling to verbalize (Fig. 5–8). Drawings of seriously ill children may demonstrate a sense of social isolation (Fig. 5–9) or feelings of being overwhelmed by the illness (Fig. 5–10). Recovery, in a psychological sense, can be seen in subsequent drawings (Fig. 5–11).

A recent study demonstrated the usefulness of children's drawings in differentiating migraine from nonmigraine (tension) headaches in an outpatient pediatric clinic. Children 4 to 19 years old were asked, "Where is your pain? What does your pain feel like? Are there any other symptoms (before or after the headache) that you can show in a drawing?" Children were then asked to explain the drawing. Features in the drawings consistent with migraine included pounding pain, nausea/vomiting, desire to lie down, periorbital pain, photophobia and visual scotoma. Sadness or crying did not differentiate migraine from nonmigraine headaches. With clinical diagnosis as the gold standard, headache drawings had a sensitivity of 93.1% and a specificity of 82.7%.

Jungian analysts emphasize the importance of colors used in the drawings and subtle changes occurring in the course of succeeding pictures as evidence of internal state changes within the child that may precede clinical changes in the course of the illness. Continuing use of only dark colors, coloring over elements and diminutive size tell us about an ill child's world vision. The drawings used in this book serve to emphasize the communicative power of these creations in identifying developmental issues, hurdles and progress.

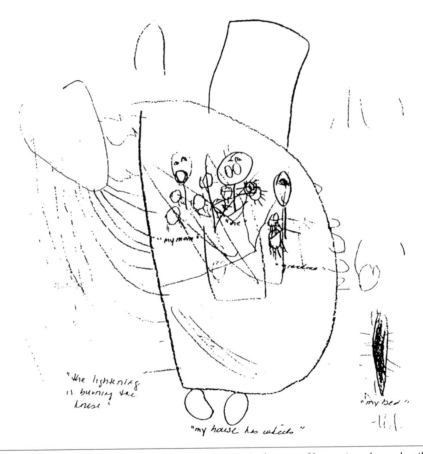

Figure 5–8 Drawing by a 6-year-old- girl with AIDS who was in the care of her maternal grandmother because her mother was ill. She drew herself in her house with her mother and grandmother during a lightning storm, as depicted by the *curved lines* on the left. She described the lightning as "burning the house … it hit the door … it's trying to get in … and it shot me," thus suggesting significant emotional distress.

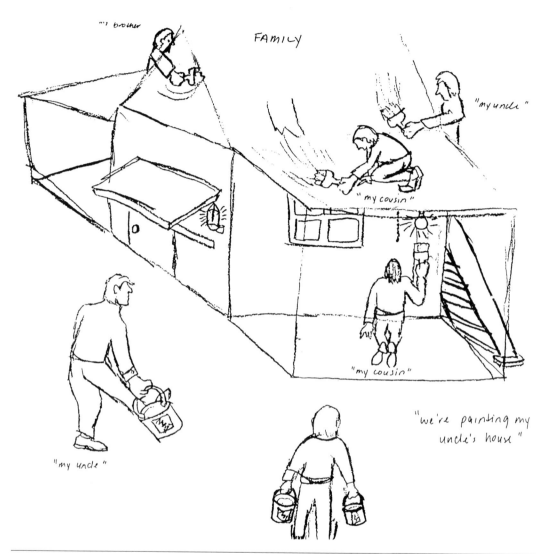

Figure 5–9 In this kinetic family drawing by a 12-year-old boy with hemophilia and AIDS, subtle barriers (the buckets and walls of the house) lie between the child and other family members, which is suggestive of feelings of separation and isolation. In addition, the absence of facial features on most of the family members, the absence of his maternal aunt (his primary guardian) and the child's depiction of himself with his back to the viewer reinforce this interpretation.

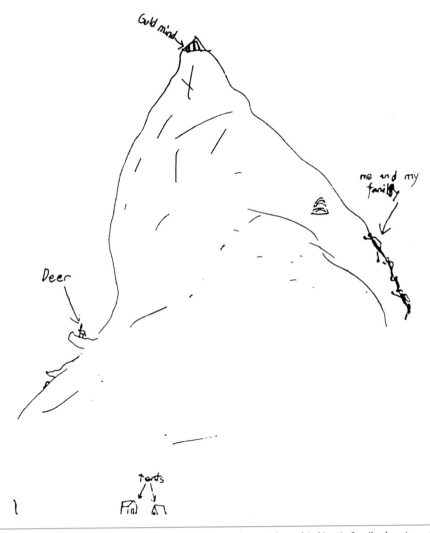

Figure 5–10   Another 11-year-old boy with hemophilia and AIDS drew this kinetic family drawing of his family on a camping trip. The minuscule sizes of individual family members (his father, mother, younger brother and himself) drawn climbing the side of a mountain toward a "gold mine" suggest a struggle against enormous odds. He rarely spoke about his illnesses during office visits and usually said that everything was "fine."

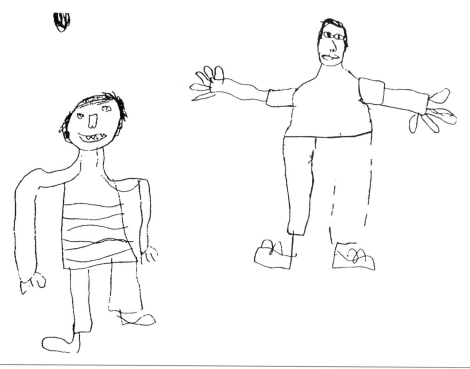

Figure 5–11 An 8-year-old boy drew the self-portrait on the *left* that illustrates his perception of his spastic left hemiparetic cerebral palsy. After treatment by an osteopathic practitioner and some improvement in function, he drew a picture of himself that reflects a different perception of his neurological impairment.

You are scheduled to see a 7-year-old boy for concerns about disruptive behavior at school and poor grades. You have established a routine in your clinical setting in which all children are encouraged to draw while they are waiting to see you. Your office assistant escorts the child and his mother into the examining room, gives the boy a black felt pen and a clipboard with several sheets of blank white paper and instructs him to "draw a picture of you and your family doing something." When you enter the examining room 10 minutes later, you notice that the boy is sitting at the small table you've placed in the corner of the room, intently finishing his drawing. He looks up briefly to acknowledge you, then returns to his task and produces the drawing found in Figure 5–4. After briefly greeting his mother, seated in a chair on the other side of the room, you approach the child and say, "What a nice job you've done with this drawing. I wonder who's in the picture and what everyone is doing." After a little more encouragement, the child identifies each figure in the drawing, but declines to say much more. You then turn to his mother and elicit information about the reason for the visit, including any relevant behavioral-developmental, family and social history.

Comment text continued

The mother reveals that her son's disruptive behavior and diminished school performance began after his parents' emotionally conflictual divorce. He had witnessed several moments of spousal abuse; his symptoms developed when his father left the home 6 months before the office visit. A brief period of counseling was recommended for behavior management and to help the boy gain a better understanding of his parents' separation, but his mother adamantly refused. The mother in the drawing is on the boy's right side, and her new boyfriend is next to her. The boyfriend's young son is at the far left. As the mother looked at the drawing, she cried for several minutes and said she could now see the need for counseling. The diminutive figure of her son was sufficient for her to recognize his poor self-esteem. The drawing was a nonverbal trigger to seek help.

DRAW-A-PERSON TEST

The purpose of the Draw-a-Person (DAP) test is to provide the clinician with an approximation of the mental age of a particular child. The test assesses three areas of visual-motor development: (1) visualization of the human figure, (2) organization and interpretation (i.e., abstract conceptualization of form, etc.) and (3) reproduction through motor skills of the visualized image as it is seen and interpreted.

The child is given a large blank piece of paper and a pencil and is instructed to draw the picture of a person. She is told to take her time and to draw as complete a picture as possible. The child is left alone to make the drawing because it is not unusual for a concerned parent to offer help or criticism. The tendency for adults to hover over the child can also produce a degree of anxiety that might cause the child to make a less complete drawing. The test is most suitable for children between 3 and 10 years of age.

Scoring

The child receives 1 point for each of the items present in the drawing. One point is equivalent to 3 months of developmental age. For each 4 points, 1 year is added to the basal age, which is 3 years. Thus, if the child scores 9 points, his mental age is $5\frac{3}{12}$ ($2\frac{3}{12}$ + 3) years. The criteria are shown in Box 5-1.

In addition to measuring mental age, the test can serve as a diagnostic aid, as previously mentioned. Very poor drawings, rather than representing low intelligence, may indicate neurological or psychological difficulties, and the child should be examined carefully for physical or neuromuscular conditions and emotional symptoms. Beyond the cognitive elements of the drawings, projective psychological elements, as described by Burns and Kaufman and as shown in Table 5-1, may become apparent (Fig. 5-12). Primary care clinicians should be cautious about overinterpreting psychological aspects in the drawings. They are not diagnostic in themselves. They open opportunities for discussion and further evaluation. Often, a parent will recognize a theme or event in the child's drawing that may trigger further discussion and assessment.

BOX 5–1   GOODENOUGH-HARRIS SCORING CRITERIA FOR THE DRAW-A-PERSON TEST

General	• Head present • Legs present • Arms present	Joints	• Elbow, shoulder or both • Knee, hip or both
Trunk	• Present • Length greater than breadth • Shoulders	Proportion	• Head: 10–50% of trunk area • Arms: approximately same length as trunk
Arms/legs	• Attached to trunk • At correct point		• Legs: 1–2 times trunk length; width less than trunk width
Neck	• Present • Outline of neck continuous with head, trunk or both		• Feet: to leg length • Arms and legs in two dimensions • Heel
Face	• Eyes • Nose • Mouth • Nose and mouth in two dimensions • Nostrils	Motor coordination	• Lines firm and well connected • Firmly drawn with correct joining • Head outline • Trunk outline • Outline of arms and legs • Features
Hair	• Present • On more than circumference, nontransparent	Ears	• Present • Correct position and proportion
Clothing	• Present • Two articles; nontransparent • Entire drawing (sleeves and trousers nontransparent) • Four articles • Costume complete	Eye detail	• Brow or lashes • Pupil • Proportion • Glance directed toward front in profile drawing
		Chin	• Present; forehead • Projection

Box continued

BOX 5–1   GOODENOUGH-HARRIS SCORING CRITERIA FOR THE DRAW-A-PERSON TEST—cont'd

Fingers
- Present
- Correct number
- Two dimensions; length and breadth
- Thumb opposition
- Hand distinct from fingers and arm

Profile
- Not more than one error
- Correct

Goodenough Age Norms

Age (yr)	3	4	5	6	7	8	9	10	11	12	13
Points	2	6	10	14	18	22	26	30	34	38	42

From Taylor E: *Psychological Appraisal of Children with Cerebral Defects.* Boston, Harvard University Press, 1961.

TABLE 5–1   Draw-a-Person: Clinical-Projective Interpretation

Element	Interpretation
Arms	Controllers of the physical environment; *arm extensions* as aids in controlling the environment may include cleaning implements (mops, brooms, vacuum cleaners), paint brushes (paddles?) and weapons; *long and powerful arms* reach out to control the environment; *lack of arms* represents feelings of helplessness; *folded arms* are usually produced by suspicious and hostile persons
Belt, heavily emphasized	Suggests conflict between expression and control of sexual impulses
Bilateral symmetry	If overemphasized, suggests an obsessive system of emotional control
Broad shoulders	Need for physical power
Buttons	Usually reflect dependency
Cartoons, clowns	Self-deprecation, defensive attitudes
Crosshatching	"Controlled shading" attempts to control anxiety through obsessive methods
Disproportionately small body parts	Feelings of inadequacy in specific areas, denial, or repression
Elevated figures	Numerous techniques will be used to elevate various figures; occasionally, a dominant sibling will be elevated or it may represent children striving for dominance
Erasures	Ambivalence, conflict or denial

Table continued

TABLE 5–1   **Draw-a-Person: Clinical-Projective Interpretation—cont'd**

Element	Interpretation
Exaggeration of body parts	Enlargement or exaggeration of parts suggests preoccupation with the function of those parts
Eyes	Facial features that refer primarily to social communication; large eyes scan the world for information, whereas small eyes exclude it and may be paranoid in their wariness or crossed out in guilt.
Facial expressions	Faces depicting various emotions were believed by Machover to be one of the more reliable signs of inner feelings
Feet, long	Need for security
Feet, tiny	Dependency, constriction, instability
Figures on back of page	Many children will have difficulty with certain figures and may finally ask whether they can put the person on the back
Figures hanging, leaning, or falling	Figures seen in precarious positions are usually associated with tension
Mouth	Emphasis may be associated with feeding difficulties or speech disturbances; in children, overemphasis is frequently associated with dependency
Neck, long	Usually reflects dependency in children; because the neck connects the impulse-laden body with the controlling mind, the neck is a frequent area of conflict expression
Omission of body parts	Suggests denial of function; conflict
Omission of figures	Conflict; the figure cannot be drawn on either the front or the back of the paper; often seen with a new baby
Precision, orderliness, neatness	Often reflects a need for a structured environment; overconcern with structure may be viewed as an attempt to control a threatening environment
Pressure	The pressure used in drawing suggests outward or inward direction of impulse; i.e., a depressed person presses lightly, whereas an acting-out individual uses excessive pressure
Rotated figures	Feelings of being different; demanding attention
Shading or scribbling	Shading in a drawing suggests preoccupation, fixation, or anxiety
Size	Size suggests a diminished or exaggerated view of self; persons who feel inadequate usually draw a tiny person
Teeth prominent	Anger

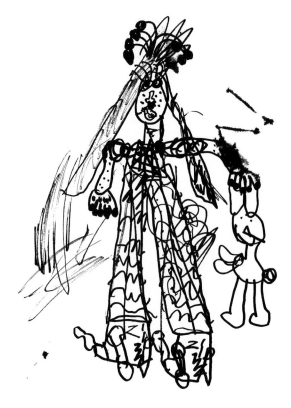

Figure 5–12 A 10-year-old girl with Asperger's syndrome draws herself in a frantic way, with incredible detail. She can hardly stop adding detail. Her anxious state and obsessive–compulsive characteristics are evident in the drawing. She was able to function better and live at home when placed on medication.

KINETIC FAMILY DRAWINGS: SYMBOLIC INTERPRETATIONS

An older preschooler or grade school child can be asked to do a family drawing as previously described. Colors can be used. The danger of overinterpretation and misinterpretation of symbols can be prevented by considering the totality of the individual who made the drawing. Viewing the drawings within the context of the child's family and sociocultural circumstances, along with a comprehensive health and developmental perspective, should prevent these mistakes. Some possible interpretations have been found to recur in kinetic family drawings. Repetitive themes may be useful for understanding a child or family when they provide suggestions and support for a diagnostic formulation. They are not diagnostic in themselves, and some drawings may have no symbolic meaning. Interpretive elements are laid out in Table 5–2. For the clinician interested in further exploration of this topic, the references will expand one's knowledge of this area of research.

SUMMARY

Children's drawings are a delightful, cost-effective, low-tech way of highlighting a child's developmental progress, emotional and social concerns and need for further evaluation. This low-cost diagnostic aid adds vitality, veracity, reflection and insight into every pediatric encounter. Facility with this tool should be in every black bag.

TABLE 5–2   **Interpretation of Elements in Kinetic Family Drawings**

Element	Interpretation
A's	Associated with an emphasis on high academic achievement
Beds	Relatively rare; associated with sexual or depressive themes
Bikes	A common activity of normal children; when overemphasized, may reflect the child's (usually a boy) significant strivings; more common in adolescents when power of the bike and motorbike becomes particularly important
Brooms	A recurrent symbol; seen particularly in the hands of mothers who put much emphasis on household cleanliness
Butterflies	Associated with a search for elusive love and beauty
Cats	Often symbolic of conflict in identification with mother; *ambivalence, conflict*
Cribs	A new baby in the family often produces jealousy in older siblings; because of their "magical thinking," they frequently insist on staying home from school out of fear that something will happen to the baby
Dirt	Theme of digging or shoveling dirt is associated with negative connotations about dirty thoughts or dirty clothes
Drums	Displaced anger
Electricity	An extreme need for warmth and love
Fire	An intense need for warmth and love; the fact that love
Flowers	Love of beauty, growth process; in girls, flowers below the waist reflect feminine identification
Garbage	"Taking out the garbage" for many children is equivalent to taking out the unwanted and "dirty" parts of the family existence; frequently found in kinetic family drawings when there is a new baby in the house or a new foster child; without young infants, garbage may reflect significant guilt about feelings of ambivalence and rivalry toward a younger sibling
Heat	Need for warmth and love
Horses	A safe comfortable sexual symbolic identification found universally in Western culture among adolescent girls
Ironing board	With an "X" by adolescent boys may reflect conflict and ambivalence toward mother; the iron may reflect the intensity of the feelings
Jump rope	Encapsulation of a rival or protection for self
Kites/balloons	Attempts to escape from restrictive family environments; escape and freedom
Ladders	Tension, precarious balance
Lamps	Need for warmth and love

Table continued

TABLE 5–2   **Interpretation of Elements in Kinetic Family Drawings–cont'd**

Element	Interpretation
Leaves	Dependency; a symbol of what clings to the source of nurturance
Light bulbs	Need for warmth and love; also *flashlights*
Logs	Hypermasculinity or masculine strivings
Paint brush	Often an extension of the hand and associated with a punishing figure
Rain	Associated with depressive tendencies
Refrigerator	Associated with deprivation and depressive reactions to deprivation; the refrigerator is a source of nurturance but is still a cold object
Snakes	An infrequent, but well-known phallic symbol
Stars	Associated with deprivation—physical or emotional; stars are usually cold and distant
Stop sign	"Keep out"; attempt at impulse control
Sun	In young children, the sun is stereotyped and has little meaning; a darkened sun drawn by older children may reflect depression; the sun's face may reflect pertinent emotions; if figures are facing the sun—the need for warmth and love; if facing away from the sun—rejection

HEADS UP–USE OF DRAWINGS

- Children's drawings provide potential insight into a child's behavior and development. Interpretation should be accompanied by other important components of a diagnostic evaluation or health supervision visit. The drawing will enhance observations of the parent-child interactions and the child's own behavior during the clinical encounter.
- Ask the child and parents what they think about the drawing. The response may surprise you and lead to areas of concern that have not been discussed.
- A child's drawing may, at times, reveal an interest, visual-motor capacity or artistic ability that is not apparent in the typical medical encounter.
- Make the drawings a part of the medical record. As the child or adolescent matures, there may be an opportunity to review the drawings with the child (or parent). Some college students have returned to the office requesting a look at their past drawings.

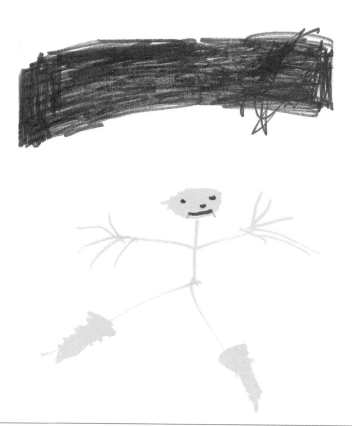

Figure 5–13 A 9-year-old boy with attention deficit/hyperactivity disorder hurries through this drawing of himself. His whole body is an electric yellow under an ominous dark blue sky. By Joshua Yudiski.

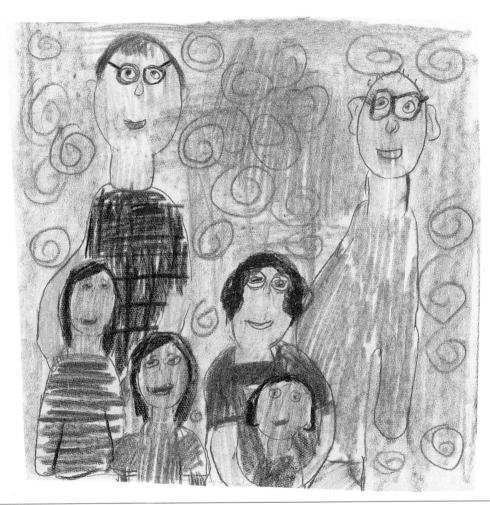

A drawing by an 11-year-old reveals that grandma was ill with cancer as she was shown without her hair. By M. D.

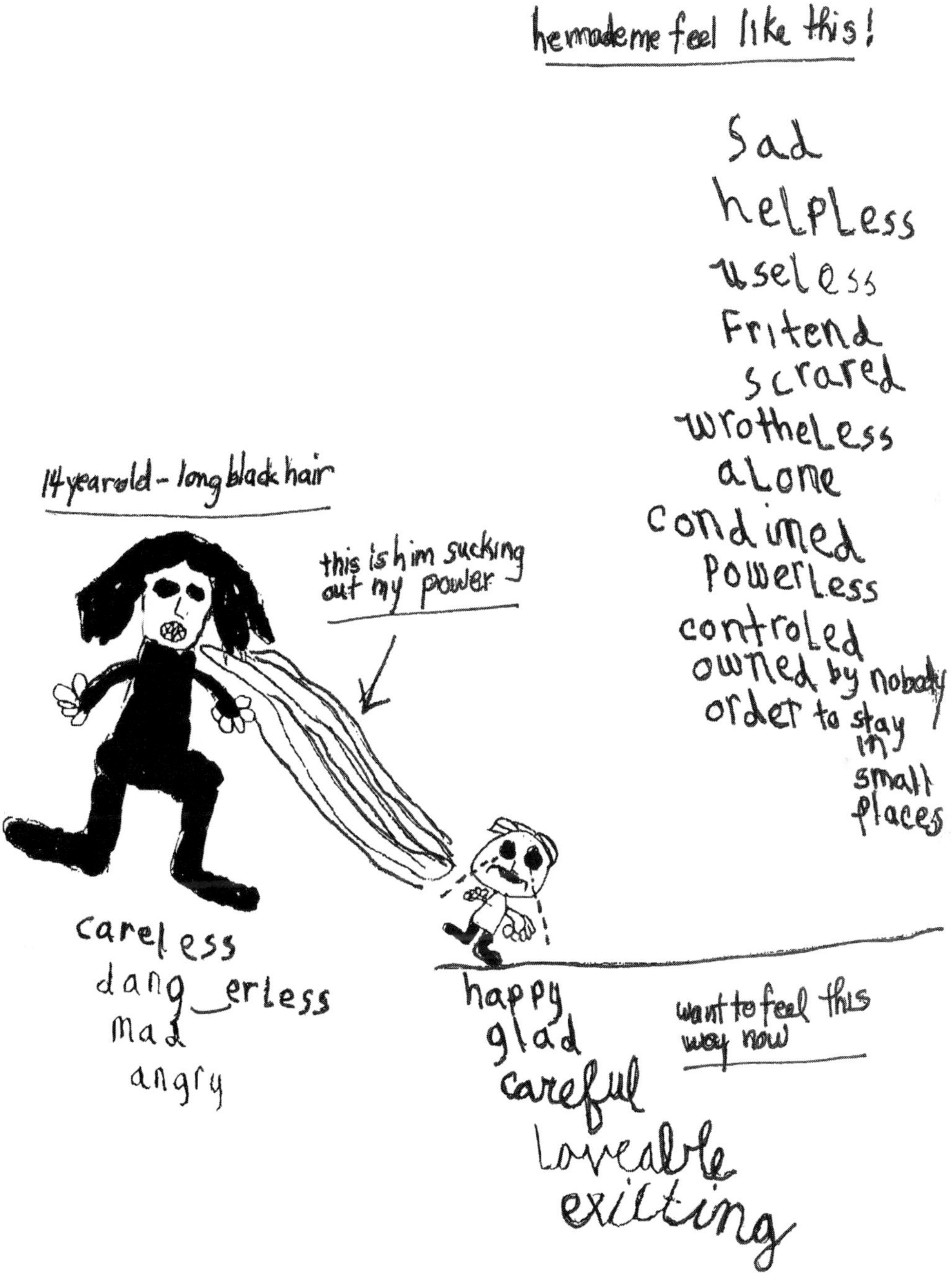

he made me feel like this!

Sad
helpless
useless
Fritend
scrared
wrotheless
alone
condimed
powerless
controled
owned by nobody
order to stay in
small places

14 year old - long black hair

this is him sucking
out my power

careless
dang_erless
mad
angry

happy
glad
careful
Loveable
exitting

want to feel this
way now

An 11 year old boy uses drawing with his therapist to open up memories of being sexually abused by a fourteen year old in a foster care years before. He identifies feelings, both current and past. He says the perpetrator sucks out his power, making him feel small, vulnerable, sad and, as shown in his depiction of himself, a bit off balance. The experience of abuse comes through powerfully. Drawings can tap into matters that are hard to discuss and also can be part of the healing process. Name withheld.

CHAPTER 6

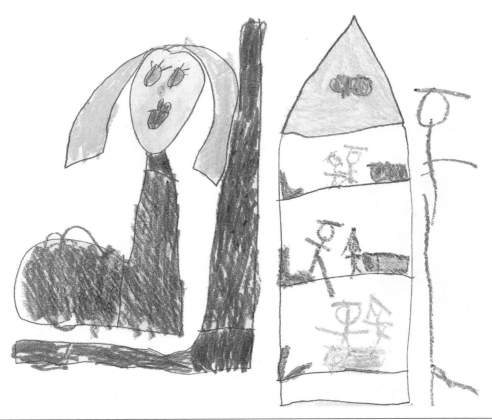

A pregnant mom with healthy baby waiting to be born. Everyone and everything is ready at home. By Briana Perkins, age 6 (her siblings were preemies).

The Prenatal Visit: Making an Alliance with a Family

SUZANNE D. DIXON

This chapter prepares the clinician to conduct an effective prenatal interview through an enhanced understanding of the adult developmental issues involved in becoming a parent. It also presents ways to acquire biomedical, social and psychological data that will be useful later.

Key Words

- Psychological Changes in Pregnancy
- Father's Involvement
- Birth of a Sibling
- Risk Factors for Attachment
- Fetal Behavior
- Breastfeeding
- Specific Health Risk

Debbie and Mark Hanson, soon-to-be parents, come in at the end of a busy day after having requested an interview to see whether they would like you to take care of their baby, who is expected in 6 weeks. Debbie wants to know whether you support breastfeeding and have evening hours for working mothers. She says she has a list of questions and wants to know whether you have any books or pamphlets. Mark expresses no immediate concerns and appears uncomfortable in the office. He says he is worried about being late for his second job helping in his dad's store.

The period before an infant's birth is a time of readjustment, concern, anxiety and some adaptive stress in a family's development. This time is the true start of the unborn child's physical and psychosocial development. It is therefore the time for the pediatric clinician to begin work. The American Academy of Pediatrics endorses the practice of making prenatal interviews part of pediatricians' practices and encourages them to become more involved in prenatal anticipatory guidance. Smart clinicians know the value of this visit to their ongoing practice. *Bright Futures 2* also lays the agenda for pediatric work to begin at this time. This type of prenatal encounter offers the unique opportunity to begin to build a strong working relationship with a family, as well as support the necessary psychological development that is demanded by the birth of a child. A unique body of information can be gathered at this time.

The prenatal visit offers the opportunity to make an impact on the child's family, even before the infant's birth. It establishes your territory, your style and your perspectives. The offering of this visit builds practices, loyalty of patients and preventive health opportunities available nowhere else.

PERINATAL RISK: BIOMEDICAL FACTORS

The data base established in the prenatal period should include an assessment of medical risk in the unborn child, as well as any familial occurrence of inherited disease, history of previous reproductive casualty or success, exposure to toxins, pregnancy events and the medical history of the parents. These factors are shown in Box 6–1. Most of these data can be gathered by questionnaire with follow-up of any specific issues. A pediatric clinician's concern for these issues emphasizes to the family the continuities in prenatal and postnatal life and allows for a focused medical assessment of the child to come and preparation for any special care needs. Because recognition of genetic disease is more common and gene therapy is increasingly promising for a variety of disorders, a detailed family profile is even more vital now than before. The prenatal period is the best time to gather a complete family history because the family has a strong reflective focus at this time. All families harbor worries about an unborn child. Your queries are more likely to give reassurance rather than prompt concern. Don't hesitate to ask these vital questions.

The pediatric perspective on these issues may vary somewhat from the obstetric perspective, with enhanced emphasis on issues affecting the fetus/infant. For example, hepatitis B carrier

---

BOX 6–1   PERINATAL MEDICAL RISK FACTORS

- History of previous pregnancy loss or infertility, previous preterm delivery or threatened preterm delivery
- Pregnancy complications such as infections, bleeding, trauma and/or high blood pressure
- Occupational exposures, risks
- Drug exposure, prescribed and illicit
- Smoking or alcohol use
- Unusual or highly restricted diet, malabsorption syndrome
- Thyroid disease, diabetes mellitus
- Hepatitis B or human immunodeficiency virus, disease or carrier status; unknown status
- Poor weight gain
- Inherited disease such as hemoglobinopathies, neurological disorders
- Prenatal identification of concerns, such as low alpha-fetoprotein
- Prenatal ultrasound abnormalities, including abnormal growth
- Family history of perinatal or early neonatal illness or death
- Previous birth interval of less than 18 months, multiple fetuses (e.g., twins, triplets)
- Maternal age younger than 15 or older than 35 years
- Maternal chronic illness (e.g., renal disease, cardiac disease, colitis)
- Breast abnormalities, past surgeries or past difficulties with breastfeeding

status in a mother requires immediate action by the child's clinician after birth and in the months following. The pediatric clinician will emphasize dietary counseling by highlighting the importance of good nutrition for the success of lactation and optimal intrauterine development of the infant. The public is aware of the danger of illicit drug exposure to a pregnant woman, but the pediatrician's specific concern may be the catalyst for maternal treatment or change. The use of alcohol during pregnancy has been shown to decrease with specific prompting by a physician. Environmental toxins are increasingly being identified as presenting risks to the long-term growth and development of the child; the pediatric perspective will put these risks in a new light.

For women involved in occupations outside the home, factors associated with occupational risks should be addressed. Additionally, questions about smoking, drug use and depression should be asked again, directly and with some context. The questioning might go as follows: "It's important that I know clearly what has been part of the pregnancy so I can check everything I need to when your baby arrives." This approach identifies a convergence of goals for parents and clinicians around fetal child health. Clinicians and parents all want to see the best outcome for the infant, no matter what the issues are during pregnancy.

Smoking cessation is particularly important for long-term child health. Although most women do cut down or stop smoking during pregnancy, many will start again after the baby's birth. Pediatric support for quitting smoking to improve fetal growth, reduce the risk of sudden infant death syndrome and decrease the incidence of respiratory illnesses should be given to both mom and dad. Alcohol and drug histories should also be taken as issues that affect the infant's health and ones for which the health care provider can mobilize help to address if needed. Vulnerability to return to drug use increases late in pregnancy and just after birth of the baby. Families should know that all these issues are pediatric concerns and that they can turn to the pediatric provider for help, most likely through appropriate referrals. A nonjudgmental attitude and an even tone of voice help in discussions about these difficult concerns. Even if all the information isn't forthcoming at this first encounter, the stage is set to bring up the issues at a later date if needed.

Previous infertility or pregnancy loss, premature delivery or delivery complications should alert the pediatric clinician to possible problems ahead, both physiological and psychological. A lingering sense of failure, loss, worry and anxiety will be present for this pregnancy in the parents' minds. Certainly, history may repeat this time as well because real risks do increase with subsequent pregnancies, although an uncomplicated outcome is likely in most circumstances. The clinician must deal with a ghost from the past, as well as real risks that may be continuing. Getting the clear history will help deal with both. Medical records will tell one story, so get a release to review these records if there is anything complicated. However, only direct, sensitive interviewing will get at the parental perceptions of these past events. Furthermore, it may be these perceptions rather than the reality that will influence the parents perspective on the pregnancy, the delivery and the child.

EXPANDING THE HORIZON: PSYCHOLOGICAL ADAPTATION

The prenatal pediatric interview is too limited if it stops merely with the data base concerning physical risk appraisal. Parents are particularly open to the establishment of a new relationship with a clinician as they reorder their views of themselves and their relationships with others.

Data are gathered with incredible efficiency at this time because of the energy a family brings to the situation and how close the adults' needs and feelings are to the surface during pregnancy. The dialogue between clinician and parents evolves into a therapeutic alliance centered around health and optimal development of the child and thereby allows the pediatric clinician to provide effective care of the child in the days after birth and throughout childhood. It will be the foundation of care, the bond of loyalty and the link to preventive care and continuity.

The range of concerns for future encounters will be established as you define your territory, which involves psychosocial aspects of development, family issues and physical concerns in care of the child. Parents can look you over to see whether your approach is in line with their expectations; a "misfit" between clinician and parents can thus be avoided.

It is vital for clinicians to understand the structure of each family, how it functions and its social and cultural dimensions to address the child's issues. Now is the time to begin that understanding and lay out your concern for the family as a whole. You will get this information through an interview that encompasses the adult development issues involved in parenting.

PSYCHOLOGICAL ADJUSTMENT TO PREGNANCY

The **adaptive psychological changes** in the parents during pregnancy have important implications for the unborn patient. Mental turbulence, an adult developmental crisis, is both normal at this time and adaptive in mobilizing the family to meet the needs of the unborn child. Some worry and anxiety are expected and healthy; after all, adults are being turned into parents, or parents of one are being turned into parents of some. Pregnancy is a time of psychological turmoil for every family and has been described as "a developmental crisis." Energy is mobilized, reordered and directed around the unborn child in a process of attachment. Anxiety, conflict, tension and fears are all normal and necessary emotional components of even the most uncomplicated gestations for mothers, fathers and other family members. It is a time for both parents to take on new roles and identities. Shifts in attention, time allocation and monetary resources follow from the process of changing priorities within the whole family unit.

Excessive stress may alter the family's ability to make these important developmental shifts. Severe psychological stress may directly affect fetal growth, normal fetal development and perhaps the psychological structures of the child. The loss of a close loved one during pregnancy is a particularly high-risk situation because the energy for attachment to the unborn is drawn off into this other "disattachment" process. Stress between spouses or between expectant parents and grandparents may be seen to some degree in every pregnant family while individuals reorder relationships. However, extremes in conflicts may draw energy away from the adaptive changes that are a necessary part of every pregnancy. Abandonment by one's partner during pregnancy is a very high-risk circumstance. The lack of a female support system may be one of the most significant risk factors for any mother undergoing pregnancy. An isolated, unsupported family has a high risk of not making the appropriate psychosocial and physiological adjustments during gestation and beyond. The whole family and the pregnancy context must be taken into account if one is preparing to understand and address a child's needs.

This process begins by a turning inward and reassessment of old relationships, particularly those between the expectant parents and their own parents. The search, either conscious or unconscious, for a role model and the need to be dependent again are all bases for this renewed focus on one's own parental relationships. Whether the grandparents of the unborn child are perceived as positive or negative, whether they are present or not, does not diminish their central psychological place in this adjustment process. Parents must work through this relationship with their own parents with each new pregnancy. Exploration of the place of grandparents is a vital part of understanding the developing family. It is important to explore who the extended family members are, how they relate and the manner in which they will fit into the life of the expected child. Whether physically close and intimately involved, occasional visitor or sources of alienation or just memories, these folks need to be accounted for in the interview.

Dr. James asked Mrs. Hanson who would come out to help after the baby was born. She said her mother-in-law, adding that her own mom "wouldn't be much help as she's really into her own stuff." Note: Dr. James needs to find out more about this maternal grandmother and her influence on what's happening.

THE DEVELOPMENTAL COURSE OF PREGNANCY

A predictable developmental course of adjustment has been described through interviews with pregnant women that were conducted as they dealt with the four major developmental tasks outlined in Table 6–1. These tasks are (1) seeking a safe passage, (2) finding an assurance of acceptance of the child by significant others, (3) binding or bonding to the unborn child and (4) learning to give of oneself.

First Trimester

In the first trimester, the inward preoccupation of the mother is largely focused on her changing body. The new body sensations, most of them unpleasant, serve to repeatedly verify the presence of pregnancy. These conflicting sensations press to resolve the disbelief that may linger around the pregnancy. The baby is not yet a real person to the family, although the mother may become attached to the *idea* of being pregnant. The fetus is viewed as a change in the mother rather than as a separate individual. Most mothers report feeling tense, edgy, nervous, irritable and occasionally depressed. For mothers with a history of spontaneous abortion, previous infertility and other perinatal problems, these feelings are deepened and complicated by fears of loss and failure.

Second Trimester

With the onset of fetal movement in the second trimester, a marked shift in psychological processes takes place. The mother starts to become attached to the child as a person. This natural process of change is suspended while the results of genetic testing are awaited when the possibility of termination is still present. Families push away an attachment and often hide the pregnancy if this decision is left hanging.

TABLE 6–1 **Psychological Stages of Pregnancy**

First trimester	Self-focus Becoming attached to the idea of pregnancy Pregnancy as a change in the mom—"I am pregnant" Ambivalence about the ability to handle the demands of (another) child Realignment of parenting issues, relationships of the past Anxiety about loss, fetal damage or mishap Emotional lability
Second trimester	The fetus experienced as a separate entity; increased awareness of the fetus Dreams and fantasies about the unborn child Making changes, readjustments, plans Maternal sense of well-being Nest building Increased dependence Interest in traditions, belief systems Sense of pride in the pregnancy; seeking acceptance by others Information seeking
Third trimester	Preparing to give up the fetus; detachment from the idea of being pregnant Seeking safe passage through labor and delivery; making plans Attachment to the idea of being a parent Fears of damage to self, the partner and the infant Looking for help and support Vulnerability to renewed alcohol, drug use Sleep changes Vivid dreams
Later	Introversion Cognitive slowing, daytime sleepiness Focus on details Fatigue, anxiety Putting things in order, cleaning, sorting

Dreams and awake fantasies about the unborn child begin at this time and are either positive or really frightening. Both are normal, a rehearsal for whatever does come. No definitive data exist yet regarding whether prenatal identification of the gender of the child changes these fantasies, speeds attachments or narrows the range of fantasies. However, preliminary work suggests that fetal imaging does "jump-start" this emergence of the child as an individual. Seeing the child moving and performing activities such as thumb sucking and seeing facial features on ultrasound make this event seem more like a child if the parents allow themselves to take it all in.

In general, most expectant parents increase their effort to solidify ties with friends, community and extended family at this time. Renewed interest in traditions, religious affiliations or hobbies is a sign of these processes. "Nest building" (i.e., thinking about and preparing a place for the baby) is a positive sign. Even in the absence of external preparations for the infant, parents are engaged in important internal preparations for the infant's arrival.

Darryl was splattered with yellow paint under his nails and on his shoes when he came in for the interview. When questioned, he said Dori, his wife, insisted they paint the house before the baby comes.

Indeed, for some families and cultures, physical preparations may be prohibited or viewed as dangerous. However, even in these cases, mothers will be preoccupied with making plans mentally for the infants and themselves. Most older children, even toddlers, now begin to show behavioral changes that indicate an awareness that their relationship with mother is changing, even if they haven't been told or cannot understand the concept of a new baby. Unexpected behavioral problems may arise because of shifts in family relationships, discussed or not discussed. It's time to begin sibling preparation (see later) if this hasn't happened before. It's impossible to keep secret the fact that something big is about to happen.

Third Trimester

The mental work of the third trimester is that of seeking a safe passage through labor and delivery. The pregnancy becomes physically burdensome, and there is an enhanced sense of vulnerability. An increase in apparent passivity and introversion peaks at 7 to 8 months in the pregnancy, combined with many underlying fears and lots of anxiety. Parents who have a pattern of coping with stress by drugs or alcohol may be vulnerable to renewed use during this time. Sleep may be erratic, lighter—changing electrophysiologically as well as behaviorally to be in line with the needs of the infant. It is often disrupted by dreams of the unborn infant, as well as by shifts to a shorter sleep cycle and less deep sleep. Psychological nest building continues through a process of inward direction of thoughts and ideations—positive and, at times, very negative. Cognitive changes also occur: women focus on microscopic details, appear somewhat disorganized and are preoccupied at this time. Prenatal interviews late in the third trimester may not be as successful as those held earlier for these reasons. The educational window closes substantially in late pregnancy, and educational programs carried out during that time appear to be less effective, perhaps because of these shifts in mental or cognitive focus. Parents may not even remember infant care advice presented at this time. Education and preparation are best done earlier if possible.

WHAT ABOUT DAD?

Although research in this area is sparse, the adjustment process for fathers in pregnancy is very real. Fathers' reactions may often be delayed and less intense, but they appear to be similar to those of mothers-to-be. An initial response of either (or both) joy and excitement or anger and disappointment follows the public announcement of the pregnancy. Emotional distancing, introspection and jealousy are often the father's second trimester feelings. A shift toward attachment, protectiveness and involvement are part of the late pregnancy changes. A father must work through his sense of loss of the relationship he once had with his wife, including the sexual aspects.

The third trimester may bring specific new anxieties about the child and the delivery. In addition, the actual cost of caring for a child may push some fathers to seek extra work and to develop new strategies for financial future planning. Some fathers will seek work to balance the anxiety that the impending delivery is bringing. Mothers may misinterpret this adaptation as "fleeing," and indeed, spousal abandonment is not uncommon if a dad doesn't feel as though he can face the role of parenting.

Do fathers make any difference in the delivery and well-being of the infant? Unequivocally yes! Research has shown that when the father is involved and present for labor and delivery, everything goes better: mothers go through labor more easily and deliveries are smoother. Indeed, the actual effectiveness of childbirth preparation classes may be realized through the medium of father participation. In a study by Parke and colleagues, 95% of the fathers reported the delivery as a positive experience. The father's presence at a cesarean section prompts greater involvement with the infant in the neonatal period and even into the first months of life. Fathers also have a role in aiding older children in their adjustment to pregnancy. In one study, fathers increased the time spent with the older child on average by 34%, and the time allocation was positively related to the ease of the older child's adjustment. The best predictor of success in breastfeeding is support of the spouse. Paternal education about breastfeeding, even among groups with low socioeconomic status, changes knowledge, attitude and support. A father's attitude in this matter is vital.

For the clinician, it is well worth the extra effort to actively encourage and support involvement of the father in the child's life before and after birth. A specific invitation to the father by the office receptionist at the time an appointment for a prenatal interview is made goes a long way in affirming the father's positive contribution to the child's well-being. Acknowledgment of the father's presence and contribution to the child's well-being is smart preventive medicine. Specific questions about the father's expectations for the delivery and his hopes and plans for the first weeks after the birth might draw him in. Few fathers readily volunteer much without a specific outreach. Specific questions directed to the father highlight the value placed on his role in the child's life.

In summary, pregnancy demands an important transition in adult development for both mothers and fathers, a process that is not complete at the time of the infant's birth. The parents who come in for the prenatal interview will not be the same as those the clinician will meet after the delivery. They are in the midst of a huge developmental shift. The pediatric clinician can anticipate the strength of the infant to mold some of the uncertainties, anxieties and mild, often adaptive disorganization seen in most families at this time. Strong, reassuring support from the clinician will be the foundation of the relationship with the parents, which in turn is the most powerful tool in one's "black bag."

ATTACHMENT—ASSESSMENT OF RISK

Attachment is defined as a strong affectional connection with another person that endures over time to make that bond. It is the psychological process that prompts attentive care, responsive nurturance and healthy mental growth for a child. Although most families will make a strong, attached relationship with the infant, the few that will need additional help should be identified early, if possible. Intervention, including a recommendation to reach out to family members and close friends, along with the support given by the primary health care

---

BOX 6–2 PRENATAL RISK FACTORS FOR ATTACHMENT DISORDERS

- Recent death of a loved one
- Previous loss of or serious illness in another child
- Previous removal of a child
- History of depression, serious mental illness
- History of infertility, pregnancy loss
- Troubled relationship with parents (i.e., the grandparents)
- Financial stress, job loss
- Marital discord, poor relationship with the other parent
- Recent move, no community ties
- No friends, no social network
- Unwanted pregnancy
- No good parenting model
- The experience of poor parenting
- Drug and/or alcohol abuse
- Extreme immaturity

---

provider and professional referrals, can prevent the long-term consequences of an impoverished emotional environment for a poorly attached child. Extra vigilance is needed when issues place family or individual parents at risk. Disorders of attachment are the basis for many common concerns in child physical and emotional health; attention to vulnerable families early may prevent many of these secondary problems. Some of risk factors for disorders in attachment are shown in Box 6–2.

OTHER CHILDREN

Adaptation to the impending arrival of a competitor is a hurdle for any young child. It's never easy. The **birth of a sibling** requires readjustment of the child's views of himself and his place in the family. The nature of that stress depends on the child's own developmental level and temperament. The parents' pregnancy adjustment processes make a child aware of a change in the family long before he is aware of its cause. In fact, concealment of the pregnancy not only is impossible but also leads to an increase in the anxiety a child may be experiencing because of all the changes that are occurring without any explanation. A young child needs to be reassured often of his parents' unwavering love and the security of his life. The child needs to know what will happen to him or her as part of this process. For a child younger than 3 years, whose capacity to understand future events is limited and whose world is largely confined to family and home, the birth of a sibling will be difficult. If changes are needed (e.g., change in beds), they should be done early to allow for accommodation. Pressure to toilet train at this time may lead to prolongation of the process. Those younger than 3 years rarely need to be told about the pregnancy until the second trimester.

Young children may enjoy feeling the baby move in utero, accompanying mother for checkups, looking at books or playing with dolls, although no data suggest that these activities ease the adjustment. Rehearsal of the specific plans for a child at the time of the delivery is helpful to a young child so that he knows what to expect. Mild regression and an increase in demands by the child are positive signs of a child's sensitivity to the pregnancy and offer testimony to the child's attachment to his parents. Parents should be congratulated for this evidence of a positive emotional bond, even if the behavior is troublesome. Pushing the child to "grow up and act like a big boy" will probably make the older child become more clingy, irritable and demanding. There is no reason to expect that having to share one's parents with another child will be greeted with enthusiasm, at least not during some period of adjustment. It's a developmental crisis for the child that can be handled with support. The central issue in the child's adjustment is the parents' continuing psychological availability.

> Tyler came in for his 3-year visit, sucking his thumb and wearing diapers. His mom reported that he's "just falling apart," whiney, clinging and not sleeping in his own bed. His bedwetting is new. She's frantic to get him back on track before the new baby arrives in a couple of months. Note: Tyler's changes should be seen as adaptive. He needs lots of hugs, some clear limits and yet less pressure to "grow up."

Parents may have significant feelings of loss in their relationship with the older child with the anticipated arrival of another and wonder whether they have enough time, energy and love to share with another child. They may need to grieve this loss to move to another level of parenting. A sense of urgency about that relationship with the older child and a feeling of pressure to do all that the parent can before the birth of the next child may be a source of additional tension in a family. The pediatric clinician should consider this family process as the basis for renewed behavioral problems, mild developmental regression or even an increase in telephone calls to the office. Addressing the adjustment issue directly may get to the heart of the matter. These issues run counter to the pulling away, inward turning of mothers at this time. An expectant mother is a new and changeable person to whom the older child must adjust. Observations in Africa suggest that this preparation time may be even more stressful for the child than the period after the birth. The same psychological shifts occur in the United States.

In the third trimester, parents can introduce books that deal with the birth of a sibling. Children's questions about the event should be answered clearly and honestly while bearing in mind what might be the *basis* for the specific question from the child's perspective (e.g., separation, loss of possessions, changes in special shared activities), as well as the child's developmental level. Medical details are usually of less interest to the child, so follow the child's lead through listening to his questions.

ATTENDANCE AT THE BIRTH

Some families will ask about a sibling's presence at the birth. Research on the effects of this experience is sparse. A consideration of the child's capacity to deal with fears and fantasy must be brought forward. The clinician may ask the parents to consider the following as they think about their older child's perspective:

- Will the intensity of the emotion be overwhelming or frightening?
- How will the child respond to an unexpected event?
- Who will be present with the *exclusive* job of support for the older child, to monitor this child's responses, answer questions and give the child permission to leave? Don't count on Mom and Dad—they'll be too busy.
- Are the parents willing and able to prepare the older child insofar as they can?
- Does the child wish to attend the birth, and will there be a chance for him to change his mind at any point?

Hospital visitation after the infant's birth may ameliorate some of the child's worries about separation from mom. Acceptance of the new baby should not be the goal of this visit; reassurance of maternal availability and intactness should be. No evidence shows that a hospital visit decreases any of the expected negative behavior at home. That rivalry appears to have to run its course.

A tool is available to assist families with sibling adjustment (Box 6–3).

BOX 6–3 HELPING SIBLINGS WITH THE ARRIVAL OF A NEW BABY

- Tell a young child that the baby is coming as soon as others are told. No secrets. Tell him as much as he wants to know and no more.
- Provide ongoing reassurance of the parents' continuing love and care. Say it again and again.
- Use books and videos made for children on sibling births.
- Include a child older than 2 years in the prenatal visits.
- Participate in the sibling preparation classes at the delivering hospital. Do at least a hospital or birthing center tour if there is not an appropriate class.
- Give a child detailed plans for where he will be and who will take care of him during the delivery.
- Include him in the plans for the new baby, such as new rooms, what the baby should wear, etc.
- Make all changes well in advance of the delivery, such as moving out of a crib, changing rooms and arranging new preschool or daycare placements.
- Help him pick out a new gift to give the baby-to-be.
- Give him a doll or stuffed animal to take care of in parallel with the new baby. Talk about his "new baby" as the parents prepare for theirs.
- Spend some alone time each day with the older child before the baby is born and afterward as well. Keep that time sacred, even if it has to be short.
- Talk about the long-term advantages of a sibling, such as having a playmate and being seen as a "big brother."
- Be patient with behavioral regressions in toileting, sleeping and eating. Keep routines as much the same as possible.
- Don't scold a child for having negative feelings for a child, but do prohibit ANY acting out against the baby.
- Praise any positive attention or any help with the infant.

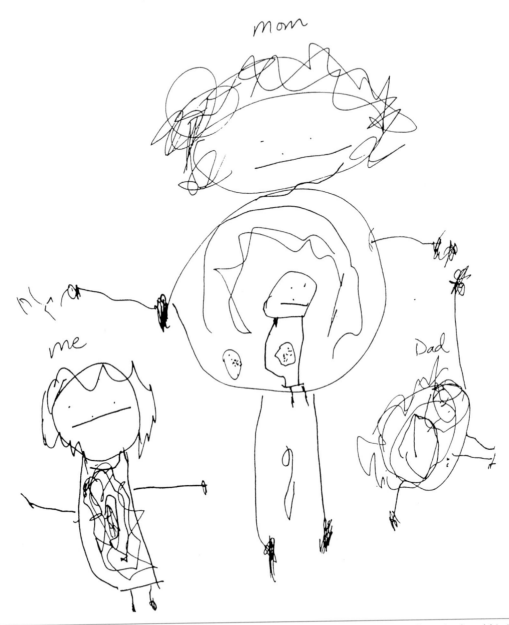

A 4-year-old girl seems uncertain about her mother's pregnancy. The father is described as aloof, and his job keeps him away from the family for extended periods.

WHAT IS THE FETUS UP TO?

Helping a family learn about the developing new life in terms of the fetus' response is a way to draw members into the idea of the infant as an important interactive participant in their lives. At least part of the visit should be a "did you know ..." recounting of **fetal behavior** capabilities. This adds fuel to the attachment process, reinforces healthy lifestyle practices and adds to understanding the individuality of the child. Importantly, it sets the stage for the newborn's arrival when these interactional capabilities will be observed directly.

These capacities are summarized by Hepper, and examples are presented in Box 6–4.

BOX 6–4   FETAL BEHAVIOR

Hearing
- Startles to loud sounds by 8 weeks
- Responsiveness to sound by the 4th month
- Turns to positive sounds by 28 weeks
- Learns familiar sounds presented after 3 weeks
- Becomes familiar with the rhythms and sounds of the parent's language by 32 weeks
- By birth will demonstrate a preference for familiar voices, music heard in utero and stories read before birth

Light
- Responds to light by the 26th week
- Will turn to light on the abdomen unless very bright—then turning away is seen

Smell/Taste
- As evidenced by heart rate changes after birth, the fetus reacts differentially to tastes in amniotic fluid, such as the spices cumin and garlic

Movement
- Movements begin at 8 weeks
- Makes postural adjustments to maternal moves and even anticipates movement in patterns by about 5 months
- May be quite still while mom is active, only to "dance" when mom wants to rest
- Hand to face, 10 weeks; yawn, 11 weeks; suck and swallow, 12 weeks
- The infant sucks his thumb, fingers, toes; rubs head; grabs the umbilical cord. He's very active in exploring his world

Response to Stress
- Maternal stress produces changes in heart rate and activity and, if chronic, changes physiological reactivity, including cortisol secretion
- May also result in preterm labor and low birthweight

Novelty and Boredom
- When a light or sound stimulus is presented to the fetus over and over, the response diminishes. When the stimulus is changed to something new and "different," the fetal response comes back.

STRESS AND SUPPORT

Families under stress bring additional risk to the developing fetus. Among others, Van DenBergh has shown that increased levels of maternal stress result in increases in fetal activity and a less optimal perinatal profile. Fetal well-being is affected by support from and integration into the community, probably through the medium of reduction in stress. Social issues during pregnancy and the health parameters of the infant are strongly related, so the former are clear pediatric concerns. Family well-being is really a pediatric concern and should be part of the factors addressed in the prenatal interview. Such an approach in turn sets the stage for ongoing appraisal of the family as part of the child health evaluation throughout childhood, the essential microenvironment for growth and development. This is family pediatrics.

Ms. Karr told Dr. Mackenzie that she hoped the baby came before March 1 so that her health coverage would be available. She just lost her job and will be moving to a smaller place soon. Note: This family is not only in trouble with health insurance but is also at general risk because of these financial stressors.

IMPROVED DEVELOPMENT THROUGH BREASTFEEDING

Breastfeeding will go a long way toward enhancing infant health and development. The decision to breastfeed is usually made in the prenatal period, so it's important for the prenatal visit to include information and enhance motivation on this issue. Strategies that have proved successful in increasing breastfeeding have been laid out by the Best Start program.* It involves building on the motivating factors of improved infant health (of which most women are well aware) and the mom's own desire to be the best mom possible and have a strong bond with the infant. Information about the physiological benefits of breastfeeding is rarely the missing piece in making the decision. Misinformation, fears and lack of role models are usually at the base of the decision. Affirmation of the positive motivators, however, goes a long way to support breastfeeding.

Psychological barriers (Box 6–5) that counter these motivators for many women should also be addressed. Although each woman has her own issues or her own angle on these barriers, they fall into predictable categories that can be specifically and briefly addressed. Notation of these issues prenatally allows the pediatric provider to address these early insights and use them as the basis for problem solving after the baby is born. At that time, the *real* concerns may be hidden. The clinician can offer targeted information and help around the barriers. This is done without being prescriptive or dogmatic and can be very brief. These short messages are a better use of time than providing a list of breastfeeding benefits. Encouragement to attend breastfeeding classes and identification of community resources should follow. Breastfeeding intervention done prenatally can lead to improved rates and duration of breastfeeding.

Ms. Daman said she didn't want the baby to be too dependent on her because she had to go back to work after 6 weeks. Dr. Marks told her that any amount of nursing would give the baby added benefits and that nursing after resumption of her work would help her feel close and connected to the infant.

---

*Best Start Social Marketing, 3500 East Fletcher Avenue, Tampa, FL 33613.

BOX 6–5 BREASTFEEDING ISSUES

Motivating Factors in the Choice to Breastfeed

Infant health

- Most women know that breastfeeding adds protection from disease for infants, but most are not as aware of the reduction of illness in the long term or the developmental advantage.

Mother-infant bonding

- Women want a special, long-lasting bond and closeness with the infant; they want to give the infant what no one else can give.

A special time

- Women enjoy the forced quiet time, the relaxed feeling and the warmth and pleasure that come with breastfeeding.
- Breastfeeding is an affirmation of womanhood.
- Women realize their physical potential and have a sense of pride in breastfeeding; they see it as a sign of maturity and responsibility.

Maternal health

- Few women are aware of the long-term benefit to themselves in terms of reduced rates of breast cancer, osteoporosis and arthritis.

Psychological Barriers to Breastfeeding

Lack of Confidence

- Fear of an inability to produce enough milk of high enough quality. Overemphasis on the need for a good diet that women cannot afford or prepare. Belief that it is hard to learn. Misinterpretation of the baby's cries.

Embarrassment

- Fear of breast exposure in public or even in the home, making the husband jealous, prompting "disgust" in other women

Loss of Freedom

- Belief that breastfeeding will cut down on an active social or work life, that she will never get to use a baby sitter, that the baby will be spoiled by breastfeeding. Often disguises a fear of bonding or fear of that bond becoming too close because of the need to work outside the home or pressure by the father of the baby to rejoin a social life unchanged by the baby

Dietary and Health Practices

- Belief that breastfeeding requires strict adherence to a special diet, giving up spicy foods and fast foods, foregoing smoking or alcohol or drug use, getting extra sleep or staying "too relaxed," which seem impossible. Perception that birth control pills cannot be used while breastfeeding. Perception that one isn't healthy enough to breastfeed

Influence of Family and Friends

- The father of the baby or the grandparents overtly or covertly discourage breastfeeding or give faulty advice.

Fear of Pain

- Perception that breastfeeding will be painful or disfiguring

From Best Start: *Best Start Training Manual.* Tampa, FL, Best Start, 1997.

DATA GATHERING

Setting the Stage

Each clinician will have a unique style of conducting prenatal interviews, and this style will vary according to parental factors as well. However, this encounter can be maximized by at least beginning with a set format. Many pediatric clinicians may be slightly uncomfortable at first without the presence of a child; a set agenda will help ameliorate this discomfort. The following are guidelines for a prenatal visit:

- Allow about 30 minutes for the interview if possible.
- Invite both parents to participate at a time that is convenient for both of them and for you. The ideal time appears to be 4 to 8 weeks before birth. The end of afternoon office hours or in the evening may provide the necessary quiet time in a pediatric practice.
- Provide at least two comfortable adult chairs in the office setting and place them in a position where eye-to-eye contact is possible.
- Ask the parents to fill out a medical history before the interview and review it before you interact with them.

Group pediatric prenatal visits are a new option for some practices and are often attached to childbirth, breastfeeding or sibling preparation classes. These sessions offer the opportunity to answer questions and to efficiently review your own philosophy and practice style. Information can be given to the group and productive discussion can take place. Many families respond to the group setting, which can lay the foundation for group health supervision visits in some situations. All such group formats should include some private time with each couple to address particular concerns and to begin to establish an individual relationship. The following are guidelines for a prenatal visit.

Observational Data

- Note who comes and why. Is dad there? Are grandparents present? A girlfriend?
- Assess the interaction between the parents as they enter the room for the interview process.
- Be aware of their general affect; some degree of anxiety and apprehension is expected.
- Determine the degree of comfort with the pregnancy through behavioral and verbal clues from both the mother and the father; for example, note the patting of the abdomen by the pregnant woman as an indicator of a positive attitude.
- Note the use of pronouns or names for the unborn child and the type and number of questions asked.

What to Ask

The format of questions outlined in Table 6–2 allows control of the interaction to flow from the clinician to the parents.

A discussion of the specifics of your contract with the family should include the following: your availability and backup plans, the schedule for seeing the infant in the neonatal period and beyond, some general statements about your own philosophy of pediatric care and your fee schedule and payment options.

TABLE 6–2   **Questions to Be Asked at the Prenatal Visit**

Question	Objective
How are you feeling?	Lay the territory to include the parent's well-being; assess the response to the situation overall
Ask how the pregnancy has gone; expand to cover medical events, life stresses, etc., as noted on the medical history form and your own individual outline (i.e., a pregnancy history from a pediatric standpoint)	Gather data for objective risk factors and the parents' perception of them, as well as assess their general response to the pregnancy and the perception of the pregnancy as high risk (whether it is by medical criteria or not)
Ask the father how the pregnancy has gone for him	Assess the father's perceptions and concerns about his wife and baby and his own adjustment to the pregnancy
Was this a planned pregnancy?	Assess the place of the child in the relationship, the parents' adjustment to pregnancy and the degree and nature of adjustment for the child's health
Do you have other children at home? What are their ages and sexes? Have you cared for an infant before? What was that experience like?	Assess the family structure; note the child's place in it; assess their experience and expectations for infant care; note the locus of control (i.e., do the parents see themselves in control of this event?); assess their preparedness and give general information on the subject; create an opportunity to give information or your own preferences about the delivery event, which may tap in on particular anxieties or fears in the third trimester; assess unrealistic or rigid expectations; when appropriate, assert that you think that the parents are in charge
How do you plan to feed the baby? (expand to include a diet history during pregnancy, preparation for nursing)	Assess realistic planning for the baby and advise; reaffirm the parents' control of this option; emphasize the importance of nurture in general; offer the opportunity for parents to say how they feel about the situation; assess maternal nutrition vis-à-vis the infant; assess specific breastfeeding preparations; do not push a decision if the family is not ready
If the infant is a boy, will you have him circumcised? (address the question to the father)	Assess individuation of the baby; bring the father into the decision-making process; open this topic for a two-way discussion by providing objective information on circumcision (i.e., the lack of clear medical indications) and the procedure itself
Have you purchased a car seat?	Show interest in safety and caretaking; assess the parents' anticipation of the needs of the infant

Table continued

TABLE 6–2 Questions to Be Asked at the Prenatal Visit—cont'd

Question	Objective
How long have you lived in this area? Where do most of your family live? Who will be available to help you after the baby comes?	Assess family support systems; assess the realignment of old relationships; tap in on parents' relationship to their own feelings
Do you have other responsibilities outside the family?	Assess the mother's other areas of responsibility and stress; what realignment of these areas is anticipated; some areas of ambivalence and concern may be discussed
Are both of you working outside your home? What are your job plans? Do you have any ideas about the time you will return to work? Are you attending school? Have you made plans for the infant's care?	Assess the psychosocial situation of the family; assess the parents' perceptions of their roles in career or education and as parents; assess realistic planning for infant care
Do you have any worries about your infant? Most parents do have some concerns about the child. Would you like to share any of those with me? Is there anything in your past history that makes you think you have some special worries about your child?	Open a discussion of concerns directly, but also use this setting to discuss normalcy of feelings and perhaps deeper concerns; provide information about common fears, fantasies and dreams during a normal pregnancy
For families with other children: How are your other children reacting to your pregnancy? What have you done to prepare them for the birth? Most parents have some worries about how they'll manage to have enough time and love for more than one child. Do you share any of these concerns? What are the specific arrangements you've made for the older child at the time of the baby's birth?	Assess the realignment of family relationships; assess the plans for readjustment around care of the infant; assess maternal and paternal feelings toward the attachment to their children who have already been born
Do you have any questions?	Set a model for pediatric visits (i.e., you are open to questions and waiting for the parents to take the lead)

! HEADS UP–THE PRENATAL VISIT

Infant Factors
- Slow intrauterine growth. Investigate the cause, and plan close follow-up
- Prenatally identified abnormalities. Identify needed evaluations, and make a note of attachment risks

Pregnancy Factors
- History of infertility, pregnancy loss, early complications. At risk for physical problems and attachment disorders
- Mom younger than 15 or older than 35 years. Pregnancy risks increase. Social issues need clarification
- Infectious disease issues. Evaluate the impact on the fetus and plan follow-up.
- Diabetes. High risk of anomalies, early monitoring required, potential for macrosomia
- Substance abuse. Needs professional therapy, monitoring, support
- Smoking, by either parent
- Maternal thyroid disease. Will need infant evaluation and postpartum treatment of mom
- Rigid plans or expectations for pregnancy, for delivery or for the infant

Family Factors
- Poverty. Increases health and development risks
- Single parenting, recent separations or spousal abandonment
- Isolated family, recent move without community ties
- Loss of job or job pressures
- Recent death of a close relative or friend
- History of or suggestion of domestic violence
- History of or current presence of parental mental illness
- Previous history of depression
- No available help after the infant arrives
- Very short parental leave from work
- Previous birth interval of less than 2 years

Special Referrals
- Call or write a note to the obstetrician regarding special concerns from a pediatric perspective. Get the records of previous pregnancies if they were complicated.
- State terms of your own availability at the time of the birth (e.g., another clinician may provide care for the baby in the hospital in some circumstances).
- Recommend prepared childbirth, breastfeeding or other parenting classes if these issues have not already been attended to.
- Refer the patient to a social service agency or a public health nurse for diagnostic aid and a support system, if indicated.
- Make a nutrition referral if indicated by the nutritional history or economic needs.
- Identify mental health professionals who work well with expectant or new parents. Refer as needed.

ANTICIPATORY GUIDANCE

• Encourage open discussion between parents of the subjects addressed in the interview.

• Advise the parents that it may be wise to plan to get help (e.g., a relative, friend or employee) in the immediate postnatal period, but to limit nonhelping visitors for about 2 weeks after the birth.

• Encourage class attendance or reading as a supplement to, but not a substitute for your own care.

• Reassure parents that fears, fantasies and feelings of loss of control are normal, adaptive and good indicators of care.

• Emphasize good nutrition and safety planning for the infant, and congratulate the parents on advance planning and responsibility in initiating the interview process.

• Emphasize that it is important to approach the birth with some flexibility so that unforeseen events (e.g., anesthesia or a cesarean section) can be weathered with adaptation and grace.

• Emphasize planning for sibling response.

WRAPPING UP

A summary statement about your understanding of the interview's content and process will allow a resolution of differences or highlight areas of omission. For example, "Although you had a little concern at the beginning of the pregnancy with bleeding, things have gone very well since. We'll send off thyroid studies on the baby right away, just to be sure, given your thyroid concerns. We'll be sure to get you the help you need to breastfeed. Dad, think about the circumcision question. Let me know what you both decide."

Your Record

Make your own assessment of this family's strengths and vulnerabilities.

• Write down the temperament or style characteristics of the parents.

• Make note of the social support. Who really are the functioning members of the family? Who lives in the house?

• Make note of any risks to attachment.

• Note things of special interest, as shown in the following examples:

Example 1 Debbie and Mark (see the case at the beginning of the chapter) are attractive, young parents-to-be.

— Strengths (+): Married 3 years. Strong extended family. Interested in learning about the baby. Committed to breastfeeding

— Vulnerabilities (−): Debbie's mom died last year. The girl will be named after her. Economic: Dad has two jobs. No boy's name. Dad does woodworking. Family history positive for congenital heart disease. Previous miscarriage

Example 2 Lydia is shy, but strong minded and has rigid expectations, She asks clear questions and is bilingual. Lydia is *not* on welfare and proud of it. She is single and wants a girl. The father of the baby is not involved.

— Strengths (+): Good parenting model. Support from family. Good job

— Vulnerabilities (−): First trimester drug use. In recovery group. Still smoking a bit. Needs to return to work in 2 weeks. Family history of early infant deaths

RECOMMENDED READINGS

American Academy of Pediatrics, Committee on Psychosocial Aspects of Child and Family Health: The prenatal visit. *Pediatrics* 97:141, 1996.

American Academy of Pediatrics: Family pediatrics. *Pediatrics* 111(6 Suppl), June 2003.

American Academy of Pediatrics: The prenatal visit. In Green M (ed): *Bright Futures*. Arlington, VA, National Center for Education in Maternal and Child Health, 1994, 2004, pp 13-17.

Dixon S: Helping siblings adjust to the new baby. In Jellinek M, Patel BP, Froehle MC (eds): *Bright Futures in Practice: Mental Health*, vol 2, *Tool Kit*. Arlington, VA, National Center for Education in Maternal and Child Health, 2002.

Fifer WP, Moon CM: The effects of fetal experience with sound. In Lecaunet JP, et al (eds): *Fetal Development: A Psychological Perspective*. Hillsdale, NJ, Lawrence Erlbaum Associates, 1995.

Stadtler A: Fostering family adjustment prenatally. In Jellinek M, Patel BP, Froehle MC (eds): *Bright Futures in Practice: Mental Health*, vol 2, *Tool Kit*. Arlington, VA, National Center for Education in Maternal and Child Health, 2002.

www.babycenter.com: Provides information on pregnancy, names, FAQs, newsletters and chats.

www.pampers.com: Provides articles, weekly pregnancy briefs, electronic monthly newsletters and FAQs for expectant families.

Zwelling E: Psychological responses to pregnancy. In Nichols F, Zwelling E (eds): *Maternal-Newborn Nursing: Theory and Practice*. Philadelphia, WB Saunders, 1997.

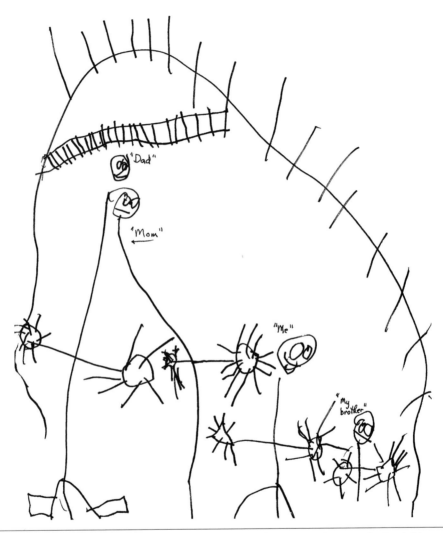

A child of 5 draws his family as he sees it when his mom, 34-weeks pregnant, is put on bed rest. Mom says she's irritable and short with the children. By Kiran Rhodes, age 5.

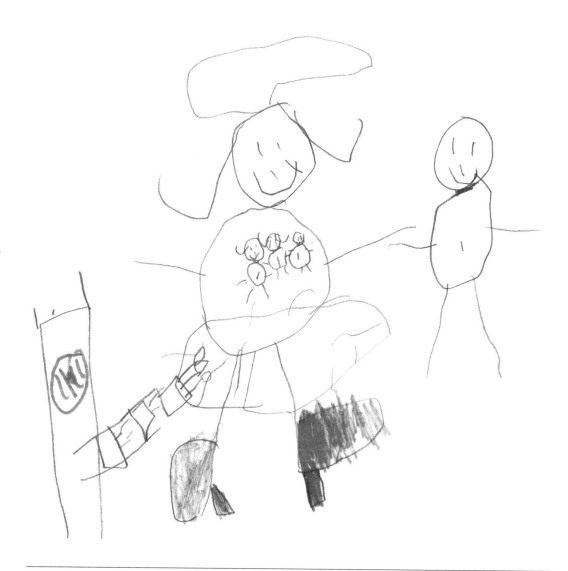

A sign of the times. A six year old portrays a family event of considerable interest to him. He draws a bride, his relative, complete with veil and her groom nearby. A wedding cake is off to the side on a table at this reception. Note the presence of triplets still to be born. By M.H.

CHAPTER 7

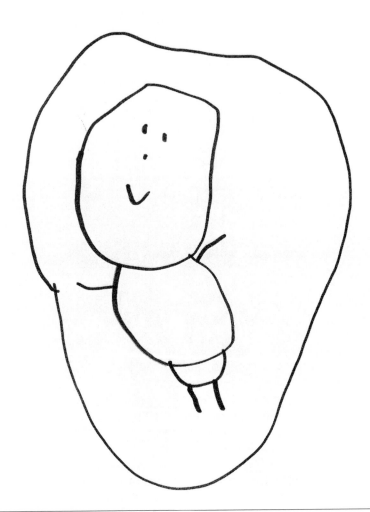

"Baby on a blanket." By Katherine Boucher, a girl aged 4 (original in a bright blue marker).

The Newborn: Ready to Get Going

SUZANNE D. DIXON

This chapter describes the neurobehavioral competencies of the newborn, the processes of adaptation to extrauterine life and the beginnings of the family/child relationship.

Key Words

- Attachment
- Reflex Behavior
- Habituation
- State Organization
- Recovery Process
- Delivery Room Practices
- Vision
- Hearing
- Taste
- Touch
- Smell

Jessica, born without complications, was to be examined at 1 hour of life. Her body was relaxed under the warmer, her hands and feet bluish. Her respirations were even. She scanned the environment with head to one side, fingers in her mouth. When her father spoke, she startled, and her eyes shifted toward him. Gradually she turned to find his face and then stared intensely at him, until her eyes crossed. She closed her lids briefly and then found his face again. Her father said he was in love already. Then she turned pale, moved restlessly and spit up mucus. Jessica's father jumped back and called for the nurse. Comment: Jessica shows the kind of alertness we expect in the first hour of life as she meets her dad for the first time. She successfully grabbed his amazement and affection. She also demonstrates the physiological "bumps" that are part of the postpartum adjustment.

A full-term human infant enters the world fully equipped to negotiate the dramatic physiological changes and behavioral adjustments required for postnatal life. These capacities enable him to begin the job of learning about his world and participating in his central interactive setting, his family. The newborn does not function solely on a reflex level; primitive reflexes are the building blocks of more complex behavior that will evolve later.

147

The goal of the newborn physical examination is to assess the neonate's general well-being and to evaluate any evidence of systemic abnormalities or illness. However, it can do a lot more for the clinician and the family in getting to know this new patient if the examination is augmented by a strong behavioral component. The full range of infant capacities can be laid out. The infant's behavior reflects both his genetic makeup and his intrauterine experience. We get an opportunity to look at both groups of factors when we evaluate the neonate. In addition, the initial visit with the newborn and his family offers the opportunity to participate in and facilitate the initial getting acquainted process for the baby and family.

By doing this exam with the parents, with an emphasis on the behavioral component, we can assure them and ourselves of the infant's wellness but can also explore what kind of person he is. This approach will help the family on the road to solid attachment and accommodation to their own child's individuality. In that sense, this visit is both an intervention and an assessment. The clinician enters into the system of the family through the shared evaluation of the infant.

The first step toward **attachment** and parenting requires assurance that the infant is intact and is successfully negotiating the postpartum adjustment. Through positive reassurance the clinician provides that emotional fuel. The second step is identifying the specialness of the infant to the family so that they can bond with the person in front of them, the real baby rather than an imagined one.

In this era, the full and complete examination of the neonate may occur shortly after birth or at a few days of age, either in the hospital or at an initial office visit. The earlier the exam, the more opportunity there is to evaluate the active processes of postbirth transition and adaptation. This overlay must be taken into account when you perform this exam, for the infant will change depending on the timing after birth. For example, in the first hour of life a healthy infant is likely to be quite alert and responsive. If you catch him later in the first day, he's likely to be a bit sleepy and slowed in his responses as he rests and recovers from birth. At about 18 hours to 2 to 3 days, he's sure to have mainly eating on his mind and seem a bit irritable when you bother him. When he's guaranteed his food supply, at about days 3 to 5, his behavior is likely to smooth out. So the timing of your initial acquaintance should be factored into your evaluation and narrated to the parents as they observe you. If you perform both an initial and a discharge or follow-up exam, the differences in performance are important for both you and the family to notice.

Researchers use formal behavioral examinations as both outcome and predictor variables in infancy research. The Neonatal Behavioral Assessment Scale developed by Brazelton and colleagues is widely used and is moderately reliable in predicting developmental outcome across infancy. Sequential exams reflecting behavioral recovery after birth are more predictive than a single assessment. Clinical adaptation of this tool has been shown to positively influence parenting responsiveness, as well as identify infants at risk for developmental concerns. Many of the maneuvers are presented informally here.

Wherever or whenever it occurs, the initial newborn examination is one of the most important ones in establishing a solid relationship with families. It is also a time to reflect on and appreciate the marvelous capacities of your new patient. Enjoy this visit.

TABLE 7–1   **Behavioral Competencies of the Newborn**

Behavior	Expected Range of Performance	Concerning Behavior
Vision	Attends to a bright object 8–12 inches away when in an alert state	No alerting to objects
	Follows an object with eyes and perhaps with head through some arc	Very brief or no following
	Follows a face or a face and voice side to side	No blink with approach
	Scans the environment when alert	Dull, flat expression
	Blinks with rapid approach of a hand	No brightening
	Hands open and close with visual attention	
Hearing	Brightens to a soft sound or voice	No alerting to sound
	Turns to parent's voice over the examiner	No turning, even with eyes
	Turns from side to side to source of the sound, a voice or rattle	
State organization	Moves smoothly from sleep to wakefulness	Stays drowsy or irritable
	Calms self when upset	Alternates from drowsy to irritable (i.e., not alert state)
		Cries with minimal disturbance
	Can be calmed by the examiner	Doesn't calm and quiet with calming techniques
	Comes to a bright alert state	
Sucking	Roots with cheek touch	Flaccid mouth
	Brings finger into the mouth	Biting
	Does bursts of sucking	Disorganized suck
	Front-to-back tongue motion	

BEHAVIORAL COMPETENCIES—THE SENSES

The newborn's sensory capacities are far greater than was previously believed (Table 7–1).

Vision

The visual system has all components, peripheral and central, present at term, but substantial maturation occurs after birth, particularly in the first 6 months. The human infant can see faces and objects when they are presented at his best focal distance, 8 to 12 inches, although his depth of focus may actually cover a wider range. Lens mobility is limited but improves rapidly. Foveal structures are less well developed, and central focus is less than in older children and adults. The neonate is quite nearsighted. At birth, vision may range from about 20/200 to 20/400. Acuity is limited primarily by retinal immaturity. Acuity and improved accommodation proceed rapidly in the first 4 months.

Extraocular movements allow for slow tracking of objects up to 180 degrees horizontally, perhaps briefly vertically, but not diagonally; this skill develops in the last quarter of the first year. Episodic disconjugate gaze is often observed in the first 6 months but is clearly abnormal after that. However, continuing, fixed limitation of eye movement is always a concern, even in the neonatal period. Full excursion of both eyes horizontally should be seen.

Infants are very sensitive to light, perhaps more so than adults, and will open their eyes only in light that is considered dim by adult standards. Automatic visual scanning occurs even in conditions of darkness or low light as the infant exercises his visual abilities. The infant clearly has the capacity to see in three dimensions, as evidenced by primitive reaching and the ability to blink as an object approaches, even when controlling for other input. This defensive response is more elaborate and less automatic than a reflex behavior and attests to the integration of visual and motor systems. Three dimensional vision improves across the first 6 months through maturation of several processes, so by the time an infant is crawling, he can clearly map his world visually in all dimensions.

Additional laboratory studies have shown that infants demonstrate differential attention to visual displays with the following characteristics:

- High contrast
- Curved lines over straight
- Bright colors rather than dull colors
- Many elements as opposed to few
- Edges and contrasting interfaces

Color detection and preference have been studied in the same way, but the results are equivocal because color is inevitably confounded by brightness and infants do prefer moderately bright objects. Infants can probably discriminate red, green and yellow, but not blue, when intensity is controlled. Cone development proceeds rapidly in the first 2 months, and color discrimination is much more reliable after 3 to 4 months.

The *human face* draws much attention from infants. Neonates will preferentially look at their mothers' faces even without sound or smile, although the concept of complete facial recognition is controversial. The hairline and the moving eyebrows may be the most salient features for the neonate in identifying his familiar care provider. By 12 weeks this capacity is clear, and the face is the most compelling sight to the baby.

The concept of newborn imitation through vision is controversial. Some researchers have demonstrated infants imitating a tongue thrust, even at 1 day of age, though with long latency. This capacity implies marvelous intersensory and motor coordination. The young infant must be in a quiet, alert state and allowed enough time, several minutes, to process the interesting display held out for imitation. Older infants imitate such displays in seconds.

The importance of visual input for the infant is illustrated by derangements in the visual system. An impairment in vision, such as that present with cataracts, may prevent the development of *functional* vision if it is not corrected during the first 6 months of life; subtle residuals of newborn visual compromise have been noted in children who have this condition even for 1 week. Without binocular input for even short periods, long-lasting impairment may result. Frank cortical blindness in the case of severe esotropia is the extreme of a continuum of perceptual compromise when vision is unavailable. The infant is vulnerable to alterations in vision even up to the third year of life. Early detection and remediation are imperative, so it is worth the time to watch the infant watch and follow you.

A newborn's visual capacities can be demonstrated at their fullest only when the infant is in a quiet, alert state and all distracting stimuli are minimized, even his own motor movements. Visual performance may be limited to brief periods and may be overridden, especially early on, by physiological events (e.g., bowel movements, hiccups). Visual processing is one of the most complex neonatal abilities and may be difficult to demonstrate in all infants all the time. It takes time and patience to fully bring out these capacities.

The newborn's higher visual processing and the coordination within the neurological system can be seen by observing the whole face and body when visual stimuli are presented. When attentive, the infant may initially startle slightly and then shut down body movements to focus on the visual display. Facial muscles will lift and the palpebral fissures will widen, thus giving the baby a bright, softened look. Brief periods of attention will cycle with periods of inattention, gaze aversion and possibly even sleep (note the opening case vignette). The infant will thereby limit the duration and the complexity of the visual events that he handles at any point in time. Gaze is a capacity under the infant's control from early in life. Maturation and recovery from birth or illness are characterized by increasing duration of these alert periods and the ability to respond to an increasing complexity of visual displays. This recovery of abilities is a very good attribute to demonstrate to families as you examine infants over the first weeks to months.

> Damien was a vigorous term infant. Dr. McDonald held him swaddled about 10 inches from his face. After a couple of gentle bobs, Damien opened his eyes and the doctor caught his attention. With a soft voice he moved his face from side to side, and the baby's gaze stayed with him. The infant's expression was bright and his whole body was quiet.

When the same visual display is presented to the infant repeatedly, he will show less and less interest in it. This process is called habituation. When something he perceives as new comes into his gaze, he'll respond to it with renewed interest and scrutiny. This characteristic demonstrates the neonate's innate ability to seek out and preferentially attend to novelty in his world. This process also allows us to test an infant's abilities to detect a difference between two objects. A decline is seen in the amount of time gazing at an object perceived by the infant as the same; renewed interest is seen if the difference in the "old" and "new" objects is appreciated. Habituation paradigms are often used in infancy research to validate the baby's ability to discriminate various stimuli: visual, auditory or other spheres. Infants who readily habituate to visual stimuli and demonstrate a strong preference for novelty are more likely to show more advanced development in infancy.

Audition

Hearing matures earlier than vision, primarily before birth, although full development continues across the first decade of life. The infant can hear and is responsive to sounds early in gestation, as described in Chapter 6. The ability to clearly direct attention to auditory input may even be seen in 28-week-old premature infants. Fluid present in the middle ear in the days after birth impairs the neonate only slightly in being very responsive to the sound environment.

An infant will respond to a pleasant auditory signal, such as a voice or soft rattle, in ways similar to his visual alerting response—an initial alerting startle, brightening of expression and diminishing of body activity. The infant may turn his eyes and then his head toward the sound after a short delay and will often search for the source of it. Female voices in highly modulated tones (i.e., "baby talk") produce the most consistent orientation response. Adults in general speak to infants in short bursts of 5 to 15 seconds, the same time unit that produces this differential auditory attention. Lower tones, such as those produced by male speakers, produce a quieting response in a newborn who is upset. Short bursts of modulated human speech produce a greater behavioral response than unpatterned speech or speech of greater or lesser duration does. Selective attention is paid to the basic elements of human speech, the phoneme or consonant-vowel combination, with particular attention to one's own language beginning in early infancy. So hearing is not only present but is clearly discriminating from birth and even before.

> Dr. Karr held the neonate horizontally at the level of his eyes. He positioned the infant's mother on the other side of the baby. As they both talked quiet "baby talk," the infant startled just a bit. Then he shifted first his eyes and then his head toward his mom. He demonstrated consistently whose voice he knew. Note: This maneuver is very powerful in letting parents know how important they are to their infant. It's well worth the time and effort.

Clearly, by 1 month of age and often in the immediate newborn period, an infant can distinguish between mother's voice and another's, as demonstrated through differential quieting and sucking responses: the infant will work harder sucking to receive the reward of a taped recording of the mother's voice than for that of another person.

Soft, low-pitched lullabies and particularly human heart tones produce decreased activity and decreased crying in the newborn. Even while continuing to cry, the infant coordinates his cry and movements with the lullaby within seconds, usually eventually quieting. Lullabies around the world have the same rhythms that appear soothing to infants. In contrast, "game songs" (i.e., lively, fast) produce either alerting or behavioral disorganization. Infants also cry when another infant cries, just as all humans seem to be programmed to experience distress when crying is heard.

The now classic work of Condon and Sander has shown that a newborn readjusts ongoing body movements to the voice patterns of those speaking around him and will do so more consistently if the speaker is his mother or at least someone speaking in the family's native language. Pure tones, runs of babble and other nonspeech tones do not produce this differential response. This "early interactional synchrony" attests to complex integration of the newborn's auditory and motor behavior, beginning in utero.

Infants fail to respond to an auditory stimulus if it is loud (e.g., hand clap) or aversive (e.g., "white noise" in a nursery) or if confounded with other stimuli (e.g., loud voice with an overly animated, close face). The infant shuts out these adverse auditory events very successfully and may even appear to have impaired hearing under such conditions. The clinician can be fooled by this inattention. A gentler approach (less background noise, soft sounds and no competing visual display) is needed to bring out these auditory capacities.

Early hearing is vital to the development of language, as well as to emotional health, because it allows us to monitor our environment and anticipate change. The world can be alarming when this sense is impaired. Deaf infants may appear hyperalert and anxious. The parent-child interaction is distorted and less positive when one of the partners is deaf.

Although major hearing loss can be identified behaviorally by the infant's failure to respond to the human voice as evidenced by at least heart rate change, there is no way to completely screen behaviorally. Risk factors for hearing loss are present only in one half the cases identified. Formal screening of all neonates with the use of various technologies is becoming nearly universal, as it should. Clinicians should support such programs and should be *sure* of the results of each child under their care before 1 month of age. Equivocal results on screenings demand prompt repeat and or a full audiological evaluation. Delay in identifying a hearing defect is clearly associated with a poorer outcome for the child. If your behavioral assessment suggests impaired hearing, a referral is warranted even if results of screening were satisfactory. Never hesitate to get a hearing test if hearing concerns are present, either in the neonatal period or throughout childhood.

Some infants will be more responsive to sound than others; visual displays will produce greater behavioral attention with other infants. These individual differences may be noted even in the newborn period and will highlight the special behavioral profile of an individual child. Some infants are listeners and some are lookers.

Taste and Smell

Studies have demonstrated that infants have a nearly fully developed sense of taste. Their taste buds are greater in number and more widely distributed across the tongue than those of an adult. Even while in utero, infants can demonstrate an alteration in sucking frequency when sugar is introduced into the amniotic fluid. Sensitivity to sweets as preferred and adverse reactions to bitter tastes are present at birth, whereas sensitivity to salty tastes develops postnatally, at about 4 to 6 months of age, the time that solids are introduced. Complex patterns of taste preference, as opposed to sensitivity, are shaped by experience during the first year of life. The infant is preprogrammed to avoid aversive tastes that in nature are largely poisonous and to seek out those that are sweet and differentially nourishing. Facial expressions of infants presented with varying tastes are similar to adults' expressions in the same circumstances. Although some infants are more sensitive to the varying tastes in breast milk based on maternal diet, it is the rare infant who truly alters his nursing pattern because of the presence of a particular taste.

Smell is well developed and well used in newborns. The infant can successfully localize odors and may demonstrate preference through differential turning away or orienting toward unpleasant and pleasant odors, respectively. Associative learning, or linking smells with other events, shows the importance of olfaction in learning about the world from early infancy.

Smell brings a family together. Infants as young as 5 days can differentiate by smell alone the breast pad of their own mother from that of other mothers. Parents, in turn, can recognize their own infant's smell after only 1 hour of exposure, thus suggesting that each infant has his own odor signature and one that is the easiest identifier for the parent to learn. Infants placed at birth on the thigh of their moms will crawl up to the breast aided only by smell. Familiar odors linked with touch prompt a positive infant response.

TRANSITIONAL BEHAVIOR

The ability to maintain breathing, heart rate and temperature and to modulate peripheral perfusion improves over the first days of life with varying speed and smoothness. Infants stressed by difficult labor, hard delivery or postnatal problems generally have more trouble with these physiological transitions. Slightly preterm infants, 36 to 38 weeks, and large-for-gestational-age babies with blood glucose irregularities take longer to get on track in this way as well. Skin color, skin perfusion, the degree of acrocyanosis and the response to stress are important to characterize and monitor for continuing improvement. The response to and recovery from undressing, handling, reflex assessment and even social interaction give us an indication of the infant's vulnerability, margin of tolerated stress and/or maturity. These vital observations can be made incidentally as part of every exam, and they add no more time but give important information on the infant's individual resilience and recovery. Infants still grappling with organization at this basic physiological level will not be as available for auditory and visual alerting tasks because these processes seem to be organized on a hierarchical level. When these measures show greater stability, the infant will be able to more readily listen and track visually. Feeding difficulties are more common in infants who are less mature or show evidence of stress at this level of organization.

STATE BEHAVIOR

Full-term infants exist in at least **six states of consciousness** (Table 7–2). These states of consciousness consist of quiet sleep, active sleep, drowsiness, a quiet/alert state, an active alert-fussy state and a crying state. They move through these states in cycles with some regularity. Responsiveness to some outside stimuli, motor tone, physiological processes (e.g., heart rate, breathing) and even **reflex behavior** based on motor tone vary with these variations in state. So the infant's state needs to be taken into account during any examination.

Clear characterization of each state and regular movement from one state to another testify to neurological competency and maturity. An intact newborn can resist outside disturbances during sleep and even awake states by shutting out any intrusive events. Noises, lights and even painful stimuli will be behaviorally and electrophysiologically ignored with successive presentation. This process is one of **habituation**, as described earlier. The adaptive, protective nature of this capacity is obvious. The infant protects his own vulnerability to overwhelming or boringly repetitive noise and light stimuli through a process of selective inattention. He will fall asleep or maintain a drowsy/sleep state if the world intrudes too harshly.

The first hours and days of life are characterized by disruption in the regularity of the state changes seen in late gestation. An alert period of about 40 to 70 minutes in a term, nondrugged neonate after birth is followed by a period of 3 to 5 hours of deep sleep. Brief, drowsy arousals occur until the newborn is about 18 to 24 hours old. Renewed wakefulness and obvious hunger with frequent feedings are the norm for the next 24 to 72 hours. Babies often feed every 1½ to 2 hours during this period. The state cycle stabilizes when the mother's milk comes in, with wakefulness occurring every 2 to 3 hours. Infants discharged at 24 hours or less

TABLE 7–2 **States of Consciousness in the Newborn**

State	Activity	Muscle Tone	Heart Rate	Respirations
Quiet sleep	Eyes closed, no eye movements, still with occasional startles	Steady, tonic	Regular	Regular
Active sleep	Eyes closed with globe movements Random, low-level facial movements; wiggles	Low	Variable	Irregular
Drowsy	Flat face; eyes closed, dully open or partially open Writhing movements, variable	Low, variable	Variable	Variable
Alert	Face bright Eyes open, following Motor movement mostly absent	Steady	First a rise, then lower than baseline	Regular
Irritable	Negative face, avoidance maneuvers, squirmy, brief whimpers or fussy vocalizations	Slight increase	Variable	Irregular
Crying	Crying, motor activity at high level	Increased level	Slightly elevated	Irregular, with crying

Modified from Prechtl HFR: The neurological examination of the full term newborn infant. In *Clinics in Developmental Medicine*, vol 63. London, MacKeith Press, 1975; and Brazelton TB, Nugent JK: Neonatal Behavioral Assessment Scale. In *Clinics in Developmental Medicine*, vol 137. London, MacKeith Press, 1995.

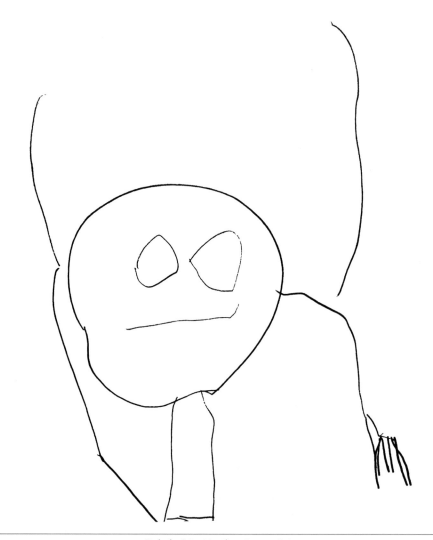

"A baby." By Heather R., age 3½.

may be perceived at home later as ill, unhappy and certainly uncooperative unless the clinician draws attention to this normal pattern of adjustment and transition.

Neurologically intact infants under the care of one caretaker will show progressive gains in state stabilization. However, some infants will remain somewhat irregular and unpredictable as part of their individual temperament profile and the slope of their recovery after birth. Infants older than 3 days (and very sleepy ones before that) will benefit from a little help in establishing a regular wake-sleep cycle through the care of a regular caregiver responding to the subtle cues of early wakefulness, wiggles and brief eye openings. Feedings geared to the infant's own shift in states are usually more successful than those attempted after a crying bout. Crying is a late sign of hunger. Regular feedings, variations in illumination and sound and close body contact with another human being all work toward stabilization of **state organization**. In contrast, constant illumination, continuous noise, many caregivers and irregular responses to restlessness, crying and distress (all characteristic of a hospital nursery) will make it more difficult for the infant to get organized with sleep, feeding and alertness. We do neither mothers nor healthy infants any favors by bringing the babies to the nursery "so mother can sleep." This is an added delay in postpartum adjustment that is to be avoided if at all possible. It confounds the process for both and may make sleep and feeding areas of concern after discharge. Because infants in a rooming-in situation cry very little, the risk is small that other mothers who are in the same unit will lose sleep. Full rooming-in should produce a quiet hospital unit, as well as an accelerated postpartum adjustment.

REFLEXES AND BEYOND

Motor behavior is built on a set of **primitive reflexes** (Table 7–3). These reflexes are indicators of general neurological integrity, and each has its own developmental course. These reflexes are based on muscle tone, which in a normal infant varies with the state of consciousness (see earlier). Therefore, in addition to noting the presence, absence or asymmetry of these reflexes, the clinician should assess active and passive tone within the context of several states, in sleep and wakefulness (Table 7–4). Relative hypotonia and hypertonia are each appropriate in different states of consciousness, but the lack of variability through several states is worrisome. For example, palmar grasp should be sluggish in active sleep, when tone is diminished, but brisk in a cry state, when tone is increased.

Abnormalities in tone may be due to transient abnormalities such as hypoglycemia or may occur as part of complex malformation syndromes such as trisomy 21. They may also be a sign of immaturity or be an indicator of a serious neurological condition. The observation of tone relative to the baby's other conditions, relative to his maturity and in the context of state of consciousness is central to the neonatal evaluation. Hypertonia or hypotonia is a symptom, like fever, that needs further evaluation.

Learned behaviors are built on these reflexes. For example, the reflexive suck becomes specific for the breast or the bottle in the first days of life. It becomes coordinated to the milk flow characteristics of each and becomes part of a complex pattern of behavior between a mother and infant. The tonic neck reflex enables the infant to watch his hand movements so that gaze and reach become linked—the first step toward volitional reach. Reflexes provide an opportunity for the infant to interact with the environment, the necessary condition for

TABLE 7–3   **Neonatal Reflexes**

Reflex	Description	Emergence	Disappears
Moro	Head back, extremities out and then in, response to head drop	28 wk, complete at 37 wk	4–6 mo
Trunk incurvation	Trunk arches to the side stroked	28 wk	4–5 mo
Placing, stepping (i.e., walking)	Infant lifts and steps when held upright touching a firm surface	36–37 wk	2–4 mo (continues under weightless condition)
Ankle clonus, or up to 2 beats	Alternating flexion and extension of the foot with rapid forced dorsiflexion	33–35 wk	1 mo
Tonic neck reflex (fencer's posture)	Arm extension when the head is placed to that side, contralateral arm flexed Legs mirror arms	35 wk, peaks at 4–6 wk post-term	7–8 mo
Palmar grasp	Fingers flex when an object is placed in the palm	28 wk	2–4 mo
Rooting	Head and mouth turn to the side where the cheek is stroked	? 34 wk	3 wk (voluntary thereafter)
Swimming	Paddling and kicking movements when the face is placed in water	? 36 wk	4–6 mo
Crawling	When in the prone position with pressure on the feet, the infant pushes forward	? 35 wk	3–4 mo
Palmar-mental	When pressure is applied to the palms, the mouth opens (i.e., the chin drops)	36–37 wk	2–3 mo

development. This "software package" helps the infant start exploring and experimenting with the world.

The manner of the execution of "random" movements gives clues to neurological competency, maturity and style. Persistent jitteriness and tremulousness, especially in both asleep and alert states, attest to neurological immaturity or irritability, perinatal stress or metabolic abnor-

TABLE 7–4 **Motor System**

Motor System	Expected in Term Infants	Concerning
Passive motor tone	Forced movement of arms and legs should be balanced, even. Return to flexion when released	Asymmetry Flaccidity Tremulousness or jitteriness on release
Active tone	Flexion of all extremities	Extension or flaccidity
Pull to sit	Head follows the axis of the trunk as the examiner pulls the hands up from laying to sitting	Head lags behind the axis or flops forward without the ability to right it
Scarf sign	Infant's hand and arm pulled across the chest, elbow coming to the midline or less	Elbow crosses the midline or elbow comes to less than the nipple line
Suspended prone position	Infant's trunk held prone over the examiner's hand. Some straightening of the trunk and head lift	Infant drapes over the hand like a "sack of meal" or extends out straight

malities. Jerky movements in arcs of 45 degrees are less worrisome in a full-term infant. Ankle clonus greater than two beats and many startles throughout the regular pediatric physical examination or with minimal handling are of similar concern in a term infant. However, these motor abnormalities do not carry predictive significance beyond the newborn period. They should be monitored over a period and be taken as clues indicating the possibility of other adjustment difficulties rather than being diagnostic or prognostic in themselves.

All in all, the infant's perceptual and behavioral repertoire is geared toward initiating and maintaining positive interactions with his world. All of his capacities enable him to reach out, to become active in eliciting responsive care.

BIRTH EXPERIENCE

The impact of perinatal events on development of the family unit is profound. Labor that is attended by supportive people, particularly the father, tends to be shorter and less fraught with complications. Advance knowledge of the events of labor and delivery allows family members to feel that they are in control of this natural process and gives an enhanced feeling of competency. Prepared childbirth training offers help on several levels, such as educating, laying out expectations, calming fears and offering the support of the educator, as well as those of other expectant families.

The role of a knowledgeable support person, a *doula*, has been shown to be helpful in smoothing the course of labor. The close physical contact that she provides seems to be particularly effective in shortening the length and stress of labor. Calm, moderately short labor is likely to result in an infant who transitions easily and raises no red flags for the child health care provider. The pediatric job is easier in all ways if the labor process is smooth. It is worth the effort to work with obstetric colleagues to create a calming birthing environment.

Long labor and epidural anesthesia can produce a rise in temperature that may be misconstrued as pathological fever. This sets up the need for medical intervention, separation and delay in discharge. The clinician should reevaluate the institution's practices to see whether they facilitate the natural processes of adaptation, acquaintance and recovery. Life will be simpler and healthier for all involved if the practices support this adjustment.

Birth is the beginning of a relationship, and as in any human relationship, it is as variable as the people involved. Sensitivity to the feelings of parents, both positive and negative, will allow the infant's physician to support this "getting acquainted" as it proceeds in its own individual way. Responsiveness to the medical needs of the infant may require that parents realign priorities; the clinician should guide and assist in this process with patient firmness.

Babies belong with their parents in all circumstances except for critical illness in the infant or mother, and even then contact should occur as soon and for as much time as possible. Advantages of contact include better and easier breastfeeding, more positive attachment behavior by the mother, less distress in the infant and perhaps some protection from sudden infant death syndrome, although such protection may be mediated through enhanced breastfeeding. Close physical contact enhances physiological stability and growth. Any separation should be considered a perturbation in the parent-child relationship and should not be considered casually.

Cesarean section, especially if it is unanticipated, may result in feelings of failure and unmet expectations on the part of parents. In addition, infants delivered by cesarean section may be drowsy, slow feeders and poorly responsive to their parents' attempts at interaction. Mothers may feel more pain from the incision and have a more prolonged recovery course than mothers of infants born by vaginal delivery. Infants delivered by cesarean section often require more time and patience getting themselves behaviorally organized in the immediate newborn period, but long-term detrimental effects on health or development have not been seen in this population as a result of the birth mode. Fathers may be even more involved with infant care after a cesarean section birth, and this has long-term positive consequences.

Medication given to the mother during labor and delivery has an effect on the infant's behavior ranging from hypotonia after epidural or spinal anesthesia or after magnesium administration to frank depression of respirations if inappropriate pain medication is given immediately before delivery. Even a small amount of drug may make a mother less alert in her early interactions with her infant, and the infant may be poorly responsive to her. Breastfeeding may take a little more time to get started. If drugs have been used, the clinician should note some of the behavioral changes related to the delivery events. This sets the stage for monitoring the expected **recovery process** with the family in the hours and days ahead.

SPECIAL CONDITIONS

- Infants of diabetic mothers tend to be slightly drowsy and hypotonic, have long latency before response during the neurodevelopmental examination and may have only brief periods of alertness. They may take longer to get on track even if their glucose levels are maintained.

- Some of these behavioral abnormalities are also seen in infants with *hyperbilirubinemia*, particularly those undergoing phototherapy.

- No systematic studies of *polycythemic infant* behavior have been performed, but many clinicians have observed that these infants tend to be lethargic, even without demonstration of frank hyperviscosity and with correction of their hematocrit levels.
- Infants born to mothers with pregnancy-induced hypertension may be behaviorally disorganized, even if not undergrown. They need more patience in the first days of life to allow for more behavioral recovery. Initiation of breastfeeding is often slower in all these situations, usually because of both maternal and infant factors.
- Infants born after long labor with a very distorted head shape may also take longer to get organized.
- Babies with fractured clavicles may experience pain with movement and when placed in certain positions. Early splinting, pain relief and avoidance of painful postures will help with adjustment.

Although these conditions are considered routine to most clinicians, many parents will see them as major deviations from their expectations. They may harbor feelings of deep disappointment and worry. This frame of mind sets the stage for "vulnerable child syndrome" (see Chapter 8).

Circumcision

Circumcision is a stressful event that predictably alters the infant's behavior, both during and after the procedure, especially if the circumcision is performed without anesthesia. Parents should anticipate that their son may be sleepy after the procedure and may need a little more prompting with feeding. These behavioral alterations appear to be self-limited. A dorsal penile nerve block provides safe and effective local anesthesia during circumcision; however, it decreases, but does not eliminate the recovery period.

Procedures and Pain

Neonates feel *pain* with the same sensitivity as older humans do. Their response may be less localized and may even be delayed. "Behavioral meltdown" in terms of physiological instability is more likely to occur after, not during a painful procedure. Physicians tend to ignore pain or undermedicate young infants. Full and complete pain relief should be given to the neonate, commensurate with what adults receive. Infants need additional monitoring and support after as well as during a painful event.

Appearance

The appearance of baby animals generally contains elements that we know prompt tender care, attentiveness and positive regard. These elements include a relatively large head, eyes below the horizontal midline of the face, a prominent forehead and a face with full cheeks. The human newborn has these features as well, and they prompt the universal "gooing" and touching demonstrated by adults around them. Across all species, malformed offspring provide a challenge to attachment; humans are no different. Minor or major physical deformities may change a parent's positive response to the infant. Every effort should be made to correct these abnormalities early, if possible. Disfiguring features may be a severe impediment to attachment, and prompt discussion and attention are therefore necessary. The relationship and the interaction are distorted by irregularities, particularly in the face.

Even without an abnormality, the baby's appearance plays a central role in his meaning and place in the family. Parents interact more with attractive babies and attribute competence to an attractive infant. The clinician should pay close attention to remarks about who the child resembles, whose eyes (temper, feet, ears, etc.) he has. These linkages may surface later in attributions of the child's behavior and course of development.

The clinician should pay attention to her own response to the infant. Compliments are due to the parents of on attractive infant, and something can always be said about a child who is less attractive.

 Dr. Cooper handed the infant back to the proud father after an exam, saying "Now that's a baby. He has a very strong nose."

Some cultural groups may be adverse to hearing specific compliments because it seems to enhance the infant's vulnerability (see Chapter 3). Nonetheless, a pleased look and positive reassurance are always welcome.

THE NEWBORN EXAMINATION

What to Observe

The infant's examination should, with rare exception, occur at the mother's bedside with both parents present. This is an intervention as well as an assessment. You should narrate your observations as part of the ongoing interaction with the family. You are there to assess the infant's neurobehavioral health and individuality. Some of the details to note include the following:

- Examination as a minor stressor for the infant—the infant's response to the procedure and the examiner can be used as an indicator of robustness, stability and maturity. The exam should be ordered with a gradient from the least stressing (e.g., observation of color and breathing) to the most (e.g., the Moro reflex).
- Where is the infant? In the nursery, in the bassinet, held by whom? Who's active in care?
- The nurses' and parents' handling of the infant—this is determined by both the caretaker and the infant. Is this infant treated very tentatively or very vigorously? What do the nurses say about the infant? Nurses readily take into account the individuality of an infant and, with any experience, have a sense of the infant getting on track.
- Your own responses to the infant—as a consistent examiner, you are registering whether this is a frail infant, an attractive one, an alert one. Do you like the baby? Why or why not? Use your response as a barometer of the infant's wellness and capability.
- Nursing record—check for sleep and crying, heart rate and breathing regularity, response to procedures (e.g., bath, neonatal screening tests) and difficulties with caretaking.

Experienced nurses know which infants "have it together" and which ones need more support. These observations are critical for **discharge planning** with a family.

- Parents' impression and handling of the infant—what do they say and do with the infant? What are their descriptions of the baby? Whom does the baby resemble?

- Maternal (and paternal) fatigue, stress and ill health—is mom moving around the room and calling friends and relatives or does she look like she's pasted to the bed? Is she crying? Can she ask questions of you or is she entirely focused on her own issues? Is dad there, involved, supportive?

What to Assess

Begin assessment at the mother's bedside, lights dim. Narrate your findings to the parents, and keep the following in mind:

- Conduct a general examination, but reorder it from the least intrusive to the most intrusive maneuvers. Observe the infant's color change, breathing and awakening as you do your assessment, starting with uncovering and undressing.

- Interrupt what you're doing if the infant becomes alert. When the infant is alert, present an object such as a ball, the stethoscope or another toy at his focal distance, 8 to 10 inches. Move the object slowly, horizontally and vertically to assess the infant's tracking and the whole performance in visual processing. The baby should stop moving and his face should brighten as his eyes and perhaps his head shift.

- Repeat the visual assessment using your face and then using your face and voice together. (The combined stimulus is more compelling than the single one for term infants; stressed and immature infants may find the combined stimulus too complex and therefore aversive.) The baby will show you that you have exceeded your limit by turning away, looking away, gagging or changing color. You and the parents will have learned the infant's limits and signaling system.

- With the infant held securely above eye level, swaddled as needed, talk softly to him. Wait for the response. Having an alert look, turning the eyes toward you and then turning the head toward you are the expected responses, if given time and a positive auditory cue.

- Repeat this process with one or both parents on the other side. Watch them fall in love when the infant turns to their voice rather than yours. Point out recognition of them.

- During this time, note the infant's irritability, changes in motor tone with state of consciousness and the amount of tremulousness and startles. Such assessment gives you an idea of the infant's maturity, neurological integrity and physiological stability. This first assessment provides a basis of comparison for subsequent assessment and thus allows you to monitor the infant's recovery. Very physiologically fragile infants will be less available socially than those who are more organized at that level.

- A full neurological examination with careful assessments of active and passive tone and the presence, character and vigor of the reflexes should be performed. This is a stressor; watch how the infant copes with it, signals distress and recovers from the distressing maneuver, including how long recovery takes.

- During periods of crying (e.g., after testing for the Moro reflex), carefully observe and assess the infant's self-quieting maneuvers and the amount of effort needed by the examiner to quiet the infant. This level of need will be replicated at home. Some infants need more help to settle down than others do. These infants should be described as "feisty, strong-minded" or other positive terms. Less perturbable infants should be described as "calm." Mildly hypertonic infants with brisk responsiveness are often portrayed as "strong." Mildly hypotonic infants may be described as "relaxed."

- The infant walk and step are reflexes that are powerful in showing the parents how much a person the infant is. Don't skip these.

- Put a gloved finger in the infant's mouth to assess oral-motor organization. An infant who is poorly coordinated, bites or puts his tongue up will need extra help with feeding.

- Cuddle the infant in the crook of the arm and at the shoulder. The infant should mold in but also maintain bend control. If not, an alteration in tone should be investigated. Floppy infants will feel as though they are falling through; hypertonic infants will push out straight and will not curl into your arm.

- Clinicians should see themselves as a barometer of the infant's behavior, now and throughout one's practice. If one feels that an infant is behaviorally vulnerable, the infant probably is, and the parents will feel that too. If the child is particularly attractive, it may be because the infant is exceptionally well organized. Pay attention to your own responses to your patients because these will be an increasingly reliable part of your clinical skills.

DISCHARGE DECISIONS AND PLANS

The timing of discharge for mother and infant is a decision that has to take into account maternal, infant, interactional and family issues. The mother must be sufficiently recovered to take independent care of herself and her infant. She must also have a safe place to go, with adequate food and shelter for herself and the infant, factors that may be inappropriately taken for granted. Support by someone with child care experience is ideal.

- *The infant must be psychologically stable* and have negotiated the postnatal physiological and behavioral transitions. The baby must be able to signal needs, have those signals understood by care providers and be able to feed well, which means that an experienced professional has seen the infant feed well at least twice and that the mother also feels comfortable with the feeding. The baby should awaken to feed, and elimination should be proceeding normally. The baby should be responsive to interactions with the environment as an index of neurological intactness. Lethargy and poor feeding are the most reliable indicators of illness or abnormalities. Beware if even a hint of these words is applied to the infant. Although these observations are nonspecific, they are key when applied by experienced health care providers.

- *Parents should be instructed in routine care* such as handling a spit up, taking the temperature and getting the infant correctly into a car seat. This should be observed, not just reported by the parent.

- *A follow-up plan should be solidly in place.* A checkup within the first week of life should be routine, perhaps coordinated with a home health visit. Problems, including breastfeeding difficulties, jaundice and poor weight gain, emerge and are more easily solved in the first week of life.

- Criteria and provisions for emergency care should be explicitly laid out. Assurance of transportation should be part of that.

- Mothers should not be discharged without the infant unless the child is in need of critical care that will be ongoing. Similarly, infants should stay with their moms if they need to stay, unless their situation is critical. Federal law now guarantees at least a 2-day stay for a vaginal delivery and 4 days for a cesarean section. However, good medical care demands that the individual needs of each family be kept in mind. These needs include behavioral readiness of the baby and the mother to thrive outside the hospital or birthing center. This is a joint decision between the clinician and the parent or parents.

Discharge Plans

Observation 1

Ms. Huttle delivered her daughter at 37 weeks gestation with a weight of 5 pounds, 9 ounces. The infant had a low temperature during transition and required two glucose feedings to keep her blood sugar up early on. Breastfeedings seem brief and are described as disorganized. On examination, the infant goes from drowsy to irritable quite readily, gets mottled by the end of the exam and is jittery even during her brief alert periods. Mom says she has a friend who will help her with the baby because the father isn't around and no relatives live in the area.

Inference: Don't be in a hurry to discharge this infant and mom because they don't really seem to be on track. Extra help with feeding will prevent jaundice and dehydration. Mom needs to learn how to support her small infant, and she needs some support herself. If discharged, a follow-up in 1 to 2 days with an office or home visit will be needed in this situation.

Observation 2

Ms. Rider delivered her second son at 39 weeks with a weight of 8 pounds, 4 ounces. At 18 hours of life he's a vigorous, feisty boy who wants to eat often and does it well. On examination his color is good, his tone strong, and he looks you right in the eye. He readily finds his hand to suck when upset and calms himself. His mom had a short labor and is surrounded by flowers, gifts and attentive relatives. She's walking everyone to the elevator.

Inference: This infant, mom and family seem intact and ready to meet the challenges ahead. Follow-up in 5 days to 1 week will allow appropriate monitoring and support.

! HEADS UP–THE NEWBORN

Infant Issues

- Infants who are small for gestational age are at greater risk for developmental difficulties, particularly those in whom length and weight are below the standard curves. Consideration of the possible cause for such undergrowth should be undertaken and close developmental tracking planned.
- Infants with small head circumferences need evaluation for infectious and/or toxic or structural explanations. Extra developmental surveillance will be needed.
- Infants with disfiguring conditions or unattractive features are at risk for altered attachment relationships.
- Infants with low tone and/or poor suck are at risk for poor feeding and need more careful scrutiny than usual.
- Any infant with unilateral weakness of an arm or leg. This is a peripheral nerve injury (e.g., a brachial plexus injury) or a herpes central nervous system infection. Evaluate and treat quickly.
- Very irritable infants need an evaluation for the cause of their irritability, as well as extra support at home for the care provider.
- Infants who alert poorly and are marginally responsive to care need close monitoring. These "too good" babies may have experienced toxic exposure or may have neurological, metabolic or infectious conditions that need attention.
- An infant whom the nurses find difficult. The parents are surely going to experience the same or worse problems. Investigate and monitor.

Parent Issues

- A parent who has experienced a recent loss (e.g., death of a close friend or relative, divorce or estrangement with a partner) is at risk for poor attachment to the infant and postpartum depression.
- An isolated parent is at risks for depression, poor parenting and both overuse and underuse of medical services.
- A parent with financial stressors may not be optimally attentive to the infant.
- A mother with a difficult delivery, postpartum infection, anemia or other compromising condition will have delayed milk production and may have decreased reserves to deal with the infant. Suspect this problem when mom looks pasted to the bed.
- A parent who wants to discuss only her issues and not the infant's is at risk for poor attachment. Parenting requires de-centering from oneself.
- A parent who wants to leave early, before the time advised. Drug issues, financial constraints, legal concerns or domestic pressures are often associated with early departure. Poor follow-up also accompanies many such forced discharges.
- A parent who attributes adult motivation to the infant. "He's crying just to get me mad."
- A parent with a substance abuse problem or history of a mental health problem. The adjustment to the demands of parenting places this family at risk for relapse. Keep close watch and consult others if needed.

QUICK CHECK—THE NEWBORN

✓ Balanced motor tone, variable across states

✓ Primitive reflexes intact and symmetrical

✓ Turns to sound

✓ Follows object visually at least briefly

✓ Clonus of two beats or less

✓ Conjugate eye movements

✓ Mottling not excessive and shows good recovery

✓ Coordinated rooting and sucking

✓ Able to organize and sustain feedings

✓ Signals hunger regularly

✓ Weight loss of less than 10%

✓ Parents demonstrate the ability to feed and care for the infant

SUMMARY

The initial newborn examination is an opportunity to assure parents that the infant is physically and behaviorally intact. Congratulations are in order for producing a lovely baby. This reassurance and an added sense of competency as being reproductively sound are necessary to begin the work of caring for and caring about the infant. It's time to introduce the real, individual infant to the family by showing the baby's unique characteristics and abilities. Unmet expectations for the delivery or for the infant or any intercurrent concerns are to be put in clear perspective so that they can be reconciled. Parents' choices in care options within the boundaries of the best care should be respected. The infant's temperament and individuality should begin to be understood in the context of the assessment, both by the clinician and by the parents. Finally, plans for ongoing care should be set up and based on an understanding of all the individuals involved.

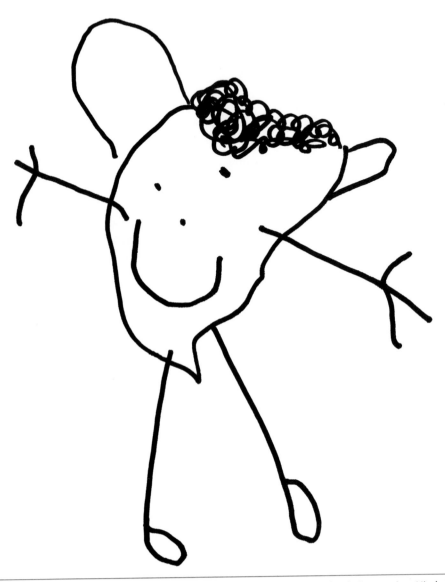

A 3-year-old draws her new little brother. His big ears and curly hair are clearly impressive. His bright-eyed reaching out to the world is more accurate than his sister knows (original in pink marker).

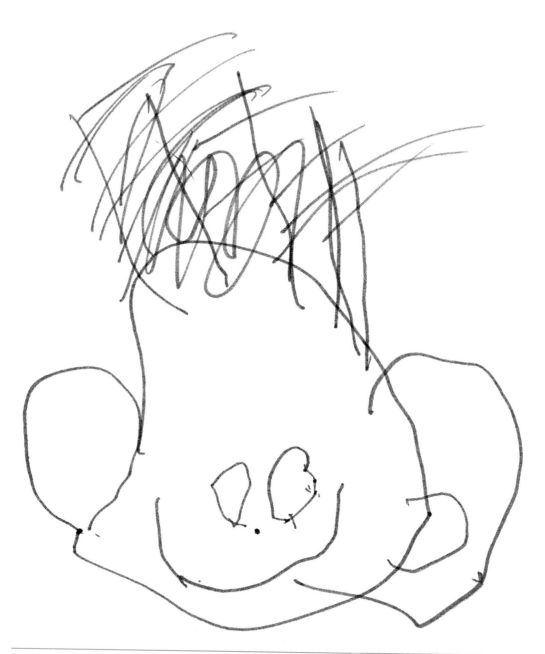

A three year old does a drawing of herself. Accurately showing that since she was born, she's been ready to take in the world with eyes, ears attuned to the social environment. By Robin A.

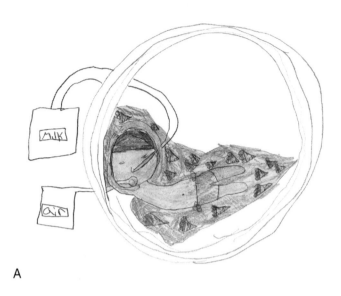

CHAPTER 8

A

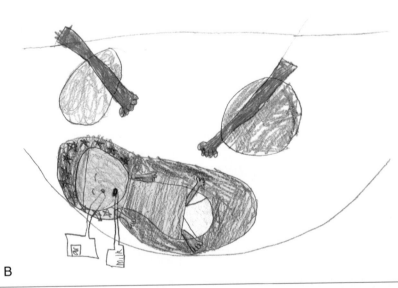

B

Nine-year-old twins draw the NICU as they see it. They were 32-week preemies themselves. Mom is now a neonatal nurse practitioner. **A**, "Sick baby. Milk and air keep her alive." By Ainsley Perkins. **B**, "Baby with problems with her heart (like her sister)." Dad's arms are in the isolette. By Alissa Perkins.

Neonatal Intensive Care Unit: Special Issues for the At-Risk Infant and Family

SUZANNE D. DIXON and YVONNE E. VAUCHER

This chapter presents the special needs and concerns of the high-risk infant and family. The concept of developmental care of the fragile infant is explained. The role of the primary care physician while the infant is in the neonatal intensive care unit and after discharge is outlined.

Key Words

- Preterm Infant's Behavior
- Developmental Course of Preemies
- Developmental Care in the NICU
- Discharge Planning
- Special Care Parenting
- Grief Reactions
- NICU Environment
- Multiple Births
- Vulnerable Child Syndrome
- Kangaroo Care

Jason Merrill, born 5 weeks ago at 31 weeks' gestation, has an adjusted age of 36 weeks and is now ready for discharge home from the neonatal intensive care unit (NICU). His parents, Carolyn and Bill, have been very involved in his care since he was born. They seem to be a competent, professional couple who have waited a long time for this infant, have visited daily and have asked many good questions throughout the hospitalization about his condition. Although they did meet the respiratory therapist as scheduled to learn about the home monitor and to review cardiopulmonary resuscitation (CPR), a discharge conference has had to be rescheduled twice, and their visiting has decreased in the last week. The nurses report that they have no more expressed stored breast milk to give Jason. When the parents came in last night, they became very angry about the dust on the windowsill beside the bassinet and the milk around Jason's mouth. The neonatologist asks you for help handling this "difficult family" and to see what you can do about the breast milk and the discharge conference. Note: This chapter will explain the nature of this difficult behavior, how to see beyond it and what to do about it.

NEONATAL INTENSIVE CARE

The advent in the 1940s of intensive care for ill or high-risk infants began an era of dramatic change for the neonate, the family and the health care provider. With increasing technological sophistication, we have pushed back the limits of viability, improved the chance of survival and increased the incidence of multiple births. Families are exposed to the NICU environment for longer and longer periods during the increasingly complex care of babies who are smaller and smaller. In the course of this progress, we have also learned a great deal about the neurological development of immature children, the behavior and developmental course of preterm infants and the impact of intensive care itself on the infant and family. Through these insights, we now have the opportunity to provide care that is not only more effective but also less stressful for the infant and family. We have become more aware and respectful of the special needs of these fragile individuals. We have refocused on the family as the ultimate intervention in the support of high-risk infants so that nurture of the family's competencies has become part of the care mission. Medical issues and prematurity per se do contribute to the long-term prognosis, particularly of very low-birthweight infants, but the ability of a parent to be responsive to a high-risk infant remains the best predictor of outcome over the longer term. We now have insight and support that parents can use to learn about and care for their high-risk infant. The role of the health care provider has expanded to include not only the technical aspects of care but also assistance to the family through the crisis of an early or complicated birth. This assistance is directed at helping parents gain skill in the special care needs of their child and to access the community resources that they will need after discharge and over the longer term. These tasks involve understanding the behavior of high-risk infants, the parent's perspectives, the NICU environment and the special follow-up care that is required for special populations.

PREMATURE INFANT DEVELOPMENT: A DIFFERENT PATH

A **preterm infant's behavior** and **developmental course** will not be the same as that of an infant born at term, no matter how smooth the postnatal course. Although behavioral expectations should be adjusted for the degree of prematurity (i.e., the adjusted age) as the best approximation, differences can be anticipated, including the following:

- Motor tone and posture will be altered. Many will have a pattern of passive hypotonia (i.e., floppiness or offering little resistance to passive movement). This may be accompanied by active hypertonia and brisk reflexes, especially of the lower extremities. Predominance of extension postures is present in many infants throughout the first year. Although most infants will resolve these differences by the second year, some will maintain an imbalance in tone that will be seen as subtle movement or postural differences.

- Much development that depends on posture and tone may take a different, often delayed path if external support is not provided to these children. *Shoulder girdle weakness* and *shoulder retraction* (i.e., shoulders rolled back) may mean that the infant has difficulty with self-quieting behavior, such as hand to mouth, and will need special help to settle in a tucked, flexed position. Without support to bring the hands forward, the natural hand regard and midline play opportunities will be diminished. This may appear as a delay in cognitive abilities or visual-motor irregularities unless intervention is provided to bring the hands forward to the midline. Such intervention can be accomplished by attention to positioning and provision of trunk support.

- *Truncal instability* results in the infant actively resisting the prone activities that are vital to learning. These babies need physical support (e.g., rolled towel under the chest) and inducements (e.g., a toy or face in front) to enable them to tolerate prone positions. Special assistance will be needed to maintain a sitting position.

- An undifferentiated, drowsy state at about 28 weeks gradually evolves into wake and sleep at about 32 weeks' adjusted age; the pattern becomes clearer over time with the emergence of active and quiet sleep at about 36 weeks. Increasing periods of alertness can be seen by 36 weeks. Full-cry states become available to the infant after 35 to 36 weeks. However, even at term, a prematurely born infant is likely to continue to have irregular sleep and variability in the quality of alertness and spend more time in a drowsy or irritable state. These difficulties are lessened if the special care environment has quiet and dark times, if the infant is not disturbed for blocks of time and if intrusive levels of light and sound are avoided. Parents often perceive the lack of wakeful interaction as rejection and regard sleep difficulties as evidence of subtle damage or poor parenting. These misconceptions need to be directly countered with realistic explanations of the evolution of social availability and state organization in this group. Alterations in wakefulness and sleep may continue even beyond the first year.

- *Visual difficulties* are common in this group, including astigmatism, refractive errors and strabismus. Retinopathy of prematurity may result in diminished peripheral vision after spontaneous resolution, as well as after photocoagulation. Careful visual follow-up and periodic reassessment should continue throughout early childhood, even without obvious abnormalities or visual complaints. Additionally, significant visual impairment precludes valid use of the usual developmental tests.

- *Alterations in motor tone*, as well as anatomical changes caused by prolonged orotracheal tube-placement, may result in difficulties with feeding and swallowing early on and articulation problems later because of structural and functional changes in the mouth and palate. In addition, orthodontic care may be needed because dental position may be altered by the architecture of the palate.

- *Recurrent otitis media* may also result from these differences in structure and function in the mouth, pharynx and airway. Eustachian tube dysfunction may likewise contribute to this problem. Vigilance and aggressive follow-up are called for. Hearing must be monitored in these circumstances.

- *Sensitivity to pain, touch of the feet and scars from procedures* may be a source of discomfort and, later, a source of unusual aversive responses. Some infants, for example, dislike feeling certain textures or having their feet touched, perhaps an association with repeated heel sticks.

- *Limited energy and oxygen reserves* result in slow growth, particularly in children with bronchopulmonary dysplasia and congenital heart disease, and often lead to additional delays in motor activities because of decreased stamina and strength. The biomechanics of movement may also be altered by these delays in linear growth.

- The emphasis on feeding and growth that is appropriate in the first year or two in this group may result in *long-term feeding issues* with origins in the baby, the parents and the interaction between them. Feeding struggles are difficult to resolve. Oral aversions and oral-motor dysfunction may be linked to prolonged intubation and result in delayed initiation of oral feeding or underlying neurological problems. Pressure to get the baby to eat is usually felt acutely by families, even if it is only implied by the health care provider.

- *Additional calories, minerals and protein* are needed by a very low-birthweight preterm infant throughout the first year to grow adequately and have appropriate catch-up growth. Nutritional requirements are even greater if the child is chronically ill. This may run counter to a family's adherence to a low-fat, low-cholesterol, low-salt regimen for themselves. On the other hand, overfeeding increases the risk of childhood obesity and its attendant long-term consequences. Expect feeding issues to emerge in one form or another.

- The infant's *self-protective behavior* of avoiding or ignoring intrusive stimuli may mean that the infant sends signals to care providers that are seen as confusing or counterintuitive. For example, gaze avoidance sends the message "Leave me alone, I'm better off without you." Confusing behavioral signals, interactional availability only in short segments and unpredictability of behavior may remain even after the baby is well. This leaves parents confused, disappointed and often frustrated. They may need an interpreter to understand their infant.

ROLES IN THE CARE OF SPECIAL NEEDS BABIES

All the differences in these preterm and high-risk youngsters, as well as those with individual conditions, mean that the roles for the parents and the health care provider are inherently altered.

The primary care clinician has dual therapeutic opportunities in interactions with a child and family under these circumstances. As important as monitoring the infant's changing capacities as he or she recovers and grows is the chance to observe and support the parents' growth into the role of caretakers of a vulnerable, special needs infant.

The single most important variable in long-term developmental outcome for these vulnerable children may be the responsiveness of the parents to the child during the first year of life. With the exception of a direct insult to the central nervous system (e.g., severe intracranial hemorrhage or meningitis), chronic hypoxemia or extremely low birthweight, the developmental outcome depends less on medical events and perinatal circumstances than it does on the family's ability to meet the needs of the individual child. Maternal education and socioeconomic status, both highly predictive of the type and amount of support and input that the mother gives the child, as well as some genetic factors, are the best predictors of outcome after 2 years of age in the majority of cases. Enhancement of the interaction between parent and child through education and support is the avenue that will positively influence development.

This is not surprising, given what we know overall about children. If a parent can learn to provide contingent and consistent interactions and appropriate responsiveness for a high-risk infant, the chances for learning and long-term developmental adjustment are augmented. If a parent continues to be unable to read the child's signals and fails to meet the child's needs on either a physical, emotional or behavioral level, the child experiences the world as noncontingent and chaotic. Emotional and cognitive growth is undermined in this circumstance. The parents' effectiveness in dealing with their own child in turn leads to stronger attachment and improved parental self-esteem.

Role of the Family

In most circumstances, the primary care clinician can do little about the particular perinatal insults that the child sustains except to help ensure optimal perinatal medical care and referral as needed. However, the primary care clinician is in a better position than a neonatologist or other medical specialist to view the broad picture of this infant and family. Less involved with the technology of neonatal care, the primary care clinician can offer a broader perspective and can see outside the walls of the special care nursery, beyond all the machines, technology and bright lights to the specific strengths and vulnerabilities in the child and family. The clinician can offer perspective and common sense in the **discharge planning process**.

Special care parenting demands that the parents see the infant as he really exists, with both strengths and weaknesses. Such a perspective implies a clear and shared view of the child's physiological and behavioral capacities at a particular point in time. From this view, the primary care provider can guide the family in supporting the development of the individual child and in accessing the special follow-up services that will be needed. This approach implies the clinician's responsibility for restoring a sense of competency and confidence in parenting inasmuch as these factors have been assaulted by the less-than-optimal circumstances of the child's birth and will need restoration.

Ms. James, a single mother, had an angry, distrustful look as she approached her son's open warmer for the first time. Then she said, "He's too small" and asked, "Who's in charge?" The nurse came forward and extended an invitation to touch the baby. She shook her head "No" but when encouraged, tentatively reached out to touch his hand. When asked, she said she had no questions.

Note: Instead of becoming irritated or getting pulled into a struggle, the clinician should recognize the anxiety and concern behind these actions and comments. The job will be to create a relationship so that energy can be directed to care of the baby, not to conflicts with the staff.

Most neonatal units actively try to include families in care. Depending on geography and training, the primary health care provider may be more or less involved in the management of acute neonatal illness but will always be involved in the important work of helping a family rebuild around the needs of a particular child after discharge. That work involves attention to details, such as the following:

- Families must have the knowledge and skills to provide physical care for the infant. If this is beyond their capabilities, specialized care and/or additional resources must be mobilized. The goal of this care should be to assist families in assuming more responsibility over time. A family resource assessment, including physical assets (e.g., a car, a phone), community support (e.g., family, friends) and psychological readiness, is the first step in planning for care after discharge.

- Judgment about the infant's needs should come from the medical and nursing staff in the NICU in conjunction with information from the primary health care provider. A home health nurse can contribute valuable insight about the home environment. Other agencies may have some input.

- Families must be able to focus on the needs of the child. Although this is a core requirement for all parenting, it is even more critical for a fragile baby who signals his needs poorly. Serious mental illness, ongoing substance abuse, extreme poverty, domestic violence and mental deficiency are some of the barriers that must be faced in making realistic discharge plans. Young teen parents require special appraisal of their family support and caretaking capacities. The infant's care must be the priority, and other drains on family energy and focus must be minimized.

- Families must have access to care that is acceptable to them and adequate to the needs of the infant. This means an in-home telephone, reliable transportation, health insurance and culturally sensitive, linguistically compatible ongoing health care. Discharge without these elements in place is likely to lead to less-than-optimal, if not dangerous circumstances. Don't send the baby and mother home without them.

PREMATURE PARENTS

The parents of a preterm infant are "premature" too because they had a baby whom they did not fully expect, with demands for care that usually go beyond their own abilities to provide. They themselves have not completed the developmental work of pregnancy, and in addition, they must put energy into resolution of the complex feelings of guilt, anger, anxiety, depression and shame that emerge as a consequence of their infant's birth. The predictable course of response to the loss of a loved one (even an imagined person in this case) has been described in classic works. The initial responses of *denial and anger* give way to depression, guilt and, finally, resolution. These same stages of **grief reaction** are apparent in the parental response to an infant born prematurely or with neonatal illness. Parents truly have lost a valued person in the form of their hoped-for or imagined perfect child. They must resolve that grief in order to attach themselves to the *real* child who is now before them. They must begin accepting this less-than-perfect child while simultaneously letting go of the idealized child. They may require extra time to even see the infant as a separate person if the baby has been born very early. Furthermore, they cannot be expected to attach to the infant until they sense a good chance for survival.

Mrs. Martin was wheeled in to see her daughter, born at 24 weeks' gestation, for the first time. She had barely looked pregnant. She sat immobilized and refused to touch the baby. She said she was tired and asked the busy nurse to get her a glass of water.

Note: This mom is still in the stage of pregnancy experienced as a change in self, an egotistical phase that is normal in early to mid pregnancy. Unfortunately, the baby's extremely premature birth interrupted the normal developmental progression of pregnancy. Mrs. Martin probably can't even believe that this has happened to her. She will need time and lots of support to see the baby as a separate individual and to focus on the baby, not herself.

Even if survival is ensured, parents may also need to cope with the long-term loss of a normal child when chronic disease or neurological disability results from the preterm delivery. Such resolution is more complex in the case of premature birth because the outcome is uncertain and will remain so for a long time. A disability such as heart disease or Down's syndrome has a predictability to it that makes for shorter adjustment in most cases. Parents may also face the actual death of their child; this is more likely in the case of multiple gestation, in which extreme prematurity is associated with increased antepartum, intrapartum and neonatal demise.

THE CLINICIAN AND THE PARENTS

Clinicians should monitor the process of grief resolution and attachment and not be surprised at the turbulence and seemingly inappropriate responses, anger and frustration that may be leveled at them or others. These are healthy, expected reactions that testify to the ongoing recovery process. Over the long run these feelings help mobilize the emotional energy that will enable the family to reorganize around the real child and his special needs. Short-term counseling may be necessary to achieve resolution of this process in some cases. Many anxious calls, trivial questions, requests for laboratory values and reluctance to be discharged from the hospital or leave the office are manifestations of this turmoil. Expect these bumps in the road. "Parental" withdrawal from the NICU as discharge nears reflects anxiety that seems over-whelming (see the opening case). One should avoid answering demands or concerns at a superficial level only; rather, they must be seen as opportunities to support a parent's recovery of competence and self-esteem and as part of the larger core process of becoming a family.

Fathers may be especially uncomfortable in the NICU environment. Personal and societal expectations place the primary responsibility for the family's well-being on the father's shoulders. Being thrust suddenly and unexpectedly into a frightening situation over which he has absolutely no control, a typical dad will have difficulty coping with his feelings of helplessness. The result may be unreasonable demands and anger directed at the staff. On the positive side, fathers are more often active in the care of their premature infants than fathers of full-term infants are. Pressed into extraordinary service early and frequently in the hospital, they remain more involved in care later. In addition, in families in which the father is supportive and involved, the mother visits more often and participates more regularly in the infant's care. A smart primary care clinician will cultivate real involvement of fathers of high-risk infants as an effective way to infuse energy into the whole family system. Grandparents and other family or community support can also add balance and energy. The clinician should look broadly for sources of help that can be mobilized. Rarely can a nuclear family manage entirely on its own.

The defense mechanism of *intellectualization* of the medical aspects of care is another frequent response in middle-class and professional families. Many families now have ready access to the Internet, an attractive, but often misleading source of unfiltered information about their child's problems. They may challenge health personnel over issues large and small. Avoid being drawn into prolonged technical discussions, intellectual nit-picking or arguments. Chasing specific concerns can lead to frustration until one pulls back to identify the underlying and unvoiced worries that are the basis for most of these discussions. On the other hand, well-educated parents may ask very pertinent, well-informed and difficult questions that the staff may perceive as directly challenging their authority and expertise. It is important for the nursing and medical care providers to give thoughtful consideration to these questions without being caught up in an emotional reaction to the perceived confrontation.

IMPACT OF THE NEONATAL INTENSIVE CARE UNIT ENVIRONMENT

The caretaking requirements of a small baby create an environment so different from the intrauterine one that it in itself provides a source of additional stress. Data suggest associations between that environment and acute physiological fluctuations. These, in turn, appear to alter important clinical and central nervous system parameters, including intracranial pressure changes, cerebral autoregulation, brain oxygenation, hypoxemia, apnea and bradycardia. Investigators have examined the sensory characteristics of NICUs along with infant behavioral and physiological responses to the caretaking activities in this environment. The **NICU environment** provides both sensory overload and deprivation. These studies found that infants experience a bombardment of stimuli from the sheer numbers of different caregivers and procedures each day. At the same time, however, very little social contact and long intervals of social isolation may also be present. From the infant's view, this may be experienced as a chaotic, nonresponsive milieu. The auditory environment is often aversive; shutting an isolette door is as loud as a rock band up close. Constant mechanical noise from equipment adds to the auditory stress. Soft talk to the infant may be minimal. Nurturing physical contact is frequently limited. Constant bright lights, noise, lack of diurnal variation in movement, light and sound, frequent painful procedures and abrupt changes in position with handling are stressful factors present in the NICU that were not part of intrauterine life.

DEVELOPMENTALLY SUPPORTIVE CARE

Caretaking can be altered to counter some of these aversive factors. Procedures and examinations should be scheduled so that quiet sleep times are uninterrupted, thereby improving behavioral organization and growth. Diurnal variation in lighting helps entrain a circadian rhythm, and noise reduction serves to minimize physiological stress for the immature infant. Gentle, gradual movements, soothing and holding after procedures and providing physical boundaries to contain the infant also help improve organization. Some activities that support this process are shown in Box 8-1.

Developmentally responsive care of infants requires that the bedside nurse be able to accurately interpret each baby's behavioral and physiological cues and fit care around them. It also means that the nurse has the power to orchestrate the baby's day for optimal well-being. The physician should respect and support this role for the primary nurse as an interface and buffer for the infant. Not only is it good for the baby, but it is also an important model for parents to emulate. They too have to learn to respect these behavioral cues as they become increasingly active in the infant's care. In addition, they must see that the necessities of life get done, but in a way that is responsive to the fluctuating needs of the individual child. Before discharge, developmentally supportive care improves feeding and growth, decreases medical support, shortens hospital stay, facilitates maturation of motor function and state regulation, improves maternal perception of both her own and her infant's competence and reduces maternal stress. In the longer term, developmental care improves neurodevelopmental outcome up to 24 months' corrected age and increases the likelihood of normal behavior at

---

BOX 8–1 COMPONENTS OF AN INDIVIDUALIZED CARE PLAN FOR A FRAGILE BABY

- Baby-specific care plans posted on each bedside, including scheduling issues, behavioral cues, likes and dislikes, stressors and facilitators
- The baby's specific nonverbal vocabulary—how does the baby signal positive or negative responses?
- Isolette covers to allow quiet, undisturbed rest
- Protected times for rest—posted and enforced
- Swaddling or positioning in a supported, flexed or prone posture
- Nesting within an isolette and the use of cloth rolls or slings to provide tactile input or containment
- Tapes of soft music or parental voices played *periodically* in the isolette
- Personalized isolette with pictures or small toys
- Family visiting plans stated and posted. Nurses may want to "save" feeding, bathing and treatments for these times if possible
- The name of the two or three nurses who serve as primary nurses and know the family and the baby best
- The baby's given name clearly posted and used in the record and in conversations
- The baby's own clothes and blanket if the infant is stable

---

5 years of age. Whether developmentally supportive care improves longer-term cognitive outcome is uncertain at this time, but it seems that the weight of evidence supports this type of care for the individual child.

BABY BODY LANGUAGE

The infant uses body language to signal both positive and negative responses to various life experiences. Even a short period of observation during the nursery rounds, treatment sessions or examinations will demonstrate many of these signs, which are listed in Boxes 8–2 and 8–3.

The behavior of a premature infant can be confusing to even an experienced caregiver. Facial expressions have a limited range, body movements may be few and cries might be nonexistent or irritating. The latency of responses may be so long that it is difficult to connect one activity with the response. Social interactions that are so exciting with a full-term infant may cause a premature infant to turn away, become mottled, hiccup or even stop breathing. The baby may actively avoid eye contact, thus sending a very negative message to those who would like to interact. At other times, an unremittingly irritable infant seems to resist all the usual consoling and comforting measures. All such behavior runs counter to what is usually expected of infants. Without some special knowledge and techniques to make sense of a premature infant's behavior, caregivers may feel ineffective, frustrated, angry, perplexed and rejected. Conversely, if the health care team can interpret some of the confusing messages and help a family develop effective caregiving patterns, parenting competency and confidence will be enhanced.

What is experienced as aversive stimuli will vary from infant to infant and will change as the infant matures. Aversive stimuli tend to be those that are physiologically overwhelming or

BOX 8–2   BEHAVIOR THAT SAYS "YES"

The following behavior signals that the baby can handle, enjoy and gain from the current interaction with the environment:

- A relaxed posture, neither hypertonic nor limp
- Easily flexed hands and feet
- Grasping movements with the hands and feet opening and closing rhythmically
- Mouthing and sucking movements when looking or listening
- Eyes widening, face lifting, lips making an oval
- Short, quiet vowel sounds—cooing
- Attending to visual or auditory stimuli—looking or listening carefully
- Decreasing body movements, wiggles, to quietly attend
- Turning toward the phenomenon, even with long latency
- Improved color—no mottling, duskiness or pallor over baseline

    The caretaker should continue monitoring for signs of distress or overload.

BOX 8–3   BEHAVIOR THAT SAYS "STOP, PLEASE"

The following behavior often signals that the interaction with the environment is overwhelming, adverse or overly costly for the infant's coping abilities:

- Extension postures—arms out, legs straightened, neck stretched
- Arching back
- Gaze avoidance
- Turning away
- Splayed hands and feet
- Grimace, lip retraction
- Furrowed brow, a worried look
- Spitting up, gagging, onset of hiccups
- Sudden limpness
- Increasing pallor, mottling, cyanosis
- Irregular breathing, apnea

    The caretaker should respond by backing off, by cutting down some aspects or intensity of the interaction and by supporting and waiting for recovery.

involve high levels of sensory input, such as bright lights, noise, pain, rapid movements and multiple, simultaneous input (e.g., movement of the infant while speech is directed at him). In addition, aversive responses emerge with rapid changes in input, even if the level of input is low. *Transitions* between one routine activity (e.g., feeding) and another (e.g., check of vital signs) may produce considerable disruptions. Even the transitions to sleep or to wakefulness may be prolonged and accompanied by much physiological instability. Times of change in activity are vulnerable periods; aversive behavior is likely to emerge at these times. Support for the infant *through* and immediately after the activity is needed if instability in behavior is to be avoided.

Ruth finished her shift in the care of Jonathan, now 31 weeks old, with a session of vital signs, physical assessment and feeding. He seemed to do well, got his diaper and shirt changed and was tucked in. As she was charting, the cardiac monitor went off because of a significant apnea and bradycardia event. The next time she held Jonathan quietly for 10 minutes after his care session while she did her charting, and no instability was seen.

Note: Most periods of instability follow periods of intervention, so care providers should not be quick to leave the bedside.

SKIN-TO-SKIN (KANGAROO) CARE AND THE IMPACT OF TOUCH

The positive role of human touch on a preterm infant is illustrated by the demonstrated benefits of skin-to-skin (kangaroo) care of an immature infant. The infant is placed prone-upright on the bare chest of the mother or father and covered on the dorsal surface by a blanket. This kind of care has no minimum weight requirement or specific time limit. It can also be used for infants on ventilators. They don't get cold, spit up or stop breathing. This approach can have a very positive impact on care and outcome. Many physiological and psychosocial benefits have been linked to skin-to-skin care and are shown in Box 8–4. Parents who can participate in this intimate care of their infant get a real sense of their own value and importance to the child. Only moms can specifically thermoregulate for their infants by adjusting skin temperature to the baby's needs, but skin-to-skin contact with dad can also produce significant benefit, including temperature stability for the infant. The primary health care provider can assist in this process by reinforcing the benefits of skin-to-skin care to the family and by encouraging the NICU staff to provide it.

Breastfeeding and giving expressed breast milk reinforce the benefits of skin-to-skin care by increasing the mother's self-esteem and confidence, the frequency of nurturing touch and awareness of her baby's behavioral cues. Additionally, it provides contingent stimuli by

---

BOX 8–4 BENEFITS OF KANGAROO CARE

- Decreased apnea
- Decreased bradycardia
- Less irritability
- Improved oxygenation
- Improved weight gain
- Improved temperature stability
- Improved breastfeeding
- Improved sleep cycles
- Faster autonomic maturation
- Better state regulation
- More positive maternal interaction

integrating maternal touch, en face contact, sucking and satiation. The smell and taste of breast milk are also sensory links to intrauterine life, where the fetus was exposed to similar odors and tastes in amniotic fluid. In addition, breastfeeding is associated with a better long-term cognitive outcome in both preterm and term infants. In turn, skin-to-skin care increases the duration and exclusivity of breastfeeding. So intimate touch and breastfeeding together are a winning combination in both the immediate and long term.

Skin-to-skin care has a positive effect on parenting and family interaction. Mothers are less likely to be depressed and spend more time touching and looking at their baby. Positive effects on parenting extend beyond discharge. Families who participate in skin-to-skin care are more cohesive, provide a better home environment and are more responsive to their infants, who in turn exhibit less negative emotionality and more sustained exploratory play and have a better developmental outcome during infancy. Skin-to-skin care may be the single most effective developmental intervention in the NICU.

An infant in the NICU is exposed to frequent intrusive, uncomfortable and painful procedures while acutely ill. Alternatively, the infant may spend large amounts of time physically isolated in an incubator while "feeding and growing." In either circumstance nurturing touch is missing. Nurturing touch is associated with more secure emotional attachment; less depression, anxiety and withdrawal; and better social competence in early childhood. Nurturing touch is integral to skin-to-skin care and can also be given by any care-taker, including nurses, doctors and "cuddlers." Gentle *massage*, a form of nurturing touch that is a daily practice in some cultures, may improve weight gain and shorten the hospital stay. Massage appears to be most effective if given by the mother herself. Co-bedding multiples in the NICU is also a safe and effective way to maximize exposure to human touch. Multiples are accustomed to bunking together and do better when allowed to continue that arrangement when out of the uterus.

Pain results in structural changes in the brain and has a deleterious effect on long-term responses to stress and behavior. Sick preterm infants are exposed to an average of 14 painful procedures every day while acutely ill. Therefore, it is important to minimize painful stimuli as much as possible and to provide physical and sensory support to reduce the physiological reactions to pain. Breastfeeding, being given expressed breast milk and skin-to-skin care, as well as sucking on a pacifier or oral sucrose, are all effective ways to reduce the distress associated with painful procedures. Specific pain medications should be used, and infants should be held and comforted whenever possible during and after all painful events.

PARENTS IN THE NEONATAL INTENSIVE CARE UNIT

The special care nursery may add to parents' stress by overtly or inadvertently giving the message that the parents are not capable of caring for their baby or that something they did caused the baby's difficulties. "Experts" such as nurses, therapists and physicians must take over because the parents "have failed." The mother feels this sense of failure especially acutely and believes that her own body has failed to protect the fetus from premature delivery or other adversity. Parents are left with little confidence and little energy to assert themselves, learn new skills, make decisions or get to know their infant. Even in the best of circumstances, the special care nursery environment itself exacerbates these feelings. This does not imply that nurses or physicians are insensitive to parents' needs; rather, the high-tech and overwhelming care

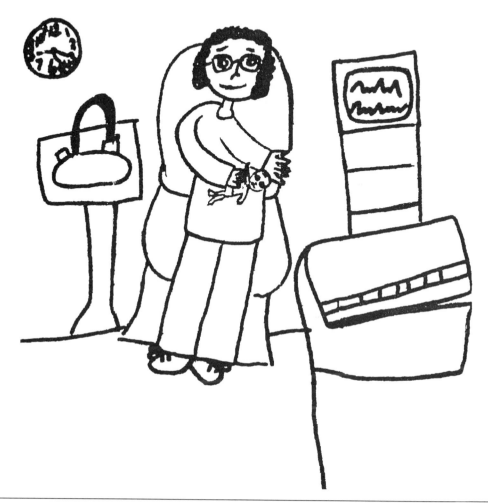

A nurse takes care of a small preemie amid the machines, strange sink and other equipment in the neonatal intensive care unit. By Carly Riehl, age 10.

requirements for sick and premature infants give these unspoken messages to families. It takes a lot of work to move away from these feelings. In addition, nurses must attach to their infant charges if they are to give the best of care, and such attachment may lead to unconscious competitiveness with parents. As a result, parents, especially mothers, may feel both emotionally and physically inadequate, even if nothing specific is said or done to prompt such feelings. An underlying competitiveness may be present, testimony to how much both parents and nurses care about the infant.

The lack of opportunity to be alone with their child or to engage in any sort of caretaking without the surveillance of the nursing staff adds stress for parents. Only 2% of the human contact in the NICU experienced by an infant was from the parents, according to one careful study, although this figure obviously depends on the availability of the parents and the willingness of the staff to encourage physical contact between the baby and family. Most families experience direct and indirect financial and time pressure associated with the care of their infants. Spending days to weeks to perhaps months in the special care nursery requires extraordinary adaptive skills at a time when parents are least able to muster these resources. Sparse visiting, lack of telephone calls, lack of initiative or angry accusations are more often maladaptive responses to these circumstances and competing demands at home rather than a measure of disattachment to the child or lack of appreciation of the expert care. The clinician and NICU staff can help interpret such behavior correctly to one another and must demonstrate considerable patience with families by granting the family latitude and time in which to recover.

MULTIPLE BIRTHS

The number of **multiple births** is increasing as a result of older maternal age and fertility treatments, which in turn are more commonly related to delayed child bearing. More than a fourth of NICU admissions now are premature multiple births. Multiple gestation increases the chance for a high-risk delivery, extremely low-birthweight babies, a prolonged stay in the NICU and the likelihood of the family facing at least one serious neonatal complication, including neonatal death.

Even in the case of term or near-term twins, the situation has higher risk and places greater demands on the parents. The process of attachment to two babies at the same time is more complicated than to one. For some period ranging from hours to weeks, families respond to these youngsters as one unit. The process of *individuation* in response and care comes on gradually in healthy circumstances and waxes and wanes. Increasing levels of recognition of individual differences, beginning with appearance and moving to behavioral characteristics, are the added dimension that should be monitored by the health care provider caring for multiples. Sharing observations of differences between the babies by the health care provider may help this process along.

Attachment difficulties get more complex if there is a discrepancy in size and vigor between the babies. Data suggest a general tendency to spend more time with the more fragile, usually lower-weight baby. This child is likely to be both more irritable and more demanding. The health care provider can assist the family in the difficult task of balancing efforts by being sure that the one who "needs the least" doesn't get left out and that the parents are able to respond appropriately to each infant's bids for attention.

Multiple gestations increase the chance of neonatal death, either prenatally (e.g., twin-to-twin transfusion, intrauterine growth retardation), in the course of early care or postnatally because of complications of illness or sudden infant death syndrome. The bereavement causes parents to pull back from the process of attachment to the surviving child or children. Fear of loss of the surviving child is a natural impediment to attachment because we don't become attached to what we think we will lose. Parents are appropriately guarded in their full psychological commitment to the survivor or survivors. Supportive care, including acknowledgment of the loss (no, the survivor doesn't "make up for" the loss of the other), patience and a longer time frame, is needed here. A mental health referral may be necessary to assist in this complex psychological adjustment.

BEHAVIORAL CHANGE WITH MINOR ILLNESS

Children who experience relatively minor complications in the perinatal period, such as intrauterine growth retardation, hyperbilirubinemia or metabolic problems as a result of maternal diabetes, sustain alterations in behavior that may affect their ability to interact maximally with their families in subtle ways. The child perpetuates the parents' perception that things are not quite right, that extraordinary care is required that may be beyond their limits of providing or that the infant is unresponsive to their caregiving. Epidural anesthesia may alter tone to the extent that oral-motor skills are compromised and breastfeeding gets off to a slow start. Maternal analgesia may also alter responsiveness so that feeding and social interaction are altered transiently. Evaluations for sepsis, observation in the NICU, blood work, placement of an intravenous line, borderline prematurity and a delay in discharge all seem minor to the clinician but may have lasting effects on the parental perception of their infant's well-being.

Even with these minor complications, the clinician should anticipate some extra hurdles for parents to overcome in spite of the clinician's own perception that things are just fine. Although this situation is not at the level of those in the NICU, clear recognition of the fragility in the circumstances overall will prompt extra care and vigilance now and in the months ahead.

Mrs. Scottfield and her 3-day-old daughter are scheduled for discharge. It had been a long labor at 36 weeks' gestation, with a final fever and sepsis evaluation for the baby, who has a heparin lock in her left hand for medication. A large cephalhematoma distorts the baby's head, and she is very sleepy. Mrs. Scottfield continues to have difficulty with breastfeeding. At the last feeding the baby fell asleep at the breast after about 5 minutes and then awoke irritable about an hour later. Earlier this morning the nurse noticed poorly coordinated sucking when she placed a gloved finger in the baby's mouth. Mrs. Scottfield is in tears. Note: Although this seems to most clinicians to be a clustering of relatively minor concerns, the parent's experience is overwhelming and frightening. Thoughtful, close monitoring and even a delay in discharge may be needed to prevent the development of distorted perceptions of the child, now and in the long run.

VULNERABLE CHILD SYNDROME

The family's perception of the child is not always directly related to the severity of the perinatal illness. Even conditions that the clinician may regard as relatively minor, insignificant or transient may set the groundwork for a permanently altered perception of the child by the family. Green and Solnit in their now classic description have highlighted the important dimensions of the "**vulnerable child syndrome.**" In this circumstance, a child with an imagined or real illness in early life is the target of altered attachment by her parents. The parents develop a long-term sense of the child being particularly susceptible to illness, injury or loss. The child is viewed as fragile and incapable of age-appropriate behavioral expectations, particularly in areas of independence. This perception of vulnerability leads to ongoing intra-familial stress, altered interaction between the child and parents and an inability to either allow age-appropriate autonomy or set limits. In our own work in a rural region of sub-Saharan Africa, the residual effects of this early impediment to attachment had long-term nutritional consequences; our observations parallel those in the United States. It appears that the consequences of perceiving one's offspring as vulnerable in early life are universal. The clinician must be sensitive to this perception in the newborn period as the basis of many later problems (e.g., problems with sleep, eating, discipline and school phobias).

Mrs. Donaldson brought in her 4-year-old because of behavior problems at home and in preschool. She said "he never minds me" and is aggressive with the other kids. He "never sleeps—not his whole life." She says he is slow in development and needs medicine. She attributes it all to his "terrible birth, when he almost died." She brings in a picture of him in the NICU. He doesn't look ill at all to the clinician. The medical record notes that he was a child born by cesarean section with a brief period of transient tachypnea and a negative evaluation for sepsis. Note: The "objective" history is very different from the "subjective" one conveyed by the mother. There needs to be a reconciliation of these views or the behavioral problems will only get worse. If family members cannot reframe their view of the child with cognitive input from the clinician, a mental health referral may be needed.

GETTING READY TO GO HOME: DISCHARGE PLANNING

As discharge approaches, parental anxiety increases sharply. The demands of unrelenting care, the lingering sense of inadequacy and the fear of further damaging the infant while at home all contribute to this increased anxiety. It may be manifested as decreased visiting, anger, accusations or the proposal of impediments to discharge. The clinician should recognize the need for the family to withdraw and consolidate before this new step, support the process, but still hold firm on the discharge plan with as specific a course as possible.

The family needs to know what the baby must be able to do to demonstrate readiness for discharge, such as the following:

- Tolerate all feedings by mouth
- Be gaining weight and maintaining body temperature in an open crib

- Have no significant apnea and bradycardia
- Have discharge assessments (e.g., eye exam, hearing screen, car seat test) and parent teaching completed

The family then knows that discharge does not occur at a specific date, gestational age or weight. Rather, it depends on the child's own maturation and recovery. If a date is given, the result will be disappointment, failure and anger if the date changes, as it often does.

Preparing a discharge notebook for all instructions, appointments, important telephone numbers and critical observations helps channel parents' anxious energy into a useful mode. Reflection on these feelings of anxiety and inadequacy as normal and as a testimony of caring will help parents put the feelings into perspective.

The *explicit* agreement of *frequent, scheduled* calls and visits after discharge appears to generate earlier independence in a family than does an ad hoc arrangement. So set this up ahead of time. It is very helpful if nursing care and parent education in the week before discharge are provided by nurses who know the infant and family well and with whom the family has developed a good relationship. After many weeks of focusing on what their baby *can't* do, a formal neurobehavioral evaluation with the parent present is an excellent way to demonstrate their infant's capabilities. This is usually a very positive and reassuring experience for parents, many of whom do not know what or even if their baby can see or hear!

The conference at discharge should be concrete. It should summarize the remaining problems briefly and focus on short-term goals, expectations and specific care plans. The primary care physician may lead or attend this conference; if that isn't possible, the clinician should receive a written summary of the discharge plans. A more expanded "debriefing" with the primary care provider should be set up 6 weeks to 3 months after discharge. At discharge the family should be given a copy of their baby's discharge summary to keep with them for future reference. It is helpful to review plans, medications and appointments and can be shown, if needed, to other health care providers unfamiliar with the neonatal history. At discharge, parents suddenly leave behind all the technology and experts who have safeguarded their baby. At home, they must assume their baby's care alone, which is often a very frightening prospect. Parents should be given explicit permission to call the NICU back for advice. The primary care nurse in the NICU is usually in the best position to offer such permission. Knowing that advice from caretakers who knew their baby well is still available after discharge, if needed, is very reassuring for parents. Social service evaluation for ill neonates' families should be routine in the NICU and should also be offered to other families who seem unable to make progress in the adaptation process after discharge. Parent-to-parent connections with families who have similar challenges can be very positive. Practical skills, access to service information and emotional support are all valuable. The clinician should facilitate such encounters because families are usually unable at this time to do much resource acquisition themselves.

Parenting groups, particularly for children with specific problems with a known outcome (e.g., Down's syndrome), may be helpful to families during this adjustment phase.

PRACTICE SESSIONS

To learn the infant's signal system, parents must spend time in the nursery watching and participating in care. The parents can be asked to monitor their own infant's response to the environment, caregiving and support (Box 8–5).

BOX 8–5   BEDSIDE OBSERVATIONS FOR CLINICIANS AND PARENTS

- Observe the infant's state.
- Can you see the cycles of sleep?
- Can you tell when the infant is waking?
- What soothes the child's upsets?
- What are the child's responses to sight? To sound?
- What things are aversive, and what are positive?
- What kinds of movement and posture are positive, and which are stressful?

Nurses should share their own observations and care techniques and note how they change over time. The goal here is not just to provide excellent care, but also to support the parents in the process of discovery about their own infant. Parents have made it with their at-risk infant when they see the baby as a special individual with communicative intent—a person who can be known and understood. Parents can reach this level only after they are sure that the infant will survive and are confident that they can cope with the child's practical care needs. Skills in CPR, monitor use and administration of medication should be seen as building tools for the parent-child relationship, as well as skills required for infant survival. Competency in skills enables parents to see their infant as manageable, understandable and lovable. It is only with these feelings that true attachment can occur.

DEVELOPMENTAL APPRAISAL

It is clear that we should make adjustments in our neurodevelopmental expectations commensurate with a child's postconceptual age rather than chronological age, beginning with a correction in the physical growth chart and how we label an office visit. Families should be reminded of this correction to adjust their expectations accordingly. For an infant who weighed less than 1500 g, this adjustment should last for 2 years and possibly 3 years for those who were born at less than 28 weeks' gestation and weighed less than 1000 g. For higher-birthweight preterm babies, the adjustment should continue for at least a year.

Mr. James brought in his 6-month-old son for a health supervision visit. The dad was worried because Derek wasn't doing anything that his cousin, also 6 months of age, did. Derek was 2 months premature. Dr. Ellis said, "This will be like a 4-month visit for Derek, given his prematurity." She then corrected the growth chart, pushing back the current measurement by 2 months. This put Derek's growth within the normal range for his adjusted age. She briefly reviewed appropriate developmental expectations for Derek. Mr. James seemed to relax immediately. Note: This is a simple, quick intervention that can change the whole family's view of things.

Formal appraisal of development should be done at regular intervals through specialized programs that offer the extended time needed to perform a comprehensive assessment of development. Appropriate referrals can be made to community-based services. This follow-up should be continued through the early school years because many problems related to prematurity are not evident until school age. Across this period, the likelihood of the emergence of particular problems changes. The early motor difficulties are rarely missed; the cognitive, organizational and linguistic concerns are more difficult to pick up in a general office setting (Box 8–6). They require specialized evaluation tools.

The best window in a primary care setting for evaluation of developmental competencies overall is observation of free play, particularly at about 8 to 9 months of corrected age. Several observations that will help assure the clinician of appropriate development are shown in Box 8–7. It may be useful and efficient to change the format for this visit entirely to look at development as the central focus.

If the clinician's observations raise concern in this unstructured setting, a more formal appraisal using a standardized assessment tool is warranted. Major developmental delays and hearing abnormalities should elicit referral for early *intervention* before 1 year, if not earlier. Significant speech and language delay at 18 to 24 months in children born prematurely warrants early referral for formal evaluation because these children are more likely to have persistent problems.

BOX 8–6 TIMING OF THE PRESENTATION OF DEVELOPMENTAL ABNORMALITIES FOR THE PREMATURE INFANT

1st Year*
- Cerebral palsy
- Severe sensory abnormalities
- Significant visual compromise
- Severe hearing loss

2nd Year
- Speech and language difficulties
- Early cognitive delays
- Subtle visual and hearing difficulties

3–5 Years
- Fine motor difficulties
- Difficulties in regulation of behavior
- Hyporesponsive or hyperresponsive behavior (i.e., attention deficit/hyperactivity disorder)
- Motor and behavioral "immaturity"

6–8 Years
- Learning disabilities
- Sensory processing problems
- Visual-motor difficulties
- Minor degrees of compromised motor coordination

---

*Probable time frames of appearance.

BOX 8-7   EVALUATION OF HIGH-RISK INFANTS AT 9 MONTHS (CORRECTED AGE)

- Baby should sit unsupported.
- Good mouthing of toys.
- Transfer of toys should be present.
- Pincer grasp should be developing and used in play.
- The child should turn to a sound behind his back.
- Stranger wariness should be present and result in going toward mom.
- Jabber and babbling should be evident with good voice quality and sounds strung together.
- Gestures and early imitation should be present (e.g., "bye-bye," "pat-a-cake").
- The child should point at objects or show them to another person.
- Some kind of movement should be present: creeping, scooting, twisting, rolling.

SLEEP DIFFICULTIES

Children cared for in the bright light and continuous sound environment of the NICU will maintain immature state regulation patterns for the first several months after discharge. It will be more difficult for these infants to settle down for sleeping, they may have long periods of irritability when awakening and falling asleep, and they may find it difficult to come to a quiet/alert state for sustained periods. Cycled lighting and activity in the NICU help somewhat but do not eliminate these problems. Once removed from the stressful NICU environment, the baby will demonstrate increasing competency at state regulation in a quieter, more predictable environment, although full normalization of sleep patterns is rarely achieved in the first year. A quiet radio and a dim light may help the baby make the transition from the NICU environment. Sleep disorders are more common in toddlers who had perinatal difficulties, and these disorders may persist. Difficulty in making transitions from one activity to another may also be impaired well beyond discharge from the nursery. Fragility makes transitions particularly troublesome. These are predictable and are not diagnostic of either poor parenting or neurological damage in themselves. Irritability and sleep difficulties should *start* to decrease at 3 to 4 months of adjusted age in most children. The individual child should be monitored for increasing regularity and predictability in sleep, with the infant's own behavior used as a baseline for future comparisons.

HEARING ISSUES

Premature or ill infants have a high incidence (2% to 4%) of hearing disorders. These difficulties can rarely be detected in office settings; they require formal assessment. A brainstem auditory evoked response screen should be done just before discharge, followed by visual reinforced audiometry or other behavioral audiometry when the child is sitting stably, at about 9 months. Otoacoustic emission techniques may be used for this population. Even normal results of these early tests do not rule out a high-frequency or progressive hearing loss, which will affect language development and school performance. Recurrent or resistant otitis media may also contribute to later hearing loss. Another preschool test of hearing is advised if any speech or language difficulties persist. An audiologist who has experience with infants and young children provides the best chance for accurate results.

DATA GATHERING AT DISCHARGE

It is assumed that the primary care clinician has been observing or has reviewed the course of the infant and is aware of the resolved or lingering medical concerns. Specific plans for these concerns need to be laid out in concrete, short-term schedules. A formal discharge summary should be made available to the primary care clinician and the family before discharge.

What to Observe

The following are examples of observations and discussions that should be part of the preparation for discharge:

- The clinician should discuss with NICU nurses the infant's awake and sleep pattern. The regularity of these state changes is an indicator of neurobehavioral integrity and maturation. It also gives a base on which to evaluate at-home change.
- The clinician should observe the parents while they are feeding and handling their infant. Competence and confidence should be evaluated. The quality of these interactions can provide valuable clues regarding future problems such as parental anxiety and depression. Supportive comments and suggestions should be offered. If not possible, notes for later conversations about these recommendations should be gathered ahead of time.
- The clinician should work with the NICU staff to identify specific training needs, such as gastric tube feeding and CPR. This training should be documented as completed before discharge.
- The infant record should indicate increasing stability of breathing, consistent feeding, steady weight gain and increasing alertness and activity. The parents should be able to describe these processes and identify the infant's individual characteristics.
- A feeding plan, particularly regarding the transition from partial to full breastfeeding after discharge and the use of supplemental formulas, should be clearly laid out at discharge.

What to Ask

Questions to be asked when the infant is nearing discharge from the special care nursery are presented in Table 8–1.

Examination

It is essential that the primary care clinician and the family examine the baby *together* before discharge or shortly thereafter. The clinician should observe the baby first in sleep and then through gentle talking, moving, undressing and examining and narrate her reading of the

TABLE 8–1   Questions to Be Asked at Discharge from a Special Care Nursery

Question	Observation
How is the baby doing?	Level of attachment—are the parents answering with a shrug of bewilderment, with a list of laboratory values or with personalized, accurate observations of their infant's response to them?
Is the baby ready for discharge?	Assess the parents' understanding of readiness issues; gather data from their perspective about the infant.
Are *you* ready to take (name) home?	Assess readiness and response—expand to include the specifics of readiness, special needs; assess parental adjustment.
Who will be at home to help?	Assess support systems, intrafamilial concerns, level of the father's involvement; assess sibling and family needs.
Do you feel comfortable with (name)?	Evaluate feelings of inadequacy; reassure parents of the normality of anxiety; evaluate specific areas in which parents' skills are inadequate.
Do you have any questions about the infant's hospital course?	Open the discussion for any questions about the perinatal events; be honest about your level of concern vis-à-vis these events.
What things would you like to see happen before you take (name) home?	Establish the locus of control with the parents; develop a plan to meet these wishes if possible, explain if not.

infant's behavior, both positive and negative. Parents should be asked to comment as well so that everyone is seeing the *same* infant. The level of stimulation that the infant tolerates should be noted. Signals of overstimulation, physiological instability and fatigue should be met with a rest period, a pulling back of stimulation and a period for recovery.

If the infant becomes alert, the clinician should demonstrate the baby's alerting and orienting to voice, then to a face and then to both together. If overload occurs, this should be pointed out to the parents as evidence of the child's limits. Considerable support for the extremities, head and trunk and temperature control may be needed to demonstrate the brief periods of alertness. The *cost* to the infant or the difficulty that the infant experiences in these periods should be noted so that this may be observed at home, hopefully to track an improving course.

The general pediatric examination, including a detailed neurological evaluation, should follow. Any areas of abnormality, as well as encouraging signs, should be clearly stated in an ongoing narrative of what the clinician is evaluating and what is observed, normal and abnormal. The clinician should carefully describe types of behavior that will represent the next step in improvement—for example, increasing periods of alertness, decreased color change with undressing and more ability to quiet self.

A summary statement by the clinician should open a discussion with the parents about the evaluation. For example, "Joey is able to really take in more of the world around him these days, and his sleep pattern is getting more regular. His legs still seem a bit tight, however, and getting a full feeding in without a break is still hard for him." An unrushed pause and encouragement may be needed for parents to convey their own observations and concerns. It is not to be expected that all issues or concerns will be laid out and discussed at this time; rather, this discussion sets a pattern for ongoing developmental surveillance, an honest partnership in observation and care and an individual perspective.

ANTICIPATORY GUIDANCE

The planning for discharge begins on admission as the clinician interprets the issues, presents them to the family and lays out a **strategy for treatment and follow-up**. This plan is expanded, revised and updated throughout the child's course. A formal conference or at least a phone call should take place at least every 2 to 3 weeks thereafter. A readiness assessment for discharge should include input from all disciplines and an assessment of behavioral maturity, as well as physiological stability. Within a week before discharge, a comprehensive discharge planning conference should be held to lay out specific plans, contacts and appointments in detail. Written documentation of these plans should always be provided to parents at the time of discharge. The goal of this conference is to review the hospital course, make plans for follow-up and review any treatment plans. The following are examples of specific components to include in the conference:

- A brief review of the medical course, anticipated problems and the need for specialized (e.g., ophthalmology) follow-up helps parents know what to expect and to ask questions or get clarification. Parents should be told that certain problems specifically related to the infant's condition at birth as a sick neonate *will not* recur (especially intraventricular hemorrhage, air leak, etc.). Many parents continue to worry that these neonatal problems could recur or be chronic, but they never ask!

- A notebook with all the infant's needs, resources to meet those needs, warning signals, appointments, medications and telephone numbers of specialists and staff can be most helpful. Most parents remember few specifics without such an aid. Highlight one or two resources, including the primary care pediatrician, to work with the parents in coordinating multiple services.

- Appropriate community agency referrals should be initiated or noted even if the services may not be needed immediately. Few parents are able to do this on their own.

- The NICU staff may designate one nurse to follow up with a call in 1 or 2 days to ease the family's transition to home.

- Parental expectations before discharge should be reviewed. The parents must demonstrate competency in all aspects of their infant's care. They should rehearse what will be needed in emergencies. Instruction in infant CPR and appropriate emergency action will relieve fears rather than generate them. Videos, dolls and pamphlets should supplement, not replace *direct* teaching in this and other areas.

- Family resources should be reviewed. A telephone should be immediately available. Guarantees of heat, electricity and basics need to be ensured.

- Families should have transportation plans laid out for both emergency and planned visits. Adjustment of the car seat, taxi vouchers and other issues should be addressed.

- Review nutritional needs, including vitamins and minerals. Very low-birthweight infants may need additional protein, electrolytes and calories in the form of special preterm discharge formulas or supplementation of breast milk with powdered preterm formula for a period. An iron-deficient infant is an irritable infant. Premature infants require additional iron supplementation up to 1 year of age. Anemia is a *late* sign of iron deficiency, which has been shown to have adverse effects on development even before the anemia surfaces. Appropriate iron supplementation should be initiated even in the absence of frank anemia. Check the hematocrit at discharge and periodically throughout the first year. Adequate vitamin D supplementation is needed to ensure optimal bone mineralization.

- Describe the infant's growth, behavior and development by the *adjusted age* so that neurodevelopmental expectations are realistic. Continue to make this correction at the beginning of future encounters. Be sure that an accurate head circumference is recorded at the time of discharge. A growth chart that includes head circumference should be started and values added at the adjusted age at each visit.

- The need for ongoing longitudinal neurodevelopmental follow-up should be discussed.

- Parents often need to be reassured that their "sleepy" premature infant will become more alert and interactive with maturity. Until they understand this, their infant's apparent response to them (to sleep) is very discouraging. The irritability that may follow it can also be predicted. Parents need to understand these aspects of typical behavior for their atypical infant.

- Routine discharge counseling includes the use of car seats and recognition of the "back-to-sleep" message. Parents should be encouraged to place their baby prone when awake to strengthen the trunk and shoulder muscles, which tend to be weaker in preterm infants and thus interfere with developmental progress.

- Discuss the need for routine immunizations in the usual amounts and at the usual times. The need and schedule for respiratory syncytial virus prophylaxis should also be addressed for eligible infants.

- An explicit invitation to call or visit the NICU after discharge is also helpful as parents attempt to separate from the nursery, the staff and the support that has been so vital.

- Parents should be encouraged to stay overnight, if possible, before discharge, or they may be accommodated for a period in nearby lodging if they are going to a rural or remote area.

SETTING THE COURSE: MAKING MINI-OBSERVATION PLANS

The construction of a developmentally supportive care plan should be part of every discharge plan. It should be developed with and guided by the nursing and consultant (e.g., occupational therapist, lactation specialist) staff who have come to understand the baby's capabilities and limits. The primary care clinician will pick one or two areas of concern or immaturity in the infant and set very small improvement goals with the family at discharge and continuing across the first year. For example, if the infant sleeps erratically, the parents might be asked to keep a sleep record to see whether sleep improves in regularity over a period of 2 to 4 weeks. Alternatively, if the infant has difficulty handling the stress of bathing, the parent and the clinician can devise supports (e.g., swaddling half the body) so that the child can begin to at least tolerate, if not enjoy the experience. By setting *specific short-term* goals, the parents and the clinician can gain a sense of progress and recovery. The parents' energy can be actively engaged in facilitating and supporting progress. Specific notes on the target area should be placed in the medical record so that the clinician can mark progress or problems at the next visit. A high-risk child will not follow the developmental pattern of a "normal" child. The clinician makes benchmarks of change for each child. This strategy allows parents to focus on their individual child rather than on comparisons with children following a typical course.

Hurdles

Soothing The irritability of many high-risk infants is a major hurdle that often emerges some weeks after discharge, often at 6 weeks' adjusted age. This behavior is sometimes referred to as "*super colic*." The development of effective soothing techniques and avoidance of overloading situations will ameliorate, but not eliminate this process. Swings, swaddling, front pack carrying, skin-to-skin care and pacifiers may all help. Respite care is often needed. Many babies settle more easily on the chest or lap of a caretaker, so additional carrying and quiet cuddles may be easier and better for all concerned.

Breastfeeding The transition to full breastfeeding is a process that takes weeks to months. Some babies never adapt to feeding directly at the breast but can continue to receive the benefits of breast milk if the mother is willing to bottle feed her expressed milk. Even if full breastfeeding doesn't occur, any amount of breast milk is of value to a premature infant in protection against disease, brain development and balanced nutrition. If formula supplementation was needed in the NICU, the mother should increase pumping to eight times daily for a period of 7 to 10 days before discharge to increase her milk supply. A *realistic* postdischarge feeding plan, developed in conjunction with a lactation specialist experienced with preterm infants, should be clearly laid out. If supplemental nutrition is needed after discharge to ensure adequate growth, it may be added directly to expressed breast milk or given as one or two feedings of an adapted preterm formula. A preterm infant should be able to nurse at the breast before discharge for part of a feeding or for all of some feedings. The recommended approach for each feeding should be

- Breastfeed at the breast
- Supplement with pumped breast milk
- Pump for next feeding to keep the milk supply up and store appropriately

Hearing and Vision Assessment The baby's vision and hearing should be monitored throughout early childhood. The first follow-up appointment for each area should be planned at discharge (Box 8–8). Parents should be told that this is routine and does not imply a special concern for their child. Specialized follow-up services are needed beyond what the primary care clinician can do.

Home Visits Home visiting, sometimes including a predischarge or postdischarge visit, is helpful if done by the NICU staff or others who knew the infant in the hospital. Discharge plans become realistic, and teaching can be focused. Follow-up and compliance are increased at least threefold when a visit is made.

BOX 8–8   ASSESSMENTS

Hearing
- Discharge hearing screen (BAER or OAE) with follow-up BAER if abnormal: VRA when sitting at 6–9 months' adjusted age
- Further follow-up if the infant has abnormal speech-language development or frequent otitis media

Ophthalmology
- If the premature baby weighs less than 1500 g, examine before discharge. The entire retina should be visualized with frequent follow-up by an experienced pediatric ophthalmologist until the retina is completely mature
- Ophthalmology follow-up for astigmatism and refractive errors at 1 to 2 years

BAER, brainstem auditory evoked response; OAE, otoacoustic emission; VRA, visual reinforced audiometry.

Planned Review

A review of the perinatal course should be added to the 6-week to 3-month visit if a discussion has not been opened by the parents before that time. Confusion about diagnoses, conditions, treatments and expected follow-up is often identified at this time. Clarification may head off the vulnerable child syndrome (mentioned earlier in this chapter), increase compliance and alleviate fears.

The 8- to 9-month visit should be expanded to allow for observation of play and a structured developmental assessment (see Box 8–7). A complete neurological examination should be performed at 1 year at a minimum.

Special attention should be paid to assessment of receptive and expressive language at 2 to $2\frac{1}{2}$ years. Preterm infants frequently have delays in expressive language. Hearing loss secondary to recurrent otitis media may contribute to language delay. Speech and language delay deserves early evaluation in a preterm infant, who is at substantially higher risk for a variety of problems affecting neurodevelopmental outcome. Oral-motor dysfunction may also result in speech articulation difficulties that may become evident in the preschool period. A preschool examination should place added emphasis on visual-motor tasks (e.g., figure copying). Disabilities in this area should trigger *immediate, specific* testing, not just a standard intelligence test.

RECOMMENDED READINGS

Bradford N, Lousada S: *Your Premature Baby: The First Five Years.* Buffalo, NY, Firefly Books Ltd, 2003.

Davis DL, Stein MT: *Parenting Your Premature Baby and Child: The Emotional Journey.* Golden, CO, Fulcrum Publishing, 2004.

Garcia-Prats JA, Hornfischer SS. *What to Do When Your Baby Is Premature: A Parent's Handbook for Coping with High-Risk Pregnancy and Caring for the Preterm Infant.* New York, Three Rivers Press, 2000.

Klein AH, Ganon JA: *Caring for Your Premature Baby: A Complete Resource for Parents.* New York, Harper Collins, 1998.

La Leche League: *Breastfeeding Your Premature Baby.* Schaumburg, Ill, La Leche League, 1999.

Linden DW, Paroli ET, Doron MW: *PREEMIES: The Essential Guide for Parents of Premature Babies.* New York, Pocket Books, 2000.

Ludington-Hoe S: *Kangaroo Care: The Best You Can Do to Help Your Preterm Infant.* New York, Bantum Books, 1993.

MedlinePlus: Premature Babies. Available at *www.nlm.nih.gov/medlineplus/prematurebabies.html*

Sears J, Sears M, Sears R, Sears W: *The Premature Baby Book: Everything You Need to Know About Your Premature Baby from Birth to Age One.* New York, Little, Brown, 2004.

Tracy AE, Maroney DI: *Your Premature Baby and Child: Helpful Answers and Advice for Parents.* New York, Berkley Books, 1999.

Zaichkin J. *Neonatal Intensive Care (Cuidado Intensivo Neonatal).* Santa Rosa, CA, NICU Ink, 2000 (in English and Spanish).

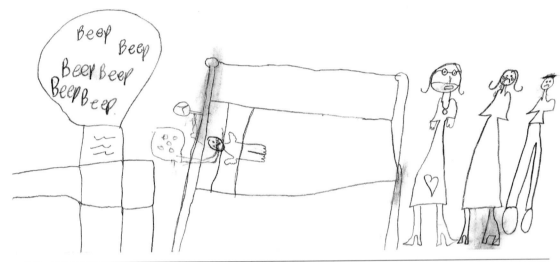

"Mom (the doctor dressed in a dress with a heart) talking to sad parents of a sick baby." The daughter of a neonatologist draws her mom at work. She clearly knows the hardest part of the job. By Katie R., age 7.

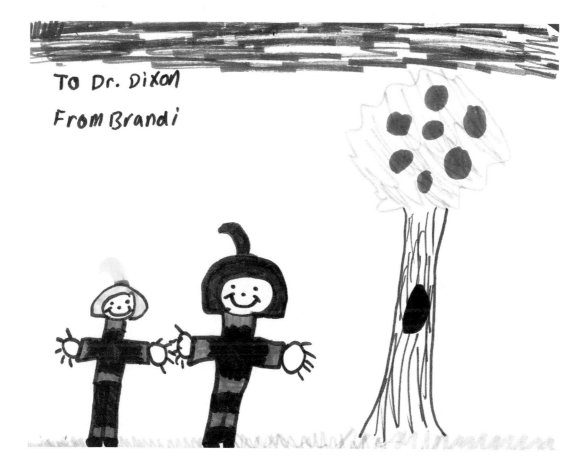

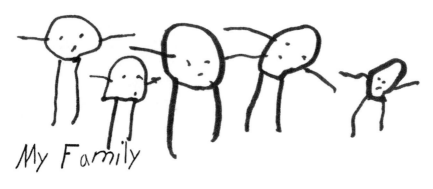

CHAPTER 9

My Family

Name: _____

Logan Henderson

A five year old draws his family, his baby sister a little tenuously at the end of the line. He's snuggled next to his mom. By Logan Henderson.

First Days at Home: Making a Place in the Family

SUZANNE D. DIXON and MARTIN T. STEIN

This chapter describes the first month of a new infant at home, the adjustments demanded of the baby and the family. Establishment of a successful breastfeeding pattern is based on responsiveness to the infant's behavioral cues and is the forum for developing contingent interaction with the infant. Postpartum depression and its effect on children are described.

Key Words

- Postpartum Adjustment
- Breastfeeding
- Postpartum Depression
- Sibling Rivalry
- Parental Competence
- Infant-Parent Interaction

Mrs. Ferris brings in her 2-week-old son, Ethan, for a weight check and is carrying him in a plastic carrier. This full-term infant has been gaining slowly with breastfeeding. He awakens very quickly when unwrapped on the examining table and immediately starts to cry. Mrs. Ferris sits quietly, mechanically getting out a new diaper for the infant. She appears pale and tired and is less well dressed than usual. Melissa, her 3-year-old, is playing with the examining room toys and throws a small car across the room. Her mother jumps up quickly and scolds her. Melissa dissolves into tears and then sucks her thumb. You notice that Melissa has diapers on. Mrs. Ferris says she's thinking of starting bottle feeding. She looks tearful. Note: Postpartum fatigue can perhaps be prompting some behavior here. Sibling rivalry with toddler regression is present. Feeding issues are a cover for basic interaction and adjustment that are not optimal at this time. The clinician must decide whether this downturn in mood is a serious concern.

The early neonatal period after hospital discharge is usually filled with turmoil and adjustments for all members of the family. These individuals must struggle to fit themselves and the infant into a family unit that has irrevocably changed. The infant is working too, using capacities for learning and adaptation to fit into his family. He must capture other family members to build a secure web of sensitive caretaking. The baby's physical and psychological needs must be met by those members who will learn to understand the infant's signals and generate appropriate responses. Each infant's particular temperament, physiological stability, stamina and behavioral characteristics determine how those needs are met. The parents' perception of the child, as it is formed during this time, is a powerful predictor of their own

201

interaction with the child over the long term, which in turn has major consequences for the child's development. Parental self-esteem and competence are built on the experiences of these early days. This period has huge implications for the child and family, and thus it is a great opportunity for the health care provider to make a difference.

The clinician's role during this first month is critical and consists of monitoring and supporting the development of synchrony in the family unit while evaluating the infant's growth and physical well-being. Turbulence is expected, as it is evidence of healthy developmental work. More serious difficulties occur in families whose members are not free enough of other concerns to make a place for the infant and develop a new role for themselves. Particularly when no extended family members are available, the clinician has a special role of support and guidance. The clinician may have to provide extra effort to help refocus the family energy on the particular needs of the infant and, indeed, those of all the family members.

This realignment within a family is done through the generation of success in each member's care of the infant. Through sensitive observations and some thoughtful suggestions on seemingly small matters of management, the clinician can ensure that everyone, including the infant, grows during the adjustment period. The processes of family realignment can be masked during routine health supervision unless the clinician brings these issues to consciousness.

INFANT SOCIAL DEVELOPMENT

The infant begins life fully equipped to interact with the environment. Evidence of the baby actively participating in social interactions includes movement in rhythm to the human voice, selective orientation to mother's milk by 6 days of age and a visual fixation on the human face that is different from that of any other kind of stimuli (see Chapter 7). The infant's early behavioral repertoire includes socially directed behavior used both to elicit and to terminate interactions. Directed gaze is important to the bonding between infant and family in the U.S. culture.

Generally, the baby's eyes widen and brighten as he fixates and tracks his parents' movements and scans their faces. This has a powerful, positive effect on the adults and locks them into a relationship with their child. Gaze aversion, conversely, is often actively used by the infant to either avoid or take a break from an interaction. In addition to gaze, the infant can demonstrate readiness for interaction with body language (e.g., smooth, cyclic movements of the extremities or slowing down of body movements, open hands and mouthing). Types of behavior that signal withdrawal from caregivers, either to modulate the level of input or to avoid insensitive or overwhelming interaction, include back arching, pulling away, hand to head, increased body tension and diffuse jittery movements of the extremities. These infant behavioral characteristics are learned almost subconsciously by most parents. They will alter their interactions in response to the infant. However, some parents may need to have such behavior identified as communication from their infant, particularly if the infant has difficulty locking in with the parents. Parents not in tune will ignore an infant making a bid for attention or continuing interaction, or they will continue to talk, shake, bounce or nuzzle an infant who is clearly overwhelmed and is signaling that he needs a break. When such dyssynchrony between the baby's body language and parent behavior is identified, intervention is warranted. A list of nonverbal communication behavior is presented in Box 9-1.

BOX 9–1   BABY LANGUAGE

Come-On Behavior

The following types of behavior signal a positive response from the infant, saying in effect, "keep doing this; this is great."

- Softening of facial expression
- Lifting of eyebrows
- Relaxed body posture
- Hands opening and closing
- Feet relaxed, "grasping" with plantar flexion
- Leaning forward with head, shoulders
- Making an "oohh" facial expression, with the mouth in an oval
- Mouthing, tongue going back and forth
- Cooing sounds

Go-Away Behavior

The following types of behavior signal a negative response from the infant, saying in effect, "Go away. Stop that."

- Arching away
- Turning the face away
- Gaze aversion
- Hands, feet splayed
- Extension of the legs, pushing away
- Down-turned face
- Lateral stretching of the mouth into a "grin"
- Spitting up, burping, passing a bowel movement
- Whiney sounds

Adapted from Als H: *Manual for the Naturalistic Observation of the Newborn (Preterm and Fullterm)*. Boston, Children's Hospital Medical Center, 1984 (revised 1997).

Attentive mothers and acoustic analysis performed in a research environment can distinguish different types of cries by the time an infant is 2 days of age. These differing types of cries include those for hunger and those expressing pain. Parents should be learning to identify these special cry features at this time.

Smiling is a powerful social "tool" that progresses from a reflexive activity to a responsive activity prompted by external events (e.g., a human face, gaze or voice) to spontaneous behavior produced to elicit response from others at the age of 6 to 8 weeks. A smiling infant changes a parent dramatically because it finally feels as though the infant is a person who is responsive to care. The first smile is a very big event in emergence of the parent-child relationship.

DANCING TOGETHER

Newborns prefer high-pitched vocal tones with lots of modulation. Parents from different cultures with different languages instinctively use high-pitched voices when communicating with a young infant. Babies begin to "answer" in the first month with cooing sounds. These soft vocalizations come out of a positive social interaction sometime in the first month. By the second month, most infants will engage in verbal "dialogues" with their mothers and fathers, going back and forth in a "conversation" that is mutually regulated by both partners.

The infant's interactional pattern begins with each parent over the first days and weeks of life. During this acquaintance period the family members develop reciprocal relationships, often rhythmic, smooth and modulated with mothers and more evenly intense and positive with fathers. This "waltzing" or "turn taking" can be observed in periods of engagement that increase in frequency and duration during the first weeks. Balanced harmony is largely dependent on the *parents' contingent responses* and their sensitivity to the child's visual, verbal and motor cues. The infant's "language" is his behavior. Parents learn to be attuned to his behavior through interactions with him. Individual variation in both infant and parental temperament is a significant factor in development of the style and form of this interaction, but not in its basic interactive structure. The infant participates in these interactions by developing predictable patterns of responsiveness; the parent participates by being a good observer and reading the infant's cues closely and by providing consistent responsiveness. This interaction is the foundation for all of parenting, so these little exchanges are not to be taken lightly.

Caretaking activities are the matrix on which this synchrony is built. Being successful in the infant's care and being able to see pattern and meaning in the infant's behavior enables the parents to grow in their role and to meet the child's physical and psychological needs. Close physical contact early helps this synchrony develop, which is essential to attachment.

The breastfeeding situation in particular emphasizes the basic interactional nature of the infant's behavior within a family. Each partner brings characteristics to this interaction (Table 9–1). The infant is born with reflexes, but they must be quickly adapted to the feeding interaction. The infant's temperament, state regulation, physiological vitality and behavioral organization all contribute to that process. Likewise, the mother's nutrition, hydration, psychological state and rate of recovery enter into the equation. In a variable time of adjustment for both partners, rhythms and behavioral patterns of individuals are melded into a

TABLE 9–1   **Interactional Nature of Breastfeeding**

Infant Characteristics	Maternal Characteristics
Reflexes	Nutrition
Temperament	Hydration
State regulation	Psychological state
Physiological variables	Recovery stage
Behavioral organization	Concepts of parenting
Residual of recovery from delivery influences	Extent and use of support
Neurological maturation	Psychosocial history Residual of pregnancy, delivery circumstances Role models

successful interaction. Within this interactional setting, both partners learn about themselves as well as the other. Personal, cultural and group differences are evident here as they are in other situations of interaction. The clinician should be *very* familiar with the practical advice and support required for successful breastfeeding because it is important for much more than the child's physiological needs (Box 9–2). Unfortunately, this is not always the case. Most

---

BOX 9–2 KNOWLEDGE ABOUT SUCCESSFUL BREASTFEEDING FOR PEDIATRIC CLINICIANS

As a result of earlier discharge after delivery, health professionals are being called on to evaluate newborns within the first few days of life. The following specific criteria will help clinicians accurately assess the success of early breastfeeding and provide timely intervention to prevent excessive infant weight loss or diminished maternal milk supply.

Schedule of Feedings

An infrequent or otherwise inappropriate feeding schedule is a common, preventable cause of insufficient milk. The mother must be prepared to nurse her baby whenever the infant signals readiness to feed, such as increased alertness, sucking motions or rooting. Crying is a late sign of hunger.

Breastfed newborns should nurse approximately 8 to 12 times in 24 hours, usually taking both breasts at each feeding. A breastfeeding mother should nurse her baby every $1\frac{1}{2}$ to 3 hours during the early postpartum weeks. A single longer night interval of 4 or 5 hours between feedings is permissible. Non-nutritive sucking on a pacifier should be discouraged until a consistent pattern of acceptable weight gain has been established. Nondemanding babies should be aroused to feed. The intrafeeding interval in days 2 to 4 of life and at any time of a growth spurt may be *very* short, an hour or so. The duration of feeding should be approximately 15 minutes per breast, during which the infant suckles actively with short pauses. Infants are unlikely to obtain sufficient milk by sucking less than 10 minutes per breast in the early weeks of life. Conversely, marathon feedings that last more than 50 minutes are usually indicative of ineffective nursing. Older breastfed babies often nurse very efficiently and take the bulk of their feeding in only 5 to 7 minutes per breast, although they may nurse longer for comfort. Very short feedings may mean that the infant only gets the thin foremilk. The high-calorie, fat-rich hindmilk follows the mother's sense of letdown. It is this milk that results in real weight gain.

Infant Behavior and Appearance

Reports of the infant's behavior during and after nursing can provide important clues about the quality of feedings. Well-fed infants should act satisfied after feedings and sleep contentedly. Hyperbilirubinemia in breastfed infants is a common marker for inadequate breastfeeding, a condition known as "breastfeeding jaundice."

Once milk has come in, a mother should hear her baby swallow regularly during feedings and see evidence of milk in the baby's mouth. These observations are somewhat subjective, however, and do not always correlate with objective measures of milk intake. Generally, a breastfed baby should appear satisfied after nursing and sleep contentedly until the next feeding. Persistent crying or excessive need for a pacifier often signifies infant hunger and suggests that little milk was obtained during feeding.

Box continued

BOX 9–2   **KNOWLEDGE ABOUT SUCCESSFUL BREASTFEEDING FOR PEDIATRIC CLINICIANS—cont'd**

Exaggerated physiological jaundice in a breastfed infant is a common marker for inadequate breastfeeding. Whenever unexplained unconjugated hyperbilirubinemia is present in a breastfed infant, evaluation of the infant's nutritional status is warranted. The baby is probably getting insufficient milk to push the bilirubin out via the gut and kidneys. Strategies to improve the effectiveness of breastfeeding should be implemented whenever "breastfeeding jaundice" is diagnosed. Formula supplements may be necessary to provide adequate nutrition, but breastfeeding need not be interrupted.

Infant Elimination

A newborn's pattern of voiding and stooling provides one of the most sensitive historical indicators of the adequacy of milk intake. Always inquire about infant elimination patterns.

Shortly after the milk comes in, a thriving breastfed newborn should void colorless urine at least six to eight times daily. With inadequate infant intake, mothers often report a "brick dust" appearance in the diaper, which is caused by precipitated urate crystals. Dark yellow, scant urine or visible urate crystals beyond 3 to 4 days of life strongly suggest that a breastfed infant is not obtaining sufficient milk. *Beginning about the fourth or fifth day of life, well-nourished breastfed infants typically pass sizable (not a small stain), loose yellow "milk stools" after most feedings.* Between about 4 days and 4 weeks of age, a thriving breastfed baby should pass at least four such "milk stools" daily, often resembling a mixture of cottage cheese and mustard. Dark transition stools, infrequent bowel movements or scant volume of stools in a young breastfed infant are common indicators of insufficient milk intake. However, beginning around 1 month of age, stooling frequency may gradually diminish in breastfed infants, although stools remain soft and easily passed.

professionals believe that they need to learn more. Within that context, the foundation for later interactions is laid down. The success that is realized with optimal nursing energizes the whole interactional system.

The American Academy of Pediatrics recognizes that support of breastfeeding has not only nutritional, immunological and infectious disease consequences but psychosocial ones as well. The first 2 weeks of life are the toughest as these patterns are established. Mothers may feel that they have been reduced to a milk machine at this point. The clinician can help them see the broader perspective, as well as provide practical management advice. The setting of family priorities (feeding for the infant, rest and good nutrition for the mother) may have to be explicitly laid out.

For mothers who decide to not nurse their infants, the basic interactional synchrony must be the basis for bottle feeding. Feeding time should provide close physical contact, attention to the infant's behavioral cues and contingent responsiveness. Nurturance in the broadest sense should be the outcome here as it is in breastfeeding. Even greater vigilance is needed if these broader needs will be consistently met because this kind of physical and emotional contact is not automatic with bottle feeding. Obviously, bottle propping is never appropriate.

Observation of the mother feeding her infant in the office offers the best opportunity to assess the synchrony that is developing between mother and infant. In addition, direct observation offers opportunities for support, specific suggestions and direct reflection on the baby's behavior. It should be a set part of the examination at least once in the first 2 weeks of life and more often if the adjustment process seems to be progressing slowly or with difficulty. An effective way to observe nursing without altering standard office routines is for the office nurse or medical assistant to suggest that the mother nurse the baby after measurements are taken, while waiting for the clinician or as the history is being taken. The clinician is then able to observe nursing. A planned office visit within the first week enables the clinician to intervene if difficulties are identified. A delayed first office visit often means that a preventable problem with feeding or an opportunity for better adjustment has been lost. Optimally, the visit should be planned within 1 week after hospital discharge for new parents and those with a rocky start and no longer than 2 weeks for mothers with previous experience. In communities where home visitation programs are available, office visits in the first few weeks may be adjusted to coordinate with the home visit. No matter where it occurs, this visit should have as its theme the issues of the whole family getting on track with the infant and themselves.

POSTPARTUM "BLUES" AND DEPRESSION

Parental adjustments to a new baby do not come automatically, nor do they emerge in a neutral emotional atmosphere. Some turbulence occurs in most families. Having postpartum "blues" is a normal, transient phase in the adaptation process for moms that occurs within the first week after birth. Crying, confusion, mood lability, anxiety and depressed mood are symptoms. They last a few hours to a few days and generally have few negative sequelae. Most women experience this phase as a mild form of depression. It may be related to exhaustion, physical depletion and hormonal shifts. Contributing factors are sleep deprivation caused by demanding caregiving responsibilities, as well as changes in role and body image. Household and other child care duties may be overwhelming. While letting go of the former relationship of "two," the couple begins to incorporate this "third person," who generally upsets most established home routines and patterns, such as mealtimes, talk times, social activities and sexual patterns. Being home all day and delaying career or academic pursuits often add to the ambivalence and role conflict many women experience. Economic uncertainty may also compound the stress. A single mother's difficulty during this time may be heightened by her sense of aloneness if supporting individuals or groups are not available. Existing family stresses usually get worse rather than better at this time.

As a result of these factors, new mothers must cope with many unanticipated feelings. They are often overwhelmed by the chaos that this new baby seems to have created. Women may feel unusually dependent on others or even intimidated by or angry with would-be supporters.

> Marcy brought in her 10-day-old for a weight check. As the nurse started to undress the infant, Marcy snapped at her and told the nurse that's not the way it's done. Later Marcy tearfully apologized for her outburst.

Many women are confused and embarrassed by their inexplicable crying, indecisiveness and fatigue during these first few weeks. The clinician may be caught up in the adjustment process as the new mother turns to her as a resource. Clinicians may be frightened, feel awkward or be uncertain about how to respond to this excessive dependency and emotionality unless they see it as a transient process of normal adult development.

The clinical features of severe depression are quite different from these "baby blues." Postpartum depression affects up to 10% of women. Its symptoms may include immobilizing indecision, impaired cognitive functioning, irritability and changes in sleep and appetite. Excessive guilt and dysphoria may also be present and last at least a week and often longer. The usual onset is within the 30-day period after birth, but it may be later. Most new mothers resolve these feelings by 6 to 8 weeks after delivery, although some studies suggest continuing symptoms at 6 months. Mothers may experience a prolonged depressive state accompanied by sleep disturbances, anorexia, constipation, agitation and a sluggish affect. They may develop an altered way of thinking that is a radical departure from the prenatal personality, such as talking about past, present and future events in a negative or unrealistic way. The mother's ability to function may be significantly impaired. Suicidal ideations, delusions and hallucinations, as seen in the most severe forms of postpartum depression, may be uncovered, both by specific questioning and by unusual responses to a routine question.

Mrs. Ferris' own behavior and her responses to her 3-week-old son and 3-year-old daughter, described in the opening vignette, are an opportunity for assessment and intervention. The clinician comments, "A new baby and a toddler are an enormous amount of work … How has it been going for you?" Mrs. Ferris' tears begin as she talks about her feelings of inadequacy as a mother, her sense of isolation from her husband and friends and her sleep deprivation.

The clinician listens without immediate suggestion. She engages the toddler with a toy, tells her what a big sister she has become and lifts her to the examination table while encouraging her participation as an observer during the baby's exam. The normal physical and developmental examination is narrated to assure Mrs. Ferris that her baby is healthy. The baby's individuality is prominent in that narrative.

Mrs. Ferris is then informed that "feeling blue" is experienced by many mothers during the first month after delivery. Then the pediatrician poses four questions to assess whether other intervention is needed (see later).

The clinician then assesses nursing by observing the baby at mother's breast. In a now calm environment, latching on and sucking appear adequate. The mother's fluid intake, need for more sleep and plans for recruiting available social support from her family and friends are reviewed. There seem to be several ways to make things go more smoothly. A 1-week follow-up is planned as an important component of health supervision. Mrs. Ferris has passed a period of postpartum depression, but a closer watch is needed to see whether these symptoms resolve or whether referral to a mental health provider will be needed.

Ongoing success as a parent with renewed self-esteem will aid in resolution of the turbulence. Help and frequent acknowledgment of maternal competencies are the tools that are available for the pediatric caregiver to assist this process. Encouragement to reach out to support systems in the family and in the community will enable the family to cope. Mothers with postpartum depression may recover faster if they participate in group health supervision visits than if they receive individual pediatric care. Many, if not most will require short-term professional counseling and/or medication, even hospitalization. Psychosis is rare, but it occurs more frequently at this time than at any other point in a woman's life, and it will be the child health provider who is the most likely professional to have the opportunity to identify this serious condition.

Persistent or severe symptoms of depression require psychiatric referral, clearly beyond what can be provided in a primary care setting. These mothers may require significant respite care, as well as psychiatric referral and perhaps medication or even hospitalization. Most studies report high rates of recovery from the acute phase of this illness.

Mothers with the following characteristics may be more vulnerable to severe depression in the postpartum period (although there is still significant disagreement within the literature on this matter):

- A history of psychiatric illness in self or in close relatives
- A history of drug abuse
- Poor marital relationship
- A recent loss (e.g., death of parent)
- A history of past or present thyroid illness
- Isolation, with other major life stressors
- Family history of severe depression

Parents of preterm, ill or disabled children are also more vulnerable. Because the pediatric clinician may be the mother's sole medical contact in the first month after birth, these symptoms may surface only during pediatric health supervision visits with specific questioning and sensitivity to these issues. It becomes the pediatric clinician's responsibility to identify the need for further evaluation, referral and possible treatment. If the mother requires psychotropic drugs, the pediatrician should evaluate the extent of the drugs' excretion into breast milk.

Assessing Postpartum Depression

Every child health care provider should have available some systematic screening process to evaluate postpartum depression or the presence of parental depression in general. There are formal screening tools such as the Edinburgh Postnatal Depression Scale (see Appendix), as recommended by the American Academy of Pediatrics Bright Future project (see Appendix).

Making it even simpler, a report by Olson and colleagues (2005) suggests that if just two questions, requiring less than a minute, posed to a parent by the primary care physician are positive, there is a high likelihood of significant depression. These simple questions regarding adult mood, stress and the enjoyment of life provide an opportunity to identify real depression. Although very large studies are needed to fully evaluate this streamlined approach, the early results are promising. Every child health care professional should be prepared to ask these questions and be ready with referrals.

Maternal depression and mental illness are a pediatric issue. Although the mother's well-being is clearly at risk in this circumstance, the baby's is too. Depressed mothers touch their infants less, speak to them less and are less responsive to their vocalizations. Even brief periods of depressive behavior have profound effects on the infant's behavior, including a decrease in infant activity, less vocalization and play interaction participation and less smiling of the infant.

Prolongation of these symptoms may have long-lasting effects on the child (see Murray and Cooper for an expanded discussion). Poorer developmental outcome and more behavioral problems are more likely in children of depressed moms. This may be indirectly caused by the lack of reciprocal interaction with the infant. The infant depends on the parent to learn about his effectiveness in acting on the world in order to begin to establish a sense of self. Many adverse child-rearing conditions, such as poverty, isolation and substance abuse, may affect the infant through the medium of maternal depression. The pediatric clinician cannot afford to ignore this condition in parents if she wants to support optimal development in the child.

REACTIONS OF OLDER SIBLINGS

Sibling rivalry is a predictable, normal and healthy response to the birth of a new brother or sister. In most families it demonstrates that the older child is appropriately attached to the parents and is responsive to a perceived threat to the parent-child relationship. It is a normal response to having your place as the baby of the family usurped. In this context, the emergence of behavior that reflects sibling rivalry should be viewed positively. Ambivalence toward the baby as evidenced by an ongoing shift between positive and negative behavior is to be expected. Indeed, its absence may be worrisome. Sibling rivalry is not a disease, but a manifestation of psychological health.

Behavioral manifestations of sibling rivalry can take several forms, such as the following:

- *Aggressive* behavior is directed most commonly toward the mother, but it may also be directed toward the baby, father, playmates, self or toys. Aggressive behavior most often occurs when the older sibling is a toddler. Increases in this behavior will probably occur when the new baby becomes more socially engaging at 4 to 5 months of age and again when he becomes mobile during the last half of the first year. Open hostility may be reduced to more subtle behavior directed at the infant, such as pulling the pacifier out of the baby's mouth or taking a toy away.

- *Naughtiness,* or doing things contrary to family rules, occurs frequently at times when the mother is busy with the baby. This strategy serves to both increase tension in the household and verify the continuing power of the toddler to alter the behavior of those around her. A careful history of when such behavior occurs may highlight to the family for the first time that it is not "random," but dependent on a particular situation.

- Some children are *overly compliant* to or overly solicitous of the infant. Perhaps the child fears being totally replaced if she misbehaves, so the child becomes "extra good" to ensure her place in the family. Then again, she may be so frightened of her own aggressive and angry feelings that she holds them tightly in check. This may become a costly strategy and may evolve into an actively aggressive pattern or an irritable, depressed mood.

- *Regressive and dependent behavior* is usually seen in the form of clinging and demanding. Other possible types of regressive behavior include sleep disturbances, stuttering, thumb sucking, bedwetting, eating refusals or demands and baby talk. These responses serve to see whether one can get the same attention and care as the infant. They are also the expected response to any stress and demand for adjustment.

Behavioral manifestations of sibling rivalry reflect a child's limited and primitive response to change in the family structure, including her own position. They generally decrease, but

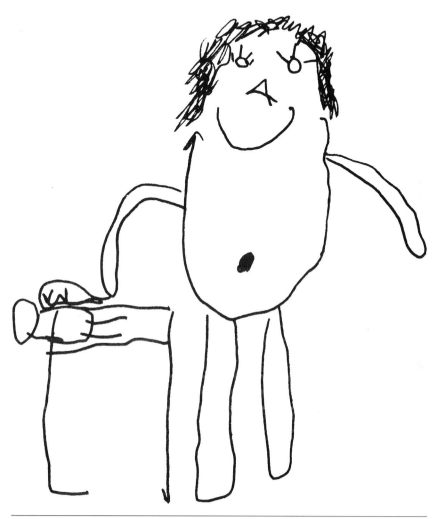

"Mom changing baby's diaper." By Eric Ries, age 6½.

may not entirely disappear during the year after the new sibling's birth. There may be periods of readjustment as the infant's abilities change. Over this period the older child becomes confident of a new place in the family, with its status and privileges. Additionally, the older sibling usually develops a separate relationship with the younger child as the latter becomes more fun, more responsive and interactive. Young babies aren't much fun and are usually quite a disappointment to a child initially.

The arrival of a younger sibling can evoke positive behavioral changes, as well as negative ones, even in the early, get-acquainted period. Dunn and Kendrick report gains in the older child's independence and mastery, particularly with regard to self-help skills (e.g., dressing and feeding). The child may gain new skills and a growing sense of competency through participation in "her" baby's care. She may be able to reflect on her own growth and development as she sees the baby's emerging capabilities. The older sibling may try out new ways of dealing with the little stranger, such as initiating and maintaining interactions in which she bears the burden of greater understanding. She will learn to laugh at the antics of the baby and grow in confidence as she learns to make the infant laugh, play games and imitate. This is an opportunity for growth if such behavior is understood and supported. Ways to support the older child are laid out in Box 9–3.

FACTORS THAT INFLUENCE RIVALRY

Some factors are correlated with a *positive* response to the infant. Enhanced signs of affection and interest in the baby are correlated with same-sex pairs in children whose mother allows the

BOX 9–3   WAYS TO HELP SIBLINGS AFTER THE ARRIVAL OF A NEW BABY

- Make time each day for the older child all by himself without infant demands. Have him decide what to do during that time.
- Be very generous with hugs, cuddles and kisses.
- Discuss the longer-term advantages of having a sibling, such as having a playmate and being the leader or the teacher of the little one.
- Don't force him to share all the toys he had as a baby. Have him decide which ones he is ready to share.
- Praise any positive attention he gives the infant.
- Provide him with a stuffed animal or a doll to hold, nurture and "baby" as his own.
- Be tolerant of behavioral regressions, but keep the rules pretty much the same. Consistency will help him feel safe.
- Invite him to participate in age-appropriate baby care; then invite him again if he initially refuses.
- Allow him to express negative feelings with words, but don't allow any physical action directed against the infant.
- Brag about the older one's accomplishments when visitors come so that the infant doesn't get all the attention.
- Bring out the older one's baby book or pictures of him as a baby so that he gets the care and attention that the new child is receiving.
- Avoid pushing him into being a "big boy." Respect his need to try to be a baby again without abandoning the general house rules.

older child to participate in the baby's care and discusses the baby's needs and behavior with her. However, an overemphasis on behaving "like a big girl (boy)," with demands for more grown-up behavior, is costly for the child and should be avoided. It is a high price to pay for continuing parental love. Parents who have an evenly warm and affectionate attachment to both children foster less rivalry. A strong, secure attachment before the infant's arrival will make it easier for the older child, but it will nonetheless be a struggle. There will still be a need to work through the inevitable negative feelings or go through at least some of the recuperative process of acting like a baby oneself.

Certain factors have been shown to intensify an older child's *negative* responses at the time of the sibling's birth:

- A very intense, tight relationship between the first child and the parents before the baby's arrival is correlated with the child's increased hostile and aggressive behavior.

- Extremely withdrawn behavior is more likely in children whose mothers experience severe postpartum exhaustion or depression.

- Evidence is conflicting regarding the effects of child spacing on the sibling's response, that is, whether a narrow age gap intensifies rivalrous behavior. There is, however, some general agreement that the birth of a sibling in the second year is more stressful than in the third year and beyond.

- Breastfeeding the second baby does not compound stress for the first child.

The child's own issues and coping strategies differ at varying ages, but an adjustment period appears at all ages. Temperamental characteristics (see Chapter 2) are also a major contributor to the nature and intensity of a sibling's response to the birth of a baby. Children who are adaptable to new situations, with positive or mild behavior changes when separated from a parent, usually have a similar behavioral response to the birth of a newborn. They come through with mild and/or short-lived reactions. Temperamentally challenged siblings who are less tolerant of change in routines or novel situations are more likely to have sleep problems and clinging behavior and to lack positive interest in the baby. They have a harder time and take longer to adjust.

Let's Return to the Opening Vignette

In response to the pediatrician's request, "Tell me how Melissa has responded to new situations since Ethan's birth," Mrs. Ferris remarked that her daughter experienced lots of difficulty. Separation experiences were intense and drawn out. When her bedroom was moved to prepare for the baby, she had frequent crying episodes, followed by withdrawal and a sullen appearance. The pediatrician saw this as an opportunity to frame Melissa's behavior after the birth of Ethan in the context of her temperament. When Mrs. Ferris was informed that Melissa's response to change was a reflection of her innate temperament (low adaptability and difficulty with novel situations), she was relieved to know that it was not a result of her parenting alone. She was also more responsive to the use of positive reinforcement as a way to prevent or redirect Melissa's responses to the newborn. Additionally, she will try to spend some time each day with Melissa on her own.

Extreme responses in younger children may be markers of long-standing family adjustment problems, not just that associated with the infant's birth. The child's clinician may be the only professional to see the family at this time of crisis, when the issues are very close to the surface. He then is able to suggest a more extensive evaluation of the family as a whole. This may be a window in time in which parents are open to getting outside help for long-standing issues.

> Madison, a 3½-year-old, was brought in 6 weeks after the birth of her brother because she was thrown out of daycare for biting three different children and being very oppositional and aggressive. She had also smeared feces on the bathroom wall after being trained for some time. Dr. Keefer asked about other changes in the family and discovered that Dad had been out of work for 3 months and the family was being forced to move. Note: This family has been in trouble for a while, but Madison's extreme behavioral change was the bellwether of the situation. Her angry response goes beyond sibling rivalry, although her brother's arrival may have tipped her and her family over the edge. Fecal smearing in a typically developing child almost always reflects severe anger.

Several parental factors negatively affect the parents' own response to the child's behavior. Such factors include the parents' ambivalence toward the new baby, guilt in feeling less attached to the new baby and mourning over loss of the previous family structure.

Parents under stress and those with a strained relationship with the older child are likely to see more rivalry. Parents may be surprised, embarrassed or disappointed to see the older child's rivalry after their concerted prenatal efforts to prevent it. Parental shame and guilt for "abandoning" the older child are confounded when the older child acts out in very negative ways. Trying to coercively control the interaction with the infant has been shown to foster a more antagonistic response between them. Certainly, the parents' physical exhaustion in caring for the new baby diminishes their ability to meet the other child's needs physically and psychologically. It is not surprising that the relationship between the mother and firstborn changes after arrival of the second baby. Second-time mothers show less affection for, spend less time with and have more confrontations with the firstborn after the birth of the infant. Conversely, father-child relationships are often enhanced ultimately. It is no wonder that birth order has a profound effect on child development.

SUPPORT FOR THE NEW FAMILY

Specific families and subcultures show wide variation in the type, extent and duration of support given to a new family. Supportive care may include emotional support, baby care or advice or homemaking tasks. The baby's father, extended family (especially grandparents), friends and neighbors (with or without children of their own) and various members of the health care team may be part of the support structure. Many studies show that the number of friends a new mother has is correlated with her success in parenting, thus attesting to the power of this network.

The amount and kind of support may be constructive or undermining. Some new parents may resent the intrusion, the "taking over" of their perceived role by others. They may have unrealistic expectations of themselves in this new role. Sometimes, support systems offer divergent and even contradictory advice, thereby leading to the new parent's sense of confusion and anxiety in feeling caught in between two "authorities." Other new parents feel fearful and overwhelmed when the support systems are withdrawn (e.g., when the grandparents return to their own home). Some visitors may take away more energy than they leave; the clinician would do well to inquire about the cost-benefit ratio of the supports. In general, the availability and use of this social network—with the family and in the community—should be encouraged.

Subcultural differences in role expectations are evident in the way that families work out the patterns of activity when a new infant arrives. In some situations, the grandmother takes over— to do less would make a mother feel abandoned. In others, relatives are expected to supply large amounts of food and clothing. Most traditional cultures have a period of at least 1 to 2 months of relative seclusion and care of the new mother after birth, whose sole role is to recover and feed the neonate. It is a very rare occurrence that a mother just "drops the baby and then goes back to the fields." Every family needs this protected time to gain strength and work through the necessary mental reorganization and physical recovery. Cultural and economic issues may dictate the form and length of this period. Parents asked to return immediately to work without this protected time may safeguard themselves against "too close" an attachment and may be reluctant to invest in breastfeeding. Clinicians should actively encourage the use of some protected time in the first 3 months.

DATA GATHERING

History

To take the history, begin with open-ended questions about the infant—"What new things is the baby doing?" or "In what ways can you tell that the baby knows you?"—and proceed to closed-ended questions, such as the following:

- Ask more focused questions regarding hearing (Does the baby turn to sounds?), seeing (Does the baby enjoy seeing things?) and feeding behavior (How does the baby act while being fed?).
- Ask about irritability episodes and soothing preferences. What seems to work best to settle the baby down? What upsets the baby? How can you tell if he doesn't like something or is enjoying something?
- Activity patterns. How predictable is he? How regular are his sleep patterns? Is he easily awakened? How long are his alert periods? Does he like his bath?
- Open-ended questions regarding the parents' adjustment are important also: How are *you* feeling? How are *you* dealing with all this? Are *you* eating and sleeping well?

If any concern appears in what is said and how it is said, have the mother describe what happened yesterday in detail. If she has a minimal response, explore further by stating possible feelings the mother may be experiencing ("Many moms describe this time as so exhausting and discouraging that they feel overwhelmed, frightened by the responsibility. Some have feelings of regret or even negative feelings about having the baby. Have you experienced any of these feelings?"). Proceed to a more structured assessment if there is any question of depression (see the earlier section "Postpartum 'Blues' and Depression").

Ask about the father's reactions and involvement. Is he there? Does he hold the baby, change diapers, help with the housework? What does he think the baby is like? This is best done directly by inviting the father's participation in health supervision visits.

The clinician should also evaluate the siblings' responses. If only positive responses are given, be suspicious. Although some sibling adaptive behavior may not manifest until months after the birth of a baby, most have some type of behavioral change or regression. Give permission for the parent to discuss possibly negative behavior with you now or in the future ("Most children show some negative reaction to the new baby at some point. This is a normal response to feeling somewhat replaced."). If negative behavior is described, pursue how it is perceived and handled by the parent.

The availability and use of support systems should be specifically explored, including the emotions that surround those reports. Ask, "How does your family feel about the baby? How is having grandparents around, positive or negative, on a scale of 1 to 10? Are there any friends or neighbors with kids you can depend on? Who is cooking, cleaning, shopping?" An alone and isolated mother or couple is at high risk for difficulties in the adjustment to parenthood.

Observation

Social Development Be sensitive to the rhythms of interaction between parents and the infant. Point out to the parents the infant's body language during the history taking and examination. This is a wonderful opportunity to inform parents about their infant's ability to communicate with them. Note the baby's responsiveness to his parents. How easily is the infant consoled? How well does the baby maintain eye contact? The clarity of the baby's body language is important. Are needs and moods easy or difficult to read? Note the parents' sensitivity to the baby's cues. Do they pick up on the baby's subtle behavior that requires parent readjustment? How do they console the infant? Note comfort in handling the baby. Keep in mind individual and cultural differences in the parents' sensory mode with the baby (e.g., talking, touching, eye contact and grooming behavior). The feeding situation offers an excellent opportunity to observe social development and interaction between baby and parent.

Note the maternal emotional state, her latency to respond to questions and the amount of physical and verbal activity on the parents' part. Note any slowing of movement or responsiveness or any evidence of fatigue.

If the older child is in the room, observe interactions with the baby and parents. Note mood changes in the child and the parents' response to him. If the father or grandparents are present, note their interactions with the baby and the mother and other children. Who holds the baby? How do they respond to the baby's distress (e.g., bowel movement, crying)? Is dad helpful and consoling? Does anyone talk for mom (e.g., giving the history, asking questions)? Provide a positive comment about the value of an extended family's presence during the office visit.

Examination

Direct the parent to sit with the baby on her lap to maximize your opportunity to observe their interactions. The infant should turn to a voice. Interact (play, smile) with the baby to evaluate response, as well as to model behavior. Observe visual and auditory responses in this context. Comment aloud about the baby's social behavior and individuality. Encourage the parent to hold and talk with the baby often at home. Explain that narrating activities with the baby encourages and promotes language development.

Give reassurance that the baby cannot be "spoiled" at this age. Holding will, in fact, decrease crying overall. Quick responses to cries, effective soothing and close human contact lead to less crying in the first and second years and improved emotional health and self-regulation. At this age, infants need close physical contact.

Ask mother specifically about her mood, feelings and behavior. Allow the mother to cry and use touch if it seems comfortable. Attempt to restore confidence (e.g., "You're doing a good job; it takes a while to adjust to this baby and to get to know one another"). Enhanced self-esteem energizes new parents. Even minor concerns (e.g., diaper rash, mild jaundice) may impinge on the parents' feeling of competence. Clinicians should be careful to put problems in a clear perspective and to be unequivocal in their praise and support of positive things about the infant, both physical and behavioral. Be explicit about your availability to discuss feelings further. If the mother seems sad, ask specifically about hallucinations or feelings of doing harm to self or others. If these are present or if the sadness appears more severe than seen in normal postpartum "blues," referral is indicated.

Reactions of Older Siblings

If an older sibling is present, acknowledge and focus on him first before you go to the infant. Ask specific, separate questions of the older child rather than only asking, "Do you help with the baby?" Give praise for any recent developmental achievements the parent may have mentioned or any helpfulness shown toward the parent and baby. Ask about the child's interpretation of the baby (e.g., "Does she cry a lot? Is she not as much fun as you thought she'd be?").

Explain to the parents the positive aspects of their older child's behavioral changes. For example, you might say, "Although I'm sure it's frustrating to see your older child behaving this way, it's actually very healthy behavior. He is clearly demonstrating that he is attached to you and highly values his relationship with you." Reassure them that no matter what preparation was made before the baby's arrival, children will have hurt and resentful feelings; this is real and natural. The goal is not to minimize the negative behavior, but to help the older child get through and gain from this experience. Some of the ways to help that happen are the following:

- Acknowledge the adjustment process that all second-time parents experience when learning to juggle their availability with the needs of two or more children. It takes time for families to settle into new patterns and rhythms. For some families, books for parents and children regarding these issues can be helpful.

- Encourage parents to continue "special time" with the older child alone on a daily basis; a realistic time frame may be 10 to 15 minutes. Emphasize the importance of physical affection or "snuggle time."

- Encourage parents to discuss the new baby's needs and behavior with the older child and to allow participation in the baby's care. Children often benefit from duplicating these activities with their own dolls; these play experiences should be encouraged.

- Plan structured activities for the older child during the baby's bath and feeding so that an attractive distraction is available for the older child.

- The child should not be expected to share all toys, even if she has outgrown them. Reserving some items that are hers alone and providing a special place in which to keep them are important. Sharing parents with the baby on a permanent basis is hard enough.

- Urge parents to minimize changes in the older child's life for a while. This is especially important for an older sibling who is temperamentally slow to adapt to change. Such changes as moving to a new bed or new room or starting nursery school should ideally occur a few months before the baby's arrival or after some weeks of adjustment.

- Displaced aggression can be released through play (e.g., with modeling clay or a foam ball and bat). As long as the younger child cannot defend himself, hitting should not be allowed, and leaving the two alone should be avoided. The intensity of the parents' message that children must not hurt others is a most powerful factor in helping children learn to appreciate others' feelings.

- The need to be tolerant of regressive behavior should be stressed. Most parents will be reassured to learn that most lapses in developmental achievements are temporary.

- Review the suggestions laid out in Box 9–3.

Support for the New Family

If the father is present, be sure to include him rather than directing comments, eye contact and questions only to the mother. Direct some questions to him specifically (e.g., "What do you think about this baby? How do you handle his fussy periods? How is the baby affecting your sleep, your work?").

If a grandparent holds the baby for the majority of the visit, ask the mother to hold the baby during the examination to allow an opportunity to observe interaction and comfort in handling. If the father or grandparent entirely dominates the visit, the clinician will need to more overtly

QUICK CHECK—FIRST DAYS AT HOME

- ✔ The infant should be alert enough to sustain feedings of at least 10 to 15 minutes
- ✔ Alertness should be brief, at least
- ✔ Fixes and follows a face
- ✔ Responds to a soft voice
- ✔ The dominant posture is flexion
- ✔ Moves all extremities equally
- ✔ The tonic neck response peaks at 6 weeks
- ✔ Hands should gradually show a more open position
- ✔ Head held up briefly when the infant is placed in a prone position
- ✔ Evaluate jaundice and hydration status
- ✔ The newborn hearing test should have been performed and the results available

HEADS UP–FIRST DAYS AT HOME

Infant Factors
- Doesn't turn to sound? Check hearing screening
- Excessive weight loss—more than 10%
- Evaluate jaundice
- Poor alerting
- Disorganized suck
- Awake/crying or sleeping excessively
- Extremely irritable and/or hypertonic child
- Lethargic and/or hypotonic child
- Any motor asymmetries on exam

Parent Factors
- Depressed (see questions and questionnaires)
- Disheveled, unkempt parent
- Illness or extreme fatigue. Excessive pain
- Discusses more of her own issues than the infant's
- Misses appointments
- Isolated family, no support
- Partner abandonment
- Suggestion of drug, alcohol use

Interaction
- Mom doesn't hold the infant or appears disengaged
- Mom asks few questions, offers few comments
- Parent cannot tell the meaning of the different cries of the infant
- Father not emotionally engaged with the baby or mom
- No joyful play or talk while caring for the infant
- Grandmother or other support person dominating the visit (except in cultures in which that is the norm)

direct some questions to the mother. Solicitous and supportive inquiry should be the goal. Judgmental comments or rigidly preconceived ideas of optimal family interactions should be avoided. Appreciation of the individual path that each family takes to adjust to the new baby enriches the clinician's professional life. Members of each family should be given appropriate support while they mark their own trail.

RECOMMENDED READINGS

American Academy of Pediatrics: The pediatrician's role in family support programs. *Pediatrics* 95:781, 1995.

American Academy of Pediatrics: The role of home visitation programs in improving health outcomes for children and families. *Pediatrics* 101:486, 1998.

Barr R, McMullan SJ, Spiess H, et al: Carrying as colic therapy: A randomized controlled trial. *Pediatrics* 87:623-630, 1991.

Beck CT: The effects of postpartum depression on child development: A meta-analysis. *Arch Psychiatr Nurs* 12:12, 1998.

Brazelton TB, Koslowski B, Main M: The origins of reciprocity: The early mother/infant interaction. In Lewis M, Rosenblum L (eds): *The Effect of the Infant on Its Caregiver.* New York, John Wiley & Sons, 1974, p 59.

Cooper PH, Murray L: Postnatal depression. *BMJ* 20:316, 1998.

Dixon S: Helping siblings adjust to the new baby. *In* Jellinek M, Patel BP, Froehle MC (eds): *Bright Futures in Practice: Mental Health,* vol 2, *Tool Kit.* Arlington, VA, National Center for Education in Maternal and Child Health, 2002.

Klaus MH, Kennell JH, Klaus PH: *Bonding: Building the Foundations of Secure Attachment and Independence.* Reading, MA, Perseus Books, 1995.

Murray L, Cooper PJ: *Postpartum Depression and Child Development.* New York, Guilford Press, 1997.

Olson A, Dietrich A, Prazar G, et al: Two approaches to maternal depression screening during well child visits. *J Dev Behav Pediatr* 2005 (in press).

Seidman D: Postpartum psychiatric illness: The role of the pediatrician. *Pediatr Rev* 19:128, 1998.

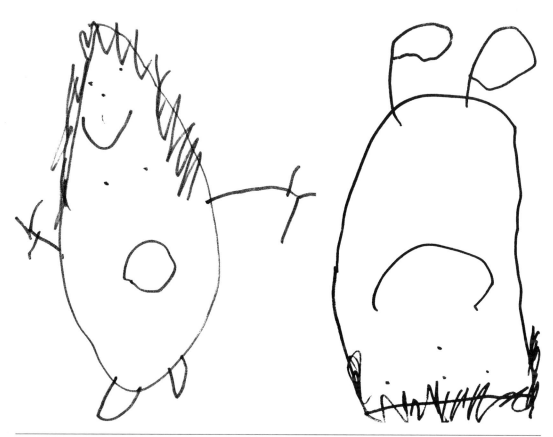

A 4-year-old draws his parents topsy-turvy. Many families feel that way with the arrival of a new child.

CHAPTER 10

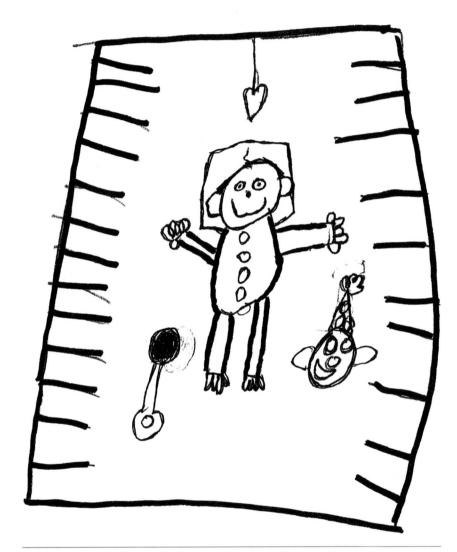

"My brother in a crib." By Abby Roberts, age 6.

One to Two Months: Getting On Track

MARTIN T. STEIN

This chapter reviews the interactions between early infant feeding patterns and the environment. Expectations for normal physical development and the determinants of inadequate growth across childhood are examined. Specific types of infant behavior (crying and night awakening) and maternal characteristics (breastfeeding and postpartum depression) are explored. The role of the clinician in ensuring adequate growth throughout childhood is discussed in the context of parent-child interactions and family relationships.

Key Words

- **Nutrients and Nurturance**
- **Consistency of Care**
- **Crying/Infant Colic**
- **Psychosocial Deprivation and Growth Failure**
- **Catch-up Growth**
- **Father's Adaptation**
- **Physical Growth**

The first few months of life are not a dress rehearsal—it's the real thing.
IRVING HARRIS

Cody's mother hovered anxiously over the scale as the nurse weighed the baby. She wanted to be sure she got the number right to place in the baby book. She asked the nurse if she should start cereal, especially to get the baby to sleep all night. Note: this is a **teachable moment**. The nurse recognizes the mother's anxiety about weight gain, helps her understand her baby's growth by showing her the growth chart and points out that her milk provides all the nutrition the baby needs at this time. She adds that feeding solid foods will not help the baby sleep longer; a note for the pediatrician is written on the chart to address this concern.

FOCUS OF DEVELOPMENTAL WORK

The period of an infant's life bounded at one end by the first month and at the other by the third month represents a transitional time. Having adjusted in the neonatal period (including postpartum physiological changes and the new extrauterine environment of the family), the second month of life is often a settling-in time for the infant and parents. Physical growth takes on new importance. As the face fills out, the chin "doubles up" and the thigh folds multiply, the baby's rapid growth organizes the parents' attention on feeding and growth measurements. Feeding the baby consumes much of the mother's time; concern about adequacy of the infant's diet occupies much of her thoughts.

The moments just before, during and after meals provide opportunities for optimal social and verbal interactions. By the middle of the second month, the parents recognize the infant's ability to smile in response to their smiles. Mutual gaze becomes a powerful form of social interaction. More frequent periods of visual attention and the onset of reproducible cooing sounds join the development of a reciprocal social smile in pulling parents into an infant's world. When feeding is managed in a secure setting and the parent is emotionally available for social interactions, physical and psychological growth move forward together. Nurturance in both the physical and psychological domains tracks together.

These early developmental strides are associated with postnatal structural maturation of the brain. Pediatric clinicians are familiar with the rapid growth in brain volume at this time; head circumference increases by 5 cm during the first 3 months of life, the most rapid period of postnatal brain growth. Formation of new synapses (synaptogenesis) occurs especially in the motor and visual cortex. Cortical maturation leads to inhibition of the more primitive brainstem functions. A spontaneous smile emerges. Maturation of the visual cortex precedes a reciprocal social smile that develops at 6 to 8 weeks of age. As the infant becomes less dependent on brainstem mechanisms, crying gradually becomes responsive to cortical control and environmental input.

Postnatal experience markedly alters brain development. The synaptic connections that are forming after birth are shaped and controlled by the infant's early experience. Adequate caloric intake and a steady flow of visual, auditory, tactile and proprioceptive stimuli act together to enhance early development of the brain. Nurturance on all levels is the theme here.

Meeting the infant's nutritional needs for appropriate physical growth requirements becomes the work of this period of infancy. Biological and environmental conditions may have an impact on either the quality of the feeding experience (e.g., difficult temperament, infant colic, maternal depression, family emotional conflict) or the outcome (e.g., failure to thrive). During this early postnatal period, clinicians become aware of the sensitive interplay between mother-child interactions, the home environment and physical growth. The positive effects of a nurturing environment or its absence are social-emotional markers for adequate growth. In addition, *consistency of care* is a critical component for successful early growth. Although it is usually the baby's mother who provides this consistency, a supportive family and a knowledgeable, available clinician add to success.

GROWTH ASSESSMENT

From birth until the age of 6 months, infants experience the most rapid rate of growth of their lives (with the exception of fetal growth) (Fig. 10–1). Several decades ago, doubling of birthweight occurred by 5 months of age; today, it is not uncommon to record a twofold increase in birthweight before the fourth month. For a breastfeeding infant, the expected weight gain from about 2 weeks to 2 to 3 months should approximate 1 oz per day. Brain and linear growth is also rapid and predictable at this age. Of course, other organ systems are growing and maturing in function simultaneously.

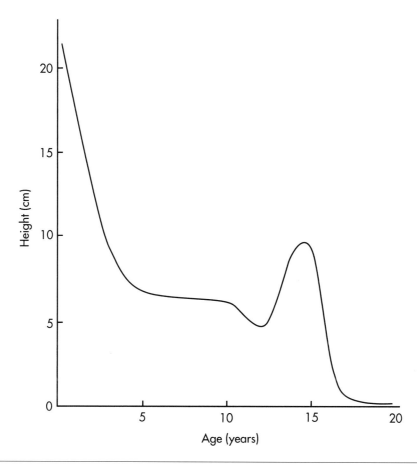

Figure 10–1 Incremental curve showing the rate of height gain. During the first years of life, the growth rate is more rapid than in other periods. (From Valadian I, Porter D: Physical Growth and Development: From Conception to Maturity. Boston, Little, Brown, 1977.)

As child health care clinicians, we monitor development as a manifestation of ongoing maturation of the central nervous system and the quality of parent-infant interactions. In the same way, physical growth can be monitored as a reflection, at one point in time, of the nutritional adequacy provided the infant and the psychological stability of the environment in which the infant grows. The growth chart reflects all of it.

From studies of emotionally neglected infants in foundling homes, a devastating effect on physical growth from less-than-optimal tactile, auditory and visual stimulation has been observed. These infants were given formula (by bottle propping) but were rarely held, spoken to or engaged visually. The effect was growth failure and an affect that appeared depressed. These infants suffered not only from caloric deprivation, but also from lack of the necessary complement of psychosocial stimulation required for optimal growth. When this condition is diagnosed early and remediated through psychosocial interventions, these infants experience catch-up growth and thrive physically and emotionally. Behavioral changes can be observed several days before the onset of weight gain, regardless of caloric intake. The body and the brain are linked in either failure or recovery.

Psychosocial deprivation and growth failure in infants remind us that adequate physical growth requires both sufficient **nutrients and nurturance**. When an infant is growing along the expected curve on a standard growth chart, it provides some degree of objective evidence that both diet and social interactions are adequate. Conversely, early signs of growth failure are clinical signals to assess not only the diet and potential organic illnesses but also the pattern of infant feeding, the temperament of the baby, the mother's psychological well-being and availability and the psychosocial condition of the family. Growth failure in early infancy has devastating effects on parental feelings of competence. The growth chart is a bit like a report card on parenting. Conversely, good growth vitalizes the whole nurturing environment. Parents see it as a positive reflection on their own care.

The behavior of a small-for-gestational-age infant and an infant who becomes underweight postnatally is altered. These infants remain hyporesponsive and stay irritable or drowsy for prolonged periods. They may show frank gaze aversion, arching, turning away or marked physiological instability. These characteristics, in turn, induce feelings of incompetency or disengagement in parents. These infants can be unrewarding for parents, even beyond the neonatal period. The acoustic characteristics of their cries differ from those of well-grown infants. Their cries are perceived as irritating by caretakers. This attitude further undermines the interaction between parents and the infant.

Standard growth curves should be used in clinical practice to assess physical growth. Accurate measurements of weight, length and head circumference (occipitofrontal measurement) are plotted on these curves at each visit, as shown in Figure 10–2. Growth curves are of tremendous value in clinical practice. They can reassure an anxious parent about the adequacy of growth. Clinicians must appreciate, however, that physical growth measurements at any one point generate a bell-shaped curve, with 5% of the normal population heavier, longer, lighter or shorter than the extremes of the charts. The infant's measurements at one time are not as significant as the rate of growth over time (i.e., the velocity of growth as reflected in the growth curve of each infant). In this way, cumulative measurements over several office visits are usually more revealing than a single measurement. The stature, weight and head circumference of the biological parents may also be helpful in interpreting the infant's growth after 6 months of age. The early growth position on the chart reflects intrauterine conditions and patterns of early feeding.

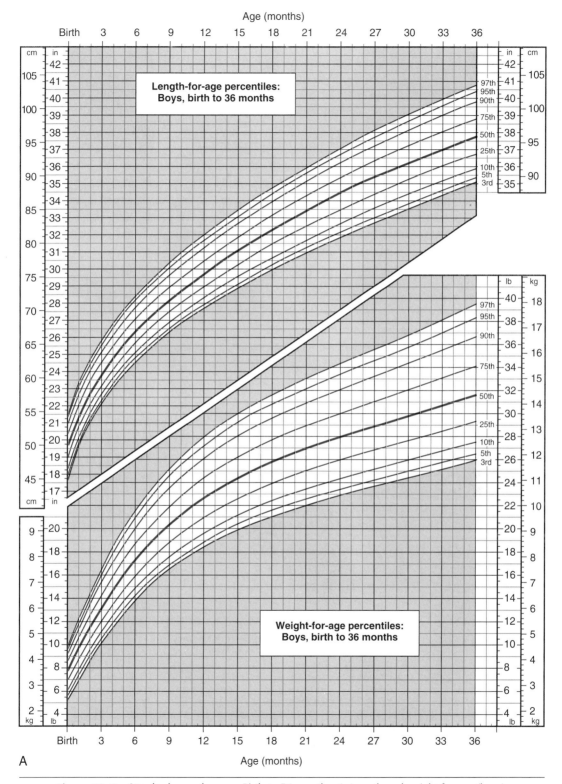

Age (months)

**Length-for-age percentiles:
Boys, birth to 36 months**

**Weight-for-age percentiles:
Boys, birth to 36 months**

A

Age (months)

Figure 10–2 Standard growth curve: Birth to 36 months. **A**, Length and weight for age (boys).

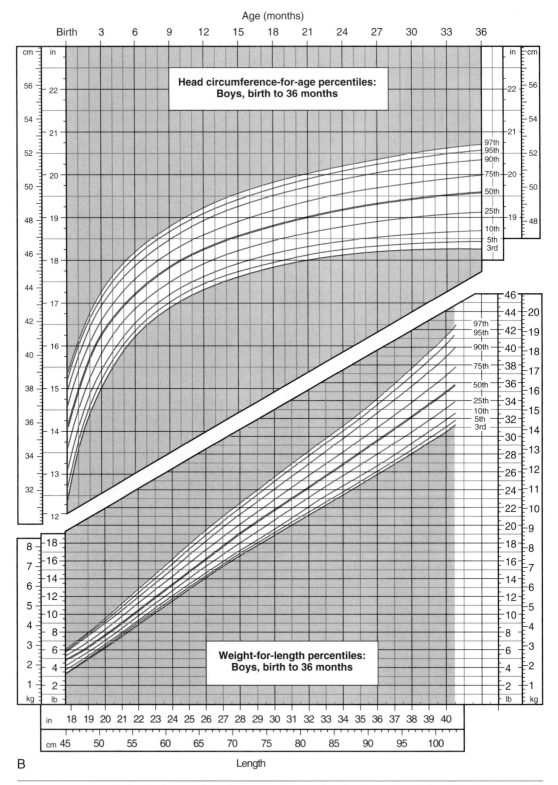

Figure 10–2 cont'd **B**, Head circumference and weight-length ratio. (From the National Center for Health Statistics in collaboration with the National Center for Chronic Disease. Prevention and Health Promotion [2000]. http://www.cdc.gov/growthcharts)

NORMAL VARIATIONS OF GROWTH IN EARLY INFANCY

Postpartum Weight Loss

Extracellular water loss may account for an 8% to 10% reduction in weight from birthweight in the immediate postnatal period. Some weight loss results from the conversion of brown fat to glucose (an energy source) and water. Generally, it is greater in breastfed than in formula fed babies and in infants born of toxemic mothers. In addition, breastfed babies may take longer to regain the weight (usually 1 week for infants receiving formula, often 2 weeks for breastfed babies). Premature babies require even longer periods to regain their birthweight; the smaller the birthweight, the longer the period of regaining. Special growth curves for preterm infants are available. Most full-term, breastfed babies surpass their birthweight before 14 days of age.

Intercurrent Illness

A brief period of illness in early infancy (e.g., gastroenteritis) is often associated with both anorexia and an increase in metabolic requirements and can thus result in a plateau in the growth curve or weight loss. In addition, a breast infection, systemic illness or postpartum depression in a lactating woman may have an adverse effect on infant growth. These maternal conditions may cause painful feedings (breast infection), decreased milk production (maternal hypothyroidism) or limited interest in nursing (depression). Too rapid a weight loss for a lactating woman means that she may not be sustaining her milk production. The effect on infant growth is the same—as the baby consumes less breast milk for any reason, the supply declines and infant growth diminishes.

An experienced mother (emergency room nurse, second child) brought her 3-month-old breastfed daughter to the office for a health supervision visit. After a normal pregnancy and delivery, the child's weight was at the 75th percentile at the 6-week examination. At the current visit, careful measurement revealed no weight gain in 2 months with normal linear and head circumference growth rates. In fact, the child looked well. Observation of nursing in the office confirmed an adequate and sustained sucking pattern.

The social history revealed that the father, previously very involved with the family, was out of town for 6 weeks on business. An 18-month-old toddler added to the burden of child care, and the mother was not sleeping well. After the results of a complete blood count, urinalysis, electrolytes, urea nitrogen and serum glutamate-pyruvate transaminase were found to be normal in the baby, the mother was instructed to supplement her breast milk with formula and to ask friends for occasional assistance with child care.

At a follow-up visit 1 week later, the baby's weight increased 1.2 oz per day in response to more frequent nursing and formula supplementation. She returned to the pediatric office the following week for another weight check and again showed gains. At this time, the mother reported that her sister, a second-year medical student, remarked that "your face looks like you have an endocrine problem." Myxedema was noted by her internist, and Hashimoto's thyroiditis with hypothyroidism was diagnosed. On thyroid replacement therapy, the mother's milk production increased and the baby thrived, now without the formula.

Box continued

Note: Postpartum thyroid dysfunction occurs in 5% of women and is vastly underdiagnosed and treated. The onset of symptoms may be subtle and overlap substantially with signs of sleep deprivation or postpartum depression. The pediatric clinician may be the only one to see the mother during this time. This case is an example of therapeutic application of the principles of "family pediatrics." Knowledge about postpartum maternal hypothyroidism and growth failure in a breastfed infant may have triggered the diagnosis by the pediatrician. Never dismiss growth failure or glibly prescribe formula without investigating the cause and planning careful follow-up.

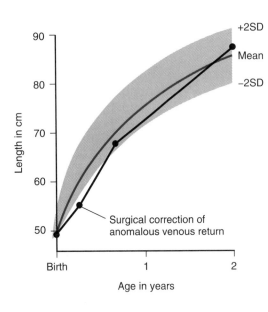

Figure 10–3 Catch-up growth after corrective surgery in a child with a congenital heart lesion associated with growth failure. (From Smith DW: *Growth and Its Disorders.* Philadelphia, WB Saunders, 1977.)

Catch-up Growth

After a period of growth failure, a healthy infant has the marvelous capacity to accelerate her growth rate during recovery. This is seen especially in the weight curve, which is most vulnerable to transient caloric depression and most adaptable by dramatic **catch-up growth**. Depressions in linear growth in infancy testify to the chronicity of the problem, thyroid disease or other long-standing organic illness (Fig. 10–3); after 6 to 12 months, growth hormone deficiency will manifest as slowed linear growth. **A child with significant prenatal (intrauterine)** growth failure may not experience catch-up growth; these children often remain small. This is particularly true of infants with a significant reduction in length for gestational age. At a later age, these prenatally growth-retarded children may respond to recombinant growth hormone therapy.

In a healthy premature infant who is not small for gestational age, postpartum catch-up growth is expected to take place (Fig. 10–4). Growth parameters in this population should be corrected for the degree of prematurity (i.e., postconceptual age for the first 2 years or up to

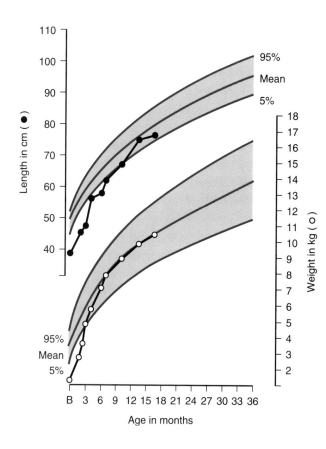

Figure 10–4 Postnatal growth curve of a 32-week appropriate-for-gestational-age premature infant. The curve demonstrates rapid catch-up growth in a healthy preterm infant.

3 years in infants born at less than 1500 g) to better assess growth velocity and relative gains in height, weight and head circumference.

Too Rapid Weight Gain

Many appropriately nourished infants in the first 6 months of life demonstrate rapid weight gain, often outstripping linear growth. They may appear chubby. Most of these infants, as long as they are not obviously overfed, will decrease their growth rate and "find" their genetic curve between 6 and 12 months of life. If an infant in this category is breastfed every 3 to 4 hours with longer periods at night (or formula-fed and consuming no more than 32 oz per day), it is appropriate to not change the diet and to reassess growth after 6 months. Even in many developing nation populations, these young infants are very "fat" by our expectations, but they eventually demonstrate a diminished rate of weight gain. This may be more normal than U.S. growth charts reflect.

Excessive weight gain is usually secondary to an intake of calories that exceeds normal growth and metabolic needs. The cause of the caloric excess may have its source in the parent (providing too much for a variety of reasons) or in the infant.

Ms. Martinez, a single mom with little experience or social support, brought her daughter in at 6 months with her head still covered, cradled in her arms. The baby's hands were covered with mitts, and she was dressed in a gown tied at the bottom. The baby weighed 22 lb and appeared pale. As soon as she whimpered, Ms. Martinez put a bottle in her mouth. Note: This mother was not aware that her baby would enjoy more open space to move and explore. Nor was she sensitive to different reasons for crying. Focused counseling about different reasons for crying and the baby's need to move and explore her surroundings resulted in a more appropriate rate of growth, as well as care in general.

Another look at the connection between overfeeding and behavior is seen in studies showing that babies rated by their mothers as temperamentally difficult and especially negative gain significantly more weight for height than other babies do. These babies are probably fed more as a way to quiet their high activity level. Iron deficiency anemia, a result of consuming an increasing amount of formula (without iron fortification) or cow's milk after 6 months, may make the child even more irritable and thereby perpetuate the cycle of overfeeding in response to crying.

SLEEP PATTERNS

Sleep-awake cycles after the first month are highly variable and dependent on the infant's temperament and satisfaction with feedings and the parents' response to periodic awakenings. This period represents a transitional time between the neonatal sleeping pattern, characterized by shorter, multiple sleep periods, and the postnatal longer sleep periods each day. Changing sleep patterns reflect central nervous system maturation after the third month (see Chapter 11). The 2–standard deviation range of maximum longest sleep time at 6 weeks of age varies from 3 to 11 hours. No wonder parents of infants with shorter sleep times seem bewildered when sharing their infants' nighttime experience with other parents!

Although a child's individual biological determinants dictate most of the variability in sleep patterns at this age, signals from the environment mediate a powerful effect. As early as 10 days of life, infants who roomed in with their mothers sleep longer at night than do those cared for in the hospital nursery.

Infants and mothers sleeping together in the same bed bring several potential benefits, such as increased total sleep time for the baby and mother, increased frequency and duration of breastfeeding at night and increased sensitivity to each other as indicated by briefly arousing to each other's movement or sounds. The sleeping environment can also have a detrimental effect on infant well-being; bed-sharing without breastfeeding combined with maternal smoking increases the risk of sudden infant death syndrome (SIDS). Other potential environmental risks of bed-sharing are a soft mattress, a couch where the infant can become trapped against the back and fall into the crevice created by a seat cushion, the baby's head being covered with a blanket and the baby slipping between the mattress and the bed frame or headboard. Parents who bed-share should be provided anticipatory guidance about these safety issues. In many cultures, both in the United States and in other countries, bed-sharing with a parent (and often with other family members) is a common practice.

Clinical studies suggest that the way a parent responds to an infant at the time of sleep induction and nighttime awakenings sets long-term patterns. Babies who are settled in a crib while partially awake learn to soothe themselves to sleep, as opposed to infants who are always nursed or rocked into a deep sleep before being placed in the crib. Associations with falling asleep may be learned at this early time. If infants experience falling asleep alone in the crib, they can reestablish that experience at predictable times of night awakening and soothe themselves back to a sleep state.

Since 1992, after review of several epidemiological studies, the American Academy of Pediatrics recommends that healthy infants be placed on their sides or backs to sleep. The data that supported this position pointed to a dramatic decrease in the incidence of SIDS associated with the "back to sleep" position. After the new recommendation, the prevalence of prone sleeping dropped from 70% in 1992 to about 20% in 2000. The SIDS rate in the United States decreased by over 50%. Other studies showed that the supine sleeping position was used less in minority populations, thus suggesting a need for focused educational programs in communities in which minority families are served. Although side and back positions are associated with a decrease in SIDS, the back position is optimal. Firm bedding, breastfeeding and avoidance of smoking are also important in SIDS reduction. Babies sleeping on their backs need to spend awake time in the prone position to strengthen arms and shoulder musculature and will also have less occipital flattening.

Positional plagiocephaly (unilateral flattening of the occiput) is a side effect of supine sleeping in some infants but is not associated with any adverse effect on brain development; most cases resolve by the second birthday. Recommendations for the prevention of occipital flattening in infants include prone positioning ("tummy time") when awake, alternating the supine head position (i.e., left and right occiput) during sleep and minimal time in a car seat when not a passenger in a vehicle.

ADAPTATION OF THE FATHER

The early infant period is an important transition in adult development for both parents (see Chapter 6). Some fathers may express a feeling that their role in the family is limited; others may restrict their contact with the baby. A physically and emotionally close feeding relationship between a mother and baby does not diminish the role of the father. Clinicians who are attentive to a father's responses may offer helpful suggestions.

After the first month when nursing is established, clinicians can point out that many fathers find pleasure and an opportunity for closeness with their babies when they take responsibility for a night feeding with either expressed breast milk or formula. Walking with the baby in an infant front carrier provides close contact. Bathing the infant followed by gentle massage with baby oil is arguably the closest physical and psychological experience for a father when compared with nursing!

INFANT COLIC

Parents are confronted with intermittent periods of fussiness in their babies at various times during the initial few months of life. Most parents describe a period of manageable irritability beginning at about 2 weeks of age, peaking between the first and second month and disappearing by 3 to 4 months. Typically, the fussy behavior begins in the late afternoon and resolves in the evening. Most parents find that if they hold, position, gently rock or feed the infant, the fussy periods resolve into comfortable sleep.

The predictability and inevitability of these events in all cultures and in varying caretaking patterns suggest that such diurnal behavior is part of normal development, probably mediated by the central nervous system. The infant wears out (as do parents!) over the course of the day and becomes increasingly unable to modulate responses to environmental stimuli. He becomes overwhelmed and needs to express that tension through crying.

Infant colic occurs in babies who are breastfed and those who are bottle fed. Boys and girls are affected equally. Premature infants may experience this behavior somewhat later in proportion to their conceptual age and may have this irritability extend to a later age. It happens in every culture in the world.

When these behavioral outbursts are either more intense or longer in duration, the term *infant colic* is used. Colic is a more severe form of the diurnal behavior seen in the majority of infants. Why certain infants at this particular age (2 to 3 weeks through 3 to 4 months) express this behavior with more intensity is unclear. Individual temperamental factors seem to be important. The intense, hyperresponsive, somewhat hypertonic infant can be spotted in the neonatal period as a likely candidate for colic. Before a diagnosis of infant colic is made, the clinician should have an appreciation for normal crying at this age. In a study of 80 infants from middle-class families, crying lasted about 2 hours daily at 2 weeks and progressed to nearly 3 hours daily by 6 weeks in normal infants. It then gradually tapered to about 1 hour daily by 3 months (Fig. 10–5). During this interval, most crying occurred in the evening. With this normal pattern in mind, Wessel's definition of infant colic is helpful. It says that "colic occurs when an infant, otherwise healthy and well fed, has paroxysms of irritability, fussiness or crying lasting for a total of more than 3 hours a day occurring on more than 3 days in any 1 week, for 3 or more weeks" (Box 10–1).

Many theories have been proposed to explain early infant colic. It was once thought to reflect maternal anxiety, but it is now clear that although severe colic may produce anxiety in parents, most cases are not caused by an overly anxious parent. Humans (especially women) are biologically programmed to respond to infant cries, regardless of individual personality differences; lack of success in calming the infant is experienced as failure. However, high-strung parents tend to give birth to high-strung infants. Colicky infants are born, not made.

Our understanding of infant temperament may provide some insight into the behavior of colicky infants. Temperament refers to an individual's behavioral style of reactivity to external events or stimuli (see Chapter 2). The normal spectrum of infant temperaments is broad. The behavior of babies with a low sensory threshold and high intensity is similar to those with colic. Babies rated by a parent at 2 weeks of age as having a "difficult" temperament were more likely to have longer and more frequent episodes of crying at 6 weeks of age.

Perhaps colic is an early infant behavior response that occurs when a baby with a susceptible, innate temperament is cared for by a parent who is less responsive (or over-responsive) to the infant's behavioral cues and may be unable to organize the caretaking environment effectively. In this context, colic is an interactional phenomenon between a baby and a parent. The acoustic characteristics and duration of an infant's cry may be viewed as a graded signal to which a parent may react with a nurturing response (relief of the infant's distress) or a non-

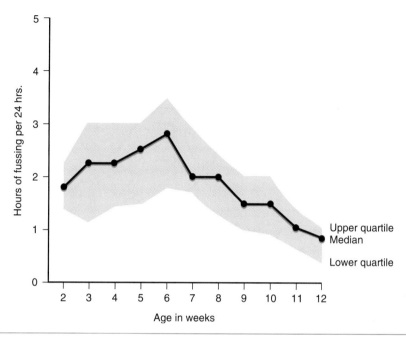

Figure 10–5 Distribution of total crying time in 80 infants from 2 to 12 weeks old; data were derived from daily crying diaries recorded by mothers. (From Brazelton TB: Crying in infancy. *Pediatrics* 29:582, 1962.)

BOX 10–1 CHARACTERISTICS OF INFANT COLIC

- Wessel's "rule of 3:" Unexpected episodes of crying lasting more than 3 hours a day, more than 3 days in a week, for more than 3 weeks
- A pattern of crying more intense and more frequent than the normal crying seen in most infants in the first 3 months
- Normal physical growth
- Usually starts in the second week and resolves at the end of the third month
- Typically occurs in late afternoon and early evening
- The duration of daily crying peaks at 6 weeks
- Occurs in breastfed and bottle fed babies
- Boys and girls equally affected
- Premature infants may have later onset in proportion to conceptual age
- Seen in all cultures

---

nurturing, avoidant response (relief of the parent's distress). Furthermore, crying patterns are culturally dependent and are related to fundamental early child-rearing principles.

Because colicky babies are observed to press their flexed hips against the abdomen during the crying episode and then pass audible flatus at the termination of the episode, it has been suggested that these babies have a form of intestinal dysmotility that produces segmental air

MOM

DAD

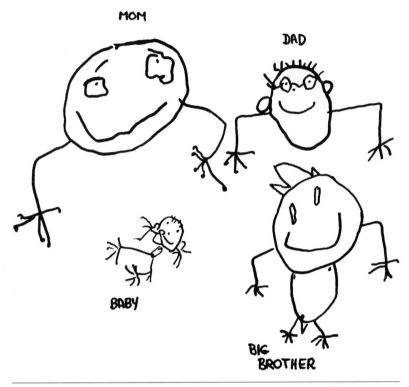

BABY

BIG
BROTHER

"Our family with our baby." By "Big Brother," age 4³/₄.

trapping secondary to autonomic dysfunction. Supporting this theory is documentation of lower colonic dysmotility in some infants. Another piece of supportive evidence is that early infant colic resolves in most cases by the end of the third month of life, which correlates chronologically with several behavioral aspects reflecting maturation of the central nervous system. For example, babies at 4 months of age show more organized sleep-wake cycles, several primitive reflexes disappear and electroencephalographic tracings reveal greater organization. It seems reasonable to assume that higher levels of central neurologic organization would be accompanied by maturation of the more primitive autonomic nervous system, which in turn might modify and regulate gastrointestinal tract motility. Research on the psychobiology of stress is beginning to describe links between different levels of reactivity and physiological responses in the cardiovascular, immunological and neuroendocrine systems. Some circulating hormones (motilin) and neurotransmitters (serotonin) that cause enterospasm have been found to be increased in colicky babies. This conceptual framework suggests that colicky infants may tend to have hyperresponsive gastrointestinal tracts that mirror their behavioral response to external stimuli.

Whatever the cause, infant colic (also known as 3-month colic) resolves by the end of the third month in almost every case. When the colic is mild to moderate, simple measures (discussed later) suffice as the parents learn to modify the behavior through various manipulations. More severe cases of colic require special attention from the child's clinician. If allowed to continue, these difficult periods of crying are taxing on parents (as well as siblings and grandparents). The potential for disrupting ongoing attachment behavior between the infant and parents exists. In this context, moderate to severe colic represents an interactional problem and requires astute clinical attention. In the presence of a vulnerable parent or caretaker, inconsolable episodes of crying may lead to the "shaken baby syndrome" (see later). In addition, crying patterns may be culturally dependent and related to fundamental child-rearing principles (Box 10-2).

BOX 10–2 CULTURAL DETERMINANTS OF CRYING IN EARLY INFANCY

"All normal human infants cry, although they vary a great deal in how much. A mysterious and still unexplained phenomenon is that crying tends to increase in the first few weeks of life, peaks in the second or third month and then decreases. Some babies in the United States cry so much during the peak period—often in excess of 3 hours a day—and seem so difficult to soothe that parents come to doubt their nurturing skills or begin to fear that their offspring is suffering from a painful disease. Some mothers discontinue nursing and switch to bottle feeding because they believe that their breast milk is insufficiently nutritious and that their infants are always hungry. In extreme cases, the crying may provoke physical abuse, sometimes even precipitating the infant's death. A look at another culture, the !Kung San hunter-gatherers of southern Africa, provides us with an opportunity to see whether caregiving strategies have any effect on infant crying. Both !Kung San and Western infants escalate their crying during the early weeks of life, with a similar peak at 2 or 3 months. A comparison of Dutch, American and !Kung San infants shows that the number of individual crying episodes is virtually identical. What differs is their length. !Kung San infants cry about half as long as Western babies, which implies that caregiving can influence only some aspects of crying, such as the duration. What is particularly striking about child rearing among the !Kung San is that infants are in constant contact with a caregiver; they are carried or held most of the time, are usually in an upright position and are breastfed about four times an hour for 1 to 2 minutes at a time. Furthermore, the mother almost always responds to the smallest cry or fret within 10 seconds. I believe that crying was adaptive for our ancestors. As seen in the contemporary !Kung San, crying probably elicited a quick response and thus consisted of frequent but relatively short episodes. This pattern helped keep an adult close to provide adequate nutrition, as well as protect the child from predators. I have also argued that crying helped an infant forge a strong attachment with the mother and, because new pregnancies are delayed by the prolongation of frequent nursing, secure more of her caregiving resources. In the United States, where the threat of predation has receded and adequate nutrition is usually available even without breastfeeding, crying may be less adaptive. In any case, caregiving in the United States may be viewed as a cultural experiment in which the infant is relatively more separated—and separable—from the mother in terms of both frequency of contact and actual distance. The Western strategy is advantageous when the mother's employment outside the home and away from the baby is necessary to sustain family resources. But the trade-off seems to be an increase in the length of crying bouts."

From Barr RG: *Natural History* 106:47, 1997.

DATA GATHERING

Observations

As you enter the examining room, observe the interaction between the infant and mother (and father, when present). If the infant is being held, observe the comfort of the mother in handling the baby.

- Does the infant seem at ease, tense?
- At the same time, observe the baby's response. Does the infant cuddle easily? Is the baby tense or responsive to the mother?
- Do the infant's posture and position appear tense with an increase in extension behavior?
- Is there evidence of visual engagement between the mother and infant?
- How does the mother talk to the baby—rhythmically and quietly or erratically and with a harsh voice?

If the baby is lying on the examining table, similar observations can be made. Does the mother maintain contact with the baby, by touching the infant or by visual contact? Alternatively, it may be important to be sensitive to the situation in which the infant has been left alone in a corner on the examining table while the mother is seated away from the infant. In this case, the clinician might want to consider whether the mother is anxious about the examination, overwhelmed by the office procedures, insecure about her mothering abilities or depressed. Careful assessment of the initial visual and verbal interactions with the mother may yield clues about how she is feeling about herself and about the infant.

The accumulation of these observations will assist the clinician in assessing the individual style, quality and intensity of the bond between the mother and infant; when the father is present, observe the way in which his presence alters the mother-infant attachment behavior. In a sense, the family's style of interactional behavior is available to you for clinical observation at this examination. These observations attain a heightened level of importance when viewed in terms of the requirements for satisfactory growth, particularly in early infancy—in other words, an emotionally nourishing bond between the young infant and its parents.

History

Table 10–1 presents questions that should be asked when taking the history and observations that should be noted during the physical examination.

MANAGEMENT AND GUIDANCE

Undernutrition

Growth failure at this age usually represents insufficient caloric intake. In breastfed infants, problems in latching on or continuously ineffective sucking are not uncommon; the correct diagnosis is usually apparent by documenting a detailed history of feeding behavior. Observing the baby feed (either by direct observation in the office or from a videotape recorded at home) may be helpful to the mother and to the clinician. Improving the mechanics of nursing often resolves the problem, such as suggesting pillow support of the baby or mother's arm, helping

TABLE 10–1 **History Taking and Examination**

History Taking	
Clinician's Question or Action	**Objective**
How is nursing (or feeding when the baby is formula fed) going?	Listen carefully to the response to this open-ended question; assess the mother's comfort with nursing; is she self-assured or does she show evidence of insecurity?
Does the baby seem satisfied at the end of a feeding? How do you feel when you are nursing?	Assess maternal satisfaction with nursing.
How often and for how long do you feed the baby? How do you know when the baby is hungry?	Assess the mother's settling in with the baby's needs and individual rhythms, as well as an estimation of the amount of milk consumed each day.
Tell me about your own diet (for nursing mothers). How much weight have you lost?	Assess a lactating mother's diet; mothers who are back to their prepregnant weight at this time may have difficulty sustaining milk supply through the anticipated increase in caloric requirement at about 2 to 3 months.
How do you manage nighttime feedings? How often and for how long is the baby fed … in a chair or in bed? Are you getting enough sleep?	Assess feeding regularity and schedule. Is the mother sleep deprived?
When the baby is formula fed, ask, "How do you prepare the formula?"	Assess the amount of milk at each feeding (calculate daily intake); assess the quantity of formula and appropriate concentration.
Can you describe your baby's personality? What is the baby like most of the time?	Assess the infant's temperament and style and the mother's attentiveness and awareness about these aspects of the baby's development.
Does the baby have a fussy time on most days? Can you describe it to me?	Assess colic-like behavior.
Do you think that your baby cries longer than most infants? What do you do when the baby cries?	Help the parent adapt to periods of difficult infant behavior; explain the expected amount of crying.
In the presence of infant colic, "What do you think causes these episodes of crying?" When appropriate, "What does your husband think?"	Assess the parent's explanatory model for the behavior; it may give a clue to the most effective therapeutic suggestion for a particular family.
Physical Examination	
Obtain accurate measurements of weight, length and head circumference plotted on standard growth curves	Assess adequacy of growth (vs. overnourished or undernourished infant); demonstrate rates of growth on chart to parent.

Table continued

TABLE 10–1   **History Taking and Examination—cont'd**

Physical Examination	
Clinician's Question or Action	**Objective**
Complete physical examination.	Although always important at a health supervision visit, performing a careful physical examination while demonstrating normal findings is particularly important to parents with a colicky baby at this age.
Assess skin texture and turgor, fat folds and state of hydration.	Evaluate nutrition.
To determine infant temperament, observe the baby at rest on the examining table and during physical examination maneuvers, when weighed and immediately following the diphtheria-pertussis-tetanus (DPT) immunization; infant temperament in response to stress can be observed.	Is this an easy baby? An overly active baby? How did the baby respond after the DPT injection? How did the mother or father respond?
If colic appears likely from the mother's history, rule out during routine physical examination the following: inguinal hernia, corneal abrasion, otitis media, or a thread wrapped tightly around a finger or toe.	Note: These are uncommon causes of paroxysmal crying at this age.

the mother encourage the infant to latch on effectively or providing a reassuring comment that it is normal for the baby to suck vigorously, followed by a brief rest period before sucking is resumed.

An insufficient milk supply may be the problem in some nursing mothers. Breast milk insufficiency may be caused by the following:

- Inadequate amount of fluid in the mother's diet—usually a minimum of 2 qt per day is required.

- Anxiety or depression—sucking during breastfeeding stimulates the maternal pituitary gland to release prolactin (a stimulant of milk production) and oxytocin (stimulates milk ejection or the "letdown" reflex). Prolactin levels are maintained by adequate breast drainage and may be diminished by maternal fatigue, stress, depression and some medications. Postpartum "baby blues" (see Chapter 9) are usually resolving around this time. Reassurance about the baby's development, coupled with frequent weight checks in the office, may be helpful. For more severely stressed or depressed nursing mothers, an appropriate mental health referral, more active involvement of the father (or other member of the extended family) or, *rarely*, formula supplementation may be appropriate. One or more of the following questions adapted from the Edinburgh Postnatal Depression Scale (see Appendix) are useful when considering postpartum depression:

Do you look forward to enjoying your baby?

Do you blame yourself unnecessarily when things go wrong?

Do you get anxious or worried when things go wrong?

Are you so unhappy that you have difficulty sleeping?

Have you been able to laugh and see the funny side of things?

- Sleep deprivation—observe for signs of fatigue, such as a tired appearance, listlessness or irritability. Always ask, "Are you getting enough sleep?" Maternal sleep deprivation is a common primary or secondary cause of milk insufficiency and growth failure. When sleep deprivation is discovered, also think about maternal depression.

- Excessive maternal weight loss—from dieting, excessive exercise or depression. Addressing the issue with compassion and knowledge may be sufficient to help the mother reorganize her lifestyle and focus on her diet or sleep-wake schedule. Reassurance about the baby's developmental progress, coupled with frequent weight checks in the office, is often helpful.

Comprehensive assessment of undernutrition in a breastfed infant includes a detailed review of the feeding schedule, evaluation of infant behavior and appearance (see Box 9–1) and examination of the mother's breasts for signs of engorgement and sore, cracked nipples. An objective office measure of the yield of breast milk during a single feeding time is available (Box 10–3).

Formula-fed babies may not be receiving enough milk at each feeding, they may be fed too infrequently or the milk may be inappropriately overdiluted. Corrective measures are simple once the problem is recognized.

With either breastfed or formula fed infants who are undernourished, it may be revealing and often therapeutic to observe the mother feeding the child in the office. Positioning of the baby, maternal-infant eye contact, comfort with feeding and the quality of the sucking mechanism are important characteristics that can be observed. Interactional difficulties can be assessed and corrected.

Less commonly, growth failure at this age is secondary to an organic disorder, either one apparent during the newborn period or one that surfaces during the history or physical examination. Laboratory assessment is seldom indicated at this age until after interactional, mechanical and nutritional problems are considered thoroughly.

Overfeeding

If the baby's weight curve is greater than 2 standard deviations above the mean, the first step is to repeat the measurements to determine their accuracy (especially length). If the data are correct and the baby looks obese, carefully review the feeding pattern of a typical day.

1. **A breastfed infant who is 1 month old is put to the breast every 2 hours** (each time she cries) for at least 12 feedings per day, each lasting 10 to 20 minutes.

Diagnosis: Overfeeding is typically the problem. However, some vigorous infants who are growing at an appropriate rate may be frequent feeders without need for intervention.

Continued

Therapy: Teach the mother other forms of soothing behavior, such as a pacifier, which can be useful after nursing has been established. "Nipple confusion" between a mother's breast nipple and an artificial nipple followed by early weaning is not supported by well-designed studies. Explain the nature and adaptive value of two different types of sucking behavior—nutritive and non-nutritive. Some babies seem to want to suck more frequently; a pacifier is very helpful in these cases. The mother may need to be taught to respond to other needs in her infant (e.g., boredom) with an expanded range of interactions. Demonstration of the use of swaddling and rocking and the use of a swing makes this a teachable moment. Assessment of the infant's temperament and the "goodness of fit" (see Chapter 2) between baby and mother may offer clues to alternative parenting responses during nursing.

2. **A large, chubby breastfed infant (95th percentile for weight) is nursed approximately every 3 to 4 hours for 10 minutes on each side at most feedings.**

Diagnosis: This apparently overweight baby is probably not being overfed. Her appetite is vigorous, and she looks big. If her length is also at or above the 95th percentile, her weight is appropriate for stature. If not, most of these breastfed infants will find their genetic growth curve (usually closer to their length curve) after 6 months.

Therapy: Reassure the mother with education about normal growth. The growth chart is an effective visual aid for parents in this situation.

3. **A formula-fed infant is consuming 40 to 45 oz each day; at 2 months she is given the bottle every 2 to 3 hours.**

Diagnosis: Overfeeding.

Therapy: Limit formula to 32 oz a day. Explain baby's nutritional requirements to the mother, along with your concerns regarding obesity. Review the concept of nutritive and non-nutritive sucking. Suggest a pacifier and other tactile soothing techniques. If the baby requires more than 32 oz of fluid a day, suggest a water supplement or, alternatively, diluting one bottle each day with water to yield 16 oz from 8 oz of formula.

Night Feedings

If you discover that the baby is awakening every 3 hours through the night, inquire how the parents respond. Parents who pick the infant up at the moment he awakes may be encouraging a long-term pattern of frequent nighttime awakenings. Point out that even a 2-month-old infant can often settle down unaided when given an opportunity. A short, fussy period will not be harmful. If necessary, a loving pat on the back while the baby remains in the crib may be sufficient to calm the child to sleep. New parents need the reassurance that brief crying periods will be neither emotionally nor physically detrimental to their baby. They will be rewarded by the knowledge that a simple behavioral intervention, initiated and sustained by them, can bring about more restful nights for the baby and parents. Parents can be taught that a young baby's cry from hunger can be distinguished from one associated with pain or the fussy cry characteristic of sleep transitions. As they learn to recognize their own infant's different cries, parents feel more comfortable letting a 2-month-old fuss for a few minutes before self-soothing behavior brings a return to sleep. On the other hand, mothers who are gone during the day and are committed to sustaining breastfeeding may choose to respond to these night wiggles and nurse the baby at that time. This is a parental choice.

BOX 10–3 OFFICE ASSESSMENT OF UNDERNOURISHED BREASTFEEDING INFANTS

Maternal Breast Evaluation

Assessment of breastfeeding should include historical information about the maternal breasts. The breasts should be inspected whenever risk factors are elicited or when adequacy of breastfeeding is in doubt.

Lactogenesis, or the onset of copious milk secretion, typically occurs 2 to 4 days postpartum. Most mothers have no difficulty recognizing the telltale signs that their milk has come in, including an increase in breast size, fullness and firmness. Rarely does lactogenesis fail to occur and infant supplementation become essential.

The leading preventable cause of insufficient milk is failure to accomplish regular, effective milk emptying once postpartum breast engorgement occurs. Many cases of insufficient lactation are associated with a maternal history of unrelieved breast engorgement during the first week. When an infant is unable to empty the breasts effectively, a rental-grade electric breast pump can preserve a mother's milk supply while effort is made to improve her baby's breastfeeding.

Once milk comes in, mothers should report that their breasts feel fuller before feedings and softer after nursing. Perceptible breast changes before and after feeding suggest that milk is being made and transferred to the infant.

Most women experience slight nipple discomfort at the beginning of feedings during the first few days of nursing. However, severe nipple pain, pain lasting throughout feedings or pain persisting beyond 1 postpartum week is atypical and suggests that the baby is not positioned correctly at the breast. Improper infant latch-on not only causes sore nipples but also impairs milk flow and leads to diminished milk supply and inadequate infant intake.

Objective Measures of Milk Yield and Infant Intake

The common practice of using clinical cues to estimate milk consumption during breastfeeding can be highly inaccurate. Several techniques are available to more precisely estimate maternal milk yield and infant milk consumption.

Determination of *infant feeding test weights* is a noninvasive, accurate method of measuring infant milk intake during a breastfeeding session. The infant is weighed under the same conditions (identically clothed) before and after nursing. The weight (in grams) before feeding subtracted from the weight after feeding equals the volume of milk consumed (in millimeters). A simplified rule of thumb for normal milk consumption in breastfed infants between 2 weeks and 2 months of age is about 1 oz of milk (28.5 mL) per hour. A relatively inexpensive, portable, user-friendly, commercial scale is available for determining accurate infant feeding test weights in the home or office.

Another option for estimating a mother's milk production is to use *a rental-grade electric breast pump to empty the breasts at a usual feeding time.* The volume of milk expressed approximates the quantity of milk available to the infant at that feeding. A pump may remove milk either more or less effectively than the baby, thereby affecting the accuracy of pumped volumes in predicting milk yield or infant intake.

Beginning around 2 weeks after birth, *the oxytocin-mediated letdown reflex becomes well conditioned, and mothers begin to experience the sensations associated with milk ejection.* Mothers typically report a "tingling," "pins-and-needles," or "tightening" sensation in their breasts in conjunction with spraying milk. The sensations usually begin shortly after the infant starts sucking, but the reflex can also be

Box continued

BOX 10-3   OFFICE ASSESSMENT OF UNDERNOURISHED BREASTFEEDING INFANTS—cont'd

triggered by hearing one's baby cry. Letdown is usually more dramatic in women with abundant milk, whereas the response is often blunted in those with diminished supplies. The letdown response can be inhibited temporarily by adrenalin.

Inspection of the maternal breast can reveal lactation risk factors, such as inverted nipples or surgical scars. Periareolar incisions for cosmetic or diagnostic breast surgery may sever lactiferous ducts and impair milk drainage. Abnormal breast development and lack of prenatal changes may be associated with insufficient lactation.

Strategies for Improving Inadequate Breastfeeding

Correct any problems identified regarding breastfeeding technique or scheduling. Improve the infant's positioning at the breast, increase the frequency of nursing if appropriate and ensure that the infant takes both breasts at each feeding.

Prescribe a rental-grade electric breast pump to augment the breast stimulation and emptying provided by the infant. Instruct the mother to pump her breasts simultaneously (using a double collection system) for 10 to 15 minutes immediately after nursing. Residual milk expressed by pump should be used to supplement the infant's sucking.

Ensure that the infant receives adequate nutrition. Use objective measures of breast milk intake (infant feeding test weights or pumped milk volumes) to estimate the quantity of formula supplement required. For malnourished babies, expect rapid catch-up weight gain, usually 2 oz a day for several days, then 1 oz a day.

Provide close infant follow-up and supervision of the feeding plan. Taper supplements *only* if objective measures confirm that the maternal milk supply has increased. All too often, infant weight falters again because supplements are arbitrarily discontinued after initial weight gain is achieved.

Have the mother continue pumping after feedings until the baby has weaned from all supplements and is gaining adequate weight with exclusive breastfeeding. Then instruct the mother to begin tapering pumping sessions over the course of a week or two.

Be willing to collaborate with the breastfeeding referral sources in your community to help your patients overcome their breastfeeding problems. Clinicians should retain their role as principal coordinator of their patients' care while using the specialized services of breastfeeding counselors and lactation centers. Other valuable resources include pump rental depots, telephone advice lines, Women, Infants and Children (WIC) agencies and mother-to-mother support groups such as the La Leche League.

Modified from Neifert M: *Early assessment of the breast feeding infant.* Marianne Neifert, MD, Lactation Program, 1719 E. 19th Avenue, Denver, CO 80218.

Supplemental Bottles

At this stage, many mothers who are nursing successfully choose to continue full-time nursing until after 6 to 12 months, as is now recommended. Supplemental feeding can be introduced when the infant can sit and learn to drink from a cup. For a variety of reasons, other mothers may choose to supplement breastfeeding with either expressed breast milk or formula in a bottle. Return of the mother to work or school, a plan to wean before the infant is ready to use a cup, the wish to have an occasional evening or afternoon out without the baby and a desire to plan for an emergency are some reasons women may have for supplementation at this time. It may be helpful to ask the nursing mother about her plans as they affect nursing. Helping her choose between expressed milk and formula, the clinician can play the role of educator rather than decision maker. When bottle supplementation is desired, waiting until after *4 or 6* weeks ensures the establishment of an adequate milk supply and gives the infant and mother enough time to form the psychological attachment and mechanical know-how to safeguard the future of breastfeeding. *What to Expect in the First Year* (see chapter references at end of book) provides detailed guidelines for supplementation, expression and storage of breast milk.

Colic ("Paroxysmal Fussing")

The following steps can assist the clinician in treating an infant with colic:

1. Begin with *reassurance,* when appropriate, that the findings of the baby's physical examination are normal. Narrating your normal findings for the parents as you examine each body part may be particularly reassuring, such as "the intestinal examination is normal, the bowels feel fine and all the organs in the tummy feel as they should."

2. Discuss *"fussiness" and crying at this age in terms of normal patterns of behavior.* A parent with a colicky baby may find it helpful to see the infant as a variation of what is expected rather than as someone who is abnormal. Showing a parent the graph in Figure 10–5 will support the concept of normal variation for some doubting parents.

3. Assist in the *alleviation of parental anxieties* that may be exacerbating the paroxysms of crying. Suggesting a time-off afternoon for the mother and brief naps during the day when the baby is sleeping may be helpful.

4. Recognize parents who may have limits on their own self-control and who may misinterpret persistent crying. *A frequent antecedent to the shaken baby syndrome is prolonged crying in a healthy infant.* The National Center on Shaken Baby Syndrome developed the pneumonic "PURPLE" as a useful educational tool to inform parents (see Box 10–4).

5. *Prevent overstimulation of the baby.* Parents of a colicky baby may be doing too much with the baby, such as too frequent feeding or picking up. Consider the following interventions:

   - Teach soothing behavior, such as swaddling, gentle rocking or use of a pacifier.
   - Demonstrate to the mother that her fussy infant can be soothed by holding the baby parallel to the floor and gently and slowly moving him back and forth; this may be enlightening.
   - White noise (a hair dryer or vacuum cleaner) placed near the crib is found helpful by some parents.
   - A mechanical swing may soothe some of the most fussy infants.
   - Formula change is almost never helpful; these babies are not allergic or intolerant of various formulas for the most part. Even the act of changing a formula may result in the mother seeing her infant as more vulnerable. A double-blind crossover study demonstrated that any initial decrease in colic after elimination of cow's milk diminished rapidly and that only infrequently was the effect reproducible. Lactose intolerance is rare at this age. Whether allergic reactions to breast milk occur is

BOX 10–4   THE COLOR PURPLE (MNEMONIC: AN EDUCATIONAL TOOL FOR PARENTS TO PREVENT THE SHAKEN BABY SYNDROME)

P—Peak pattern: crying peaks around 2 months
U—Unpredictable: crying can come and go unexpectedly with no apparent reason
R—Resistant to soothing: crying continues despite soothing efforts of caregivers
P—Pain-like face: healthy infants can look like they are in pain when crying even though they are not
L—Long bouts: crying can go on for 30 to 40 minutes and longer
E—Evening crying: crying occurs more often in the afternoon and evening

Parent Action Steps to Prevent Shaken Baby Syndrome
1. Discover ways to comfort baby: carry-walk-talk responses to crying.
2. If crying persists and you get frustrated, it's okay to put the baby down in the crib and walk away for a brief time.
3. Never shake or hurt your baby.
4. More information for parents: www.dontshake.com.

controversial. Some nursing babies seem to improve when cow's milk is removed from the mother's diet. Other studies have not supported such an association.

- Occasionally, elimination of caffeine, chocolate (xanthine) or stimulant medications consumed by the nursing mother will alleviate episodes of colic. Maternal use of fluoxetine has also been associated with excessive crying.

- Reflux esophagitis as a cause of intermittent fussiness and crying should be considered when symptoms occur after meals. It is an unlikely diagnosis when the crying pattern is diurnal, as seen in infant colic.

- Many of these interventions have not been studied extensively. They are part of the folklore for colicky babies and seem to help (parent, baby or both) in some cases. Two recent reports demonstrate the creativity and caution found in treatment studies:

    When parents played a recording of a baby's favorite music, gave extra attention to the baby at quiet, calm times and turned the music off and left the room briefly at the start of a crying episode, crying was significantly decreased in colicky babies.

    Babies without colic whose parents were instructed to hold them for an extra 2 hours each day cried significantly less than a control group of babies; when the same research team conducted a randomized, controlled trial of extra carrying time as a form of colic therapy, increased carrying was not effective.

6. *Review feeding practices.* Encourage quiet feeding times when the mother is comfortable with herself and the baby. This may require a darkened room away from the center of activity in a busy house or apartment. Babies who are nursed more frequently overall show significantly less crying and fretting behavior of the episodic or colicky type.

7. *Medication should not be used as a treatment of infant colic.* One exception is for the most severe cases of infant colic in which the baby's behavior has produced a significant level of parental tension that threatens healthy, trust-building interactions between the child and parents. These situations may be apparent before the office visit as a result of frequent telephone calls about crying and feeding dysfunction. Before medication is

used, the measures discussed earlier should have been tried. The use of a mild sedative or antispasmodic preparation for a brief period (a few days to 1 week) in this situation serves to temporarily break the cycle of a crying baby leading to tense parents leading to a dysfunctional family. It may allow the parents a period of rest and an opportunity to try out other soothing behavior with a more comfortable infant. A medication that may be used is hyoscyamine sulfate (Levsin), four to six drops three or four times daily. It should be emphasized that although rare cases are suitable for a brief course of medicine, the majority of fussy babies should not receive medication. Sedatives and dicyclomine should never be prescribed, and simethicone is not more helpful for colicky babies than a placebo.

8. *A positive and optimistic approach is required and beneficial.* Parents must be told that the baby is normal. Some measures can be tried, and improvement and resolution will occur. In all but the most severe cases, this conservative approach is rewarded by improvement. It often means that the parents have discovered new ways to relate to and settle their baby. Frequent follow-up telephone calls are essential, usually helpful and serve to enhance the therapeutic relationship.

The time invested in a colicky infant and the family is well worth it. The parents will come to understand that this intensity is part of their own infant's style and that this characteristic is one that the child must learn to handle. They must be taught to respect and appreciate their infant's vitality, vigor and excitement. If these broader perspectives are not achieved at this juncture, a colicky infant will come back to haunt the clinician in another guise (sleeping, feeding or discipline issues).

But what am I?
An infant crying in the night:
An infant crying for the light:
And with no language but a cry.
　　—LORD ALFRED TENNYSON (1809–1892)
IN MEMORIAM

QUICK CHECK—1 TO 2 MONTHS

- ✓ Hands becoming open, unfisted most of the time
- ✓ A tonic neck peaks at 6 weeks and then decreases
- ✓ Head up in the prone position
- ✓ Symmetrical motor movements, arms and legs when the head is in the midline
- ✓ Visual tracking to 180 degrees horizontally, briefly vertically
- ✓ Alerts to pleasant sounds
- ✓ Cooing sounds
- ✓ Spontaneous smile
- ✓ More awake time during the day; moving the longest sleep time to night
- ✓ Alert periods increase in length and predictability
- ✓ At 6 weeks, the range of the longest sleep time is 3 to 11 hours

HEADS UP–1 TO 2 MONTHS

- *A full-term newborn*, determined by examination of gestational age (38 to 42 weeks), who weighs less than 2500 g or is less than 45 cm in length is small and has suffered intrauterine growth retardation. Linear growth depression reflects second trimester growth failure. Absolutely or relatively underweight babies with normal length have usually experienced late gestation weight loss as a result of placental insufficiency from one or more causes.
- *Small-for-gestational-age babies* who have the genetic capacity to catch up to the normal range usually show accelerated growth in the first 6 months. Failure to show catch-up growth in the first 6 months generally means that growth will continue at a slow rate. Examples might include children with alcohol-related neurodevelopmental disorder, congenital infection and maternal hypertension.
- *Postpartum weight loss: up to 8% to 10% of birthweight.* Breastfed infants regain birthweight by 2 weeks, formula-fed infants by 1 week.
- *After the reacquisition of birthweight*, most babies will grow at approximately 1 oz per day. Weight increases much greater than 1 oz per day are often associated with overweight infants or those undergoing catch-up growth. Weight gain that is less than 0.5 oz per day is usually inadequate. Premature infants (less than 38 weeks' corrected age) may sustain weight gain velocities consistent with expected intrauterine growth, higher than those of infants beyond 40 weeks' conceptual age.
- *A head circumference* of less than 32 cm in a full-term newborn represents microcephaly; more than 38 cm represents macrocephaly. Evaluations should follow from these determinations.
- *Head circumference measurements* in the first 6 months of life typically conform to the following pattern of growth: birth to 2 months, 1 cm per 2 weeks; 3 to 6 months, 1 cm per month.
- *Breastfed infants who have a decelerated growth rate* after 1 month should draw attention to maternal diet and rapid maternal weight loss during this time (i.e., dieting, illness or strenuous exercise).
- Occasionally, a baby with a *head circumference* in the usual or upper range at birth rapidly crosses percentile lines in the first few months and is at or above the 95th percentile. When this curve is maintained in the absence of any evidence of increased intracranial pressure, it usually represents familial macrocephaly, a benign, dominantly inherited condition. Measurement of parental head circumference will suggest the diagnosis.
- Maternal hypothyroidism and postpartum depression have many similar symptoms at this time.
- Young infants are at the highest risk for shaken baby syndrome in the first 3 months. Unsupported, stressed families and irritable infants are at greatest risk.
- Any emerging motor asymmetry is abnormal and suggests an upper motor neuron problem (possible perinatal stroke) or a previously undetected peripheral nerve injury.
- Any dysconjugate eye movements should be transitional; fixed strabismus needs evaluation.

RECOMMENDED READINGS

For Clinicians

American Academy of Pediatrics: Changing concepts of sudden infant death syndrome: Implications for infant sleep environment and sleep position. *Pediatrics* 105:650, 2000.

Barr RG, Hopkins B, Green JA: *Crying as a Sign, a Symptom, & a Signal: Clinical, Emotional and Developmental Aspects of Infant and Toddler Crying.* London, Cambridge Press, 2000.

Carey WB, McDevitt SC: *Coping with Children's Temperament: A Guide for Professionals.* New York, Basic Books, 1995.

Jellinek MS: *Bright Futures in Practice: Mental Health.* Washington, DC, National Center for Education in Maternal and Child Health, 2002.

Shonkoff J, Phillips D (eds): *From Neurons to Neighborhood: The Science of Early Child Development.* National Research Council, National Academic Press, 2000.

Stein MT, Colarusso CA, McKenna JT, Powers NG: Cosleeping (bedsharing) among infants and toddlers. *J Dev Behav Pediatr* 18:408-412, 1997.

For Parents

Ferber R: *Solve Your Child's Sleep Problems.* New York, Fireside Books, 2004.

Murkoff H: *What to Expect the First Year,* 2nd ed. New York, Workman Publishing, 2003.

National Center on Shaken Baby Syndrome: *http://www.dontshake.com/.*

Weissbluth M: *Healthy Sleep Habits, Happy Child.* New York, Ballantine Books, 1999.

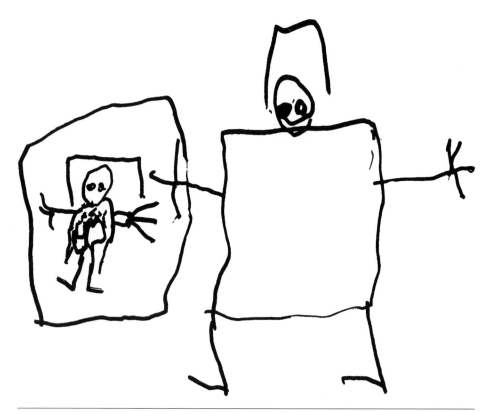

"Dad goes to comfort baby in cradle." By Colin Hennessy, age 4.

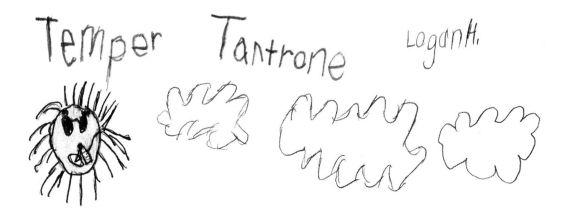

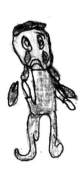
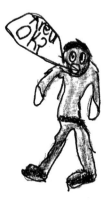

An older boy captures the spectacle of a temper tantrum in a younger family member. Even the sun has on blinders. By L. H.

CHAPTER 11

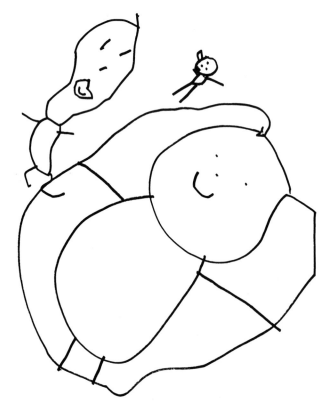

"Happy baby on a blanket with family all around." By Katherine Boucher, age 4½. Clearly the baby's presence is large and everyone is gathered around.

Three to Four Months: Having Fun with the Picture Book Baby

SUZANNE D. DIXON

This chapter examines the role of social interactions in early child development. The importance of learning how to play interactive games as a core prompt to cognitive and emotional development is explored. The profound impact of maternal depression on the development of a child is discussed. The emergence of night awakenings at this age and across early childhood is explained.

Key Words

- Night Awakenings
- Social Interaction
- Games
- Maternal Depression
- Sleep Organization in Infancy
- Social Play
- Spoiling
- Smiling
- Temperamental Differences

Mrs. Martin brings her 3-month-old daughter Anna in and asks what formula to buy for the infant. She was previously breastfeeding but says that the baby doesn't like to nurse any more. She is tearful and says she wonders if it is time she went back to work. She is also concerned because everyone in the supermarket comes up to play with the baby, and he will not go to sleep when they get home; "the whole day gets messed up." She says she has not been sleeping well herself, but the baby "gets along fine without her" all night long. Anna smiles broadly, waves her arms and pulls the clinician into a nuzzle. Note: This case demonstrates the huge neurobehavioral shifts that occur at about 3 months and make the baby a different person. It requires an essential shift in parenting from the early days at home.

A child 3 to 4 months of age is a delightful, cherubic, engaging creature. A big shift in responsiveness, an expanded behavioral repertoire, social needs and a real personality serve to draw people into interaction with her. A decrease in reflex-determined behavior and more predictability in routine should free up everyone for the next level of parenting, which includes real social interaction and play. If a mother isn't going along with this shift or isn't having real fun with a baby this age, something is off track. Parents should be enjoying the baby, and this should be a delightful visit for the clinician. If this one isn't fun, there are problems here. An emphasis on the importance of play and social interaction should be the main focus of this visit.

SLEEP PATTERNS

By the third or fourth month, the state organization and the wake-sleep cycles of the child have shown increased stability and reliability. Most infants have shifted their longest sleep time to nighttime hours and have developed reasonably set nap times. This may be called "sleeping through the night," although a 5- to 6-hour stretch is more usual. Most children do not require a night feeding at this age and can learn ways to settle themselves. Routines for settling to sleep have usually developed between the child and parents, and this predictability gives parents a sense of competence, as well as less fatigue. The child, if left alone, can usually settle back to sleep after the periodic awakenings that occur every $1\frac{1}{2}$ to 3 hours during sleep times. Individual, biologically determined differences are now manifested in these sleep patterns: some children are short sleepers and some are long sleepers. They are likely to maintain these characteristics through the life span. An infant at this age usually has two to four naps per day, gradually moving toward two naps throughout the first year and consolidating to one regular nap per day from 18 to 36 months, or longer if a strong environmental push to a nap at midday exists. This pattern varies a lot. Total sleep time, including nighttime and naptime, decreases gradually across toddlerhood, but the actual amount varies from child to child. As kids give up naps, their nighttime sleep increases. Sleep at this stage of infancy is less automatic than it was earlier, and its patterns are now altered by care practices. This neurological change means that the family is at a critical juncture at which parents have choices about where and when their child sleeps.

Regularity in the environment helps with sleep organization; a regular bedtime, a regular ritual and clear expectations are helpful throughout childhood, beginning now, in facilitating good sleep organization (Box 11–1).

Premature infants, even those without serious perinatal complications, will have less regular sleep and will be more difficult to quiet throughout the first year. Some active children are predictably wiggly at night, and others have a pattern of difficulty settling to sleep. These children need a little more support from the environment, but *not* qualitatively different interventions. Good sleep hygiene applies to all.

Ms. Johnson comes in looking very tired, complaining that she just can't get Aidan "on a schedule" like her other kids were at his age. He's now 5 months old, but he was a 34-week preemie with an easy course during a 3-week postnatal hospitalization. He still wakes up frequently at night. His weight gain and development have otherwise caused no concern. Mom still feeds him several times at night. Note: Individual differences are prominent within as well as between families. A lingering sense of vulnerability on mom's part may prompt her to feed Aidan more frequently and respond more readily to each little wiggle. Neurology and psychology nest in this situation. Part of mom's frustration may be that many parents regard "sleeping through the night" as a measure of their own competence. It is not.

BOX 11–1   ASSISTING SLEEP ORGANIZATION FOR YOUNG INFANTS

- Put the infant to bed when he is drowsy, not fully asleep, so that he gets used to fully settling himself.
- Don't feed an infant to sleep. Otherwise he'll expect room service all night long.
- Put the infant to sleep where you want him to sleep all night long. Falling asleep in one place and trying to get back to sleep in another is confusing.
- Be consistent as possible with sleep times and places. Start a routine.
- Don't respond to the baby's every whimper at night. Give him a chance to settle back down on his own.
- Make your evenings calm and relaxing.
- Examine your own nighttime behavior. Does your vigorous handling and talk give the infant the idea that it's play time? Calm, quiet responses are best. Avoid lifting the infant out of the bed if he sleeps on his own.
- Awaken the infant after a 2-hour nap and awaken from all naps after 4 PM.
- Be generous with a bedtime feeding, but limit middle-of-the-night feedings (unless you are consciously strengthening breastfeeding with nighttime nursing). This is a type of trained night wakening.
- If you cosleep with an infant, he'll expect that every night. Discuss your plans with your partner because consistency is what the baby needs. Make a plan. Never cosleep if drugs or alcohol is involved.
- If the infant is an early riser but sleeps 6 hours or more, consider a later bedtime. Shift gradually, 30 minutes earlier every 5 days or so.

Up at Night

Sleep is usually disturbed by periodic awakening at all ages. Some children are able to quietly settle themselves back to sleep without awakening their parents. These children are said to sleep through the night. Individual differences exist in children, in parents, in families, in household layouts and schedules and even in cultural expectations. In the United States, we usually expect infants to demonstrate substantial independence in the matter of sleeping. Being awakened by an infant at night is a violation of these expectations, of the infant and the parent, who it is felt should be able to get bedtime organized. Therefore, infants who do not "sleep through the night" are viewed as defective, or at least developmentally delayed, and certainly as a source of stress, if not a sign of "parenting failure." In other cultures, where schedules are more fluid and independence is not a goal in child rearing, "sleep problems" do not exist. **Night awakenings** are the usual occurrence in all groups because awakenings are biologically based. The introduction of solid food *does not* result in longer sleep times. Most infants by 3 to 4 months of age do not *need* to be fed during the night to maintain nutrition, although many of them and their parents may choose to provide nighttime feedings. Parents can prolong the awakening and sustain this pattern of waking others by responding with an elaborate interaction with the infant at that time. Talk, activities and game playing will all communicate to the infant that this is a time for play. Quiet comforting, perhaps a quiet feeding, dim lights and silent rhythmic soothing (e.g., patting, rocking) will signal the infant that this is the time to sleep.

Sleep at 3 to 4 months of age becomes more vulnerable to outside disturbances (e.g., the telephone ringing). The excitement of the day's activities may infiltrate sleep time, so settling in for the night or staying asleep may be a new problem when there is a change in routine or household excitement.

Some parents who do not get enough time alone with their infants during the day may choose, consciously or unconsciously, to use the night as a private time to get and stay close. For working parents, those without partners or parents who've experienced a lot of loss, this is likely to be a separation they cannot stand. They must be willing to invest the time to quiet the infant back down and to realize that this will be an expectation of the infant every night. Inconsistency on their part will make it hard for the child to organize his own behavior.

Cosleeping with infants is common at this age. This may be the *least* disruptive pattern for some families to manage sleep and is very common, even into the toddler years. Cautions about soft bedding and cosleeping while under the influence of drugs or alcohol must be discussed. Some clinicians advise against cosleeping to avoid rollover deaths, although others feel that the risk is overstated. Safe bedding and no alcohol or drugs should be present.

Some parents may choose to maintain breast milk supply through a pattern of nighttime feedings, which are thought to be even more important to the physiology of lactation. Each family must decide a sleep management plan with each child. The clinician should offer information on infancy sleep issues and options and should support families in the development of their own solutions. Questions about what's been going on sleep-wise up to now and the sleep traditions and expectations of the family and the culture are important. The clinician should find out the sleep goals for each so that assistance can be given to reach these goals. This leads to the important choices parents have at this juncture. The age of 4 months is the time to highlight this decision point because a change in pattern will be much more difficult later. A prescriptive approach is to be avoided, but a choice will be made, either actively or by default (see Box 11–1). Consistency in the expectations and the environment is the key from the child's perspective.

READY FOR PLAY

Neurological Maturation

The central nervous system changes occurring at this time prompt both shifts in sleep and new social skills. Increases in myelination, synaptogenesis (the establishment of connections between neurons with the formation of new synapses) and maturation of the electro-encephalogram attest to these processes. Increases in the mobility of the lens in the eye and better optic muscle control mean that the baby can see and track a person close up and across the room. She can watch her own hands and their actions in the environment while experimenting with distance, size and depth perception. Refinements in vocalization and facial movements allow a wider range of emotional expressiveness. As noted psychologist Hans Papousek has stated, there is "a marked qualitative change in higher nervous function at the third month." This new organizational level enables the child to interact with the family in new and elaborate ways.

Cognitive Growth

New cognitive skills are evident in the infant's ability to momentarily delay gratification and to make linkages in life events. For example, a child of 3 months will stop crying when placed in the nursing position and may hold back on vigorous sucking at the breast for a few minutes until milk letdown begins, content in the anticipation of the reward. The infant may smile while being eased into a front pack, linking that event to an expected adventure, and may flex the hips readily when placed on a changing table. All such behavior indicates that the child has been mentally active in assimilating events that occur consistently. He is observing patterns of association and can anticipate and wait. This behavior can be observed easily during dressing, feeding or a play session.

Social Skills

The human drive for **social interaction** is never more obvious than in the behavior of a 3-month-old infant. The presence of people is more compelling than any other phenomenon. A 2-month-old infant participates in social exchanges; a 3-month-old can actively *initiate* the interaction with wiggles, smiles and soft cooing—a whole range of social behavior. The infant draws people into play because that is the fuel for his development.

> Marisa is in her infant seat as you enter the examination room. After a brief, wary look and a subtle startle, she gives you a big grin and some delighted wiggles. She stares at you intensely as you move closer. As you reach for her, she puts her head and arms forward in anticipation of being picked up. Note: This observation of less than 5 seconds allows you to appreciate these core developmental gains at this age.

Although studies of parent-infant interactions confirm that infants know their specific parents from the earliest weeks of life, a 3-month-old infant offers very dramatic testimony even to the most skeptical parent. At this age, the child will visually search a room until he finds familiar care providers, will move all extremities in excitement and will arch forward with outstretched arms to urge them to notice, talk and touch him. Even a temperamentally quiet infant will stop all activity and increase visual regard in his parents' presence. Vocalizing in different ways, such as squeals, laughs and phony coughs, serves to initiate and sustain an interaction. A 3-month-old has a whole new series of facial expressions to indicate an expanded range of emotional responses and individual personality: pouting, coyness, disgruntlement, teasing, wariness, appearing to be insulted, fearful, bored and so forth. The infant explores the caregivers' faces through looking at their facial components and then swipes, pokes and pulls toward them. Parents' clothes, hair, glasses and skin offer new, safe opportunities to explore the most important part of the environment, the family.

The Game

In an interactive setting, an infant has incredible abilities to respond to subtle behavior (e.g., glances away for fractions of a second) or underlying emotional tones (e.g., frustration, tension).

A baby is like a sponge for the emotional tones of the environment. This awareness and sensitivity set the stage for more complex patterns of interaction. The development of "the game" as a concept is strong at this age and is a foundation for later cognitive and emotional growth. A child learns how to prompt and respond to reliable exchanges with the caregiver. Finding the world predictably responsive is the key at this age. Verbal, tactile, vestibular and motor games are the elements through which the child learns about affecting the behavior of others and that his own behavior has meaning and effectiveness. The infant is developing a sense of self through seeing the results of his actions on people and objects. Social game interactions, delivered in the context of caretaking and as individual as the players involved, are the main event of the infant's day. Responsive caretaking is essential for cognitive and emotional growth. The infant needs ready partners for all these games, day in and day out. There's no idle chit chat here; it's all essential for development.

Rhythms, styles, content of games and the intensity of interactions vary across individuals, socio-economic groups and cultures and subcultures, but the basic pattern of game playing with its reciprocal nature, mutually regulated, seems to be a universal pattern of human development.

Infants work hard at **social play**. They are motivated to attend to the social behavior around them and modify their own behavior in response. Familiar people call forth the most attention; unfamiliar adults elicit wariness, an initial unbroken gaze, a tentative bright smile and then avoidance behavior such as gaze aversion and head turning. A baby will make new relationships with regular interaction, so this is a good time to introduce alternative care providers. A baby will hook new adults into a relationship at this age without the stranger anxiety that will come later. Any caretaker should be attentive to the baby in this need for social interaction, as well as for care. The caretaker should be physically nurturing, promptly attentive and constant. Rarely can a caregiver provide that while caring for four or more infants, which is what occurs in some daycare settings.

Maternal Depression and Altered Interaction

Infants who do not experience this contingent responsiveness have an altered developmental course, either temporarily or permanently. Depressed moms are unable to respond to their infants, and the babies' behavior offers quick testimony to this missing component of their lives. These infants smile less, frown more and are more withdrawn and less responsive. This sparse interactional pattern carries over to their behavior with nondepressed adults (e.g., health care providers). Infants of depressed mothers are at risk for developmental compromise because this reciprocal interaction is not available, some or all of the time.

Maternal depression may be the final common pathway of developmental morbidity in circumstances of poverty, family stress, economic decline and other difficulties; these conditions are known to have an adverse effect on a child's development. Conversely, even depressed moms can learn how to be more responsive in play interactions, and the babies can show behavioral recovery through better eye contact and decreased distress. These observations make it vital to identify and intervene with a parent and infant who are not having fun with each other. Joy in the interaction is a vital observation; its absence is a signal for prompt intervention. This is probably the core evaluation to be done at this stage of infancy.

Mrs. Neilson is in a chair by the window in the exam room while her daughter is in an infant seat on the exam table. Mom's face is flat as she says she has no concerns or questions about the baby, that everything is going fine. The baby also has a flat expression and an intense stare as you begin to examine her. She's not very active during the exam and is very still when you pick her up at your shoulder. When she cries, mom quickly puts a bottle in her mouth. You notice that the baby's weight is above the 95th percentile, her length is at the 50th and there is occipital flattening. Mom would like to be sure that the Women, Infants and Children (WIC) form is filled out. You can't wait to get on to the next patient.

Note: Both mother and baby are depressed. Your own reaction is a good indicator of this altered emotional climate. Pay attention to it. Something's very wrong here, and an intervention is needed promptly. "I notice that you seem a bit down today" or a similar inquiry will start a discussion of this child's greatest developmental risk factor: maternal depression.

"Spoiling" Baby

For game playing to be successful and mutually enjoyable and to meet the infant's needs for responsive caretaking, some elements are required. The adult must be convinced that these affectionate interchanges are worthwhile. Playing with the infant and holding, massaging, moving, talking to and nuzzling her are not "**spoiling**" the child (i.e., making the infant more dependent or demanding). Babies at this age don't act with premeditation to manipulate and can't disobey. In fact, the more that caregivers play with the baby, the more the infant will learn ways to amuse herself. Play is a way of learning, building basic trust and improving self-esteem. Prompt and appropriate responses build self-sufficiency, not dependency. The world is experienced as a safe, responsive, predictable and exciting place to be. Parents or care providers who continue to "feed and cuddle only" or who leave a baby to "cry it out" don't support development.

Meals Will Never Be the Same

The extent of the infant's drive for social interaction is very evident in feeding behavior at this age. The baby simply cannot resist looking around, **smiling**, cooing and poking at mom's face during a feeding. Distracted by every sound or sight, the child may even stop nursing just to look around. This is very frustrating for moms and the danger is that nursing will be discontinued at this time. The mother may interpret the infant's social behavior as indicative of a desire to wean at this time. She herself may not be ready to change her parenting from the "symbiosis" or tight biological bond of the early newborn period. Parents must make this shift and appreciate needs as social times, not just physical nurturance.

Mrs. Martin asks what kind of formula to buy because the "baby doesn't like breast milk anymore." She says the baby pulls away from the breast whenever anything happens, such as a loud noise from the TV, the cat walking by or her older brother going through the room. Your notes say that it was Mom's intention to breastfeed for the first year. Note: Mom is misinterpreting the baby's signals for social interaction. Playmate as well as feeder is a new role demanded of mom at this time.

An intervention can turn this situation around. The child's new social interest should be highlighted, as well as the tendency to overdose on excitement if given the opportunity. At least two feedings per day should take place in a quiet, darkened room without distractions. Nighttime feedings will also sustain the milk supply and maintain a sense of closeness for both the mother and baby, although the feedings are not needed for nutritional requirements. Other types of vigorous social interactions should be enjoyed at other times. The social agenda has to be added to the feeding one. Families should adjust to these new demands and see the interactions and the games with the baby as being vital as food. This is a basic change period or "touchpoint" in development, when changes in abilities require changes in parenting.

Overdosing on Fun

The seductive behavior of a 3-month-old infant is hard to resist. The baby's orgasmic smiles, laughs and total body wiggles are a terrific reward for a few tickles or a play face expression. Some parents, probably most parents some of the time, will really push the infant beyond the limits of what the child can tolerate in the way of excitement. Overstimulation is a very real danger if the infant's body language is not heard, particularly for a neurologically, physiologically or temperamentally fragile child. The parent must be sensitive to the infant's behavioral cues, that she is on "overload" and play must slow down. This pause allows organization of the experience, recovery of attentional energy and some physiological rest. The required pause may be seconds or hours. Each child manifests stress and overstimulation in different ways. Some children will be more clear in signaling their overload than others. Sensitive adults respond to these behavioral signals and pull back; others need help in understanding the baby's needs.

Many anxious, depressed or stressed parents push too hard, interact very intrusively and don't read the baby's "back off" signals. The baby disengages and may even cry, leaving such parents feeling as though they are a failure. They often push even harder and a losing cycle starts. The clinician can demonstrate a play interaction that is more responsive to the individual baby. This change in approach will help parents be more successful.

> Ms. Jones put her face close to the baby's as she vigorously undressed her for the exam and spoke in loud baby talk all the time. Then she lifted the baby, bounced her at the shoulder and nuzzled the infant in the neck. The baby turned away from her mom, and her left arm extended out, fingers splayed. You feel suddenly claustrophobic in the room with them and hardly know where to begin. Note: Your own response to a situation will tell you something is wrong here. Pay attention to these feelings. Demonstrate how a quieter approach with pauses gets the infant's attention and positive response.

Young children who are brought for long periods to large gatherings, on prolonged trips to large shopping centers, to siblings' schools or on long car rides may have a markedly decreased capacity to handle further stress. Sleep and feeding difficulties are predictable in these contexts. Letting infants at this age "cry it out" may only exaggerate the frenzy at a time when the infant is least able to handle it. Quiet containment by a calm adult helps the infant get back under control. This kind of responsiveness restores energy to the child; it does not "spoil" him. Parents who are upset themselves by the episode should put the baby down or hand him over to another person if they feel out of control.

Infants this age love active play, but "flying baby," roughhousing, bicycle seats and joggers are not safe at this age. The "shaken impact syndrome," as well as behavioral overload, can result from such vigorous play activities.

Temperamental Differences

Temperamental differences in infants' personalities make some babies' bids for social interaction difficult to interpret. For example, one infant may signal interactional readiness by serious regard and be overloaded by all but the most gentle play. This child may be perceived as negative, dull or unappreciative of the parents' efforts at interaction. The parents may even feel that the child doesn't like them. This situation may evolve into a "difficult" or "slow to warm up" style that will continue to challenge parents and clinicians in the days ahead. Sensitivity and low-key responsiveness ought to be pointed out and a subtler style modeled. Reassurances about the child's normalcy and competency must be given.

Ms. Galen says she is worried because her baby never smiles at her. She's dropped out of the play group because she's ashamed that her baby doesn't seem as happy as the rest of the infants. She's given up her career to be with the baby and wonders what she's doing wrong; she plays with her all day. Emma, the baby, regards you very seriously and is very still as you approach. You smile at her without a word or a touch, and she smiles back very tentatively. As you move the stethoscope across her field of vision, her face brightens and she follows it very intently. You feel yourself slowing down with the baby, a welcome relief after a busy morning. Mom scoops her up and starts to bounce and pace. Emma gets fussy. Your notes from the prenatal interview say that Dad is a very serious and busy businessman. Mom did all the talking and was in the local theater group. Note: The temperamental differences between mom and baby are the source of disappointments in the relationship. Mom will need to appreciate the child's individuality if they are to "fit" together now and in the long run. The parallels with Dad's style and personality are helpful and may have been missed without the early interview.

For most infants, classic "colic" has disappeared by this age, but what may not have disappeared is the highly responsive, intense and overly reactive characteristics in a previously colicky infant. This temperamental profile is now seen as an infant who is easily overwhelmed by exciting days, who handles change in scheduling poorly and who may have difficulty in falling asleep or restless, disturbed sleep. Vomiting may follow feedings that are frantic and fast, or feedings may be full of wiggles and distractions. The need to anticipate and bypass these buildups, give support at the time of change in routine and provide quiet times for winding down is evident now. Such actions will establish the healthy interactional patterns that will be needed later. Individual differences get clearer every day as a child's temperament unfolds. The earlier these profiles are understood, the smoother things will go (see Chapter 2).

THE FAMILY AT 3 MONTHS

Parents should be having fun with their infants at this time, and if they are not, something is wrong with the child, with the parents or with the interaction between them. The parents should be on or moving toward a new level of parenting—that of attention to the individuality of the infant through playful responsiveness and care. Parents should both enjoy and appreciate the infant as an individual at this time. Feeding in response to every whimper is not enough. Single parents, parents of ill or preterm infants, overly isolated or stressed parents or some daycare providers may hold on to the earlier pattern of carrying and feeding as the only responses. Overfeeding may result and may be a clue to this "development arrest" in family development. Maternal depression will now affect the infant's behavior immediately and profoundly with long-lasting results. A flattening of responsiveness, lack of joy in the interaction and lack of social engagement with the baby may be clues that the parent needs a mental health referral. Often the child health care provider is the only professional who sees the parent at this time and thus is in a position to make this vital referral.

Siblings may reach a new level of organization at this time as well. The baby is now able to enjoy the older child's antics and bids for interaction, provided that they are not too vigorous or overwhelming. The infant will prefer to watch the other child if not overloaded or stressed. The infant's sleep stability and the parents' more rested state allow a little more time for the older child's separate time with the parents. The infant should be adding energy to the family at this time in the form of love, delight and active appreciation of the life around him or her. If not, something is wrong.

> Devin, age 3, marches into the exam room ahead of his mom and baby sister as he carries the diaper bag. He says he wants you to check "his baby." He pulls out a small car and shakes it in front of the baby, making car noises. The baby smiles broadly and nearly wiggles out of mom's arms. Mom laughs and says that the baby watches everything that Devin does. Note: This looks like a healthy family. A 5-second observation shows appropriate responsiveness for the infant, a positive sibling response and a joyful mom. Your core observations are done before you ask the first question.

SUMMARY

The visit at 3 to 4 four months is about joy, delight and fun. This is not a frivolous agenda. When we look at the essential tasks of infancy—the development of trust, a sense of self-effectiveness and a positive emotional state for learning and growth—this visit gives us a chance to look at the emergence of these core developmental tasks. With these insights we have a chance for long-lasting positive intervention. It is through parent-infant exchanges that these vital forces for growth are activated. As stated by Stanley Greenspan in a reflection on the importance of these early interactions in infancy:

The self now exists in relation to others. It is aware of shared pleasures and joys and even of loss and despair, as when the caregiver doesn't return the infant's overtures ... the consciousness that (now) embraces the human world—the sense of shared personhood as critical to the development of an individual's feeling part of the human community—flowers out of these early and enduring interchanges.

The clinician has the chance to observe, support and even participate in these most vital processes.

DATA GATHERING

What to Observe

- Does the parent enjoy the baby?
- Does the parent look and act happy?
- Does the parent's and the baby's personal appearance show the parent's ability to care for the basics?
- Is undressing, holding and waiting sprinkled with game playing, dialogues and toy object play?
- Does the infant visually scan and auditorially monitor the room with a bright, active search?
- Does the infant monitor your approach and initiate an interaction on a smile cue alone?
- Are the infant's hands open, active and meeting in the midline?
- Is the infant beginning to make verbal exchanges with the parent?
- How many "games" are played as the infant is undressed, weighed, examined, etc.?
- Does the baby invite interaction? How does he show it? What's his style?

What to Ask

The following are questions the clinician should ask the parents during the visit:

- Are you enjoying the baby?
- What games do you play together?
- Describe the baby's personality. Is he like you? Like his dad?
- Has the baby's schedule changed? Describe it.
- Has your schedule changed (e.g., returning to work)?
- Can you predict the infant's behavior from day to day?
- What things does the baby do to settle into sleep? What are your bedtime routines?
- Can he amuse himself for a time?
- Can he wait for feedings if you call to him or pick him up? Does he stop crying just with anticipation?
- How regular is his schedule?
- Does he awaken during the night?
- What does he do to settle himself back down to sleep?
- Has he discovered his hands, feet?
- Does he play with both hands together?
- Does he respond to sound and visual objects easily?
- Does he bat at things?
- Can he hold onto simple toys?

Examination

During the examination the clinician should ask herself the following questions:

- Is this baby fun to deal with?
- Does he coo (ahs, ows, i.e., open vowel sounds with the beginning of labial consonants), smile, laugh? Does he do this without a prompt?
- Are his hands active? When visually regarding things, does he swipe, reach, grasp at things? Does he delight in doing so?
- Are his reach attempts symmetrical?
- Have the primitive reflexes disappeared (e.g., tonic neck reflex, grasp reflex, Moro reflex and walk-in-place reflexes)?
- Can the child lift his head and hands up when prone?
- Does he repeat a behavior that produced an interesting event (e.g., place a rattle in his hand and see whether he understands that his own activity causes the interesting sound)?
- Does he look at and follow you across the room?
- Is the baby positioned so that he can look around the room? Are his hands free?

Modeling of play interactions during the examination may be particularly important to parents. Point out the baby's smiles as social elicitations. Develop a verbal or tactile game with the infant to see the response. Point out the infant's signs of overload or avoidance during the course of the physical examination or even with undressing. Does the child look away, dampen her expression, arch her back, change color to pale or mottled or get fussy or frantic in movement? Consciously stop, pull back and point out the infant's behavioral recovery. When is the baby ready to deal with you again?

QUICK CHECK—3 TO 4 MONTHS

- ✓ Waves hands and arms at the sight of a toy
- ✓ Bats at object (such as a stethoscope) and may grab it
- ✓ Holds onto a toy placed in hand. Shakes a rattle
- ✓ Holds his head steady when held in a sitting position
- ✓ Head up to 90 degrees when in a prone position, up on hands
- ✓ Rolls back to abdomen
- ✓ Laughs and squeals
- ✓ Initiates smiling
- ✓ Symmetrical postures and movements
- ✓ Follow a person across the room with eyes and head
- ✓ Brings toy to mouth
- ✓ Alerts or turns to sounds at the sides
- ✓ Holds and examines his own hands, scratches, clutches at clothes or exam table paper
- ✓ Has a variety of facial expressions

⚠ HEADS UP–3 TO 4 MONTHS

Infant Issues

- Be alert to any asymmetry in movement. Hemiparesis shows up at this time with asymmetrical arm or leg movement.
- A hypervigilant infant may have compromised hearing. Check the neonatal screen, test sound localization with your voice but without vision and order a hearing test if there is any doubt in any of these.
- If babbling shows a decline instead of an increase, also consider hearing loss.
- Hands should be open and all extremities in an easy, flexed position. If not, consider abnormalities in the neuromotor system (e.g., cerebral palsy).
- The infant should have enough head control to come up with a pull to sit and should maintain head control in a supported sit position.
- The infant should notice and follow a person across the room. Consider visual or generalized neurological concerns if not.
- The infant should be having his longest sleep at night with a pretty predictable schedule overall. If not, discuss care practices, expectations.
- If the infant is getting too heavy for length, consider whether there is a "developmental arrest" in the family development described earlier. Is overfeeding an issue?
- Infants are too strong for infant seats at this age and may flip out. These seats need to be retired.
- Infants with a very late bedtime or prolonged night awakening may have a "phase shift" disturbance in which they sleep too much during the day and not enough at night. Limit naps, and wake from a nap by 4 PM.

Parent Issues

- The parents should be enjoying the infant. If not, investigate.
- We expect parents to be somewhat rested and put together, generally positive and interactive at this visit. If not, look into issues described in this chapter.
- Parents should be comfortable leaving the infant with a trusted sitter for an evening out. Perceived vulnerability may be present if they are not comfortable. Investigate.
- Daycare: If the child is in group care, there should be no more than four infants per adult. More than that suggests that the child's emotional needs are unlikely to be consistently met.
- If mom is planning to wean the infant, discuss her motivation and real desires.
- Propping the bottle doesn't meet the child's needs for interaction, and nighttime cereal doesn't make the child sleep through the night. Check feeding patterns from the interactional angle, as well as from the nutritional point of view.
- Parents who complain about sleep problems need to have this situation assessed and some intervention performed. Sleep issues will only get worse if they are a problem at this time. They can be manifestations of attachment issues, maternal depression, vulnerable child syndrome and parents grieving and making up for daytime absence. If simple interventions and education don't work, a look at deeper issues is warranted.
- Does the parent respond specifically to the infant's style and behavioral cues? Observations during weighing and measuring and after immunizations may reveal the parent's response to various minor stresses.

ANTICIPATORY GUIDANCE

The clinician can offer parents advice and assurance about a variety of issues that arise at this age:

- Some active infants may jettison themselves out of infant seats at this time of increased activity. Therefore, the old seat should be retired. The crib should also be lowered at this time.

- The importance of the child's own active exploration of the world, particularly her own actions, should be emphasized.

- The infant is still too young for joggers, bike seats or vigorous throwing-around games. The baby may be ready for a backpack for walking, not jogging, with an adult if the infant's head control is good.

- Parents should be cautioned about overstimulation in toys, social interactions and stressful events. Excess fatigue because of loss of the ability to handle environmental disturbances is a pitfall to be avoided. In considering any changes, think of ways to make the least number of alterations.

- The surge in activity often produces an increase in appetite and growth. It also means feedings may be more disrupted by wiggles and giggles.

- Emphasize the importance of holding and playing. Infants cannot be spoiled at this age. The baby should be near someone whenever awake.

- Siblings should receive cautious permission to interact with the baby under supervision. Help them learn what is too much.

- Breastfeeding turbulence is to be expected at this time. Explain its origin and options for management. A vulnerability to early weaning appears at this time.

- Babies at this age do not need to be fed at night, although their moms may wish to do so to maintain milk production.

- Good sleep rituals begin at this age. The baby should be put to bed in a drowsy state without a bottle and with a quiet, calming song, poem or pat.

RECOMMENDED READINGS

Anders T, Sadeh A, Appareddy V: Normal sleep in infants and children. *In* Ferber R, Kryger M (eds): *Principles and Practice of Sleep Medicine in the Child.* Philadelphia, WB Saunders, 1995.

Field T: Infants of depressed mothers. *Infant Behav Dev* 18:1, 1995.

Howard B, Wong J: Sleep disorders. *Pediatr Rev* 22(10):327-342, 2001.

Zeanah CH: Disturbances of attachment in young children adopted from institutions. *J Dev Behav Pediatr* 21:230-236, 2000.

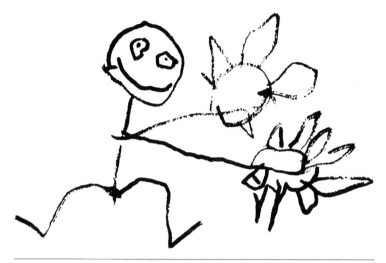

"Smiling kid." By girl, age 5½.

CHAPTER 12

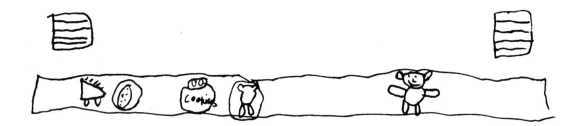

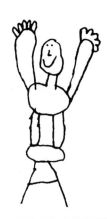

"Reaching out." By boy, age 7.

Six Months: Reaching Out

SUZANNE D. DIXON and MICHAEL J. HENNESSY

The chapter describes the general principles of motor development and tracks the emergence of reaching, grasping and hand movements from infancy to the preschool period. Sitting, stimulation programs and the importance of self-feeding are discussed.

Key Words

- Motor Development
- Reach
- Grasp
- Ontogeny of Reach and Grasp
- Self-Feeding
- Motor Asymmetry
- Sitting
- Fine Motor Skills
- Handedness
- Infant Stimulation Programs

Nicholas, brought in on time for his third set of immunizations, is a roly-poly, quiet boy. His mother is concerned because he uses his left hand too much and puts everything in his mouth. She thinks she gives enough formula and cereal but wonders if he is still hungry. She wants to know when she can feed him foods like crackers and breakfast cereal bits. She says her brother is a "lefty" and always had trouble in school; she wants to know if Nicholas will have the same kind of trouble. On examination, Nicholas does reach first for your stethoscope with his left hand but will extend his right hand if the left is restrained. He grabs your pen more accurately with his left hand, shaping his hand before he touches the object. On the right side, his reach is less well directed, and its form doesn't anticipate the pen's shape as well. Note: This observation allows us to look at the emergence of hand movement and hand-eye coordination. The small amount of asymmetry in Nicholas' reach requires more observation of the motor system.

Now that the baby has visually discovered his hands and has a simple grasp, the 5- to 6-month-old goes on to learn what to do with these new skills; sights can be explored in an active way. The texture, temperature, shape and malleability of objects become new dimensions of the world that add interest and excitement to the child's life, as well as enhanced learning opportunities. The eyes, hands and mouth work together in this exploration. Reaching and grasping have a direct link to cognitive growth because such skills allow for the active learning that is fuel for mental growth in infancy. The specific way that the skills of reach and grasp are refined during infancy and how these changes make interaction with the external world possible are the focus of this visit. Hand watching at this age and beyond will not only tell us about motor development but also allow us a window on cognitive development and social engagement with the environment. Knowledge of the workings of the hand allows the clinician to monitor not only motor skills but also cognitive changes. This chapter is designed to build clinical skills in the monitoring of manipulative behavior in early childhood.

BASIC PRINCIPLES OF MOTOR DEVELOPMENT

The pattern of acquisition of skills in this area illustrates several observations about **motor development** in general:

- *Primitive* reflexes must disappear before *voluntary* behavior appears. For example, the grasp reflexes must be gone before voluntary grasp begins. Whether these reflexes are subsumed into voluntary patterns or disappear to set the stage for non–reflex-driven behavior is debated. However, the sequence of events is not. During the overlap period, grasp reflexes still influence hand behavior as volitional grasp emerges.

- Development follows a *proximal-to-distal* progression. This is evident in control proceeding from the shoulder to the fingers. **Reach** precedes **grasp**. Control moves from the shoulder down to the fingers and from the hip to the ankle (see Chapter 14).

- The emergence of motor skills follows a relatively rigid sequence, but the timing and style show variation from child to child. Some environmental supports or constraints influence this process, although the sequence remains constant.

- Variation in motor development occurs in the *rate* of maturation of skills, with the timing at each stage being poorly predictive of the time at which the next stage will emerge.

- *Pronation precedes supination.* Palm-down maneuvers, such as picking up objects, occur before palm-up maneuvers, such as putting objects in the mouth or transferring objects.

- *Action and movement precede inhibition.* A child holds onto objects before being able to release them. Inhibition of a movement already started is harder than never moving in the first place. Once a reach is initiated, it is difficult for the child to stop. Once an early walker takes off, it is hard for the young child to readily stop. Starting and moving come under the child's control before stopping or changing course.

- The *exact* way a skill (e.g., grasping, forward progression) is completed each time varies; every attempt is a new behavior in that sense. In fact, *lack* of variability in such behavior, with rigid or stereotyped patterns of reach, is characteristic of a child with motor disabilities rather than typically developing children. The ability to modify motor actions in an ongoing process of learning and adaptation is a characteristic seen in infancy and throughout life in the course of skill development.

CHANGED PERSPECTIVES ON MOTOR DEVELOPMENT

The process of motor development is no longer conceived of as the inevitable rolling out of skills based on neuromotor competencies. Rather, along with these evolving neuromotor competencies, changes in the biomechanical dimensions of the body and the child's internal motivation and drive to mastery create new movement possibilities and patterns. The environment provides challenges to adaptation, differing circumstances and external motivators. Growth or change in one or more of these four areas (size, neural maturation, sparkle and skills) creates an imbalance in the movement system. This imbalance in turn leads to a mini-reorganization at a higher skill level. New skills emerge when balance is restored across all these contributing factors. Old skills evolve into new skills as all these forces work together to prompt change and growth. One level blends into the next in an ever-changing, dynamic way. This view of a *dynamic systems approach* to motor development allows us to see the vital interplay between child and environment in the emergence of motor skills (see Chapter 2). Support for active practice of skills with prompts to adapt to mildly challenging conditions means that caretaking practices can make a difference in this area. Opportunities to exercise and use new skills in ever-changing ways and circumstances are created by a supportive environment. This is quite different from the idea of practice, which is repetitive, rote and, in some cases, passive. Children develop motor skills by using internal drive, maturing motor competencies, changing physical characteristics and environmental prompts. Adaptation is specific to the mix of these factors within each child. *The importance of active interplay with the environment is a relatively new view of motor development in general.*

THE REFLEXES

The grasp reflexes have been described in the classic work by Twitchell and are presented in Table 12–1 and Figure 12–1. The timing in the appearance of these reflexes testifies to neurological maturation and integrity. These reflexes have a predictable course that allows us to "date" central nervous system (CNS) maturation. From the child's vantage point, these

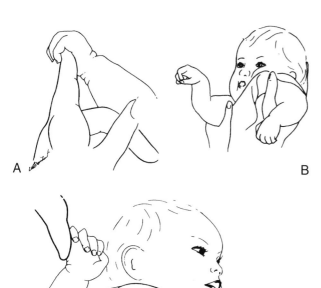

Figure 12–1 Grasp reflexes. **A**, Reflex palmar grasp. **B**, Traction orientation grasp, type B, ulnar. **C**, Instinctive orientation grasp.

TABLE 12–1   **Types of Grasp Reflexes**

Reflex	Elicitation	Response	Emerges	Disappears
Mental	Touch chin	Hands close	Birth	At 6 wk
Palmar	Touch palm between thumb and index finger	Hands close	28 wk of gestation	2 mo
Traction	Stretch shoulder adductors and flexors	All joints of the arm flex	2–3 wk, weakens at 6 wk	Up to 5 mo
Instinctive grasp reaction, orientation A	Light touch to radial side of the hand	Open and supinate hand	3–4½ mo	4–5 mo
Instinctive grasp reaction, orientation B	Light touch to ulnar side of the hand	Open and pronate hand	5½–6 mo	6 (?) mo
Groping	Light touch to hand on the side	Hand will move toward stimulus	6–7 mo	7 mo (onset of reliable volitional grasp)
Grasping	Light touch to side of the hand	Hand will grasp object	6–7 mo	7 mo (onset of reliable volitional grasp)

reflexes help him start feeling the world (Fig. 12–2). They are like prepackaged software that gets the user (the infant) started.

The asymmetrical tonic neck response, which peaks at about 6 weeks of age, facilitates the infant's exploration of his own hands. The infant is able to see what interesting things the hands are by turning his head to the outstretched hand even before having the strength and coordination to bring his hands before his eyes in the midline. The influence of the tonic neck reflex either before its full peak or after it wanes is such that muscle tone increases on the side of the body to which the head is turned. This means that all neurological maneuvers should be done with the head secured in the midline. Consistent asymmetry in reflexes or their persistence beyond the expected departure date should cause the clinician to evaluate the CNS in general and the child's overall development.

ONTOGENY OF REACH AND GRASP

Early Infancy

The precursors of reach and grasp are in the form of coordination of visual processing with hand activity, the presence of grasp reflexes and some early reaching behavior. A newborn in the quiet/alert state who visually fixates on a pleasant sight will begin to have mouthing

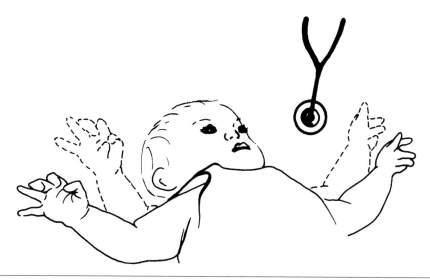

Figure 12–2 Early infancy contains the earliest elements of reach and hand-arm and foot-leg activation with the presentation of interesting sights.

BOX 12–1 REACH

- Arm and hand activation: 6 weeks–2½ months
- Closed hand reaching: 2–3 months
- Hands open with reach: 4 months
- Accurate reaching: 6 months
- Anticipatory hand shape and movement: 9 months
- Coordinated timing of hand closure with reach: 13 months

---

movements, his hands will open and close, and after considerable latency, the infant will swipe toward the midline with the hand and arm working as a unit. The feet and toes may also be activated in this process, closing and opening. A neonate will reach up to touch the breast while nursing, a skill that goes away at a month or two. Infants as young as 4 weeks respond differently to objects that are in their range of reach than to those that are beyond that range; they will swipe at reachable and touchable objects but not at those that are out of range. Such behavior shows a primitive visual-motor linkage. Infants may even show the ability to differentiate their manual approach to two dimensional versus three dimensional objects with a curved swipe to the latter and a flat swipe to the former. Coordination of systems is present from the start, even though accurate completion of the task and efficient control of hand movements may be months down the road (Box 12–1).

In this earliest form of infant reach, vision may initiate the reach but does not control it accurately: the infant cannot make ongoing corrections of efforts toward an object after starting a swipe toward it. This lack of fully mature coordination ability makes success very unlikely at this stage. Additionally, a young infant will reach out in the dark for a pleasant sound, using his mouth, hands and feet, although success is unlikely here as well. In later infancy, reach becomes more finely tuned with vision and more adjustable based on visual input. Reach in the dark without vision will rarely occur after 6 months of age.

An infant initially swipes with the whole hand and arm as a unit, with initiation of movement at the shoulder. Hand grasp will occur only if the hand touches something. This early type of volitional reach disappears at about 7 weeks of age. In a typical clinical setting, we rarely see it because we do not wait out the long latency period needed for this behavior to emerge, unbind the infant's arms or provide the truncal support that is needed to see these skills. Moms may note that the baby reaches up to touch the breast and will comment on swipes at a mobile or toy while the infant is lying in a crib or in an infant seat. The **ontogeny of reach and grasp** is detailed in the following milestones:

- *Mutual hand grasp* comes in 2 to 3 months after a decrease in the tonic neck response. The infant really starts to explore his hands when this happens. Wrapping and propping so that the hands come together facilitate this process. Shoulders need to be held forward to get the hands to consistently find one another.

- By 5 months of age, the automatic grasp responses to objects touching the hand have largely disappeared, although remnants may linger for years. *Volitional grasp* is prominent now and acts independently from reach (i.e., the hand moves separately from the shoulder). Increasing bulk and control of the shoulder musculature, as well as truncal strength and stability (i.e., sitting with slight or no support), enable reach to be more reliable at this age as well (see later).

- Fixed-extension postures at the shoulders or weakness of the shoulder girdle musculature, often present in a premature infant, may prevent the child from using reach and facilitating skill in this area. Applying external support with an increase in flexion at the shoulder (e.g., a rolled towel or small blanket behind the shoulders) often helps this group of youngsters develop these reaching abilities. For children with persistent truncal hypotonia, external supports may be needed to free up the hands for exploratory work.

- By 3 to 6 months the hands should be loosely fisted at rest and both hands activated when the infant attempts to reach. Repeated failure to see one arm or hand move when the other extends is cause to consider perinatal stroke or peripheral nerve damage. Tightly fisted hands, with thumbs tucked inside, are at this age generally a sign of pathological hypertonia and delay.

- By 6 months the child should *reach across the midline* when the contralateral hand is restrained, although both hands are usually activated when a reach is started.

- By 6 months the *thumb fully participates* in grasp, although full thumb opposition may not be present until 2 to 3 months later.

- A few simple items in the office allow the clinician to be a good hand watcher with minimal effort. For a child in an alert state and comfortably supported, these observations are easy to set up (see Box 12–3).

Grasp Development

Volitional grasp matures with increasing control at the wrist and with increasing use of the fingers as separate units. A grasp with the whole hand is used for medium objects, and a raking

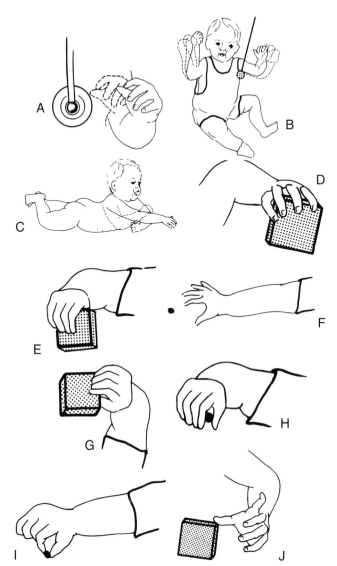

Figure 12–3 Progression of reach and grasp. **A**, Nondirected swiping, 1 month. **B**, Swiping, about 4 months. **C**, Corralling, about 4 months. **D**, Ulnar–palmar grasp of a cube, 4 to 5 months. **E**, Radial-palmar grasp of a cube, 6 to 7 months. **F**, Raking of a pellet, 6 to 7 months. **G**, Radial-digital grasp of a cube, 7 to 8 months. **H**, Scissors grasp of a pellet, 7 to 9 months. **I**, Pincer grasp of a pellet, 9 to 10 months. **J**, Voluntary release, 9 to 10 months.

grasp is used for small objects at first. Then control of grasp moves to the fingers as a unit, including the thumb, which is kept to the side of the hand; the result is an "inferior pincer" for small objects and a flat rather than cupped-hand grasp for the latter. When the tips of the fingers are used to deftly pick up a small object with the thumb across from the index finger ("opposed"), this is termed a pincer grasp. The pincer grasp is used naturally only with visual coordination; we all revert to raking for small objects in the dark, and blind children must be taught to use a pincer grasp (Fig. 12–3).

Even before the complete pincer grasp is evident, the *index finger* takes the lead in grasping and exploring objects. Poking at things, particularly into holes at 8 to 9 months old, testifies to

TABLE 12–2   **Progression of Grasp**

Age (mo)	Term	Pattern Components
1	Nondirected swiping	Arms and legs activated, often beginning with a startle; long latency; hands and mouth may open
3–4	Swiping	Moving arm up and down in an attempt to contact objects
4	Corralling	Reaching out with an entire arm and hand and sweeping the arm toward the body
4–5	Ulnar-palmar grasp of a cube; rotates the wrist	Fingers on the top surface of an object press it into the center of the palm, thumb adducted, wrist flexed
6–7	Radial-palmar grasp of a cube	Fingers on the far side of an object press against the opposed thumb and radial side of the palm, wrist straight
6–7	Raking grasp of a pellet	Raking an object into the palm with an adducted, totally flexed thumb and fingers
7–8	Radial-digital grasp of a cube	Object held with opposed thumb and fingertips; space visible between
7–9	Scissors grasp of a pellet	Object held between the ventral surfaces of the thumb and index finger
9–10	Pincer grasp of a pellet	Object held between the distal pad of the thumb and index finger
9–10	Voluntary release	Drops objects when desired

Modified from Bayley N: *Bayley Scales of Infant Development.* New York, Psychological Corp, 1969; Erhardt RP: *Developmental Hand Dysfunction: Theory, Assessment, Treatment.* Laurel, MD, RAMSCO, 1982; and Knobloch H, Stevens F, Malone A: *Manual of Developmental Diagnosis: The Administration and Interpretation of the Revised Gesell and Amatruda Developmental and Neurologic Examination.* New York, Harper & Row, 1980.

this maturation of specific finger skills and is usually coincident with the pincer grasp. It also means that electrical outlets, buttons, cracks and other dangers become very attractive for this exploring first finger.

Grasp of medium-sized objects, such as small blocks, shows a similar progression from use of the whole hand and palm at 7 months to increasing use of the fingertips and finally to use of the index finger and thumb to stack the blocks "deftly and directly" (see Fig. 12–3). The hand goes from a flat approach to a cupped position as the thumb moves down and around an object and the fingers splay out around the object.

The child shows increasing ability to anticipate the shape and weight of an object (Table 12–2; also see Fig. 12–3). That is, as the child begins consistent grasp or reach, near the age of 6 to 8 months, the hand position and the arc of movement of the arm and hand reflect the shape and distance away from the object sought, as shown in Figure 12–4. As the baby begins to go

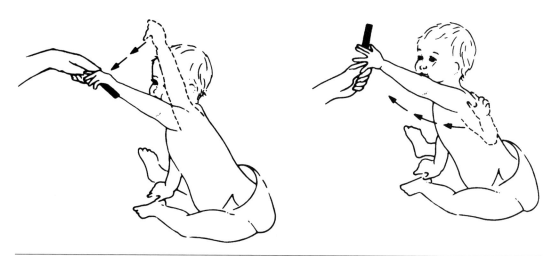

Figure 12–4 Child anticipates the shape of an object. Reach is initiated with the hand in position to grasp the object, dependent upon the object's shape and position.

after an object, the hand position, angle of arm movement and postural adjustment show that the properties of the desired object are understood and that these concepts are transferred from the visual system to the motor system. This system coordination, vision and reach, and the higher level of integration that it implies can be seen even in children who cannot successfully execute a reach or a grasp, such as a child with athetoid movements, weakness, hypertonicity or an arm in a cast or splint (see Fig. 12–4). Again, the clinician should look at the *quality* of the grasp attempt and the basis for it even when task accomplishment remains incomplete for reasons such as those just stated. Although difficulties with visual-motor tasks will be more obvious as the child becomes capable of drawing tasks (see Chapter 5), they may be evident at this age if the clinician watches these aspects of reach and grasp.

After 6 months of age, reach and grasp are separate. That is, the child can grasp a nearby object without a reach and can first reach for an object and grasp it only when it is near. This uncoupling is an example of the increasing efficiency of the motor system with maturation.

Between *5 and 7 months*, visually directed corrective movements can be seen in patterns of grasp. That is, the child watches his hand and alters its moves to more closely accommodate the object's shape, distance and texture, even if these change as he is reaching. These ongoing corrections affect both the direction and the velocity of movement. Grasp is more specific, efficient and smooth.

Volitional reach at this time is two handed and symmetrical, at least at its start. The child "misses" and "overshoots," occasionally getting the object batted into the opposite, available hand.

Between *7 and 11 months*, diminishing dependency on bimanual reach can be demonstrated and consistent single-hand reach becomes evident. The transfer of objects is an outgrowth of these midline activities (Fig. 12–5).

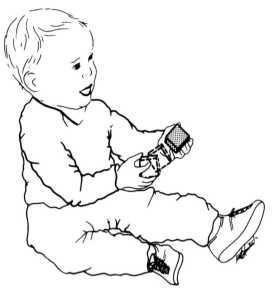

Figure 12–5 Transfer of objects from one hand to the other.

BOX 12–2 GRASP

- Regards toy: newborn
- Activates with reachable toy: 1–4 weeks
- Holds onto toy: 1–2 months
- Hands open: 2½–3½ months
- Grasps toy near hand, palm: 4–5 months
- Two-hand grasp: 4–5 months
- Rotates wrist: 5–7 months
- Unilateral reaching: 6–7 months
- Grasps two things in each hand: 7–8 months
- Scoops (rakes) a pellet: 6–8 months
- Inferior pincer: 6–10 months
- Pincer: 7–12 months

Wrist movement comes in after 1 year and wrist rotation at about age 2. Doorknobs and other latches become vulnerable after that time.

The interest and vigor in the infant's investment in the manipulation of objects at this age make it both easy and exciting for parents and clinicians to begin to be "hand watchers." A dangling stethoscope, a red ball of yarn or even a pencil can be used to watch the emergence of these hand and hand-eye skills throughout the first year (Box 12–2).

USE OF TOOLS

The use of tools to extend, amplify and specialize our hand movement distinguishes humans from most lower animals. After a child learns how to use the hands well—reaching, grasping, transferring, manipulating—she learns to extend the functions of the hand through the use of objects. These instruments or tools allow her to reach farther, to act on things in new ways and to do things that would be impossible through the use of hands alone. Although this seems like just a progression, it is conceptually an enormous step that allows for much more elaborate exploration of objects. It is, at the child's level, the dawning of the age of technology. Progression of the *use of instruments* at this new age is shown in the following stages:

- First comes the discovery that banging one thing against another makes an interesting sight and sound. Putting objects together in the midline and banging one object on the table demonstrate this first step.

- The second stage is to see that an object extends reach, such as seeing that a stick can get a toy that otherwise would be out of reach. The instrument becomes a *hand extender*, doing the same thing as the hand, only farther afield.

- The next stage is to see that a tool can do something *different than the hand*. This progression goes on through childhood with increasing agility with specialized tools that do more and more complex things, farther removed from the simple actions capable of the hand alone. For example, the child discovers that a spoon can scoop stuff that would otherwise squish between the fingers on the way to the mouth. Children start to use spoons at around 1 year, but they are rarely adept at doing so until closer to 2. Forks do things very differently than hands do and are generally used by 3 to 4 years of age. Skill with a knife, which requires both hands doing very different but coordinated actions, will take years, into school age at 5 to 6 years. Scissors are used at 3 years.

- The child's hands become more adept at using these specialized tools, with more coordination between the hands, increasingly separate use of the fingers and each hand separately and differently threading objects; the use of simple musical instruments is an example of these "tool tasks."

Frustration, fatigue and stress cause children to go backward in the demonstration of skills. For example, they may use their hands to eat or may tear something rather than cut it with scissors. In general, a slight gender difference arises in these visual-motor tasks, with girls being more skilled after 2 to 3 years of age. Facility with preschool craft projects and some copying of letters or numbers may emerge slightly earlier in girls.

The developmental course of figure copying and other paper and pencil tasks is presented in Chapter 5.

ENVIRONMENTAL FACILITATORS AND DETRACTORS

Several factors may influence both the emergence and the demonstration of reach and grasp behavior, including distraction, past experience with particular objects, temperament and general state of the child (e.g., sick, tired or hungry). Characteristics such as texture, shape, thickness, distance and density of the object will also play a part because these factors will either prompt interest and adaptation or cause the child to withdraw from the task. Objects

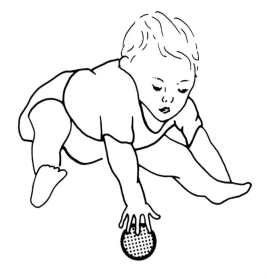

Figure 12–6 Sitting steadily with the hips abducted enables a child to stretch to the limits of his play space and use vision effectively in going after objects of varying size and texture. Adjustment to the size of the object will only occur when the child actually touches the object.

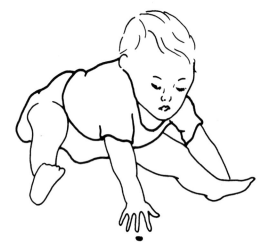

with varying shapes, colors and characteristics that can be perceived as novel by the child have been shown to provoke the most manipulative behavior by infants (Fig. 12–6). As in other areas of mental development, *moderate novelty* elicits more activity on the child's part. An environment filled with a variety of safe, reachable, graspable objects provides fuel for development in this area. For some children who are more sensitive to all or some textures, this means a gradual, gentle approach to the consistent presentation of a variety of types of these objects.

Populations of preterm infants, even without significant perinatal complications, may show specific delays in visual-motor activities even though other areas of development are normal. The lack of self hand monitoring in this population as a result of shoulder girdle weakness and retraction may be at least part of the basis for such delay, although CNS dysfunction may also

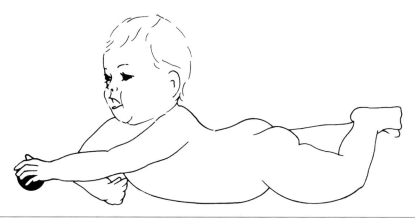

Figure 12–7 The importance of truncal stability in the prone posture is seen in situations in which the child is unwilling or unable to assume this posture. Reach and grasp are facilitated in the prone position.

play a role. The clinician should pay particular attention to visual-motor coordination in this population from infancy into school age. Assisting the infant in ways that bring the hands into the visual field may preclude any secondary deficits. Practice with hand/eye tasks should be included in any intervention program for this group.

New "back to sleep" recommendations mean that day or awake tummy time is essential to develop good visual-motor skills. This position is illustrated in Figure 12–7. This may mean specific supports for infants who have truncal weakness, instability or hypertonicity or for those who just resist this posture after weeks of being cared for in the supine position.

MOUTHING BEHAVIOR

Mouthing of and at objects should be expected in the majority of young children because it is an integral part of the infant's early exploration of objects, as part of the reach and grasp sequence. A child at 3 to 5 months and beyond goes after things with hands and mouth together, sucking at things that look interesting and bringing everything to the mouth when able. No evidence has shown unsatisfied oral gratification as the basis for such behavior. As reaching and grasping skills mature, children learn to explore their world with increasing hand-to-mouth activity. Luckily, this produces a lot of drool to coat toys with antibody-laden saliva. Within limits of cleanliness and safety, it should be praised and encouraged. With cognitive growth, the child learns more specific and complex ways to explore particular objects, and mouthing behavior disappears in typically developing children (Fig. 12–8).

Feeding provides the optimal exercise for these emerging fine motor skills (Fig. 12–9), but hunger or lack of food is not the usual reason for mouthing. Foods with varying texture and size are a great way to get a child interested in **self-feeding**, as well as in learning more about the world. As soon as a child can sit with stability and is eating solids, self-feeding should become another laboratory for cognitive growth. If this period of maximal interest in hand activities and hand-to-mouth behavior passes without such an opportunity, a long-term diminution in hand-to-mouth behavior may result. Self-feeding will then become a struggle rather than an opportunity.

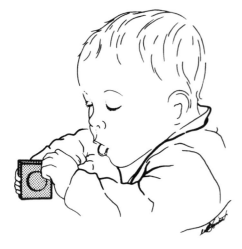

Figure 12–8 The hands and mouth work together to explore the world, independent of hunger and adequacy of the feeding situation; this is to be encouraged.

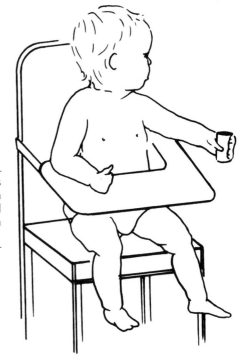

Figure 12–9 Self-feeding is best initiated when sitting is steady, reach is unilateral and grasp is at least scissors in type. The multiple sensory inputs in this situation and opportunities for exploration make it an exciting (though messy) part of the day.

ASYMMETRIES

Children with **motor asymmetry** of reach or grasp in the first 3 to 4 months of life are likely to have a peripheral nerve deficit (e.g., Erb's palsy) or some bone or joint impairment or injury (e.g., fractured humerus). Central lesions (e.g., perinatal stroke) will be manifested between 3 and 6 months by increasing asymmetry of spontaneous arm and hand movement, an asymmetrical residual Moro reflex, exclusive use of one hand or asymmetries in movement when the child is upset. Differences in the maturation of reach and grasp between one side of the body and the other, from reflexes to volitional movement, may also signal a central lesion. Such differences may be observed in free play and exaggerated when the child is crying. Failure to use both hands to pull a cloth off the face also adds to evidence of central dysfunction in this age range. Asymmetries of this type should always be evaluated. By 6 months both hands should be used in this maneuver, perhaps with one predominating or leading as part of the early emergence of **handedness**. The lead hand can usually be identified by careful observation, but clear hand dominance before 18 months is not typical and calls for additional evaluation because being "hanedd" before that time is pathological.

HANDEDNESS

A child gradually comes to use one hand more frequently than the other; this hand is termed *dominant*. There are many ways to define dominance. A practical definition for the pediatric clinician, though somewhat arbitrary, is that the dominant hand is the hand used consistently to hold a spoon, preferred to stack blocks, hold a crayon or throw a ball. It may or may not be the strongest hand.

Handedness is the most commonly observed manifestation of lateralization in the CNS. Though not commonly observed in clinical settings, subtle signs of lateralization are evident in very young infants. In a child between 1 and 3 years of age, the dominant hand becomes more and more apparent. Dominance appearing in the first 18 months most often indicates impaired peripheral or central control of the other hand (see earlier). Normally, clear and consistent handedness is not fully established until 4 to 6 years of age, with most children being right-handed. Mixed or indeterminate dominance is seen in a higher proportion of children than adults, thus suggesting a continuum of increasing lateralization with age. This process is related to differential functional maturation of the cerebral hemispheres. About 15% to 18% of children will still not have established clear dominance of one hand by school entry.

Left-hand dominance is believed to represent the consequence of less distinct cerebral lateralization, particularly in children and adults who write overhand with the left hand. The whole body participates in this laterality of function (e.g., eye, leg, arm, ear), but we focus on hand function because of its central importance in fine motor functioning.

A strong genetic predisposition to dominance exists. Only 2% of children of right-handed parents are left-handed, whereas 42% of children with left-handed parents are left-handed. Higher-level cerebral functions are better in left-handed individuals with left-handed relatives than in those without such a familial pattern. This again suggests that there is "normal" left-handedness and another type that is "abnormal."

Preterm infants and children with learning disabilities have a higher than expected rate of left-handedness, thus suggesting that this may be a subtle manifestation of CNS maturational dysfunction. The observation of an increased frequency in twins, regardless of zygosity and chorion type, may also reflect this process or may be related to some other unknown factor in CNS development.

A left-handed child of a right-hand–dominant family pedigree warrants *careful* evaluation. A detailed neurological examination should be performed at school entry or earlier to look for subtle signs of asymmetry in tone and reflexes, perseverance of mirroring activities and tremulousness or overshooting. Although the majority of these children may demonstrate normal neurodevelopmental skills, in a few, left-hand dominance may be an early or subtle clue to a mild central motor disability. Hand preference should be placed in the global assessment of an individual child's health and development, not as a pathological indicator by itself.

SITTING

To be 6 months old is to sit, at least usually. This proceeds from propped sitting to an increasingly upright, independent posture.

With increasing truncal strength and stability, a child is able to sit upright with decreasing amounts of support for increasing amounts of time. As **sitting** evolves, the spine increasingly straightens and the hands are used less and less for balance and support. When the hands are needed forward for balance and support, the position is called a *tripod sit* (5 to 7 months); this gradually emerges to an independent, stable sitting position, first on a regular surface (6 to 8 months) and then on an irregular or soft one (6 to 9 months). As soon as independent sitting is established, the hands are freed to manipulate objects, with gravity as a help rather than the hindrance it was when the baby was confined to his back. So object manipulation takes off when sitting is established. These two milestones are intertwined.

For children with truncal weakness or with hypotonic or hypertonic postures, a delay in the ability to sit means that the learning opportunities provided by object manipulation are curtailed. Devices and activities that give the child support while sitting are worth pursuing for these youngsters so that these play opportunities are available to a physically disabled child. Secondary cognitive difficulties might be avoided.

The visual world changes greatly when sitting is established. The child has at least a 90-degree horizontal horizon. As he gradually learns to pivot, it may extend to as far as 270 degrees. Truncal strength and flexibility allow him to increasingly control what he looks at and what he reaches for. This milestone is also dependent on biomechanical factors: large children or those with weakness may have a struggle to keep the balance required for maintaining this position.

When sitting is well established, the child begins to map three dimensional space. The child turns to follow and then get a toy going behind her (8 to 9 months), provided that pivoting is stable. Turning to get an object behind with only a sound cue takes place at 8 to 9 months, as does throwing toys from a high chair to see where they go and, of course, who will retrieve them (Fig. 12–10). Increasing gross motor competency, including stable sitting and hand control, sets the stage for new learning opportunities and novel ways to interact with the environment.

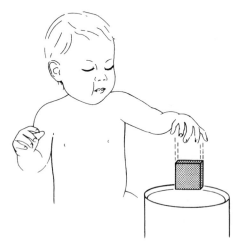

Figure 12–10 Active experimentation with objects serves the important cognitive work of play. Simple objects allow basic principles to be clear to a young child.

TABLE 12–3 **Reach Progression**

Action	Age
Visual object pursuit	Birth
Arm/body activation (long latency)	2 wk–2 mo
Sustained hand regard	2–4 mo
Arm swipes, bilateral	2–3 mo
Alternating glances	2½–4 mo
Unilateral arm activity	3 mo
Reliable reach to midline	4 mo
Reach for object disappearing beyond the visual field	4–5 mo
Unilateral reach	4–7 mo
Hand-to-hand transfer	5½–6 mo
Finger poke	8–10 mo
Plays midline games	8–12 mo
Visual anticipation of object shape	9–10 mo
Throwing objects	9–18 mo

SUMMARY

The emergence of voluntary reach and grasp is the time to look at motor competency, visual-motor coordination and the appropriateness of the environment in exploring the object world.

DATA GATHERING

What to Observe

Age-appropriate milestones as delineated in Table 12–3 can provide an assessment scale, along with the following:

- At 1 to 2 months, does the child move his hands and mouth to go after an object?
- At 2 to 3 months, does the infant increase motor activity (wiggle) when looking at a novel object nearby?
- Does the baby hold his hands together?
- At 4 months, does the child bring his hands to the midline?
- At 6 months, does the child rattle the paper on the examination table or grab his feet?
- At 7 months, does the child explore and manipulate toys, such as hitting them on the table or banging two blocks together?

- At 10 to 11 months, does the child hold a toy out to show you?
- How does the child use his hands and mouth in exploration?
- Does the child use both hands and arms equally? Are the movements smooth?

During examinations from birth through the third year, the examiner should present objects toward which the child can reach. Four objects are suggested (Box 12–3): (1) dangling stethoscope; (2) 1-inch cubed blocks with up to six available, beginning at 2 months; (3) a raisin or round cereal bit, beginning at 5 months; (4) an unsharpened pencil, beginning at 4 months.

The **raisin** offers the child the opportunity to demonstrate fine motor activity with increasing use of the fingers. The pincer grasp should be seen by 8 months. The use of both hands equally during the course of this play should be seen.

An unsharpened pencil or stick can be presented in the midline horizontally and then vertically to induce reach. A 4-month-old should have a bimanual reach and close the grasp if contact is made. A 6-month-old should anticipate the shape at the beginning of shoulder movement by shaping her hand to an accommodating posture. After 1 year the child will readily transfer the pencil and will begin to direct it downward to write. Going from a fisted grasp to an increasingly mature finger hold should be mapped across this time. By 5 years of age, if not earlier, a mature "writing" grasp of the pencil may be the single best predictor of adequate **fine motor skills** for school achievement. Motor tone, the child's posture and strength and control in the trunk, shoulders and extremities should be noted throughout the course of the examination. Disappearance of the reflex grasp should be noted to follow the course outlined in Table 12–1.

A dangling **stethoscope** should elicit increasingly smooth tracking with activation of the mouth, hands, arms and lower extremities in the newborn period. Swiping should begin at 3 to 4 months of age. Reach should be reliable by 5 to 6 months of age, with both arms participating and the hands opening on contact. With one arm restrained, the child should reach across the midline. By 9 to 10 months of age the reach should be quite unilateral, although mirroring will be common. Reaching across the midline may not be seen reliably until the second year of life. Movements should be increasingly smooth with increasing use of the elbow and wrist.

A small block should be placed before the child on a surface while the child is sitting on the caretaker's lap. The grasp efforts should proceed as shown in Table 12–2 and Box 12–2. This activity can be done during the history taking. In the second year and beyond, this activity can move along the continuum of stacking blocks and building imagined structures, bridges, trains and then stairs.

Observe delays or abnormal patterns of the infant's fine motor behavior. Persistence of primitive reflexes will interfere with the emergence of purposeful fine motor skills.

In addition to observing laterality, observe what the other hand is doing. For example, at 7 months, are the hands equal in skill? At 10 to 11 months, is the other hand mirroring the active hand? At 12 to 13 months, is the other hand passive but fisted during a manipulation? At 4 to 6 years, is the other hand passive during a manipulation?

What to Ask

The pediatric clinician should inquire about the infant achieving developmental milestones for reach and grasp as indicated in Tables 12–1 and 12–2 and Box 12–3. These are minimal

BOX 12–3 REACH AND GRASP BEHAVIOR SEQUENCE: USE OF SIMPLE OBJECTS IN ASSESSMENT

Raisin Behavior

5 months: regards, mouthing, activation

6 months: rakes

7 months: inferior pincer

9 months: pincer

Pencil Behavior

2 months: follows with eyes horizontally

3 months: activates hands, follows vertically

4 months: bimanual reach, opens hands if touching

7 months: anticipates shape with hand opening at the start of reach

8 months: unilateral grasp

9 months: reaches across midline

12 months: makes marks on paper

18–24 months: imitates stroke on paper

30 months: imitates circle

3–5 years: mature hold on pencil

Stethoscope Behavior

2 months: regards across midline, follows vertically

3 months: bimanually swipes; brings to mouth if caught

5–6 months: reliable reach, hands open on contact

6–7 months: reaches across midline if restrained

9–10 months: unilateral reach, with mirroring movements

13 months: unilateral reach with contralateral opening/closing

Block (1 × 1 × 1 Inch) Behavior While Sitting

3–4 months: waves at block on the table, holds onto one if placed in the hand

4–5 months: brings both hands to the block

5–6 months: brings block to mouth

6–7 months: picks up with one hand; holds onto one in each hand

7–8 months: bangs block on table

9–10 months: bangs 2 blocks together

10–13 months: stacks 2 blocks

15 months: stacks 3 blocks

18 months: stacks 4 blocks

24 months: stacks 7 blocks

36 months: stacks 10 blocks

competencies, not average. Failure to achieve these milestones calls for further evaluation. The following are questions to ask parents during office visits:

- At 1 to 3 months, does the baby look at his hands?
- At 4 months, does the baby swipe at objects within his visual space?
- At 5 months, can the baby reach for and hold onto toys?
- At 6 months, can the baby transfer an object from one hand to the other?
- At 7 to 9 months, does the baby feed crackers to himself?
- At 9 to 11 months, can the baby pick up a pea, raisin or a cereal bit between the thumb and forefinger?
- Are there any imbalances, weaknesses or asymmetries that caregivers notice?

ANTICIPATORY GUIDANCE

Play Activities

The child should be provided with a variety of safe materials to see, touch and mouth. Parents can facilitate this through positioning the child in a variety of ways in different surroundings with a few simple, safe items to reach for. The office should model this activity with safe, washable toys. With the advisory now to place children supine for sleep, it is even more important to provide prone time while awake to encourage object manipulation.

- When solid foods are introduced after 6 months, the child should be free to explore them with his hands. When the pincer grasp appears, the child will participate in self-feeding and effectively reach for and consume small, soft pieces of cooked vegetables, dry cereal, cooked rice and pasta and cheese. Failure to start allowing participation in and relinquish some control in this area spells the beginning of feeding difficulties.
- Every room in the house should have some evidence of the child's work—a play place, the child's own magazines to tear up, a container of simple objects and safe places to explore.
- Asymmetry of reach or grasp should be taken very seriously because it may signal underlying neurological difficulty. Although subtle differences may be apparent, very evident persistent or worsening differences must be investigated. Parents should provide ample opportunities for the child to use the "less mature" hand. However, if these differences persist for 1 to 2 months, further evaluation is indicated; a short reevaluation time is needed in these matters.
- A premature infant or any child with altered tone or strength should be placed with forward shoulder support to allow for good visual monitoring of hand activity. Prone positioning is particularly important in these groups, even though it may take the child a while to accept this position. Chest support will help. When the child is seated, a towel under the thighs flexes the hips, thereby relaxing the trunk and facilitating hand movement.

SPECIAL ISSUES

Stimulation Programs

Parents should be cautioned about **infant stimulation programs** that promise gains in cognitive development through a specific series of activities or through the use of specific devices. No program can provide a curriculum that is any better than the baby's own drive to use newly emerging hand-eye skills in productive ways. These programs may perpetuate a feeling in some parents that they must teach their children developmental skills. This is the wrong perspective. The parental role as primary teachers for their child is one of facilitating the child's own efforts through careful observation and developing a safe environment for the child's own free exploration. Many "developmentally appropriate" toys are available for purchase, but they do not possess magical qualities in themselves. Good toys are simple, safe and brightly colored (e.g., blocks and balls) and provide a variety of textures and actions. They also leave room for the child's imagination.

Excessive concern about stimulation equipment and programs should alert the clinician that such parents may be anxious about their child, feel incompetent as play companions and teachers to their child, cannot appreciate their own child's play needs or have a distorted view regarding what fuels a child's own development. The clinician should take these questions seriously and address the underlying parental issues. Motor competencies depend on the child's motivation (which can be supported through positive, but not overwhelming response) and an opportunity for exploration of objects with her hands (a setup parents can provide).

QUICK CHECK—6 MONTHS

- ✓ Sits with minimal support
- ✓ Bears weight on feet when held upright
- ✓ Rotates wrist
- ✓ Picks up a cube from the table
- ✓ Rakes a pellet
- ✓ Reaches and grasps an object
- ✓ Transfers objects from hand to hand
- ✓ Grasps and brings feet to his mouth, lying supine
- ✓ Makes the phonemes "ba," "ga," "da"
- ✓ Up on arms when in the prone position
- ✓ Makes sounds with objects (shake, rattle or bang)

! HEADS UP–6 MONTHS

Motor Delays at This Age
- No prop sit. If a child has such poor truncal tone and/or head control that he cannot be maintained in a sitting position with support at the hips only, he's behind in a motor sense. Central and peripheral causes need consideration, as well as general physical well-being and strength.
- Both hands should be active, and there should be accurate reaching in the midline.
- Objects should be manipulated in the midline.
- Asymmetrical reaching suggests hemiparesis on a peripheral or central basis.

Other
- Babbling, or sound units with a consonant and a vowel, should be heard at this age, perhaps even strung together in "phrases." Watch a child who has not said any "ba's" or "ma's."
- Any child with a decrease in vocalizations at this time (or any other) needs a hearing test.
- Children at this age should have a wary look when strangers first approach. Failure to "glare" raises the question of delay in social development (perhaps because of cognitive delay) or an attachment disorder.
- Six-month-olds should be very interested in and going after interesting people and objects in the environment. A "too good" child who sits quietly may be delayed or even chronically ill or depressed.
- Naps should be consolidated into two periods. Sleep should be solid at night because no night feedings are needed for nutrition. Separation and attachment (too much or too little) may be at the basis of a delay in sleep pattern maturation.
- Dysconjugate gaze should be resolved at this time. If not, an ophthalmological referral is indicated.
- Solid foods should be started now if not before. If tongue thrust persists at this age after 2 to 3 weeks of solid feeding, a closer look at pharyngeal function and development is generally necessary.

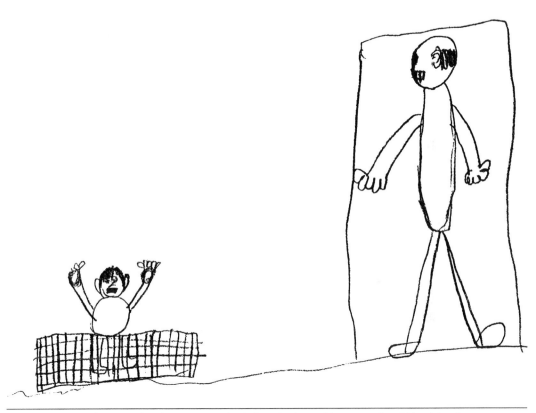

"Dad goes to the playpen to get the baby, who is reaching up to signal his wishes."

CHAPTER 13

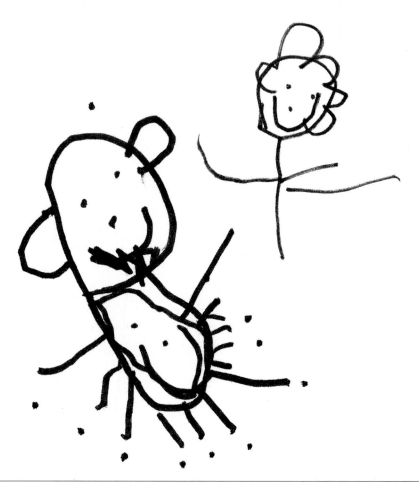

The active movement of a young child is conveyed by the use of multiple legs. Mom looks on, dancing herself to keep up. By Katherine Baucher, age 4.

Eight to Nine Months: Exploring and Clinging

MARIA TROZZI and SUZANNE D. DIXON

This chapter discusses the social and emotional changes occurring in early childhood that produce stranger anxiety, night wakening and a shift in parent-child interaction. New motor skills and cognitive abilities at this age create new safety issues, as well as the requisite shifts in parental care and vigilance. Specific, simple play activities are presented as ways to probe a child's development in clinical settings, at this age and beyond.

Key Words

- **Stranger Anxiety**
- **Attachment**
- **Play**
- **The Strange Situation**
- **Separations**
- **Advances in Play**
- **Accidents**
- **Transitional Objects**
- **Crawling**
- **Night Wakening**
- **Safety Based on Developmental Skills**
- **Self-Feeding**
- **Object Permanence**

Hailey, 8 months old, comes in for removal of sutures from her forehead. She had fallen out of her highchair during a struggle to lock her in. She screams and digs into her mother at your approach. Her mother says Hailey just started these "tantrums" and is worried that this injury has made her fearful. She says that even Hailey's grandmother cannot take her without protest anymore, and Hailey is waking up crying at night. She believes all this "bad behavior" was caused by the laceration. Mother says she will just step out quietly while you remove the sutures because Hailey cries even more when she is in the room. Besides, she is really tired, having been up three to four times a night with Hailey, who has just started awakening again. Note: This case illustrates the expected emergence of stranger anxiety at this age, the nighttime disturbances that appear to be prompted by cognitive shifts and the new safety requirements needed with new motor capabilities.

The landmark of social development described by Rene Spitz as "stranger anxiety" is reached after the midpoint of the first year. This change from the all-trusting, happy-to-be-with-anyone baby to the screaming, fearful child does not appear to be a developmental advancement when first encountered, but it really is. This confusing behavior calls for some explanation, requires awareness by all who care for and make decisions about children and testifies to the huge leaps in cognitive development that occur at this age. Play at this age is particularly interesting and important and offers a window to look at these new cognitive gains. The environment should be reviewed because the baby's new motor and mental skills bring the potential for getting into more trouble. We will explore safety from this developmental perspective.

STRANGER RESPONSES

The child has been sensitive to the differences between parents and strangers since the earliest weeks of life and has shown real preference for the company and games of parents and other predictable adults. This continuum of development makes a quantum change in the second half of the first year. Real fear of being touched or picked up when approached by a stranger occurs at about 6 months; it elicits more discomfort than just seeing a stranger. However, a more apparent and overtly negative reaction known as **stranger anxiety** begins to appear around 8 months and continues in its fullest form until about 18 to 24 months. This encompasses the period during which the child can envision and miss regular care providers (a cognitive skill we call **object permanence** for people), but does not have the linguistic and social skills to quickly negotiate a relationship with new people, the strangers. Although children much older than 2 are still appropriately wary and worried about strangers, the degree and intensity of stress are much less than during this time frame around the first birthday. In addition, other cognitive capabilities such as the ability to categorize and remember allow the child to notice very quickly and become acutely distressed by the appearance, sound and touch of unfamiliar people. Well-established routines of interaction and care are now in place, and the child becomes exquisitely sensitive to any differences from these expectations. Usually, the more dissonance from the expected, the greater the initial distress in a new circumstance.

The child needs reliable features of the environment as she starts to venture out to explore new territory, a scary proposition. The child can now change position in space (see later) and investigate things that were not possible to get to before. Familiar care providers are treated as safe sources of comfort in the midst of these little journeys; they serve as a **secure base** from which to explore. The presence of the familiar care provider allows the child to take risks in moving away—creeping, crawling, rolling or scooting—and later walking. When the child gets too far away or perceives a threat or danger, she counts on being rescued by care providers or on having them available to return to.

As Dr. Mason stooped down to pick up Megan, an active 9-month-old, she glared at him, quickly crawled to her mom and hid her face in mom's legs. Note: Mom is a secure base for Megan, a healthy sign.

If separated from a parent, particularly if left in the presence of strangers, the child becomes, justifiably from her perspective, very upset. This reliance on care providers is evidence of attachment to them, as well as the child's new cognitive skills in visualizing them and wishing they were present when they are not. Cross-cultural work provides evidence of this process being universal in healthy human development. The intensity and form of the behavior may vary around the world, but this pattern between child and care provider has been observed everywhere it has been studied.

WHAT IS ATTACHMENT?

Attachment is the enduring emotional bond that humans feel toward special people in their lives. It encompasses trust that the other will be attentive and responsive to one's needs and emotional state. It leads to types of behavior that keep us close to the attachment figure. Absence from that person creates distress to some degree, and reunion brings relief from that distress. The work of the first year is to develop an attachment to one's care providers. This forms a model for other attachments throughout life. It is the foundation for healthy emotional development.

Becoming attached is the core work of infancy and serves as the foundation for building a sense of self and establishing a healthy emotional life. Although a child begins to become familiar with his primary care providers even before birth, it is in the last quarter of the first year that this process becomes very clear and at the center stage of development. Attachment behaviors that give testimony to the underlying emotional state are similar across the life span. Such behavior includes seeking to be near the attachment object (a person), showing distress when separated, displaying happiness when reunited and orienting one's actions to the object of attachment. This means checking in with that person, sharing objects and observations and doing things with and for that person. Although these are lifelong patterns, the foundation is laid down in the first year.

 Logan held a cookie out to his mom. He wanted to have her come near and to give it to her.

THE STRANGE SITUATION

A predictable response in a young child who has experienced responsive care allows child development specialists to evaluate attachment by using an experimental paradigm called **"The Strange Situation."** This procedure (abbreviated) is outlined in Box 13–1. This experimental paradigm has been applied widely and helps us understand the nature of a child's relationship to care providers.

By making us aware of the range of possible responses to this laboratory situation, this task can assist us in identifying kids who are poorly attached. We can also ask focused questions about a child's behavior at home, on outings or in other situations that involve separation. Developmental psychologists have identified varying profiles in this lab setting that have clinical parallels.

- A *securely attached* child of 8 to 24 months plays eagerly with new toys when mom is present but looks wary at the approach of a stranger and will turn or move away with

---

BOX 13–1   THE STRANGE SITUATION

- The mom* is seated and the child plays in a room of toys.
- A stranger enters the room and talks to the mom.
- The mom leaves.
- The stranger attempts to comfort or play with the child.
- The mom returns and greets and comforts the baby.
- The stranger leaves.

---

*Any familiar care provider may be in this role. The word *mom* is used because most experimental work has been done with moms. Work done specifically with involved fathers shows similar behavior.

---

approach or touch. The child will protest, may or may not cry and will try to follow the departing parent. On the mother's return, the child will go to her for comfort, perhaps after a brief "punishment" of ignoring her. Crying is immediately reduced when the parent returns.

- An *avoidant* child seems unresponsive to mom and demonstrates little distress when she leaves. The child reacts to the stranger in the same way as to the parent, and at reunion she avoids the parent or is very slow to approach. The child may resist being picked up and does not cling. Although this behavior may be caused by cultural or temperamental differences, such a pattern suggests to the clinician that more attention should be placed on monitoring the child's physical and emotional environment.

- A *resistantly attached* child clings to the parent and doesn't explore the room at all. The child becomes very angry on separation and shows it on reunification with hitting, pushing and failure to be comforted easily when picked up. This behavior is worrisome and calls for more investigation of the child's environment.

- *Disorganized* attachment is evident in a child who looks flat throughout the procedure and shows little response to mom leaving or returning, often failing to cry or crying at odd times. Gaze avoidance with mom may be seen. Little or no toy exploration takes place. This is a very concerning observation that suggests a significant lack of attachment in this child's life. This behavior corresponds to infantile or anaclitic depression and has long-term implications.

Experimental work in this country and around the world has substantiated these observations as being universally present. The first type of child, one securely attached, appears to signal the optimal response in all settings. The other patterns indicate some form of attenuation of attachment, although other factors may influence this type of behavior.

VARIATIONS IN ATTACHMENT BEHAVIOR

Clinical use of attachment observations requires that some confounders be taken into consideration when evaluating a child's response to separation and reunion, particularly in clinical rather than experimental settings. The following are factors that influence attachment behavior and color observations:

- *Temperament.* An intense child may show a dramatic response to separation, whereas a mellow child may use more subtle behavior to show distress. A positive-approach child may be more intrigued by the stranger, whereas a child who usually withdraws from something new will be more quiet and clingy in this situation. However, temperament makes only a modest contribution to the response to strangers. Parent issues rather than individual child differences (see later) have stronger correlations to this behavior.

- *Cultural issues.* Although the strange situation test has been used around the world with similar results—the secure pattern being the most frequently seen response—cultural values influence behavior in varying circumstances. For example, in Germany, a common response tends to be the "avoidant" pattern. Parents in that culture value early independence and discourage clinging, so this might be expected. Japanese infants more frequently reveal a "resistant" pattern, but they are rarely out of the mother's sight, and she fosters a dependent pattern of care in line with cultural values (see Chapter 3).

- *Degree of familiarity.* A situation or care provider who is very different in style, appearance or voice from a familiar one is likely to elicit more distress than if the circumstances are only moderately discrepant from the usual. A child at home will be less distressed than one experiencing separation away from home.

- *Fatigue, illness, injury, pain.* We're all at low tide to cope with stress under adverse circumstances, and so are children. The most valid observations are made when the child feels well, is rested and is in no pain.

Individual infant temperament modifies the course of this response. Some children sail through this period with a mild behavior change over a short period. Other children have predictable and dramatic fear responses that continue full-blown until the end of the second year. Dramatic negative responses are not the result of bad experiences in the past or lack of love in the regular environment. These infants are likely to be shy, sensitive and somewhat slow to warm up as part of their individual makeup. Transitions with people and events may require additional time and support for these children, in the first year and beyond.

Cross-cultural investigations suggest that infants of all groups studied have the onset and the first peak of stranger anxiety at about 8 months of age. However, in cultures in which infants are regularly exposed to many caregivers, the response was less intense, was more easily overcome with a familiarization time and lasted for a shorter period into the second year. In all cultures studied, even those described as "polymatric" (many mothers), the strongest protests came with separation from birth mothers. In the United States, infants attach to their parents, even those working outside the home full-time, if the parents' care is responsive and if time spent with the parents early in the infant's life has helped a relationship to start.

Does scrutiny of these attachment patterns have any predictive value? Yes! Well-attached children have a brighter future as a group. Securely attached children have more elaborate play and enthusiasm in the preschool years. They demonstrate more flexibility and persistence in problem solving. As they approach school age, they are seen as more socially competent and empathetic. By middle school they have more and stronger friendships and better social skills.

Attachment, or the lack thereof is very important in altering the life course in infancy and throughout childhood and the adult years.

Factors That Alter Attachment

The following are core influences on attachment:

- *Responsive care.* Ongoing sensitivity to the child's needs and emotional states is most important. This is played out in the course of everyday care. Social and emotional attunement is the critical element. This means appropriate and prompt response to needs, consistency and tender and careful holding. An avoidant response may result when care is too intrusive, too controlling or overstimulating or, conversely, very unresponsive or intermittently neglectful. A resistant pattern may follow from inconsistent, negative or rejecting care. Decreased physical contact, awkward handling or a rough "no nonsense" approach suggests this type of interaction.

- The parent needs to have an *internal working model* of responsive care. This means that the parent has experienced strong attachments in her own childhood and emulates that kind of care. Parents who did not receive such optimal care can create a healthy internal model with effort and good models. It is most important in these cases that the parent has come to some understanding and resolution of the deficits in her own care and has the insight to go beyond that experience. A new model of care can be constructed from others, from interactions with people outside the family. Mentors, friends and other respected individuals can contribute to this model and can repair a negative history in a parent. Interventions for families at risk are probably most effective when they set up these models through relationships. When parents continue to harbor anger, resentment or ambivalence, the "ghosts from the nursery" will haunt their care of their own children. Inconsistencies in responsiveness and a fluctuating emotional climate will make it more difficult for the infant to attach. Therefore, a parent's childhood history is important to the baby's emotional growth.

- An *altered mental state* will affect care. Parents with major mental illness, such as severe depression, bipolar disorder or schizophrenia, cannot be attuned to the baby and the baby's needs. Depression, in particular, may be the final common pathway for many adverse circumstances to have a negative impact on child health and development. Substance abuse fits in here because the fluctuating mental status and availability that are part of the drug use pattern do not support good attachment. Because many women who use illicit drugs self-medicate their depression and because those on stimulants may experience serious depression when they come off drugs, drug use often makes a family at risk for poor attachment between parent and child. A baby's well-being has to be at the center of the family's care and focus. Conditions that marginalize the baby's care are not conducive to good attachment. Rote care, awkward handling, expressions of resentment toward the child and little physical contact may be seen in clinical settings when attachment is poor.

- *Family and social stressors* play a role. A family with financial stresses, joblessness, unwanted moves, food insecurity, dissolved or troubled marriages or a variety of other pressures may not be consistently available to the infant either physically or psychologically. Furthermore, a lot of changes in care or less-than-optimal care because of cost or parental absence creates stress. It is no surprise that resistant and avoidant attachment patterns are seen much more commonly in families struggling with such circumstances.

These conditions dramatically alter the interface between the child and parent. This situation recalls Bronfenbrenner's social ecology model of development (see Chapter 2).

Dr. Ogdahl noted that Ethan, previously a roly-poly and jolly baby, seemed quiet and subdued at the 9-month-old checkup. He was sitting quietly in his mom's lap but didn't turn to her at all. Because it was 10:00 AM, Dr. Ogdahl asked how Lisa, Ethan's mom, had gotten off work. She said she'd been laid off. As a single mom, she had no family support. She said she was looking for work. Ethan's weight was down a little, and he looked pale. Note: Ethan and Lisa are probably both depressed, and Ethan's emotional development is at risk. A mental health referral is needed here, as well as help with financial matters. Ethan needs his mom's responsiveness and care.

ATTACHMENT OBSERVATIONS IN CLINICAL SETTINGS

Awareness of the meaning of these types of attachment behavior allows the clinician to make observations of attachment incidentally. Every visit can invite the child to explore, includes the approach of a stranger (the clinician) and may include some separation. An attuned mind makes such assessment easy and automatic.

The quality of the reaction to strangers is influenced by the infant's developmental age (remember, this tracks with cognitive development), temperament, presence of illness or fatigue, the stranger's demeanor and the presence or absence of familiar figures. Conditions that heighten the fear response are unfamiliar surroundings (e.g., an examining room), active approach by the stranger (e.g., moving in quickly to examine the child) and close proximity to the stranger, especially with eye-to-eye contact. In addition, the response to the stranger is more dramatic when the mother is present but not in physical contact with the infant (e.g., mother in chair and child on examining table).

Factors that lessen fearful behavior include a position close to or in contact with the mother or father, familiarization time in a new setting and a stranger who approaches with toys and whose behavior is responsive to the infant's cues. Children who are exposed to many adults during infancy usually have less dramatic responses to strangers. Strangers who are similar to the parents in their responses to the child will elicit less anxiety than those who are different, no matter how "good" (i.e., sensitive) they are with children in general. Other children elicit less anxiety than adults do in children older than 1 year, although the erratic behavior of a toddler may frighten, as well as delight, an infant.

SEPARATION ASSOCIATIONS

Infants are sensitive to the patterns associated with leave-taking, so separation can be anticipated, and anxiety builds before the actual **separation** occurs. This anticipatory response may explain some behavior in infants. Although these rituals will eventually be an anchor and help for a child, they may initially trigger anticipatory anxiety.

Dylan crawled toward his mom and screamed in what sounded like pain as she picked up her purse. Whenever she did so, he sensed that her departure was imminent. She picked him up for a good-bye hug and wondered if his long-time baby-sitter wasn't taking good care of him any more. When she returned, he seemed very happy and came to her eagerly for comfort. He grabbed her purse and threw it down. Note: Dylan's protests don't come from anticipation of unresponsive care. They are a testimony to his attachment to his mom. He has linked her purse to her leaving. Dylan is anxious because of separation from a person on whom he has relied to orchestrate his life. This behavior is evidence of an attachment that is based on his emotional needs being met by his mom. Eventually, it is the appearance of these same leave-taking and returning rituals that will help build the skills to anticipate return. The more clear and consistent the pattern, the easier it will be for him to become less anxious with these brief separations.

Dylan's mom learned to take her wallet in her briefcase and leave her empty purse with Dylan, putting it on the shelf before she left the house. "Mommy will be right back. See, I've left my purse. I'll get it when I come home." Dylan liked to bring the purse into his room when the sitter put him down for his nap. He was also very clear that he needed his "blanky" right with him for sleep and when he went on an outing.

Transitional Objects

Bowlby and Winnicott have pointed out that a young child's attachment to a cuddly object, which they called the **transitional object**, is part of the developmental process of becoming independent, of separating from parents psychologically. These first treasured possessions are frequently capable of filling the role of an important, though subsidiary attachment when the primary attachment person is not there. The object is a substitute that is sought, especially when the child is hungry, tired or distressed, just as the parent is sought. These props stand in for the absent parent.

Transitional objects, or "loveys," are effectively used by children to shut out environmental stimuli and to calm themselves when upset. Selection of a special object may occur as early as 7 to 8 months but usually takes place between 1 and 2 years of age. Two thirds of children in the United States have a transitional object; other cultural groups have a lower rate, perhaps because the cultural drive for and value of independence are less than in this country. This object may take many forms—a blanket, doll, toy or piece of the child's or parent's clothing. Although most children discard the transitional object as they approach 3 or 4 years of age, when the separation process is farther along and peer pressure mounts, some children retain these attachments into their school years without evidence of psychopathology.

Some parents may perceive the ever-present cuddly object as a weakness, a crutch rather than a strength. Embarrassment may develop if they view it as a negative reflection on their parenting or on the child's ability to cope. The parents and the child may also receive pressure from extended family or child care providers to "give up that thing." The child's clinician can help parents appreciate their child's resourcefulness and emerging independence. Having a duplicate for washing or replacement is wise because these treasured items get heavy use.

Comfort Habits

Most children rock on occasion (usually when falling asleep), do some head banging or later twirl hair, pull at their ears or rub their faces. These comfort habits, along with the use of "loveys," or transitional objects, are healthy ways to settle down, to cope with stress or to fill in quiet time. These are positive steps in learning ways to solve life's little problems. Use of these comfort habits is healthy most of the time, but may be a concern if any of the following are true:

- The child prefers the lovey to people and spends more time alone with the lovey than with people.
- The child will not usually stop to acknowledge or respond to a parent when using the lovey or comfort routine.
- The child often leaves an activity to go to his lovey.
- The child hurts herself with the lovey or other comfort habit.

If any such behavior is noted, further evaluation of development and the environment should take place.

INFANTILE DEPRESSION

Infants do become depressed when there is a significant alteration in the availability of a primary caregiver. A change in demeanor, eating, sleeping and activity can signal this.

Rosalie was a 13-month-old, a third child who was brought to her clinician because "she's changed." Her parents reported that 5 months ago she was babbling, cruising around furniture and very active. Now she "just sits," hasn't progressed to walking and has very little to say. The growth chart shows a falloff in growth, from the 90th to the 50th percentile in weight, the relative height declining just a bit and head circumference maintained. The parents date the change to a car accident Rosalie experienced with her mom. Mom's car was hit from the side. Rosalie never left her car seat, and examinations then and 2 weeks later by a pediatric neurologist showed no neurological injury to the child. Mom had a dislocated shoulder, facial lacerations and a sprained ankle. She stayed overnight in the hospital. She says, "I was a basket case" and developed symptoms of posttraumatic stress disorder. Mom's sleep was poor and the family routines fell apart. Rosalie's exam at this visit was normal except that she had a flat affect, refused to explore any of the toys in the office and screamed frantically when the examiner picked her up. Mom was referred for mental health services and was started on an antidepressant. On a return visit, both mom and Rosalie were brighter and more interactive. Rosalie was noisy, moved easily around the room and took a toy from the clinician, although she toddled back to her mom immediately. Note: This child was profoundly affected by the change in the mental and physical states of her mother and demonstrated signs of infantile depression. Mom's facial injuries and change in mobility were probably the first factors noted by the infant. Restoration of the well-being of mom led to emotional recovery of the child. Although mom was not physically absent from the child, she was emotionally, psychologically unavailable and had an altered physical appearance.

Coming and Going

As new motor competencies are discovered and practiced, the child can move away from a parent by crawling, scooting and eventually walking. This can be both exciting and alarming for a child. Mahler and colleagues called this new emotional state "hatching" (see Chapter 2). It refers to the realization by the child of being separate from mother, that the mother can leave or the child can leave her and that proximity is not a guarantee during exploratory movements. The internal drive for mastery and discovery is tempered by the realization that approaching new things or people in the environment increases one's distance from familiar providers. *Internal security is needed to go forward on these adventures.* A child who is anxious will not explore as widely, as often or as confidently. Such a child needs to "hatch" in order to grow developmentally. Being free to explore requires that the relationship with the parent be secure. The parent's presence must be seen as a reliable place to which the child can return physically and psychologically if he needs safety and assurance. A child with an insecure attachment will be less willing to venture out.

Another peak of stranger anxiety often occurs at 18 to 20 months of age, usually just before the development of real language competency. The toddler relies heavily on the nonverbal communication patterns established with his parents. Strangers are not immediately a part of this individualized communication network. The emotional state of this second peak of stranger anxiety has been called *rapprochement.* It is observed when a previously secure toddler intermittently checks in with a parent, either running back to a secure base or visually making contact across a room. This allows reassurance and refueling for more adventures.

Michael ran out of the examining room and down the hall. He stopped as the clerk at the desk greeted him. He quickly ran back and buried his head in mom's lap. Note: This simple observation shows the healthy tension in this child's life between discovery and security.

This resurgence of stranger anxiety at 18 months diminishes gradually as the child's mastery of language skills allows communication with unknown people. By 2 to 3 years of age, the child begins to show decreased distress and increased friendliness with strangers. This process of increasing socialization and independence is gradual and very individual. As the preschool child explores new people and objects, he continues initially to draw closer to mother or father and plays less when encountering strangers. Children who are well attached to their primary caregivers use them as bases to venture out in ever-widening circles of exploration; children who are poorly attached do not venture out as readily, or when they do, they don't look back to check, to share a discovery or to point to something of interest, an act of shared social attention. Children who remain extremely shy and clingy beyond age 3 or those who are not becoming more and more willing to explore when they are given familiarization and support are worrisome. They are developmentally delayed, emotionally and perhaps cognitively, or are very insecure in their attachment to care providers or so temperamentally withdrawn that it is an impediment to ordinary childhood experiences. These children need a second look by a mental health professional.

Noah is in his second year of daycare but still stays very close to Miss Julie. He refuses to go to the sandbox by himself and rarely initiates an interaction with another child except to "claim" a toy the other child possesses. Note: Noah and his parents need a closer look by the clinician and perhaps referral to a professional skilled in working with young children. This degree of withdrawal after this much time in a responsive environment is not typical.

Assimilating Strangers

The opportunity to interact with adults outside the immediate family offers the infant new perspectives and the chance to learn about other people and self through these social interactions. The child's world is richer because of what others can bring to it. Friends, relatives and other children add vitality to a child's life. The child learns that other adults can be trusted and enjoyed. This is not to displace the parents from their central position, but to expand the child's horizons.

Alternative caregivers (grandparents, baby-sitters, etc.) can be introduced in a way that supports the child's efforts at social expansion without unduly stressing the child. A time of familiarization with the new caretaker, maintaining regular routines and place (if possible) and the initiation of leave-taking routines all make brief separations easier. The most important element, however, is an unambivalent attitude in parents. Parents must be comfortable with separation before the child can be because the child takes cues from them. Children are very sensitive to a parent's distress and worry even if the parent attempts to disguise it.

Separations that are unplanned, prolonged or accompanied by exposure to a caregiver who cannot meet the child's needs for consistency and responsiveness should be avoided at any age, particularly from about 6 to 18 months, when these emotional issues are dominant. Family vacations, visitation schedules, change of placement, business needs and career decisions must take these needs into account in balancing family priorities and minimizing stress for young children.

Mark and Sharon wanted to go on a long holiday with Sharon's folks. Alissa, 10 months old, was an active child, and her grandparents weren't excited to have her on the month-long trip. Alissa's parents decided to forego the trip, go on a long weekend vacation by themselves and then spend a week at a camp that had child care for Alissa.

When Families Come Apart

Divorce is hard on kids at any age, but it is particularly stressful at times of enhanced stranger anxiety. Separation from the noncustodial spouse will be a stressor, and changes in the emotional climate, financial pressures, moves and alterations in routine are very problematic to kids. The more things change, the harder it is on kids. Shared physical custody of a young child is especially difficult at this time and should be avoided at all costs because it requires too much change in every aspect of life—bed, play space, feeding and so forth. The child doesn't have the cognitive and linguistic skills to understand explanations of the situation and has no sense of time to understand when Daddy or Mommy are coming back. The family should look for other solutions to keep both parents involved without requiring the baby to absorb the great separation stress precipitated by changes in family structure.

Shifts in foster placement and adoption are to be avoided at this time for similar reasons. A child's attachment to familiar people is the foundation of a sense of self. To blow that apart at this critical time will be detrimental even if the placement overall is better. Wait until age 2 to make these shifts if unable to do so before 6 months. Clinicians may have to be advocates for young children with social service agencies and the courts regarding shifts in care during this critical interval.

See Chapters 25 and 27 for more detail on these topics.

The Institutionalized Child

Chronically or repeatedly hospitalized children are at risk for poor attachments because their world changes from shift to shift and they do not have a chance to develop relationships with their parents because of the many demands and constraints of such a situation. Although hospitalization these days is less frequent, shorter and rarely without some parental involvement, many children suffer emotionally from these experiences. One can identify a child with no real attachment to anyone in an institutional setting, one who is in serious trouble emotionally, by seeing which child goes to anyone, is carried around by everyone and rarely cries or turns to anyone special for comfort. This child is detached, a shallow and dangerous emotional state in which the child guards against any investment in anyone. Children raised in institutions that lack individualized care, such as some international adoptees, are at risk because of this lack of attachment. The "pet" of all may be a child who is very damaged emotionally. The child not only is in trouble now, but will also have difficulties in the future with social relationships, personality problems and perhaps delinquency. Healing must include the development of a relationship with a primary attachment figure, in the institution or somewhere else. This is a behavioral emergency.

Daily Situations

Separations, strangers and mild stresses are a part of life; they are opportunities for growth through widening social experience, the development of coping strategies and the re-energization of parents. The clinician can identify the child's perspective by participating in discussion of family management decisions that involve separations. The clinician thus serves as the child's advocate by promoting expansion of the social experiences and lessening any detrimental impact of prolonged separation. Data on daycare experience suggest that it is the quality of responsive care that is critical to healthy emotional development. A quality daycare experience can be enriching for any child, particularly children born at a disadvantage.

On a daily basis for most families, leave-takings should be brief, affectionate and accompanied by a clear statement of return, even for a child who does not understand words or have a sense of time. These patterns should be clearly established in infancy and maintained throughout early childhood. Parents should never sneak out, lie about a return time or promise gifts at each leave-taking. Trust is violated and brief separations are seen as either punishment or an extraordinary event.

BABIES WHO MAKE NOISE IN THE NIGHT

Night wakening that awakes others often returns at this age. Some believe that the basis for this is the ability to miss the parents because the child can now envision them when he wakens (i.e., he has the cognitive ability called object permanence). The child cries out to call them. In addition, the ability to pull to stand means that the child can really wake up completely by trying out these new motor skills at night. If the child is worried or aggravated about being unable to get down or just wants to share the adventure, he will cry out for attention and reassurance. To parents, this feels like a big step backward; a solid night's sleep is gone. The distress is genuine, but what to do? Answer: go back to the basics:

- Form a simple, but consistent bedtime ritual that involves putting the child to bed while he is still awake (see Chapter 11).
- Be sure the child has a "lovey" for cuddling.
- When the child awakens and calls out, wait a minute or two to provide the opportunity for the child to get back to sleep on his own.
- If the cries are frantic, go in silently and tuck the child back in, using the same procedures that were done originally.
- Avoid taking the child out of bed unless you want to do that all night long.
- Reassurance delivered in a quiet, nonplayful way with brevity will help the child learn how to settle himself down and go back to sleep.

Sleep means a separation, particularly as we set things up in the United States. From the child's perspective, he is in his own bed, away from others, in the dark and alone until he wakes up. Going to sleep means saying good-bye for a while. This, like other separations, creates a little stress for a child, so it's no wonder that sleep concerns are so common. For parents too, putting the baby to bed is a separation, and they may not come to the task without ambivalence. For this reason, when the clinician counsels families about sleep problems, the underlying issues are how everyone feels about separation, what they can tolerate and what do they really want. Family inconsistency and failure to follow advice about sleep concerns usually come down to an underlying attachment-separation issue that should be addressed before dealing with the specifics of sleep problems. The following groups are likely to have trouble around this sleep separation issue.

- Parents of a small, sick or prematurely born baby, who are still concerned about losing the child even if the child is not physically ill. Often, the parents themselves are not aware of this underlying worry
- A family who has lost a previous child
- A divorced, separating or single parent
- A working couple who are away from the baby all day
- A family with a history of loss issues, particularly recent ones (e.g., a move, a death in the family, loss of a job)

For these families, night wakening is perceived as a bid for closeness and help rather than a manifestation of developmental change. These parents cannot let the child solve this issue on his own. The motivations and emotional needs of the parents must be addressed openly if night wakening is frequent and problematic. Temperamental issues in the child and particular cultural or family issues may also be the source of barriers to achieve the stated sleep goals.

The clinical management strategy is to allay anxiety while supporting the child's own efforts to go back to sleep. Too vigorous an intervention just further awakens the child and makes settling down all the more difficult. No evidence shows that bringing a child into the parents' bed is either uncommon or leads to disturbance. Some families choose a family bed and cosleeping. Breastfeeding may be enhanced in that circumstance. This will not harm the child as long as the following are true:

- The child's bids for independence are met in other ways.
- The child doesn't become exposed to sexual activity, which may seem violent to a small child.
- The adults aren't under the influence of drugs or alcohol, which can make them forget that the child is in the bed.
- The bedding is firm and the mattress fits the bed so that a child cannot get caught between the mattress and frame (i.e., entrapment).
- Cigarette smoke is not in the environment.

AROUND AND ABOUT: MOTOR SKILLS

At about 9 months of age, children learn to use the index finger as a separate "pointer finger" and to use the index and thumb together in a "pincer grasp" (see Chapter 12 for a discussion of the emergence of hand skills). Opposition of the thumb sets the stage for the sophisticated use of the hand characteristic of humans. In the immediate sense, this ability allows the child to pick up very small objects and explore them in very complex ways. Moreover, the ability to put one thing into another that emerges at this time sets the stage for much more elaborate ways to play and explore.

Moving in space somehow is the motor milestone that comes in at this age. Although each infant solves the problem of getting around his environment in his own way, exploration of the world becomes his goal. Some children roll, others scoot along while sitting, others creep by pulling with their arms and still others eventually get up on hands and knees and crawl. The manner of movement in itself is not important, but the exploration of space is vital to cognitive growth. Interesting sights at a distance, objects that disappear and just the joy of moving prompt this forward progression. After a year of age, an unseen sound producer will prompt movement. Getting a chance to move and explore opens up opportunities to refine these motor skills and to learn from these explorations.

EXPLORING AND SAFETY

Madeline Jones, a 9-month-old obese child, was brought to the emergency room by her frantic mother. The child had a small scald burn on her left forearm and a large "goose egg" on her forehead, but appeared alert as she whimpered in her mother's arms. Mrs. Jones said her daughter had pulled the coffee pot over and spilled coffee on herself. Mrs. Jones said she didn't even know that Madeline could go that far or move as fast as she did. She really had not been crawling until recently. Madeline sat quietly at her mother's feet, playing with some papers from the desk while her mother got out some tissue.

With each new developmental competency, a child has the chance of getting into trouble in entirely new and surprising ways. The clinician can put into place the general concept that **safety** has to be linked to each new developmental gain. If the parents can see the world from their child's perspective at each new juncture of enhanced competence, they can anticipate how to make the environment safe while offering the child the chance to explore and learn to use the new skills. This is a broader perspective than merely a list of safety issues or a checklist given at each visit (see Table 13–1).

TABLE 13–1   Age-Appropriate Safety Guidelines

Age	Child's Activities	Dangers, Risks	Questions and Suggestions for Parents
0–6 mo	Swimming reflex	Drowning, water intoxication, stress	Counsel on early swimming lessons
	Immobile	Fire, smoke dangers	Place a smoke alarm near the infant's sleeping quarters
	Rolling over	Falls, rolling off a table	Use appropriate bathing facilities, restraints, safe changing area, padded floor
	Attempts to sit up	Flipping out of infant seat (3 mo)	Keep the child restrained in the infant seat; remove the infant seat at 3 mo
	Sucking and mouthing objects	Ingestion, aspiration, strangulation from a pacifier string or other objects	Keep toys clean; avoid letting the child mouth keys
	Motor excitement	Slipping while bathing	Lower the temperature of the hot water heater (<120° F)
	Reaching for objects	Burns, cuts	
7–12 mo	Crawl, pull to stand, cruising	Burns; falls down stairs, into toilet bowl or into tub	Block stairs; eliminate walker
	Increased curiosity	Ingestions (medicines, plants, chemicals, household cleaning agents)	Have poison control phone numbers and available; lock cabinets
	Pincer grasp	Aspiration of small objects such as marbles and toy parts, pills, seeds, plants	Keep older children's toys (with button eyes, removable parts) and other small objects out of reach
	Puts everything in mouth	Electric cord bites	Keep cords out of reach

Continued

TABLE 13–1   **Age-Appropriate Safety Guidelines—cont'd**

Age	Child's Activities	Dangers, Risks	Questions and Suggestions for Parents
	Goes after hidden objects	Aspiration, strangulation (cords)	Look under tables, chairs, beds for dangers
	Pulls objects down	Hot liquid burns, objects on tables	Put heavy or hot objects out of reach
1–2 yr*	Walking, running	Traffic accidents	Does the child have access to the street?
	Loves to be chased (18–24 mo)	Runs away, into streets	Block doors, walkways; use automatic gate locks
	Climbing (tables, desks, counters)	Ingestions, falls, burns	How are medications stored? Put chairs away from counters
	Goes after hidden objects	Ingestions, electrocution	Are medications in purse? Are outlets covered?
	Increased independence and curiosity	Ingestions, burns, drownings	Is access to a pool blocked?
2–3 yr*	Expanding world (backyard, garage, friend's house)	Ingestions	Is there access to garage, backyard, safe play equipment?
	Imitative behavior	Climbs, follows older children, ingests pills	Keep medications locked up and out of reach
	"Swim" classes	Drowning, drinking pool water with hyponatremia	Avoid. Be sure of full parent participation. Do not expect the child to be drowning proof
	Introduction to adult foods	Aspiration (nuts, popcorn, chewing gum)	Avoid access to nuts, popcorn and chewing gum at this age
	Resists constraints (e.g., car seats)	Car accidents	Possess, install correctly and use a car seat
	False maturity leading toward less parental supervision (2-yr-olds)	All accidents	Keep under constant observation

TABLE 13–1   **Age-Appropriate Safety Guidelines—cont'd**

Age	Child's Activities	Dangers, Risks	Questions and Suggestions for Parents
3–5 yr	Improved motor development: reaches high "safe" places	Ingestions, burns, falls	Supervise play
	Tricycles, big wheels	Spoke injuries, traffic accidents	Provide safe places to play
	Expanded world (school, neighborhood)	Car accidents, falls	Has traffic safety been taught?
	Continued drive to discover world	Burns (matches)	Discuss fire safety
	Role playing, superhero imitations	Burns, ingestions, falls	Keep play areas safe; regularly supervise; discuss role models
	Resists constraints (e.g., car seats)	Car accidents	Possess, install correctly and use car seat
6–14 yr	Independence, spends time away from home	Bike, skateboard and car accidents; drownings	Child should wear a helmet; skateboard off streets, hills; use inline skates with wrist, elbow and knee pads and helmet; swim in groups under supervision; take swimming and water classes
	Unsupervised activities	Burns (fireworks and matches), alcohol and drug exploration or overdose	Talk to the kid
15–17 yr		Car accidents; drug and alcohol use	Make sure the child takes driver education. Discuss peer-proofing and other drug education programs. Apply reasonable curfews. All parties should be supervised

*Highest accident rates of all groups.

The Child's Point of View

This general dictum aside, at 8 to 9 months, dramatic changes in the child call for safety inspections in a lot of new ways. This time is ideal to put the new parental mind-set into place: a change in the child's abilities demands a new safety review. The emergence of mobility in one form or another and the more adept use of fingers and hands mean more fun, learning and potential trouble. Parents should be told to get on their hands and knees and go around the house to see the world as the baby sees it. The lurking dangers, as well as the temptations, are more obvious with that activity than merely by going through a checklist.

It is also a good metaphor for seeing things from the child's perspective as one tries to anticipate or solve child-rearing problems. Many times it is the clinician who has to evoke the child's view of things for the parent to see the way through to problem solving. Starting in the first year, on their knees to check out safety issues, parents get a good start on seeing things from the child's viewpoint. It is a handy exercise for the clinician to suggest.

When the baby can creep, crawl, roll or scoot on her bottom, the child can change her placement in space. Now the sphere of safety widens to wherever the child can move. A whole room has to be made safe, and some spaces have to be blocked off because they contain too many things that can get the child into trouble. **The goal here is not to discuss every safety issue, but to put forward a strategy of looking at safety issues that are triggered by developmental change.** Then, whenever new skills emerge, a parenting pattern can be set up. For example, when the child can climb, what about the surface under play equipment? When the child rides the bus to school, what safety measures are needed?

Box 13–2 shows some of the maneuvers that are appropriate for a newly mobile child who can now change location.

Because children are more adept with their hands working together at this age and in using the index finger and the pincer grasp, what they can grab and what they pull toward them must be considered. Exploring discoveries with the mouth is to be expected, so that should also be considered.

Box 13–3 shows some of the safety issues to keep in mind about a child who now has enhanced manipulative skills.

BOX 13–2 SAFETY FIRST FOR BABY ON THE MOVE

- Cupboard doors should have safety stoppers.
- Household cleaning products should be put up out of baby's reach.
- All stairways should be blocked by attached gates.
- Outside doors should be closed tightly, perhaps with plastic sealers, or for older children, high hooks.
- The crib mattress should be at the lowest level.
- The diaper-changing area should be safe in the event of falls, which may mean a pad on the floor or on a low bed.
- Baby walkers should not be used at all.
- The car seat should be adjusted for size and never ignored. Watch for the child wriggling out of it.
- The garage and bathroom should be off limits unless an adult, focused on the child, is present at all times.
- Sharp corners of tables and cabinets should have protectors on them.
- Poisonous plants should be removed from house and yard.
- Attached gates at staircases and to block off rooms.
- Bathroom should be off limits.
- Any body of water should be removed or blocked. A bucket and a toilet are bodies of water.

BOX 13–3 SAFETY FIRST FOR ACTIVE HANDS

- All electrical outlets should be plugged or covered.
- Electrical cords should not hang down.
- Protective caps should be put on faucets to prevent kids from turning them on.
- All breakables should be put away.
- Residents' and visitors' purses should be placed out of the child's reach.
- All medicines must have safety caps that are kept on.
- All siblings' toys with small pieces should be put away.
- Pets and babies are a mix ready for trouble.
- All houseplants should be checked for poisonous components and removed if present. If safe ones are kept, be ready for pruning that you didn't count on and roughage (i.e., dirt) for the baby that you didn't plan.
- Cat and dog food should be kept out of the child's reach.
- Anything tiny should be kept off the floor.
- Sandboxes, beaches and playgrounds should be inspected for tiny undesirables such as cigarette butts, coins and buttons.

FEEDING AND EATING AS EXPLORATION AND SEPARATION

No better classroom exists for learning about the world and exerting just a taste of independence than eating does. With each new developmental gain, the child can explore **food** in new ways and take greater and greater charge of what goes into her mouth. This is a messy process. Parents have to be able to tolerate this and be ready to hand over some control to the child. This is hard if the parents are anxious about the child, have a need to control or don't like the mess and uncertainty that self-feeding involves. At 8 months, with development of the pincer grasp and improved eye-hand coordination, the child should be allowed finger foods that she can handle and be allowed to explore the feel and texture of food. If the child is not given that opportunity, eating will be less interesting later or will turn into a battleground between parent and child. Furthermore, it's a battle that parents never win. If there are struggles around food, there are likely to be struggles around a lot of things in the interaction between parent and child.

Rayna was an obese, placid child who moved around very little during the 9-month visit. At every whimper her mother took out a bottle and gave it to her, cradling her and covering her head while feeding.

Rayna was found to be anemic and was drinking about 48 to 52 oz of milk per day. Her mother reported that Rayna didn't want to feed herself and was "too little" to drink from a cup.

Note: Rayna's mother is still treating her like a newborn, not responding to her developmental gains. Anemia and obesity are only part of the problem here—a "developmental arrest" in feeding interaction overall exists. The clinician should show mom what Rayna can and should be doing with feeding at this age and should explore why mom needs to keep this baby as a newborn. A mere prescription for feeding is unlikely to work here.

With each change in the child, the feeding-eating situation should change. Table 13–2 presents the developmental course of feeding. If the child can't carry out age-appropriate self-feeding, the clinician should explore whether the baby has developmental delays, oral-motor difficulties, unusual taste and touch sensitivities or other difficulties. If these problems are not the case, the interaction between parent and child should be explored. Sometimes this means having the mother bring in food and try to feed the baby in the office. Although this may seem time-consuming at first, it can be efficient in identifying the source of the problem.

NOW YOU SEE IT; NOW YOU DON'T

A child's ability to use his hands in more complex play with objects and his ability to move around in space prompt a whole new level of cognitive ability. The world becomes for him a three dimensional universe that stays put even if he can't see its features or be near them at all times. A very young infant acts as though objects cease to exist when he can't see them; now, a child will pursue a disappearing object—uncovering a block, moving to get a car behind a chair. Such behavior is called object permanence, a key cognitive building block. A very young infant treats the world as a movie that turns off when he closes his eyes. A 9-month-old knows that the drama goes on even if he's not observing it. Disappearing people need to be followed; hidden toys need to be found. He loves peek-a-boo at this age because this game plays into this new mental ability, to remember and to anticipate. He'll nearly shake with anticipation when dad disappears behind a screen, just waiting for dad's reappearance. In fact, his own play at this age will include experiments with hiding and finding, putting one thing into another and then retrieving it. Play, at this age, as at all ages, reflects the newly emerging mental abilities.

PLAY AS AN ASSESSMENT: CHANGING THE AGENDA OF THIS VISIT

Children will demonstrate the cutting edge of their developmental competency in their **play** if we give them just a few props and a lot of support and protection from stressors. The 9-month visit, because it occurs at a time of great developmental change and before real mobility and stranger anxiety make the child take flight at every encounter, is the perfect time to really look at how the child plays. Referrals for additional evaluations and enrollment in early intervention programs can all be completed before the first birthday if concerns are found at this assessment. So change the agenda: play first; examine later. You'll learn more and your focus will realign a family's interest in the infant's development when you make a different agenda for this visit.

Formal assessments are done by only a few primary care clinicians. Most are left to specialists, special programs or clinics. However, the concept of "developmental surveillance," to which the clinician should be committed, demands specific observations that inform the situation with a given child. Some evaluation formats (see Appendix) are useful to back up parental concerns or ones evoked by general observations in the clinic. However, certain "essential" play activities inform the observer quite readily of where the child is on the developmental continuum, from newborn through adolescence, and such aids should be kept in the clinician's pocket or exam room drawer:

TABLE 13–2 **Behavioral and Developmental Abilities Related to Feeding**

Newborn–2 mo	Primitive reflexes (rooting, sucking, swallowing) facilitate feeding and quickly become organized into a wide pattern of behavior; a hunger cry initiates feeding interaction; minimal vocal, visual or motor activity during feeding
2–4 mo	More alert and interactive during feeding; explosive cough to protect self from aspiration; beginning ability to wait for food; associates mother's smell, voice and cradling with feeding; hand-to-mouth behavior quiets infant, increases interest in mouthing activities
4–6 mo	Readiness for solids; excellent head and trunk control; reaching for objects; raking grasp; increased hand-to-mouth facility; loss of extrusion reflex of the tongue; may purposefully spit out food as part of food exploration; adaptation to introduction of solids may be affected by infant's temperament
6–8 mo	Sits alone with a steady head during seated feedings; chewing mechanism developed; holds bottle; vocal eagerness during meal preparation; much more motor activity during feeding
8–10 mo	Finger food readiness; thumb-forefinger grasp (i.e., inferior pincer); grasps spoon but cannot use it effectively; feeds self crackers, etc.; enjoys new textures, tastes; emerging independence
10–12 mo	Increasing determination to feed self; neat pincer grasp; drops food off highchair onto floor to see where it goes; holds cup but frequently spills it; more verbal and motor behavior during feeding
12–15 mo	Demands to feed self without help; decreased appetite and nutritional requirements; improved cup use (both hands); uses spoon, fills poorly, spills, turns at mouth; can use spoon as extension of the hand; messy play
15–18 mo	Eats rapidly, with short feeding sessions; wants to be physically active (too busy to eat); fairly good use of spoon and cup; enhanced ability to wait for food; plays with or throws food to elicit response from parent
18–24 mo	Feeds self with combination of utensils and fingers; verbalizes "eat, all gone," asks for food; negativism emerges, says no when really wanting offered food; wants control of feeding situation
2–3 yr	Uses fork; ritualistic, repetitive at mealtimes; food jags, all one food at a time; dawdles; likes to help set and clear table; may begin to help self to refrigerator contents
3–4 yr	Spills little; uses utensils well; washes hands with minimal help; likes food preparation; reasonable table manners while eating out
4–5 yr	Serves self; choosy about food; resists some textures; begins to request foods seen on television ads (especially junk food); makes menu suggestions; likes to assist in washing dishes; helps in food preparation
5–6 yr	Uses knife; assists in preparing and packing own box lunch; can be responsible for setting and clearing table; aids younger siblings' requests for food or drink
6–8 yr	Does dishes independently and willingly; increases pressure to buy junk food; interested in, often critical of and attempts to negotiate about daily menu; manages money for school meal ticket
8–10 yr	Enjoys planning and preparing simple family meals; wants supplemental spending money to buy snacks when away from home; more reticent about trying new foods; resists kitchen chores

TABLE 13-3 **Stethoscope Play Continuum**

Action	Age
Regards in the midline	Birth–1 mo
Follows to at least 90 degrees	2–6 wk
Swipes at it	2–4 mo
Reaches for it	4–5 mo
Brings it to the mouth	5–8 mo
Reaches across the midline	6–8 mo
Pivots to get it while seated	8–11 mo
Unilateral reach	9–11 mo
Examines parts of it	12–15 mo
Imitates use	15–19 mo
Pretends with others	2 yr
Knows where the heart is and perhaps what it does	3–5 yr

- Blocks (1-inch cubes)
- Stethoscope
- Markers for drawing on paper

With these few items and the structure to characterize the child's response, you can get a fairly accurate estimate of development across childhood with minimal time expenditure. For children with unknown developmental status, block play is a good place to start. Blocks can be brought out at the beginning of the visit, while you are talking to mom or dad before any procedures; you will have real data on the child before the conversation is finished. Then you can decide whether you or another professional should spend more time on an evaluation with more formal tools and structure. Tables 13–3 and 13–4 lay out these structures. The drawing progression is presented in Chapter 5.

DATA GATHERING

Observation

On entering the examination room at the beginning of the office visit when the infant is 8 to 9 months old, you may observe either a wary expression on the child's face or a sobering infant. Observe the child's *social distance*—the limits of proximity that the child allows before showing signs of distress. These "extra data" are obtained without special effort, merely the systematic observation of the child as you begin your encounter. Within the visit, pay attention to the following kinds of observations:

TABLE 13–4 **Block Play**

Action	Age
Regards the block at 8–10 inches	Birth–1 mo
Follows the block to at least 45 degrees while supine	Birth–2 mo
Mouth, hands and feet activate, go after the block	1–3 mo
Swipes at the block	2–4 mo
Holds the block placed in the hand	3–5 mo
Holds 2 blocks	5–7 mo
Bangs 2 blocks together	7–8 mo
Releases the block to put it in a cup	11 mo
Builds tower of 2	15 mo
Builds tower of 6	20 mo
Builds tower of 8	25 mo
Builds bridge of 3	30 mo
Builds stairs of 6	35 mo
Counts 1 block	36 mo
Knows 4 different colors of the blocks	$3\frac{1}{2}$ yr
Counts 5 blocks	$4–4\frac{1}{2}$ yr
Can add 2 sets of blocks (i.e., 2 + 3 = 5)	5–7 yr
Can calculate take away to 10	7–8 yr

- The parent's response to the child's distress will reveal the interactive style of the mother or father.
- Are the child's needs for comfort easily met (e.g., during the physical examination, when the child is being weighed or at the time of an immunization)?
- Be aware of the signs of infantile depression in children who have experienced prolonged or particularly stressful situations.

History Taking

Several issues can be addressed while taking the child and family's history by asking questions such as the following:

Stranger Anxiety

- How does the baby respond to seeing new people?
- Has the baby begun to be a bit wary of people seen infrequently?
- If the baby cries vigorously at these encounters, how do you respond?

Transitional Objects

- Does the child have a "lovey," a special toy or object?
- Ask whether the parent notes any pattern to the child's associated behavior when she wants the object (e.g., fatigue, hunger, stress).
- How do you feel about use of the object?

Other Care Providers At this office visit or earlier, the parents' activities outside the home should be discussed in terms of their impact on the child:

- Is the child left with a regular care provider?
- What is the leave-taking routine?
- Is the baby's response different now than before?
- What helps the baby with these transitions?
- Do you plan any changes in the future?

Observation

Sitting down on the floor or with the child on some surface will get you ready to look at how the baby explores the world. At 8 months of age, in a *free play session*, we would expect the child to do the following:

- Sit without support
- Reach around the side to get a toy
- Reach for objects with both hands
- Anticipate the shape of an object with shaping of the hand while reaching. Use a pencil or the stethoscope
- Transfer objects from hand to hand
- Stand while holding on (i.e., weight bearing)
- Move in some way—scooting, creeping, crawling
- Use a pincer grasp for small objects
- String phonemes together, such as "mamamama," "dadadada"
- May do pat-a-cake or wave bye-bye
- Hold a cube in each hand
- Bang cubes together
- Go after the stethoscope with one hand at a time, may imitate the dangling
- Be unable to let go of a cube to put it in a cup or hand
- Look wary at first approach

- Cry when the parent leaves or moves away
- Require help to sit and stand
- Try to put the ball and the cube together

QUICK CHECK–8 TO 9 MONTHS

✔ Sits: Gets there, sits steadily, pivots

✔ Moves forward: Scoots, creeps, crawls, rolls, cruises or walks

✔ Says: Phonemes, strung together, jabbers, gestures

✔ Understands: Name, "no," familiar objects or people, "bye, bye"

✔ Games: Peek-a-boo, pat-a-cake, waves "bye, bye"

✔ Finds a hidden object she has seen disappear

✔ Hands: Shapes hands to objects, transfers, has pincer grasp, pokes with fingers coming apart, used separately

✔ Stranger response: Wary, worried or distressed

✔ Feeding: Feeds self with hands, fingers

✔ Sleeping: 1–2 naps. Expect night wakening

HEADS UP–8 TO 9 MONTHS

Signs of Attachment Concerns
- A child who shows no differential response to strangers by 1 year of age
- A child who is extremely fearful and clingy in all circumstances and doesn't change by age 2
- A child who becomes so upset with a brief separation that she repeatedly refuses to eat or to stop crying
- A child who doesn't notice or become upset with departure of the parent or care provider
- A child who never checks back with the parent when exploring a new environment
- A child older than 8 months who goes to anyone without preference
- An extreme response to a stranger, e.g., extreme fear
- A young child in foster care, adoption beyond infancy or any unusual caretaking circumstance

Note: The child's current caretaking environment and medical, developmental and social history should be explored if such responses are present. Children with developmental delays have a delayed onset of stranger awareness in line with their cognitive level. Those with disorders in the autistic spectrum will have both delayed and atypical responses to separations.

ANTICIPATORY GUIDANCE

The cognitive basis for emerging stranger anxiety should be clearly explained. This puts it in a positive, normative framework; it doesn't mean that the child has been abused or poorly cared for. The clinician can offer guidance for dealing with separation issues:

- Children should never be forced to show affection for a new person if they are distressed. This protest behavior must be seen as developmentally based and protective. Give children a chance to see the stranger in a familiar context for a period.

- Leave-taking rituals should be well established by this time. A routine helps children cope with separations. This includes sleep; bedtime rituals are vital.

- When moving from room to room, parents should keep voice contact with children and reappear regularly.

- Baby-sitters should be introduced while the child is in the parent's arms, should approach slowly and should give the child a chance to look them over.

- Parents should never sneak away or go out after the child is asleep if possible. The child's protest should be expected and tolerated rather than the parent violating the child's basic trust.

- Discuss separation issues as parents plan trips, vacations and other separations. Discuss what can be done to support the child at times of necessary separations.

- Tell the family to avoid changes in the child's placement or custody between 6 and 18 months if at all possible.

- If a child needs a medical procedure, encourage the parent to stay with the child. The child may cry *more*, but the stress of the situation will be *less*. Decreased crying is not necessarily the desired endpoint.

- Suggest sharing of the infant's care with other adults if no other adults are regularly in the family. The child needs to be introduced to friendly strangers as opportunities for growth.

- Advise the parents to hold the child close after a separation until *the child* signals readiness to play or move away. This may mean that dinner preparation, laundry or the mail should wait after a day at work.

- Discuss the night awakenings often seen at this age. Discuss management through allowing the child opportunity to get back to sleep.

- Suggest establishing falling-asleep rituals that can be replicated by the child when he awakens in the night. Tell the parents that they should not put a child fully to sleep by holding unless they are prepared to do so all night long.

- Suggest support in choosing a transitional object for a child or family who is having trouble with separations.

- Beware of a chronically ill child who "likes everybody" in the hospital or a foster child who goes too easily to your arms. These children may have a serious derangement in attachment and may need extensive remedial work.

ACKNOWLEDGMENT

Previous versions of this work benefited from the contributions of Pamela Kaiser, PNP, PhD.

RECOMMENDED READINGS

Ainsworth MDS: Infancy in Uganda: *Infant Care and the Growth of Attachment.* Baltimore, Johns Hopkins Press, 1967.
Bowlby J: *Attachment,* vol 1. New York, Basic Books, 1969.
Kagan J, Kearsley RB, Zelano P: *Infancy: Its Place in Human Development.* Cambridge, MA, Harvard University Press, 1978.
Rutter M: Separation experiences: A new look at an old topic. *J Pediatr* 95:147, 1995.
Stein MT: Common issues in feeding. In Levine MD, Carey WB, Crocker A (eds): *Developmental-Behavioral Pediatrics,* 3rd ed. Philadelphia, WB Saunders, 1997, pp 392-396.

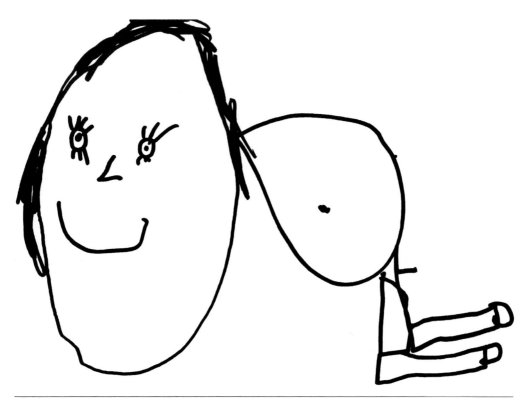

"My brother crawling." By Anne Atkinson, age 5½.

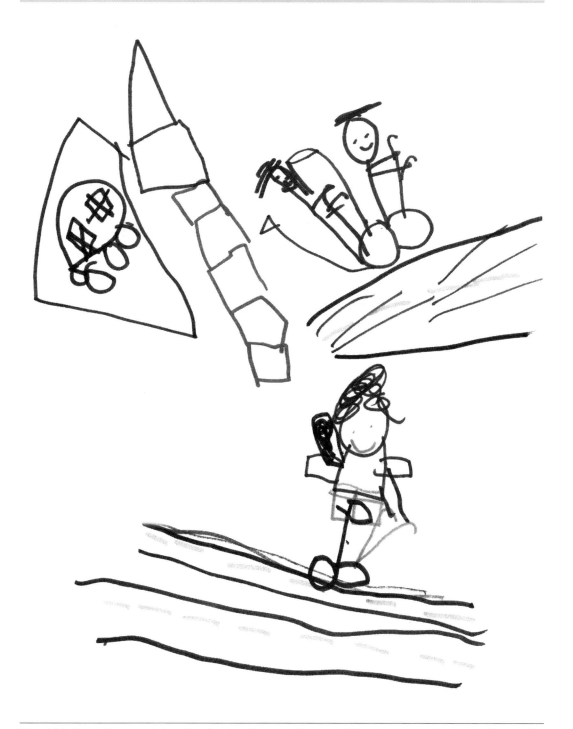

This child shows the expanded world of exploration available to a child as she grows. Freedom to discover the world on your own terms begins in infancy with a secure attachment to care providers. Note the house, the walk and the garage with car form a secure base for this child as she moves out with a parent and sibling on the back of a bike. By Hannahmarie Zambroski, age 8.

CHAPTER 14

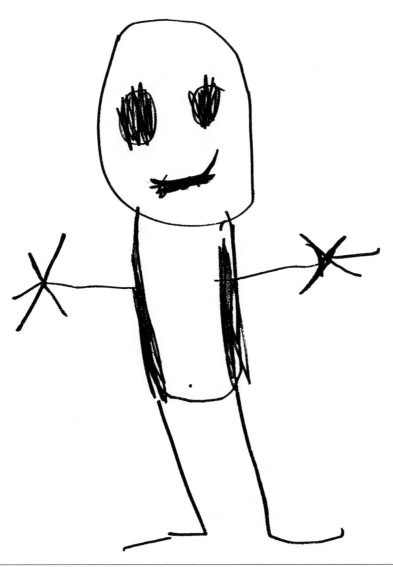

"Getting up on your own two feet" gives a sense of independence and an urge to explore. By Colin Hennessy, age 3½.

One Year: One Giant Step Forward

SUZANNE D. DIXON and MICHAEL J. HENNESSY

This chapter explores gross motor development broadly with a special focus on the emergence and refinement of walking as it progresses from infancy into middle childhood. Complex motor skill development is explored. The changes in the child that are prompted by the ability to walk are explained.

Key Words

- Walking
- Gross Motor Development
- Gait Cycle
- Running
- Infant Walkers
- Atypical Motor Development
- Evolution of Sports Activities
- Shoes

Marshall's mom looks very glum as she comes in for his 1-year-old visit. She says that her mother-in-law wants Marshall's legs checked and wants her to get advice about shoes. Mom admits that they're all concerned about Marshall not walking yet. His older brother walked at 9 months. Note: This case illustrates the heightened importance of walking for a family, as well as some common misconceptions about legs, shoes and the variation in motor development.

The developmental milestone that parents focus on most prominently is the age at which the child starts **walking**. Independent gait is greeted by parents as a source of pride and assurance of normality; any delay in its appearance may trigger worry and dire prognostication. Clinicians are also more likely to note and record this developmental landmark than any other.

The child's perspective on the world and on himself changes dramatically when he can alter location, so he's a different child after walking. The visit of a 1-year-old offers the opportunity to look at the development of ambulation and **gross motor processes** in general that emerge both before and after the start of walking. The goal of this chapter is to see this area of development in the broader context of the whole child and its importance to the family. The manner of emergence of this milestone provides great insight into a child and family from more than the motor vantage point. This view of the processes in and around motor development gives the clinician an expanded perspective on these readily observed and reliably noted milestones.

Some of the earliest perspectives on the regularities of early childhood development came from the observations of gross motor milestones made by Arnold Gesell, Myrtle McGraw and others. This sequence came out of careful longitudinal and cross-sectional observations of normal children. The pediatric perspective on development in general has been strongly based on these schemes of motor milestones following from a neuromaturational model (see Chapter 2). Although we now know that not every aspect of gross motor development can be accounted for by this model, the regularity and the readily observable nature of these motor achievements form a core of basic developmental appraisal, as shown in Figures 14–1 and 14–2. Physical milestones in infancy are presented in Table 14–1. These milestones are easy to observe, readily reported by parents and easier than most to remember. Through a chronicle of regular achievement of these skills, clinicians are assured of the child's neurological adequacy.

MOTOR SKILLS: GENERAL PRINCIPLES

Walking must be seen in the context of other gross motor accomplishments. These all share, in addition to their regular sequence, certain characteristics:

- These skills are built on *neuromotor tone*, the base that determines behavior, skills and patterns. Hypotonic children, from whatever cause, will have delays in postural maturation and skill acquisition. Hypertonic children, with prominence of extensor postures, will have predictable "pseudo-accelerations" (e.g., rolling over, weight bearing on legs and pull to stand) and delays (e.g., sitting).

- *Volitional behavior is preceded by reflex behavior.* For example, the newborn reflex patterns of reciprocal kicking and automatic stepping clearly foreshadow the movements of walking seen near the end of the first year. These early patterns usually disappear clinically at approximately 2 months of age, only to later reappear in the progressive emergence of independent gait, although they can be elicited under certain conditions. This sequence is thought to result from increasing suppression of the primitive reflexes by maturing cortical centers and their subsequent reorganization into volitional movement patterns. Concomitant with increased strength and improved balance, the child learns to control the reflex pattern and use it in a more complex and flexible pattern.

- Alternatively, it has been suggested that *evolution of a more continuous movement pattern* characterizes motor development, thereby avoiding this adaptation of the primitive reflex model. A delay in the disappearance of early infant reflexes is associated with a comparable delay in the emergence of voluntary motor skills and can be anticipated by the clinician, although the mechanism of association is unclear. The sequence is clear, even if the description of the linkage is not. For example, the parachute reflexes, first the upper and then the lower, appear at about 9 months. Independent walking starts about 4 months after these reflexes appear, which suggests some orderly adaptation to the inevitable stumbles that early walkers experience.

- *Maturation entails increasing efficiency in the energy expenditure that is required to move through space.* The child becomes an increasingly efficient movement machine. The biomechanical parameters ensure that with maturation and practice, forward movement is achieved with less change in the center of gravity, less overall joint movement and refinement of muscle movement. This means more efficient movement.

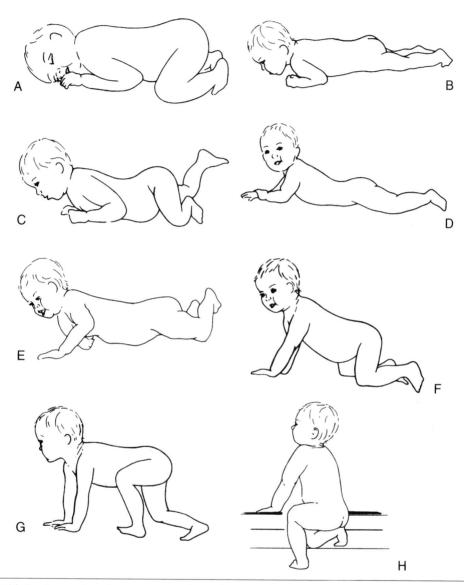

Figure 14–1 Progression of prone posture. **A,** Newborn in a flexed posture. **B,** Infant at about 1 month of age, head up briefly, some extension at the hips and knees. **C,** Infant about 1 to 2 months old, head up to about 45 degrees, active legs. **D,** Infant about 3 to 4 months old, up easily on forearms, head steady and able to be turned with minimal bobbing. **E,** Infant about 5 to 9 months old, up on hands; may use arm to pull self forward; may push with thighs and knees, creeping. **F,** Infant 7 to 11 months old, crawling; reciprocal movement of legs and legs with hands. **G,** Crawling on feet. **H,** Child 8 to 18 months of age, climbs stairs.

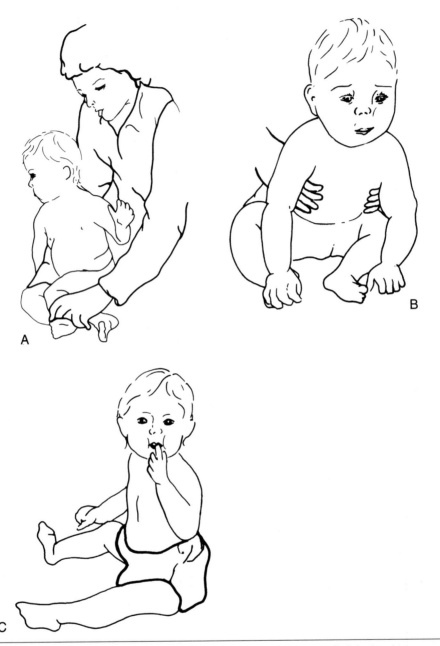

Figure 14–2   Sitting progression. With each time period, steadiness and control of the head increase, the back becomes straighter from the upper portion down, and the arms are held naturally further back, with external rotation at the shoulder. **A**, Age 1 to 2 months, sits with truncal support, head and shoulders steady, lower part of the back still rounded. **B**, Age 4 to 7 months, sits in a pivot position with slight truncal support; all energy is directed at maintaining posture. **C**, Age 5 to 9 months, independent sitting, back straight, able to pivot without losing balance.

TABLE 14–1 **Physical Milestones in Infancy**

Behavior	Age Range (mo)*	Average Age (mo)
Raises self by arms while lying face down	0.7–5	2.1
Sits with support	1–5	2.3
Sits alone momentarily	4–8	5.3
Sits alone 10–30 seconds or longer	5–8	6.0
Rolls from back to stomach	4–10	6.4
Sits alone quite steadily for long periods	5–9	6.6
Stands up holding onto furniture	6–12	8.6
Walks while adult holds hands	7–12	9.6
Sits down after standing	7–14	9.6
Stands alone	9–16	11.0
Walks alone	9–17	11.7
Walks sideways	10–20	14.1
Walks backward	11–20	14.6
Walks up stairs with help	12–23	16.1
Stands on left foot alone	15–30	22.7
Jumps off floor with both feet	17–30+	23.4
Stands on right foot alone	16–30+	23.5
Jumps from the last stair step to floor	19–30+	24.8
Walks up stairs alone with both feet on each step	18–30+	25.1
Walks a few steps on tiptoes	16–30+	25.7
Walks down stairs alone with both feet on each step	19–30+	25.8
Jumps from the second stair step to the floor	21–30+	28.1
Walks up stairs, alternating forward foot	23–30+	30+

*Fifth to 95th percentile.
From Bayley N: Motor scale record. In Bayley N: *Bayley Scales of Infant Development,* Psychological Corp, 1969, 1994. Used by permission.

- *The progression of control is from more proximal joint movement to recruitment of more distal movement.* This usually means a refinement, a fine-tuning of movement because the more distal joint can make adjustments with less movement and more accuracy, as seen in the development of reach (see Chapter 12). Control of reach moves from the shoulder to the wrist; control of gait is transferred in part to the knee and then to the ankle with

BOX 14–1   WORRY MARKERS*

- No rolling prone to supine by 7 months
- No rolling supine to prone by 9 months
- No unsupported sitting by 10 months
- No independent steps by 18 months
- No running by 2 years
- No jumping by 2½ to 3 years
- No pedaling of a tricycle or big wheel by 4 years
- No bike riding by age 10

*These time frames should alert the clinician to problems that clearly call for more evaluation.

maturation. This is an example of the general principle of cephalocaudal direction of development that began in fetal life.

- *The child increases in both speed and accuracy of movement with time.* These last characteristics (gains in efficiency, accuracy and speed) are demonstrated in the specific developmental course of gait. Overshooting or undershooting and less well directed movements are characteristics of immature movement. Fewer mistakes and greater accuracy evolve with maturation.

- *Moving is easier than stopping; going up is easier than going down.* Acceleration, in biomechanical terms, is less complex and matures earlier, whereas deceleration requires more energy and organization. In simple language, kids develop a gas pedal before brakes.

MOTOR MILESTONES: THE TIME COURSE

The incredible importance placed on walking is curious. The age of independent ambulation, unless it is delayed beyond 18 months, poorly predicts other areas of development. Accelerated motor development in general does not testify to superior mental skills. Delayed walking in children with perinatal difficulties is associated with an increased incidence of broader developmental delay, but without this history of risk, the age of walking has poor prognostic value (see Box 14–1).

Aiden, age 16 months (corrected age of 14½), shows no sign of pulling to stand and is resistant to his dad's efforts to help him walk. He's quite content to sit. Note: Worry about this child because he's missing the precursors of walking, as well as walking itself, and has perinatal risk because of prematurity.

WALKING: A CHANGE IN PERSPECTIVES

New motor competencies dramatically change the child's view of herself and the world. Placement in space is now under the child's own control, and her hands are free to explore the new sights. The child can now choose (within limits) *what* to explore, not just *how* to investigate the objects within vision or reach. These skills allow the child to perceive, learn and experience in entirely new ways by movement through space, such as choosing to go away from or toward caregivers. That new option is both exciting and scary. Everything changes because of this new perspective. Selma Fraiberg describes the overwhelming world and self-view changes that a child experiences when he or she learns to walk:

In the last quarter of the first year, the baby is no longer an observer of a passing scene. He is in it. Travel changes one's perspective. A chair, for example, is an object of one dimension when viewed by a 6-month-old baby propped up on a sofa. ... It's when you start to get around under your own steam that you discover what a chair really is.

The first time the baby stands unsupported and the first wobbly independent steps are milestones in personality development, as well as in motor development. To stand unsupported, to take that first step is a brave and lonely thing to do.

All development is fueled by the ability to change position in space and to move away from a completely dependent vantage point. Or as pointed out again by Fraiberg:

The discovery of independent locomotion and the discovery of a new self usher in a new phase in personality development. The toddler is quite giddy with his new achievements. He behaves as if he had invented this new mode of locomotion and he is quite in love with himself for being so clever. From dawn to dusk he marches around in an ecstatic, drunken dance, which ends only when he collapses with fatigue.

A physically slow or disabled child suffers secondary disabilities because of limitations in visual, perceptual and tactile experiences when compared with walking, moving peers. That child also misses the energizing sense of competency that follows from the acquisition of motor skills. Seen in this context, therapies, surgical procedures and external supports and braces should be considered for these children or evaluated from the perspective of their impact on these areas of development. Just normalization of position or posture is not enough if real mobility is not clearly improved.

THE ONTOGENY OF GAIT

Adult human ambulation is remarkably consistent and regular in terms of angles of displacement of the joints involved; the mathematical relationships between cadence, stride length and velocity; and the timing of these events through the **gait cycle**. Figure 14–3 illustrates the gait cycle of events that occur from heel strike to the next heel strike. These biomechanical events have specific durations, timing of muscle group firing and shifts of weight that mature over time, as shown in Table 14–2. The observation of gait throughout these phases allows a more accurate characterization of gait in both normal and abnormal conditions. The observation, "He walks funny," can be given more specificity if we understand what the parts of the gait cycle are and what to expect developmentally.

TYPICAL NORMAL WALK CYCLE

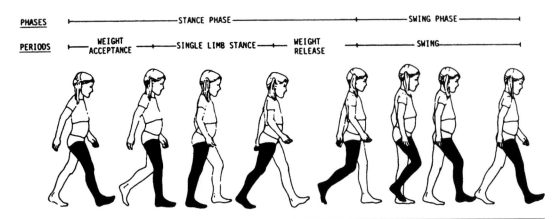

Figure 14–3 Phases of the normal gait in childhood. (From Hennessy M, Dixon S, Simon S: The development of gait: A study in African children ages one to five. *Child Dev* 55:844-853, 1984.)

TABLE 14–2 **Walking Chart**

Stepping movements	6–12 mo
Walks holding onto furniture	7¼–12¾ mo
Walks with help	7–12 mo
Walks independently	9–17 mo
Walks well	11–14½ mo
Walks sideways and backward	10–20 mo

All these gait parameters are geared toward maximal displacement in space with a minimum of energy expenditure. The body's center of gravity moves forward in nearly a straight line in a mature gait, the path of least energy expenditure. Extremity movements work together toward that end. Each of these parameters has its own developmental course, as demonstrated by high-speed film analysis coupled with floor force plate measurement and analysis of electromyographic (EMG) data. These highly technical studies have allowed a more complete and refined description of gait; they specify what the clinician can learn by careful observation. These techniques are also useful in children in whom gait is abnormal and surgical correction is being contemplated. The following are characteristics of walking in a young child (Figs. 14–4 to 14–6):

- A toddler's stance is *broad based*. As the child matures, the stance will narrow in absolute measure and in proportion to leg length. The narrower the base, the more mature the gait.

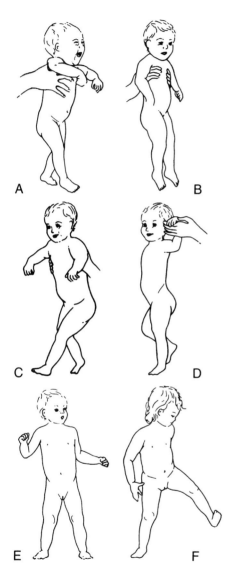

A

B

C

D

E

F

Figure 14–4 Progression of gait development in toddlers and preschoolers. **A**, Reflex walk of the newborn, which usually disappears at 3 to 4 weeks of age. **B**, Before 3 months, an infant bears little weight on his legs. **C**, After 7 months, an infant will walk with much truncal support. Excessive hip flexion with a forwardly displaced center of gravity means that the child is not ready for walking. **D**, Near 1 year of age, a child's center of gravity is over the hips, and the child can walk with help. **E**, During the toddler years, the position of the child's arm and feet testifies to the level of maturity of gait. **F**, It is not until 3 to 5 years of age that a child can balance steadily on one foot with all the reciprocal truncal, hip and arm adjustments that are required.

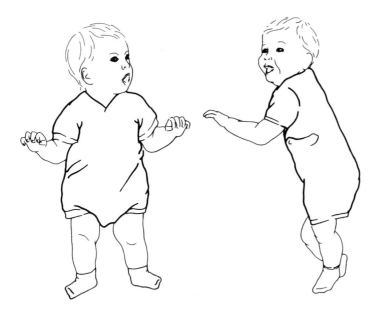

Figure 14–5 Toddler's gait: wide based, flexion at the hip and knees, abducted feet and arms up and fixed.

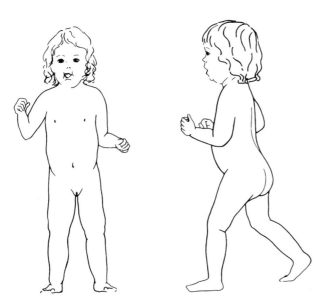

Figure 14–6 Gait of an older toddler: arms still used as part of balance, feet turned out and relative lordosis with the trunk over the hips.

- A young child's *knees and hips are flexed,* even while standing, and remain so as the toddler waddles with one leg forward and a twist of the trunk and a swing of the hip. Hip movement involving alternating flexion and extension and a locked knee will emerge with maturation.

- A child's belly and bottom stick out because of the increased lordotic curve of the lower part of the back. This provides balance in an immature walker. As the hips straighten (i.e., extend), with time the child will tuck in the tummy and straighten the back. The "S" curve of the body viewed from the side will become less pronounced.

- Ankle movement is minimal at first with flat-footed foot placement. As a child matures, the ankle will dorsiflex and plantarflex. The child will develop a consistent heel strike to start his step after 30 months and a reliable lift-off with the forefoot and toes after that. A toddler's foot moves very little in early walking but becomes active during walking between 2½ and 3 years. *Toe leads are never part of normal gait progression.*

- When the child is first walking, the arms are abducted (out to his sides) and flexed at the elbow. The arms move little throughout the gait cycle, providing balance only. The arms first come down, the hands go from fisted or splayed to relaxed, and then reciprocal arm movements are added. The higher and more fixed the arms, the less mature the gait.

- Feet go out nearly sideways at first. With maturation they turn more straight ahead— from a duck walk to a people walk.

- The center of gravity in a youngster just starting to walk shifts markedly up and down and side to side, an observation you can note if you just watch the umbilicus move throughout the gait cycle. This movement stabilizes throughout gait maturation, and truncal rotation decreases. At first the whole body goes back and forth, up and down, side to side. With maturation, the movement is more and more isolated to the extremities. Watching the belly button helps identify this maturational point.

- Angles of displacement at all joints decrease with time. Less overshooting or excess movement occurs. Things become smoother, targeted and graceful. Lurching, waddling and swaying become less as this joint movement is minimized.

- Acceleration forces are stronger than deceleration forces, so forward momentum is hard to check at first. Stopping is much harder than starting for a young child. Only later can stopping be combined with a pivot.

- For the same reason, going down an incline is much harder than going up. A child cannot check his speed.

- Step length and walking speed increase, and cadence decreases with time, gradually approaching a fixed mathematical relationship between these biomechanical aspects of gait. Older children take fewer steps to walk at a given speed, largely because of an increase in step length. This, in turn, is related to leg length; shorter children have a faster cadence, whereas those with longer legs have a slower cadence.

By 5 years of age, gait has matured to nearly adult patterns clinically and biomechanically (Fig. 14–7). EMG tracings show adult patterns of muscle firing by this age as well. Although increasing refinements emerge slowly and allow for more complex movements to develop, the mature biomechanical aspects of gait are established by school age.

Running emerges about 6 months after independent walking is well established. This involves a reduction in stance time (time with weight on both feet) to less than 50% of the gait cycle. Young children don't increase their stride length when they run as toddlers; they just take more steps to go at a running speed. They keep the knees at a fixed flexion and don't use their feet to initiate a lift-off. Hip movement is as inefficient with running as it is for walking

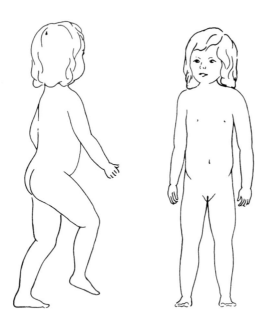

Figure 14–7 Gait of a preschooler: biomechanically, nearly at adult patterns; heel strike present; and neck, shoulder, hips and knees nearly vertical.

in the younger ages. This means that running requires a lot of effort for a toddler, although most find the effort worth it. All of the run parameters gradually shift to more mature forms across the preschool years. Children will learn how to increase stride length, will add a "flight" phase when they lift off the ground briefly and will learn to use reciprocal arm movement to propel themselves forward. With less extraneous movement the run is smooth and straight and has much less sideways movement in an older child. Running should be very smooth by school age.

PREWALKING

The biomechanical precursors of gait are the reciprocal hip and leg movements of a kicking and crawling child, not standing or pulling to stand. These early spontaneous movements have the biomechanical characteristics, interrelationships, coordination and rhythm of gait. However, not every child will crawl, and this does not reflect either motor or cognitive development. In fact, crawling may be the most overrated motor milestone in the first year. However, all typical children will demonstrate ongoing reciprocal movement of the lower extremities that becomes smoother and more rhythmic and efficient from 9 to 12 months of age (Fig. 14–8). Spontaneous "swimming" movements are seen during bathing at about 9 months. These spontaneous movements are important to monitor (e.g., when a child is supine on an examining table) during the first year rather than merely checking off specific skill acquisitions, a process that can be misleading. These back-and-forth movements are the precursors of gait. Practice walking has not been shown to accelerate or decelerate the emergence of walking. Freedom to move in the prone position and enticements to explore in space by whatever means form the prompts for walking.

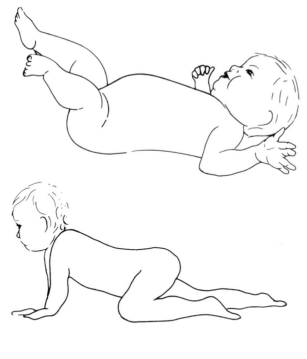

Figure 14–8 Spontaneous reciprocal hip movements take a variety of forms. Practice opportunities are provided in the prone position.

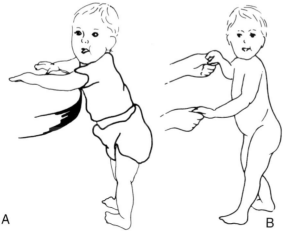

Figure 14–9 Getting upright, cruising. **A,** Cruising on one's own provides opportunities to practice and explore. Most children do this by 12 months. **B,** Walking with help. Many families enjoy this activity. No evidence shows that walking with help harms the child or accelerates walking. Some children resist holding on with both hands.

A   B

GETTING STARTED AND REFINING SKILLS

Most children will cruise by 12 months, walking while holding onto objects at shoulder height, as shown in Figure 14–9. Some children may resist any attempts at stepping if their hands are held up because this eliminates the usefulness of arm position and truncal rotation, which provide stability. Cruising *on one's own* provides opportunity for real practice and the development of firm prototypes of movement that can be applied to varying demands, such as walking on a carpet versus walking on grass and going up the stairs or down an incline versus walking on a flat plane. The child is experimenting with new approaches to motor activity rather than simply repeating fixed actions. It is not rote repetition of a single activity in a single circumstance many times over, but the accumulation of experiences that demands the ongoing accommodation that forms the basis of gait development. For example, an adult could not claim competency in skiing after going down only one hill no matter how expertly that hill had been skied. Learning the skill (in the child's case, walking; for the adult, skiing) includes actively assimilated experiences in many circumstances and conditions. Passive practice or repetitive exercise of motor skills in isolation has no effect on skill acquisition, although range of motion at the joints may be maintained in a disabled child. *Self-initiated actions, active movement and exploration of the possibilities of movement are the necessary components of motor development.*

The specific process of walking is shown in Table 14–2. Note the overlapping ranges of these refinements of locomotion. Indeed, the definition of walking may vary from family to family. Some mark down the very first step alone, whereas others wait for a self-initiated trip across the room.

Dynamic system explanations posit that separate abilities must be put together in complex systems of action (see Chapter 2). Central nervous system (CNS) maturation, movement options, goals and motivation in the child and environmental supports all contribute. This changed perspective means that even motor skills thought to be so internally determined are the product of interaction between the child and the environment. Changes in one of these components demand adjustments in the others. Walking, as an example, is not like turning on a switch. The movement possibilities change with body proportions, so infants learn to walk over and over, with altered biochemical constraints. There is a burst of cortical electro-encephalographic activity and changes on magnetic resonance imaging studies that occur with the onset of walking. New connections are made that go beyond the motor cortex. The biomechanical aspects of gait in a child younger than 2 years may vary widely from child to child and will change from month to month. This is as dynamic and wobbly a process as the version of the early walker suggests. It's like each child finds his own course and reinvents himself over and over.

In spite of our own expectations, most children are *not* walking on their first birthday. The mean age for walking is about 60 weeks, with a 2–standard deviation range of 9 to 17 months. The misconception that a child will walk by age 1 leads parents to feel worried and disappointed if the first steps haven't appeared by the first birthday. The clinician should mention the real norms if the child isn't walking, regardless of whether the parents bring up the issue. Many cultural groups will seek remedies for perceived weakness, bone problems or foot irregularities in a child who is not walking by the first birthday. As long as the child is moving in space somehow, has tone within a normal range, demonstrates unrestricted joint movement and has shown some reciprocal leg movements, patience is all that is needed.

 Mrs. Rodriguez asked Dr. Martin for vitamins to build up her Jorge's blood. "He's already 1, and his legs are weak and turned (bowed)." Note: Time to correct some misconceptions if the exam is normal.

INFANT EXERCISE CLASSES AND TREATMENTS

Infant exercise programs for children without disabilities do not enhance motor development except as they energize the child and family through the enjoyment of movement and time spent together. Therapy programs that rely on *passive* movement may keep disabled children's joints flexible, but they do not ensure or augment skill acquisition. *No* evidence shows that repeated practice of motor movements (i.e., patterning) has any effect on the development of a handicapped or learning-impaired child. Therapies should be designed to liberate the child from constraints based on tone, irregularities, weaknesses or the preservation of premature reflexes to allow for active exploration and self-initiated movement. Furthermore, there is *no* evidence that such programs are needed to "reprogram" a child with (any kind of) developmental difficulties. These approaches are quackery.

Mrs. Jordan wants to enroll her 9-month-old in swimming classes so he'll be safe around the pool in the summer. Note: Bad idea. The child won't learn to swim (although he'll demonstrate primitive swimming moves in the water), and he's at risk for water intoxication and hypothermia. Wait until after 4 to 5 years of age.

INFLUENCES ON WALKING

The range of perception of achievement with **skill appearance** (i.e., doing the activity in any way or form), as well as **competency** (i.e., being able to do it without seeming to choose to exercise that skill, doing it regularly and automatically), is quite marked and is related to temperamental, familial, ethnic and, to some degree, experiential factors.

Although regularity in the sequence of gross motor development offers support for a prominent neuromaturational component in this area of development, a clear role is played by environmental factors as well. Neuromaturational readiness, physical factors such as leg length and strength, motivation of the child and opportunities to hone and practice skills all play into this. Motor skills develop through an integration of previously acquired and practiced skills. This *dynamic systems* view is in contrast to the previous notion of motor skills developing nearly automatically and environmental supports having no role at all.

Expectations and timing of these events may vary by culture and family. Familial patterns of walking may be related to the temporal aspects of nerve myelinization, to an inherited behavioral style or to the degree of emphasis on gross motor activities. Basic neuromotor precocity and these individual factors may be the basis for the observed early acceleration of motor development in several groups, including African, Mexican, East Indian and Middle Eastern children, when compared with that of white Americans. Subgroup differences exist in the average age of achievement of motor milestones. A basic motor competency appears to be present at birth in these groups, which propels the infants forward at a faster rate and also leads to different patterns of handling that build on this early competency.

Mr. Jackson, an African American, proudly held his 7-month-old son Miles' hands and walked him across the examining room to Dr. Strain. The baby bubbled with delight, squealing with every move.

Mrs. Williamson, a white American, held her daughter Melissa with strong support in a sitting position, her pale skin, delicate frame and feathery hair making her seem younger and more fragile than her 9 months. She delicately moved a toy back and forth without a sound, watching it and all the people in the room with an intensity that was almost alarming. Note: These differences are due to child, parent, cultural and environmental differences.

Severe experiential deprivation is necessary before any significant delay in motor development is noted. Dennis' study of Hopi Indian infants placed on cradle boards demonstrated no alteration in the maturity or timing of walking, and more recent studies have confirmed these classic findings. These Native American children, in spite of some early confinement (usually when sleeping), had ample opportunity for free movement and developed normally. Specific training of motor skills (e.g., climbing) appears to have no effect on the time of emergence of these competencies.

The new advisory on infant **sleep position** has resulted in a slight shift in the timing of some **motor milestones**, such as rolling prone to supine, creeping and crawling and pull to stand. Walking age shows no difference based on sleep position. Importantly, infants placed on their backs to sleep also had more awake time in that position, so it is unclear what contributes to this shift of less than a month in these motor landmarks. Experience may play a role in the development of these skills. Tummy time while awake and back to sleep at night are good practices to recommend.

The use of **infant walkers** in particular does not improve, but in fact delays motor and mental development. Safety may be seriously impaired in children using these devices, and injury and death may occur. They are *not* recommended. Extensor postures may be solidified in children with lower extremity hypertonia, thereby undermining rather than facilitating walking in these youngsters. If a parent insists on using a walker, it should be wider than 36 inches, too wide to go through a door. Stationary activity centers contain a child without risk of injury, so these are preferred as a safer alternative to walkers.

INDIVIDUAL DIFFERENCES

Peripheral nerve myelinization and cerebellar growth increase rapidly from 6 to 12 months, and these changes appear to coincide with the movement changes that occur during that time. These processes in the CNS set up basic readiness. Physical growth factors such as height and leg length may influence patterns of motor development through biomechanical relationships that are necessary to get walking going. Any condition that delays growth, undermines nutrition or produces muscle weakness will probably delay motor achievement. Balance and strength are important as well. Obese children may have later gross motor skill acquisition because of these biomechanical factors; they just have more mass to move.

> Brady, a 15-month-old weighing 28 pounds, was not yet walking and actually moved very little in the course of play. He was quite content in a playpen. However, he moved quickly in a crawl as he tried to grab the cat while he was on the floor. Note: Brady needs a nutritional intervention but is unlikely to have neuromotor difficulties.

A maturational readiness seems to be inherent within a child, so motor skills emerge within a supportive, but noninstructive environment. The environment alone can take little credit or blame for gross motor achievements, but it acts with other factors synergistically. As stated by Wolff, "Neither intrinsic developmental timetables nor experience is a sufficient condition for motor skill acquisition. At every stage motor development depends not only on experience and quality of the stimuli, but also on brain mechanisms that assimilate and organize information from the environment and from action in progress."

An internal consistency within a child allows some anticipation of gross motor skills. For example, a late sitter is likely to be a late walker. Alterations in general tone, though still within the range of normal, may set the stage for this delay.

The style with which a child approaches motor skill development is also consistent. Some children charge ahead to pull to stand, cruise and walk with lots of energy and lots of falls. Others will take a more contemplative approach: they study the task well, wind up slowly and feel assured of each step before trying the next. The clinician will learn more about a child by monitoring *how* she achieves gross motor skills than by focusing exclusively on the timing of such behavior.

> Madison is a tiny, wiry child. She was up on her feet by 8 months and was charging around the house at 10 months. The sitter nicknamed her "Crash" because she was always bumping into things, falling and just getting going too fast. Note: We can expect this daredevil to provide some safety and discipline challenges.

GAIT ABNORMALITIES

Though awkward at first, the gait of a young child should follow the sequence described previously and should show symmetry. A parent saying something is wrong with her child's walking should be cause for careful evaluation. Some specific concerns are laid out in Box 14–2.

BOX 14–2   OBSERVATIONS THAT TRIGGER WORRY ABOUT WALKING

- A "limp" at any time
- Gait asymmetry, including asymmetry of the arms
- Persistent toe walking or the appearance of toe walking after 2 years
- A decline in performance, ability, coordination or endurance
- A persistent waddling gait
- Refusal to walk or bear weight
- Persistent forward falling

In response to the question, "Do you have any other concerns?" asked at the end of a health supervision visit, the mother of 12-month-old Caleb exclaimed, "His left foot looks odd!" The developmental history revealed normal motor, language and social skills in a child who took a few unaided steps 1 week before the visit. The physical examination was normal. The left foot was moderately inverted when standing; it was thought to be secondary to a mild positional deformity. The mother was reassured.

At the 15-month visit, she reminded the clinician that "the left foot still looks odd!" Examination revealed a normal foot and leg when examined passively but inversion of the foot when standing and walking. To the pediatrician's surprise, the left calf circumference was 0.5 cm smaller than that on the right side, and the left foot exerting muscles were weak. Strength, tone, sensation and deep tendon reflexes were otherwise normal and symmetrical. A magnetic resonance image of the spine demonstrated congenital syringomyelia. Surgical exploration, drainage and shunting prevented further neurological deterioration.

In another scenario,

Logan's mom said she couldn't keep any shoes on him and those she tried just didn't seem to fit. His foot came out of them. In addition, she says he's always getting "goose eggs" as he's falling on his face frequently. On exam, Logan clearly had tightness of his Achilles tendons, hyperreflexia in the lower extremities and some limitation in foot dorsiflexion. Dr. James hadn't noticed this before but he did recall Logan's rocky start in life with meconium aspiration and respiratory problems. Note: This is a case of subtle cerebral palsy that was missed initially. Logan may need a tendon-lengthening procedure if therapy and bracing cannot improve his foot position. Early walkers fall, in the main, with their bottoms hitting first. The prominence of facial bumps should also raise suspicion about unbalanced muscle tone.

A SPECIAL WORD ABOUT PREEMIES

The predictably altered motor tone of a preemie and enhancement of extension postures in this group of infants result in greater risk for motor difficulties. Even correcting for gestational age, preemies walk later and also seem to lack some of the coordination and efficiency that is age appropriate. These factors in themselves do not predict other areas of development, but all children born prematurely are generally at risk for developmental concerns. Although they might even show early standing, the reciprocal hip movements, the experience in the prone position and tightness at the hips and knees may make walking more of a challenge. Truncal weakness, any degree of slow weight gain, reductions in linear growth and the stress of chronic illness mean that strength and truncal tone will compromise walking further. Steady progress and gradual closing of the gap between expected and observed competencies should be parameters to monitor in this group.

ALTERED PERCEPTUAL DEVELOPMENT: CHANGES IN MOTOR TIMETABLE

The impact of perceptual input on gross motor development is illustrated through the motor development of infants with congenital **blindness**. These infants demonstrate all the postural readiness (e.g., excellent truncal tone) and acquisition of static skills (e.g., stepping in place with support) at the same time as sighted children do. However, they are predictably delayed in any movement through space, such as crawling, walking and climbing. These skills do not begin to emerge until the child can reach toward sound cues alone, a landmark met by *all* children between 10 and 15 months. Some children with blindness will not crawl at all, won't walk until they are 2 or older and may even begin sitting or standing late, although they may have the ability to maintain these postures. Until these children are able to use perceptual input other than vision to map their environment and are able to understand the consistency of three-dimensional space, they seem unwilling to risk moving about. In addition, the fueling that walking typically receives by way of visual input does not sustain the efforts of children with blindness through all the falls and uncertainties of early movement. It is a lot of work to walk, and the rewards must be there. Enhanced feelings of independence, greater perceptual input and the attainment of goals (e.g., getting a toy) make the effort worthwhile. Perceptually handicapped children lack these incentives even if they have neuromaturational readiness. This emphasizes the role of internal motivation in the process of gross motor development; it is not purely a neuromaturational process.

When to Worry

Motor milestones are not usually missed in clinical observation, but one needs a clear backstop about when to be worried after the average age of achievement has passed. Motor delays accompanied by alterations in motor tone—hypotonia or hypertonia—are generally more worrisome than a delay in one or more landmarks alone with normal tone and reflexes. Postures or positions not seen in the normal sequence should elicit concern, such as a frog-leg position in the supine posture. Late integration of primitive reflexes with delays in several areas is of more concern regarding slowed central CNS maturation. Finally, some milestones should be weighted more than others. *Unsupported sitting* is a strong indicator of general developmental progress because it involves balanced truncal tone, good hip flexion and abduction and excellent head control. In contrast, creeping and crawling are poor indicators because some children never perform these activities and the timing and form are highly variable. With these general considerations in mind, some clinical precision points may be considered (see Box 14–2).

Later Motor Development

Although we often place the greatest emphasis on gross motor development in the first 2 years of life, this sequence continues beyond walking. These competencies are based on an increasing ability to *balance* on one side and to *lateralize* more and on other varying motor activities (Box 14–3). Children should be able to ride a big wheel adeptly at 4 years of age and should be able to ride a bicycle at 7. Skateboarding and in-line skating, activities we can neither

BOX 14–3   LATER GROSS MOTOR SKILL PROGRESSION

2–3 Years
- Both feet on each stair, up and down
- Full arm swing
- True run begins
- Jumps down a step
- Jumps up stiffly
- Hops 1–3 times
- Throws ball with forearm extension only
- Catches ball with fixed, outstretched arms
- Pushes riding toy with feet, no steering

3–4 Years
- Alternates feet up stairs
- Walks in a straight line
- Jumps, using arms
- Broad jump, about 1 foot
- Hops 4–6 times, arms and body helping
- Catches ball against chest
- Pedals and steers tricycle

4–5 Years
- Alternates feet down stairs
- Smooth run
- Gallops and does 1-foot skip
- Hops 7–9 times on one foot smoothly
- Throws ball with shift of body
- Catches ball with hands
- Rides tricycle very well

5–6 Years
- Gallops and skips smoothly
- Jumps up 1 foot
- Broad jumps 3 feet
- Mature throwing with shift of weight
- Adjusts body, arms, hands to catch
- Rides bicycle

Modified from Berk LE: *Infants, Children and Adolescents*, 3rd ed. Boston, Allyn & Bacon, 1999.

condone nor stop, can usually be done by 7 to 9 years, although perhaps not safely. Observations of jumping, hopping, ball catching and throwing, as well as specific questions about the handling of stairs and the type of vehicular travel that a child can handle, will usually give you all the data you need on gross motor competencies. Therapeutic implications and considerations are based on these increasing skills. For example, a big wheeler *may* be able to walk with crutches; certainly, a biker can learn to do so if needed. A child who cannot hop will have difficulty using crutches because both skills require lateralization at about the same level (see Table 14–3).

LEARNING COMPLEX MOTOR SKILLS

Motor skills do not exist in isolation. Cognitive competencies have an impact on when and how a child learns new motor skills. It is not until midlatency or even adolescence that a youngster can use preknowledge of outcome to improve motor performance; younger children must experience the outcome of their motor activities to alter them, and they need considerable practice before they can do that. The ability to sequence concepts parallels the ability to sequence motor behavior; only an older grade-schooler or high school student can do this reliably if the sequence is longer than two to three movements. This has implications for participation in classes and coaching of **sports**. Children can refine movements only through practice and through suggestions made *while the child is engaged in the activity*. Lengthy

TABLE 14-3 **Gross Motor Development: 3–15 Years**

Age (yr)	Gross Motor Development
3	Stands on one foot; walks upstairs by alternating feet
4	Pedals tricycle; runs smoothly; throws ball overhand
5	Walks downstairs by alternating feet; skips; marches with rhythm; catches bounced ball
6	Hops; jumps
7	Pedals bicycle
8	Has good body balance
9	Engages in vigorous body activities, especially in team sports
10	Balances on one foot 15 seconds; catches fly ball
12	Motor awkwardness secondary to uneven bone and muscle growth
15	Gradual correction of motor awkwardness

Modified from Sahler OJZ, McAnarney ER: *The Child from Three to Eighteen.* St. Louis, CV Mosby, 1981.

discussions of sports skills may not be useful for young grade school children. Sports activities, both individual and group, should be accompanied by individual and direct feedback to each child during the action. Complex group play can be often only understood when there is a "run-through" (probably several), with each child experiencing the way all members should act together. Coaching from the sidelines is helpful only when closely associated with the child's own action. Very young children cannot use verbal input to put together a motor sequence. They can imitate a short sequence (e.g., a simple dance step) but cannot be reliably taught skills such as swimming until late preschool or even school age. So formal classes and coaching should be limited during the preschool period and parental expectations adjusted.

A WORD ABOUT SHOES

The role of **shoes** is to protect the child from sharp, rough, hot or cold surfaces. They do not shape the foot or assist in gait development. Barefoot walking best develops the lower part of the leg, foot and particularly the arch, and thus avoiding shoes when it is safe to do so is best. The arch develops with foot movement, so rigid shoes do not further this process. In typically developing children, high tops, wedges, inserts and other expensive foot devices are not needed. Shoes should be changed frequently to accommodate rapidly growing feet. Those made of soft material that allows flexing by the child and monitoring of fit by the parent are best. Orthotics for children should be reserved for those with clear neuromuscular problems and should be used only with the advice of a clinician or physical therapist trained to evaluate and monitor these conditions.

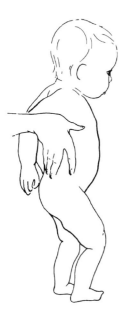

Figure 14–10 Parenting support should be gentle, well placed, but not compelling.

THE DRIVE TO WALK: THE RIPPLE EFFECTS

The drive to mastery that energizes all of development is never more obvious than in a child just learning to walk. The revelation that one's placement in space can be changed while visually monitoring and even holding onto an object is so overwhelming for a child that all else pales by comparison. Routine things such as feeding, diaper changes and sleeping are terrible interferences with this new activity from the child's viewpoint. A child's new interest in motor activities may even invade sleep time with wakefulness and restlessness. The child may pull to stand and cruise around the bed with every night wakening. Difficulties, as well as regressions, in other areas of functioning should be anticipated at the time of learning to walk. The child may be less interested in learning new words or engaging in sustained toy play. The expression of joy in accomplishment and tangible excitement should be apparent in every child, even if accompanied by looks of panic and wariness.

PARENTS' ROLE

The sparkle of joy testifies to a walking child's own sense of internal reward for a growing sense of competency. This sparkle is generalizable to other areas in which a child achieves mastery. An internal reward system is fueled as the child learns walking for walking's sake. An external reward system cannot have the energy or longevity of the internal one. The parents' role is to encourage, ensure safety in exploration, prevent overtiredness and enjoy (Fig. 14–10). It is not to exercise, instruct or smother the child with excessive acclaim. A parent's praise is welcome if not overwhelming, but it isn't the key motivating factor.

Walking changes a child's perspective of self and those around him or her. It literally makes the child a new person. A sense of independence and ability to separate from parents is enhanced by this accomplishment. Some parents are thrilled. Others are surprised and many are sad. Most have all these emotions. The child can play by roaming the environment with clear planning and direction and is no longer as dependent on caregivers to deliver toys and orchestrate his whereabouts. The child can get into more trouble and can have more fun. The ability to ambulate independently heralds a whole new era. Parents must change in response to the child's new level. The child will soon discover temper tantrums, the word *no* and the thrill of running away. The infant becomes a toddler.

DATA GATHERING

What to Observe

The following are actions the clinician should observe to track the development of motor skills:

- At every encounter during the first 5 years, the child should be allowed free movement so that the clinician can observe the child's motor competencies. Place the child both supine and prone on the examining table to observe increasing head control, truncal stability, arm support, movement at the hip and the smoothness and rhythmicity of the movement. Symmetry in movement is a vital observation.

- A line on the floor provides guidance for the child's directed walking. An area of some reasonable length (e.g., a hallway) must be provided for free-walking assessment. A child won't be able to follow a line exactly until age 2 or older.

- Observe the amount of support the child requires to do other things, such as reach for a stethoscope. Note a decreasing need for support with sitting and increasing weight bearing on the lower extremities across the first year.

- Observation of the child walking with help and then alone should begin when the child is 9 months of age and continue until school age or beyond if there is a question. The walking base, the foot position, truncal rotation and movement at the knee should be observed and should change along the lines presented earlier. The hand and arm position should change over time. The child's stopping and pivoting should improve. Rising to stand, stooping and recovering will become smoother with time.

- The style, interest and excitement of a child with motor activities should be noted at every encounter.

- At 3 years of age, knee and ankle motion should be good, and heel strike should be present.

Climbing A simple two-step climbing device kept in the examining room against the examining table can provide observation of increasing motor competencies. This apparatus will allow demonstration of lower extremity movement, proximal muscle strength and coordination in climbing. Walking up and down stairs should follow age expectations (see Box 14–3).

Parent's Handling A parent's handling of a child can give clues to both the child's competencies and the child's motor abilities. A parent who carefully supports the infant's head at all times when the child is 3 months or older may rightfully anticipate that this infant's head control is poor. Children around the world will be ready for upright packaging with or without attachment (e.g., backpacks, wrapping on the hip or back, cradle boarding) by 3 to 4 months. If a child is being carried like a neonate, something is wrong, either in the child's development or in the parent's ability to alter caretaking based on the child's competencies.

Parents who cannot allow a 4-year-old to climb up on an examining table may anticipate that the child will be unsuccessful or awkward. Excessive "coaching" of a child during the motor assessment may also be a clue that the parent has a worry about functioning in this area.

What to Ask

Parents will usually find reporting of gross motor skills the easiest of all areas of development. In addition to asking what the child can do, ask *how* the child approaches the task (i.e., with caution at one extreme or with abandon and impulsivity at the other). The manner or style in which these skills are performed may reflect the emerging personality, family expectations or difficulty with motor coordination.

The parents' response about the child's accomplishments may provide data about any underlying anxiety or specific worries. By beginning questions at a lower level of functioning than anticipated, the clinician can find the floor of the child's performance and convey the importance of individual expectations in motor development.

Children readily practice newly emerging skills in motor development, as well as in other areas of development. The relatively invariant order of motor skill acquisition allows a clinician taking the history of a child whose development is generally normal to simply ask what kind of new movements or activities the child is doing. The internally regulated and self-fueling nature of this area of development is highlighted in this approach.

A child whose motor development is not synchronous with other areas of development or is delayed beyond levels of normal variation (see Box 14–1) needs a more detailed history. Disorders of movement versus disorders of tone and posture can be specified through the history, coupled with a careful examination. Perinatal difficulties must alert the clinician to the need for careful evaluation of gross motor competencies, particularly if walking is delayed beyond 18 months.

Examination

Most of the gross motor examination is best moved to the end of the assessment because these activities usually energize kids, who are then difficult to calm down. Doing activities that require child involvement while you are filling out forms is an efficient management of time. The following are other things to keep in mind about the examination:

- The clinician should assess the passive motor tone of all extremities throughout the first 3 years. Move all four extremities as part of a playful game.
- Both slow and rapid motions should be applied to the limbs to elicit any lowered threshold to a stretch reflex.
- Deep tendon reflexes should be monitored.
- Asymmetries in tone, reflexes or movement, provided that the child's head is in the midline, should receive very careful follow-up. Persistence of these signs may require further neurological evaluation.

- Early evidence of spastic cerebral palsy is tight heel cords with limited dorsiflexion of the foot or a "catch" in the Achilles tendon.

- Scissoring of the lower extremities when the child is held upright reflects adductor spasm.

- A limp requires complete neurological and orthopedic assessment by an experienced specialist.

- Head and truncal tone should be assessed through the pull-to-sit and prone positions, as well as the position of a child being held over the hand. In addition, the child's head and body control when being held upright, at the shoulder or under the arms in front of the examiner should be assessed during the first year. Truncal tone is often reflected in how the child responds to handling and holding by the examiner. It's a perfect excuse to hold and handle the baby as part of every assessment until that is too troublesome, often at 15 to 18 months.

- Placing the baby both prone and supine offers the chance to assess increasing shoulder girdle tone and strength, as well as control of the lower part of the body.

- Alternating hip movements appear at 5 months of age, but they significantly increase in some form after 9 months.

- Weight bearing on the feet is observed in children from the age of 5 months to walking.

- Persistent standing on tiptoe is abnormal after 9 months.

- Walking with help should be attempted after 9 months but may not be present until after the first birthday.

- Climbing up stairs is seen from 8 to 18 months. After the age of 2 years, children will attempt to do this with feet only, two feet on the step. Only after 2 to 3 years of age do children alternate feet on steps.

- Gait should be observed during the second through the sixth years and beyond if indicated. As the toddler begins to walk independently, gait is typically wide based, accompanied by waddling hips and intermittent toe walking. With each observation, the base should narrow, the arms should come down and reciprocal movement should be added. Waddling at the hip should decrease, the knees should move a bit more, ankle movement should increase and heel strike should be present at the age of 3 years. By the age of 5 years, a sticker placed below the umbilicus should move very little except forward as the child walks. Forward movement, either walking or crawling, should be smooth and rhythmic by and large. Any asymmetry in gait is always cause for concern.

- Children can stoop about 6 months after independent walking. They bounce to music at 15 to 18 months of age. Getting up to sit or stand should be accomplished by a smooth roll to the side by 15 months.

- A soft foam ball provides an easy way to assess catching skills (see Box 14–3). This game can be done at the end of the exam or as part of the weight-measure procedure of the nurse.

- Children who are consistently 3 to 6 months behind on motor skill acquisition need a second look. Muscle tone, deep tendon reflexes and the persistence of primitive reflexes and postures should be evaluated carefully. Cerebral palsy, hypotonia and muscular and metabolic diseases must be considered. Through a careful history and assessment over time, the primary care provider may determine whether the delays are global or confined to the motor area. Further evaluation and intervention can become more focused with this in mind.

QUICK CHECK—1 YEAR

- ✓ Pulls to stand, cruises and takes (maybe) a few steps
- ✓ Refined pincer grasp; points with the index finger
- ✓ One word plus "mama" and "dada"
- ✓ Waves "bye, bye"
- ✓ Tries to pull off clothes
- ✓ Feeds self, with hands
- ✓ Drinks from a cup
- ✓ Imitates vocalizations
- ✓ Understands simple requests, phrases and familiar objects
- ✓ Points at objects desired (proto-naming)
- ✓ Watches and imitates older children and adults, single actions

ANTICIPATORY GUIDANCE

- The clinician can support the parents' feelings of assurance and pride in their child's motor accomplishments and can highlight the individual **temperamental characteristics** of the child that affect all areas of development, including the style of motor achievements. Careful assessment should appropriately diffuse anxiety about individual patterns of development and confirm the child's integrity.

- Parents support development of gross motor skills by providing opportunities for free exploration of the environment within safe limits. Excessive practice (adult perspective) and even overwhelming praise squelch the child's own innate drive for mastery and competency.

- A safe play area and encouragement of daily gross motor activities for girls and boys in nonrestrictive, unfussy clothes support development.

- Playing on the floor, wrestling sessions and ball playing are good activities for both sexes if they are done in a relaxed, social manner. Baby gymnastics, swimming classes and therapy programs are fine if they are done with these principles in mind; the activities themselves do not magically enhance development.

- Swimming lessons in particular may be dangerous for young infants, and it is unrealistic for children to reliably sequence and coordinate the motor activities of swimming before the age of 4 years. Primitive reflexes are the basis for most behavior in the water at younger ages.

⚠ HEADS UP–1 YEAR

- A child who is not moving in space in some manner needs evaluation, including a broad assessment of development with emphasis on the neuromotor system.
- Asymmetries in movement must be taken seriously at this age. The arms and hands, legs and feet should be working in a parallel, balanced way. If not, hemiparesis must be considered. "Oh, he's just a lefty" or similar comments are not acceptable at this age.
- A child who cannot pick up a raisin or pellet needs an extra look at this age. This may indicate general delays or specific neuromotor concerns.
- Children should be pointing at objects. If not, suspect language problems. A child with an autistic spectrum disorder will also not bring toys to show or share. Pulling a parent's hand to an object is not the same as pointing.
- Children who only bang or mouth toys are at an earlier stage in development and need an evaluation. The play should be specific to the toy.
- A drop-off in the amount and complexity of vocalizations may signal hearing loss or appearance of the autistic spectrum of disorders.
- Poorly attached children show either no or a frantic response to separations, cling to or avoid the parent or are "too friendly" to strangers. Delay in stranger anxiety may also signal general cognitive delays.
- Children not feeding themselves at this time are headed for feeding problems. If they can't feed themselves, suspect developmental delay. If they're not allowed to feed themselves, there is a parenting problem.
- Sleep should generally extend through the night and naps generally consolidated to one a day. If not, investigate because a sleep problem is about to emerge.
- Lead exposure becomes a real possibility as children become mobile. Evaluate risks. Even low levels depress cognitive abilities.
- Uneven gait or a limp always needs evaluation for hip and structural problems, intra-articular pathology or abnormalities in neuromotor functioning. Toddling should be symmetrical.
- Early walkers generally fall backward and land on their bottoms. A consistent "forward faller" needs evaluation of motor tone and Achilles' tendon tightness.
- Bruises on early walkers are on the bottom, forehead and, occasionally, the anterior tibial surfaces. Investigate atypical bruise patterns or injuries because nonaccidental injury must be suspected.
- A 1-year-old should be exuberant, active, avoidant and wiggly—in other words, very difficult to examine. If your exam is too easy, look again at developmental competence, social/emotional processes and family issues.

- Beginning walkers are very energy inefficient. They require about 1200 kcal/day to sustain their new activities. This has to be delivered in six small meals because toddlers cannot usually sit still long enough for larger meals. Clinicians can anticipate these changes in feeding for parents. Children younger than 4 years should never be allowed to eat and walk at the same time because of the danger of aspiration.

- In spite of its name, an infant walker may *not* enhance a child's ability to walk. Head injuries are common in young children in walkers. Children with lower extremity extensor hypertonicity do very well in walkers. However, that posture only exaggerates the children's own abnormal preponderance of extensor tone. These children need to be on the floor, moving freely and practicing reciprocal hip and knee movement. Every child can push a walker out doors, down stairs and out into streets. Walkers contain children poorly and thwart prewalking progression. Individual therapy programs may include walkers for specific children in order to stabilize the trunk. Other than in that context, it is better to actively discourage their use.

- Programs based on the concept that *all* learning is facilitated through an integration of motor activities have no basis in science and have had no demonstration of effectiveness. These programs prescribe a rigid series of motor activities to be done by the parent so that patterns, either accelerated or remedial, can be established in the child. These activities consume up to 8 hours per day of "therapy" by the parent. Failures are attributed to noncompliance. These programs, under several names throughout the country, victimize parents of handicapped children, who are looking for anything to improve their child's outcome. No evidence shows that this "patterning" is important for development at all, certainly no evidence that learning to crawl has anything to do with learning to read. Secondary gain from increased parental attention, social interaction and fun may have some benefit for some children in some circumstances, but the formal activities of these programs are incidental to these processes. Clinicians should be informed of what programs are operative in their communities and examine them carefully. Parents should be offered the clinician's professional input.

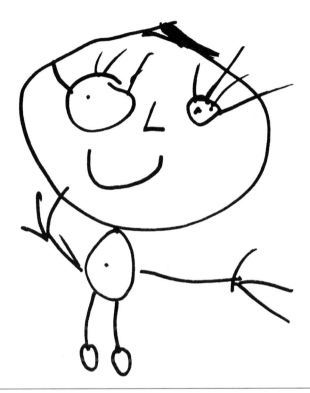

"A girl-baby walking." By Anne Atkinson, age 5.

CHAPTER 15

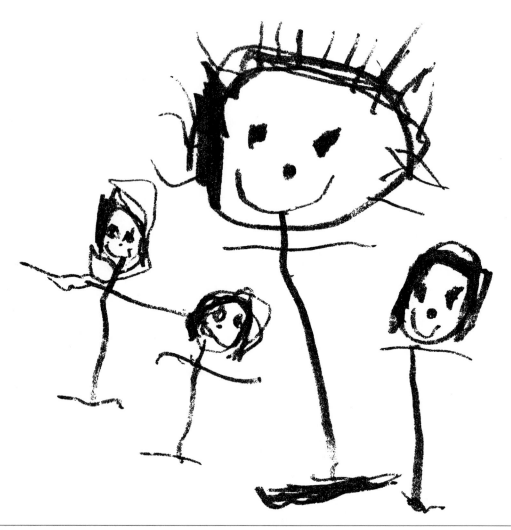

This picture shows the preschooler's perspective on the world, a healthy self-importance. This girl shows herself as the largest and central figure. Mom and Dad are shown close and well aligned, though smaller and looking a bit frazzled. Her older sister is off to the side, next to Dad. A sense of independence and a need to be in charge are balanced by a need to stay close and safe with the family. By Louise Dixon, age 3½ (original in brown marker).

15 to 18 Months: Declaring Independence and Pushing the Limits

MARIA TROZZI and MARTIN T. STEIN

Temper tantrums, temporary regressions in development and other negative behavior should be interpreted in the context of a toddler's quest for autonomy and independence. Experience with toilet training, discipline and learning self-feeding skills are discussed in the context of changes in cognitive development and the drive to independence. Early recognition of autistic spectrum at this age is reviewed and supported with specific screening tools.

Key Words

- **Autonomy**
- **Attachment**
- **Discipline**
- **Regressions**
- **Self-feeding**
- **Rapprochement**
- **Transitional Object**
- **Behavior Modification**
- **Autism**
- **Temper Tantrums**
- **Toilet Training**

Maria's mother asks her pediatrician if she should be concerned about her 18-month old daughter's preference for a bottle—during the day and at bedtime. The pediatrician responds, "A child this age no longer needs her bottle. It's bad for her teeth and may increase the rate of ear infections. My advice is to take it away and let her drink from a cup. She's a big girl now. She needs to grow up!"

An alternative approach would encourage a response based on more information about Maria's developmental skills. Recognizing that maintaining a preference for the bottle represents holding onto an earlier, more dependent stage of development, an exploration of other milestones that reflect her level of autonomy might be useful. Focused questions to the mother, as well as office observations, reveal that this toddler feeds herself independently with a spoon and drinks from a cup, soothes herself to sleep each night with minimal fussing and responds to her parents' verbal restraints at times of conflict. She enjoys the care of a regular baby-sitter and does not cry when her parents occasionally leave her at night. In the office, she plays by herself with toys. Periodically, she

Continued

checks in with her mother and then returns to the toy box. She seems happy and able to move back and forth between the security of her mother and independent, self-initiated play.

Maria's development demonstrates a strong attachment to her mother while she is simultaneously becoming more independent in social and motor skills. Although use of a bottle may be viewed as a residual symbol of infancy, perhaps this remarkably healthy girl needs a temporary "crutch" in the form of a bottle to negotiate the more demanding achievements of the second year.

The discrepancy between what a parent tells you about behavior and development and what you observe in the office setting is perhaps most striking when the child is in the middle of the second year. Although a parent may describe a child as one who now feeds herself, has the capability to express needs, can follow simple directions and is a "delightful child," the clinician frequently observes someone quite different. In the office the same child may be suspicious of the clinician's kind and gentle approach, cling firmly to the parent, scream at any touch and resist initial social interchange with a toy or an examining tool. How can this behavior be understood in a way that provides useful insight into a child's development for the clinician and for the parents?

The behavior of a typical 1½-year-old does contain many contradictions. The child seeks to be more independent by using newly attained skills but needs additional nurturance to refuel the push toward **autonomy or personal self-governance**. Children need parents for additional security but at the same time seem to be always assertive in pulling away. The resistance and the negativism of this age try the patience of parents. Simultaneously, these forces supply the energy the child needs to act more independently. It's this push-pull behavior that is confusing and trying.

The toddler appears to have an innate resource of energy to master new skills in an even more complex world. Unfortunately, attention span, cooperation with playmates, motor dexterity and, perhaps most significantly, tolerance for frustration are limited. Although drive for mastery of the environment appears to be built in (some parents describe the toddler's efforts as driven, striving or searching), the child's abilities inevitably apply limits and precipitate conflicts as the child reaches out for more independence. Frustration is a fact of life for a child struggling to do more things, explore more places and push at the limits of behavior.

An 18-month-old has developed a strong emotional tie with his parents; events in the outside world are measured against that link. At this age, the child frequently checks back with a parent as if to say, "Is it safe? Can I continue to play … to move forward?" Parents are a secure base from which to explore. This behavior can be seen in daycare centers and playgrounds when the toddler is brave and independent and then suddenly searches and runs to a secure area when the social environment changes or becomes threatening. For some toddlers, even the benevolent approach of a physician or nurse threatens a fragile internal stability. In the office, the child runs quickly to the parent, seeking a sanctum and security. The same child might have appeared more secure with the clinician during the first half of the second year, but by 18 months a "rapprochement" with the parent and outer world produces what on the surface appears to be more infantile behavior (clinging to a parent, crying in the presence of a stranger or refusing the approach of a playmate). Maturational change in the central nervous system generates greater awareness of the external world (e.g., other children, other adults, toys, furniture), and this awareness now comes into conflict with a previously secure, parentally modulated environment. Cognitive skills have matured enough that a child can imagine a threat and appreciate more subtle dissonance with what is familiar. Emerging language informs the toddler that communication is important, but an 18-month-old cannot effectively communicate with strangers. The toddler is lost without parental translation and interpretation. It is the gaps in cognition, memory, language and sense of self that set the stage for this challenging behavior.

Helping parents through this period is easier when the clinician's observations and expectations of behavior are informed by these developmental phenomena. The parental patterns of interaction with the child that are established at this time have considerable longevity. Parents must see the struggles for mastery and independence as both inevitable and a positive sign of the child's emotional and social growth. Such an outlook will sustain them through this "first adolescence." Anger, anxiety, overcontrol and overprotection at this time do not allow room for the psychological growth that is appropriate at this age.

Three aspects of behavior and development often surface at this age, either in the questions parents bring to the office visit or in what a clinician observes in the office setting: (1) discipline and temper tantrums, (2) toilet training and (3) changes in feeding patterns. All of these issues can be seen within the context of a drive for independence.

DISCIPLINE

Isabella was an "easy" child in her first year. She reached each new developmental milestone with apparent joy in her achievement. Between 15 and 18 months of age, her parents reported a significant shift in her behavior. She refused new foods, often throwing the food over the highchair table; she would not use a cup, preferring only breastfeeding or a bottle. Sleep patterns were erratic, with frequent night awakening. Temper tantrums were becoming more frequent. Note: the shift in parenting that is prompted by this "strange" behavior means that Isabella is likely to be brought in for a health assessment. It seems at first glance that everything is going downhill.

The newly discovered capacity to walk, run and climb opens up new pathways of exploration for the toddler. Not only can she get to things through curiosity and self-discovery, but she can also manipulate objects into new forms that follow from imagination. Fine motor and visual-perceptual skills allow the toddler to shape, invent and explore objects; these manipulations give definition and form to the child's world. Simultaneously, receptive language function is developing rapidly; the child now *understands* many words, follows simple directions and can even point to some parts of the body when a parent sounds its name.

These new skills emerge rapidly and must be incorporated into a psychological framework that was previously dependent solely on caretakers' manipulation of the child's environment. The awareness that through language, motor and perceptual skills the child can shape and pattern his own world brings about inner conflict for most children. These conflicts can be seen when a tower of neatly stacked blocks falls; when a playmate, benign and cooperative at one moment, commits the awful sin of touching a child's toys momentarily; or when a parent removes a child from one enjoyable activity and moves her to another place (e.g., from playing

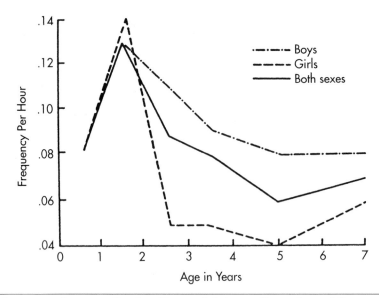

Figure 15–1   Frequency of anger outbursts, with a peak between 18 months and 2 years. (Modified from Goodenough FL: *Anger in Young Children*. St. Paul, MN, University of Minnesota Press, 1931. Cited in Helms DB, Turner JS: *Exploring Child Behavior: Basic Principles*. Philadelphia, WB Saunders, 1978.)

with toys to the dreaded highchair). The toddler can now make a choice about a toy, a playmate or a meal. Infringement on these choices produces inner disharmony that may lead to anger and aggression. A young toddler does not possess the psychological structure to delay gratification, to suppress or displace angry feelings or to manage these difficult situations through verbal communication. The child cannot wait, see things from another's point of view, anticipate compound effects of actions or cope effectively. An explosion is predictable.

Seeking alternative responses consistent with developmental capacities, the child pouts, cries, becomes morose or has a temper tantrum. Behavior outbursts by an 18-month-old can be viewed as developmentally predictable (Fig. 15–1). The frequency and intensity with which an individual child manifests such behavior is dependent on many factors, including (1) the type of attachment to parents, (2) the toddler's individual temperament and way of adapting to new and stressful situations and (3) the parents' style of responding to various behavior in the child.

Attachment (the enduring emotional bond that people feel toward special people in their lives) directed to parents is a major goal of the first year of life; in the second year, children need to be encouraged to broaden the focus of that attachment and become more independent. (Some observers of human development have suggested that the guiding psychological goal throughout life after the first birthday is to detach from one's parents!) Parents can be encouraged to allow self-play, mistakes, mishaps and consequent frustrations in their child. Piaget pointed out that children at this age learn through the experience of their own errors and successes in problem solving and exploration. "Mistakes" during play give clues about how children work to understand their experience with others and objects.

If a parent is too protective and limits the development of independent skills by providing an overly protective environment, infantile attachment behavior becomes more locked into an earlier phase of development. New situations—without mommy or daddy or when frustration is inevitable—become intolerable. When a toddler is allowed, even encouraged, to experience moderate amounts of frustration during the course of play, the child learns to manage angry feelings, feelings that may be directed toward parents, play objects or a playmate. These kinds of experience assist the child in the gradual journey to becoming more independent from parents and more self-regulated.

A toddler's *temperament* is reflected in the style of response to conflict with self, others and the environment. Toddlers vary significantly in the energy released when a frustrating experience arises. A youngster with a high level of adaptability to change and a positive approach to new stimuli will probably move quickly from a conflictual situation to one that is harmonious. At the opposite end of the spectrum is a child with intense expressions of mood and withdrawal responses to new situations. This child may be easily frustrated at seemingly minor disruptions. The intensity and duration of crying, screaming and the level of consolability will, in part, relate to these innate aspects of temperament. Although most children are somewhere between these temperamental extremes, a clinical appreciation for them can be helpful in assessing a particular child and the parents' responses to that child.

Parental styles of responding to a toddler's tantrums affect the resolution of the episode, as well as the nature of future tantrums. Children are sponges of adult attitudes and actions at this age. They learn how to handle their own anger, aggression and frustration as they observe parents and other caretakers. Frequently, parents who seem able to manage toddler tantrums are less threatened by their child's aggressive moments and emerging independence. They do not get drawn into the struggle themselves. They recognize, often unconsciously, the strengths of this autonomous act and can freely assist the child in handling his own feelings. Other parents may feel challenged or threatened by the child's bids for independence and respond only with anger. Styles of parenting the child at this age often reflect a parent's own sense of self-effectiveness and own experiences from childhood. A toddler can call forth feelings and responses that many parents did not even know were within them. Parents may become unrecognizable to themselves when faced with toddler challenges.

Discipline at this age means teaching, guiding behavior and showing the child how to cooperate. It's not simply the parents' response to a tantrum. When viewed constructively, discipline can be seen as a process of teaching the toddler to place limits or boundaries on behavior within family and cultural expectations, to learn to "use words" to express anger, to feel comfortable with feelings of anger and to learn to cope with the inevitable frustrations of normal life. It may be useful to compare tantrums with a blown fuse. The tantrum serves a purpose in itself; it releases tension by providing an exit for bound-up energy that momentarily finds no other outlet. Occasional toddler tantrums viewed in this manner can be accepted, understood and allowed to occur by an understanding parent. In a healthy toddler, occasional tantrums cannot usually be stopped and should even be seen as helpful.

From another perspective, "discipline solidifies the boundaries, as well as the core of the ego" (see Brazelton and colleagues, 1984). It offers the child a way to manage conflictual feelings and unacceptable behavior. Because the fragile ego is developing a sense of self at this time, conflicts directed at parents, peers, siblings and toys are necessary. These conflicts collectively define the child's emerging ego, or sense of self (Who am I?). Simultaneously, the child needs an adult to define acceptable limits of behavior. Pushing and testing these limits may be the only way to be sure of their firmness. The push-pull process of a toddler's development is now seen in terms of both the child's behavior and the parental response to such behavior.

TOILET TRAINING

Four milestones must be reached before a toddler is ready to master bowel and bladder control. They are a result of neurological maturation, increased attention span, attachment to a caretaker whom they want to please and the emerging ability to sequence events (Box 15–1).

These milestones of development reflect mastery of the motor, social and language skills that usually come together after the second birthday. For some, it may be a few months earlier; for others, developmental readiness may not be apparent until 3 or more years of age (Table 15–1). From the child's viewpoint, toilet training that is too early or too rapid has no advantages. Indeed, from a child's perspective, there is not much to be recommended in stopping play, going to the toilet, giving up part of yourself and then watching it summarily flushed. The process may be detrimental if it creates expectations the child cannot handle. When viewed from the standpoint of the child's needs, toilet training demands a level of complex, multi-stepped, voluntary control that could not be obtained previously. Motor, social and receptive

---

BOX 15–1   DEVELOPMENTAL PREREQUISITES FOR BOWEL AND BLADDER CONTROL

- Maturation of the central and peripheral nervous systems to the degree that voluntary control of the anal and urethral sphincters is possible; ability to sense and signal the urge to go
- Ability to sit on a potty seat quietly for a moderate amount of time with the conscious intent to have a bowel movement or urinate
- Desire to gain satisfaction from the successful completion of defecation and urination and recognize the pleasure in the supervising parent and within oneself through growth in competency as a form of positive reinforcement
- Ability to understand the sequence of requirements of the task

Drive to imitate greater than drive to oppose parents

At her second birthday, Janelle's parents initiated potty training, but Janelle refused their efforts. She balked at sitting on a brightly painted potty seat. When her father read a book to her, she would sit on the seat but would neither urinate nor defecate. She popped up and ran out of the bathroom as soon as the story was finished. When Janelle's pediatrician inquired about the parents' attempts, they said that they were not sure she made a connection between sitting on the potty seat and a bowel movement. At 30 months of age, Janelle seemed to enjoy sitting on "my potty" and defecating with ease. At this time, Janelle's facial expression demonstrated pleasure when her parents congratulated her on her new skill. Note: This case demonstrates the enormous difference that is seen when the process is presented once a child shows individual readiness.

TABLE 15–1   Guide to Toilet Training Readiness: A Developmental Approach

Child's Behavior/Competencies	Parental Response
Complex, multistep behavior; completing household tasks; completing tasks in sequence	Narrate the process while the child is watching a parent or siblings at the toilet
Undresses self	Allow child to undress self; loose, easily removed clothes are preferred; praise the child while mentioning that he will soon use a potty seat
Shows interest in a potty seat Demonstrates an ability to understand the requirements of various tasks	Keep a potty seat in a regular place in the bathroom; let the child know that he can sit on it and what it is used for; some children can learn about the seat initially by sitting on it with a diaper on
Points to, looks at or announces a BM in his diaper	Put the diaper/BM in the seat; dispose of it later; acknowledge the production
Increasing periods of daytime dryness	Use training pants during the day
Ability to sit quietly on the potty seat for a moderate period	Praise the child for knowing about the seat and discuss its use; encourage sitting on the seat
Shows satisfaction in having a BM	Praise moderately by showing pleasure in completion of the task
Asks to use the potty seat or uses it in a self-directed manner	Encourage use of the potty seat after a meal (gastrocolic reflex) or (for some children) at a time when the child usually has a BM
Desire to please by imitating parents	Praise the child by pointing out that "my big girl is now ready to use her potty seat"
Partial voluntary control of anal and urethral sphincters, as demonstrated by having a BM or urinating at a planned time on the potty seat	Show pleasure in task completion while expecting setbacks, both at times of stress and spontaneously
Interest in successful use of a potty seat	Try training pants; encourage the child to remove the training pants by self

BM, bowel movement.

language skills come together to make this a big event in a child's life. It is an opportunity for growth and increased feelings of self-esteem.

As a form of anticipatory guidance, it is helpful to discuss toilet training at the visit when the child is between 15 and 18 months old for three reasons: (1) to prevent parents from rushing into training before the child is ready, (2) to bring out the developmental significance of training as a way to assist parents in understanding and responding to the broader developmental events at this age and (3) to help parents begin to set the stage for this process later on.

Clues that a child is physically and emotionally ready for potty training may be observed some time between 18 months and 2 years of age in most children. The following are examples of such clues:

- The child will demonstrate having made the connection between the feeling (muscular contractions) of urination or defecation and what is produced. This connection is communicated to the parent as the child points or looks at the urine or bowel movement.
- The child has increased periods of daytime dryness (i.e., increased bladder capacity and sphincter control), tells the parent after having a bowel movement or urinating and can sit quietly for a period.
- The child shows interest in the toilet, shows imitative behavior in other areas (e.g., dressing, household tasks), is interested in compulsively putting things away and is not violently negative.

At this time, parents can be encouraged to introduce a potty seat, explain its function to the child and make it available. Parents must take the child into the bathroom and discuss and demonstrate the process. Having the child sit on a potty chair (initially with the diaper attached) is a first step in getting acquainted with the chair. The parents should be positive toward the behavior and the product (feces). The child will see the bowel movement as a part of self; parents should not regard it as "yucky." Parents can be encouraged to show their pleasure at a successful movement, but overenthusiasm is not warranted because this exaggerates the importance of using the potty chair, thereby adding stress to the child and inviting negative behavior. Conversely, parents whose 2-year-old does not seem interested in a potty chair should be encouraged to wait a few months. It is often helpful to point out to parents that just as some normal children do not walk until after 15 months, some toddlers require more time to attain consistent voluntary sphincter control and to be willing to exercise it. It is not a measure of intelligence on the child's part or of adequacy of child rearing on the parents' part.

Initiation and continuation of toilet training are dependent on the child's personal health and environmental events. External events such as intercurrent illness, birth of a new sibling, a family vacation or absence of a parent for a prolonged period can be expected to delay or cause a setback in the mastery of toilet training. When some of these events are predictable, potty training may be delayed by the parents. **Regressions** without any explanations should also be expected. The child's self-respect should be preserved in these circumstances. Parents should be informed that other less predictable changes in family function may delay mastery of this new skill. Boys generally train 2 months later than girls. Firstborn children train 1.7 months later than children born later. In most families, the whole process will take months. The later one starts, in general, the shorter the duration of the training period.

FEEDING AND SELF-DETERMINATION

As fine motor manipulations and visual-motor coordination advance, an 18-month-old learns to use these skills and enjoys the use of a cup and spoon. Self-feeding represents a significant form of mastery in the use of an instrument to extend and expand the abilities of the hand and in the honing of visual-motor skills (Box 15–2). It is also another psychological separation from dependency on parents. It is helpful to point out to parents that although messy and seemingly disorganized, allowing a child the freedom to feed herself assists development and mastery at several levels.

BOX 15–2   DEVELOPMENTAL SKILLS ENHANCED BY SELF-FEEDING

- Fine motor skills
- Hand-to-eye coordination
- Independent actions yielding an enjoyable response
- Learning to choose and enjoy different food textures and colors

As with any new skill, learning may progress at different rates in children of various temperaments, and setbacks (or regressions) may occur after intercurrent events in the family. As with most new experiences that require mastery, feeding is particularly vulnerable to individual differences and fluctuations. Particular attractions or dislikes for certain foods are frequently seen at this time. Prolonged periods of refusing one food group are common (i.e., food jags). Excessive intake of juice or milk at this age can satisfy a toddler's appetite, discourage the intake of more caloric-dense foods and lead to failure to thrive or anemia. However, as long as the child's physical growth has not been compromised, parents need reassurance that fluctuations in diet are normal and self-limited. Demonstrating the child's rate of growth on a standard growth curve is often reassuring to a parent who perceives the toddler as "starving herself." Food refusal provides an opportunity to explain to parents the importance of self-directed feeding in terms of a child's need for emotional independence and, eventually, better eating habits.

Robbie was known to his pediatrician as an engaging and socially interactive infant. At his 18-month-old health supervision visit, his clinician observed that he was walking around the room with a bottle of juice. Even block play did not distract him from a firm grasp of the bottle. Robbie's mother listed only a single concern on the previsit Q card (see Appendix)—his refusal to eat most foods. She tried to make meals that he might like and spoke to other parents about their children's food interest. Nothing seemed to help.

Robbie's physical exam and developmental assessment were normal. In fact, he had achieved mastery of independent skills in several areas of development, including falling to sleep by himself, playing with toys for an extended period and showing a few early signs of readiness for toilet training. However, his growth chart revealed a decrease in the velocity of weight gain, most likely a result of inadequate caloric intake caused by excessive juice consumption. Robbie's clinician not only made use of the encounter to counsel about the need for calorie-rich foods and significantly less juice, but also saw an opportunity to point out to his mother that exchanging the bottle for a cup would also give a boost to Robbie's development. The cup, similar to self-feeding, becomes a symbol of growth and self-reliance.

The more the clinician can do to assist the parent of a toddler in understanding these new skills as a reflection of mastery and "separation" from infantile dependency on the parent, the better equipped the parent will be for "letting go" through continued guidance and surveillance without squelching further growth. A parent has never won a feeding battle with a child! Ingenuity and patience are required to set up feeding as a source of good nutrition, physical and psychological.

Some parents remain anxious and overfocused on a thriving toddler's food intake even after pointing out the adequacy of his nutritional intake and normal growth pattern. Pediatric clinicians should be attuned to an overanxious parent whose exaggerated concern about eating may lead to forced feeding. The velocity of growth slows in the second year, so the parental observation that he eats less than before is likely to be accurate. As long as he's growing well and is not a juice or milk addict, his nutrition intake is adequate for growth. The fast-food French fry habit is also a risk at this age as food preferences get solidified.

Transitional Object

About two thirds of toddlers will have an inanimate **transitional object** that is used for comforting, especially when they are falling asleep and at times of stress. Some parents need the reassurance that these old, threadbare blankets, dolls or toys are a reasonable way to find the security required at certain moments in each day. Their use may persist until the third or fourth birthday and occasionally later. Developmental assessments at 10 years old in which children who used a transitional object were compared with those who did not possess an obvious one showed no significant differences in behavioral or educational outcomes. Some youngsters seem to need a transitional object.

Summary

The "push-pull" process that characterizes this stage of development can be viewed as one of daily increments of psychological growth achieved by mastery of more complicated skills. These skills require adequate maturation of the toddler's nervous system and the parents' ability to simultaneously stimulate and pull back, that is, to encourage self-feeding, potty seat recognition and creative play while letting the child master these objects and events independently. To be sure, it is a delicate balance that requires parental skill that will vary in different families. The child's clinician can point out the developmental necessity of this balance. It can be demonstrated with a "teachable moment" during the physical examination with toys or examining instruments or when observing the child's play during the interview with the parent.

AUTISM: EARLY DETECTION MAKES A DIFFERENCE

Alex was a "happy baby" in the first year of life. His mother commented to the pediatrician on several occasions that he seemed so easy to care for in comparison to her friend's children. At the 12-month visit, the pediatrician noted that although he could babble interactively, Alex had not expressed any words. At the 15-month health supervision visit, Alex's only word was "ma," and there was a question of whether he understood directions. His mother felt that he had good hearing (passed a newborn auditory screening test). The physical examination was normal, but the pediatrician found it difficult to engage Alex's interest in either toys or himself. Alex preferred to be left alone and play with a toy car.

Autism is a neurodevelopmental disorder that includes many conditions, all of which have three core features: impairment in socialization, impairment in verbal and nonverbal communication and restricted and repetitive patterns of behavior. Kanner described the first group of children with autism in 1943; they had an atypical developmental course exemplified by the following:

- Delayed acquisition of language and atypical use of language (noncommunicative and echolalic)
- Social remoteness, unrelatedness
- A preference for repetitive, stereotyped, nonimaginative play patterns
- A need for sameness or rituals

The average age at the diagnosis of autism in the United States is 3 to 4 years. There is now sufficient empirical research to demonstrate the effectiveness of early, intensive behavior modification programs when they occur for at least 2 years during the preschool period. Recent studies demonstrate improved outcomes in most young children with autism, including progress in speech, social skills and intellectual performance. *The challenge for pediatricians is early recognition of the core features of autism in the second year of life.* The characteristics of autism are measurable by 18 months of age and stable through the preschool period. The 15- and 18-month health supervision visits should include specific observations and questions directed to parents that screen for autism.

The development of most children with autism appears normal to parents and clinicians in the first year of life. However, when home videotapes of first birthday parties in infants with autism were compared with those of infants who had typical development, four aspects of behavior correctly identified over 90% of the autistic infants:

- Diminished eye contact
- Lack of orienting to their name being called
- Infrequent pointing with a finger to indicate interest in something
- Not showing an object by bringing it to a person

Delays in pointing and showing are early signs of atypical development in "joint attention" behavior that are seen in toddlers with autism. Indications for immediate referral for further evaluation during the second year of life include

- No babbling by 12 months
- No gesturing (pointing, waving bye-bye) by 12 months
- No single words by 16 months
- No two-word spontaneous (not just echolalia) phrases by 23 months
- Any loss of any language or social skills at any age

Parental concerns that are "red flags" for an early diagnosis of autism and specific questions that may be asked during a health supervision visit are found in Tables 15–2 and 15–3. Screening instruments with good validity and sufficient sensitivity and specificity include the Modified Checklist for Autism in Toddlers (MCHAT), which is designed to screen for autistic spectrum disorder at 18 months (see Appendix), and the Pervasive Developmental Disorders

TABLE 15–2   Parental Concerns that are RED FLAGS for Autism

Communication Concerns
  Does not respond to name
  Cannot tell me what the child wants
  Language is delayed
  Doesn't follow directions
  Appears deaf at times
  Seems to hear sometimes but not others
  Doesn't point or wave bye-bye
  Used to say a few words but now doesn't

Social Concerns
  Doesn't smile socially
  Seems to prefer to play alone
  Gets things for himself
  Is very independent
  Does things "early"
  Has poor eye contact
  Is in his own world
  Tunes us out
  Is not interested in other children

Behavioral Concerns
  Tantrums
  Is hyperactive/uncooperative or oppositional
  Doesn't know how to play with toys
  Gets stuck on things over and over
  Toe walks
  Has unusual attachments to toys (e.g., is always holding a certain object)
  Lines things up
  Is oversensitive to certain textures or sounds
  Has odd movement patterns

Absolute Indications **for Immediate Further Evaluation**
  No babbling by 12 months
  No gesturing (pointing, waving bye-bye, etc.) by 12 months
  No single words by 16 months
  No 2-word spontaneous (*not just echolalic*) phrases by 24 months
  ANY loss of ANY language or social skills at ANY age

From Filipek PA, Pasquale JA, Baranek GT, et al: The screening and diagnosis of autistic spectrum disorders. *J Autism Dev Disord* 29:6, 1999. Used by permission.

Screening Test–Stage 1 (PDDST-1), a parent questionnaire designed for use in primary care settings for infants and toddlers up to 36 months of age.

  Early diagnosis followed by an appropriate referral will have a significant impact on a child's development and bring a tremendous sense of accomplishment to the clinician.

TABLE 15-3 Screening and Diagnosis of Autistic Spectrum Disorders

Ask specific development probes: "Does she or he ..." or "Is there ..."	
Socialization	Cuddle like other children? Look at you when you are talking or playing? Smile in response to a smile from others? Engage in reciprocal, back-and-forth play? Play simple imitation games, such as pat-a-cake or peek-a-boo? Show interest in other children?
Communication	Point with his finger? Gesture? Nod yes and no? Direct your attention by holding up objects for you to see? Anything odd about his/her speech? Show things to people? Lead an adult by the hand? Give inconsistent responses to name? To commands? Use rote, repetitive or echolalic speech? Memorize strings of words or scripts?
Behavior	Have repetitive, stereotyped or odd motor behavior? Have preoccupations or a narrow range of interests? Attend more to parts of objects (e.g., wheels)? Have limited or absent pretend play? Imitate other people's actions? Play with toys in the exact same way each time? Have a strong attachment to a specific unusual object?

From Filipek PA, Pasquale JA, Baranek GT, et al: The screening and diagnosis of autistic spectrum disorders. *J Autism Dev Disord* 29:6, 1999. Used by permission.

DATA GATHERING

Observations

Watching an 18-month-old child, both during independent play and while interacting with the parent, provides insight into the developmental goals of this age. As the history is recorded, helpful observations include the following:

- Does the child play independently, making use of toys in the examining room?
- Fine motor dexterity and visual-motor skills can be observed through play. Does the child play spontaneously with toys in the office, make a tower out of four cubes, scribble spontaneously or try to remove clothes by himself?
- Does the child have a transitional object? Was it brought to the office? If so, how is it used by the child?
- Does the parent allow the child to move around the examining room independently, to experiment with the available toys?
- How does the parent modulate the child's play, verbally and nonverbally?

- When you walk into the room, what is the child doing? Does the activity change in your presence?
- What is the intensity and duration with which the child clings to the parent? How does the parent respond?
- What is the content and style of the parent's verbal interactions with the child?
- Assess the child's response to your examination.

History

To determine the point on the developmental pathway from dependency to autonomy for a particular toddler, the clinician may ask a parent to describe a typical morning at home with the child. Motor, language and social milestones are documented. Feeding styles, behavior, response to disciplinary and play content are often discussed spontaneously by looking in detail at one time interval. If not, focused questions can be directed to the parent or parents, with the goal of assessing psychological independence:

- Does the child play alone for short periods? What kind of toys are of interest? Does the home have safe places for exploration? Is there a place for the child in every room?
- Does the child experience temper tantrums? What appears to set them off? When do they occur? How intense are they? What are your usual responses? How do they make you feel?
- Do you and your spouse agree on expectations for and management of the child's behavior?
- Does the child have a favorite thing to carry around or take to bed? How do you feel about it? Do you always make it available?
- When the child is doing something that is off limits, how do you respond? What do you say? What do you do?
- Many parents of toddlers find it hard to say *no* so many times each day. How do you manage to change behavior without always saying *no*?
- Have you thought about toilet training? If so, what ideas do you have about when and how to accomplish it?

Examination

Approach the child cautiously. If when you enter the examining room the toddler is on the floor or at a table playing with toys, you might bend down to the child's level. Sitting on the floor and engaging the child with a ball or other toy may yield a temporary alliance and permit effective interaction with the child. A simple, brief comment about the toy the child is playing with or a color (or pattern) on clothes may be helpful.

Frequently at this age a toddler may react with alarm at your entrance into the examining room, usually seeking out the mother and either clinging to her or sitting quietly on her lap. Reassure the parent that this is normal and expected behavior at this age. In fact, it represents an emotionally close attachment between the child and parent.

The physical examination is usually performed optimally with the child in the parent's lap. Stranger awareness is lessened in this more secure position. Physical abnormalities can be assessed accurately while the parent holds the child. In the same manner, assessment of language, motor and social skills can be successful when the child is sitting on the parent's lap. The extent of the stranger awareness response will determine how much developmental information can be observed; other data can be obtained from the parent's history.

Because the move toward independence is in progress at this stage, coupled with an unfamiliar examining room where the assessment is done, development at the age of 18 months can appear more delayed than it is. Explaining this to parents is helpful. They should not feel embarrassment when their toddler screams and clings to mother at the clinician's approach. A comment such as, "Maggie certainly knows who is important in her life!" will go a long way to ease any tension the mother may experience.

ANTICIPATORY GUIDANCE

The pediatric perspective for parent education at this examination should focus on the following:

1. Anticipating behavioral or developmental problems based on the clinician's findings during the interview and physical examination

2. Assisting parents with the next developmental stage by pointing to new milestones and anticipated behavior

The child's temperament, behavioral responses to new situations, progress in self-directed feeding and independent play will guide the discussion of anticipatory guidance. Not every visit at 18 months will require the discussion offered in these guidelines. For some parents, reassurance that development is on track will suffice. However, insight into broader meanings of new skills is appreciated by all parents.

Behavioral and developmental education for parents of an 18-month-old may include the following topics:

Concept of Rapprochement

Rapprochement ("reconnection") refers to the normal transition from independent play and exploratory activity to a period of clinging to the parent in the presence of other children and adults. It is usually seen between 18 and 24 months and may last for a week to several months. It is age appropriate, transient and, for some children, a developmental necessity before achieving greater independence in play, language and motor skills. Rapprochement reflects the cognitive gains of this age. The child is now able to form expectations for control in shaping his environment, and he is understandably irritated when these expectations are threatened.

Self-feeding as an Expression of Control and Independence

The clinician can help parents see mealtime as important in the child's growing expression of control and independence.

- Talk about feeding time in terms of the *child's* needs, not only the need for nutrients but also the need for self-directed mastery over an important part of the environment.
- Point out that appetites are often erratic at this age, but that toddlers do not starve themselves.
- Let parents know that the appetite control mechanism in the hypothalamus is well developed and that given the availability of nutritious foods, an 18-month-old will choose adequate nutrients over time.
- Discourage forced feeding or battles over food intake. Redirect the discussion to help the parents view feeding in developmental terms, as an expression of learning to be satisfied through a self-directed task.
- Let parents know that messy feeding behavior is both expected and appropriate at this age.
- Praise parents for allowing the toddler to exercise new visual-motor skills that provide the hand-eye coordination for successful use of a cup and spoon. Socially accepted eating patterns are nurtured over time by a positive approach to these social situations.
- Explain that foods that the family eats should make up most of the toddler's diet.
- Tell parents that throwing food and screaming mean that the child is done eating and should be put down.

Toilet Training Readiness

This examination (usually the last health supervision visit before the second birthday) is an ideal time to anticipate the parents' expectations, knowledge and plans for the initiation of toilet training. Readiness skills have been discussed earlier. Ask the parents, "What are your ideas or plans for toilet training?" Providing developmentally appropriate information at this time in terms of motor, social and receptive language skills goes a long way in preventing either a too rigid or a too lenient program for the child. Table 15–1 provides guidelines for the early stages of the process. It is helpful to teach parents that learning to use a potty seat is an important milestone in the toddler's ability to take control of the environment while gaining a sense of mastery and feeling good about oneself. The focus should be on the *child's* control, not the parents'.

Anticipating Disciplinary Problems

Assisting parents in understanding the expected development of negative behavior in the form of emotional outbursts is a significant task for the child's clinician at this time. It should be explained and interpreted in terms of the toddler's striving for psychological independence while the ability to manage anger and frustrations is limited by both language and attachment to parents. It is the child's bid to have a say in what is going on, to have his or her perspective appreciated.

The mother of an 18-month-old who has been brought to your office for a health supervision visit is surprised to discover a poster and brochure in your waiting room that encourages alternatives to spanking. Just as you do as part of each patient's visit at this age, you mention the poster and ask the mother what she thinks about it. "What's so bad about spanking? We spanked our two older kids when they needed it. When the kids get wild or don't mind, a quick swat on the behind lets them know what's right. I don't do it a lot, but all kids need a spanking sometimes," she responds.

This situation is both an opportunity and a challenge for the clinician. Several different responses are possible:

A. "You should never spank your child. It is an act of violence that gives your child the wrong message. I'm sure you don't want to teach him that physical violence is a way to solve conflicts. Such behavior will encourage physical responses when he gets angry as an older child or teenager."

B. "There are other ways to manage your child when he is angry or out of control. I'd like to show you some of these methods, especially what we call distraction and time-out. I'd also like to talk about preventing tantrums by showing you the value of praising your child when he does things well or when he behaves well."

C. "You seem to have learned that spanking gets a quick response." Pause, wait for a response; or,

"Can you give me an example of your child's behavior that is usually followed by spanking?" Pause, wait for a response; or,

"What do you hope to accomplish when you spank your child?" Pause, wait for a response; or,

"Many parents who use spanking as a form of discipline tell me that they were spanked by their parents. Can you tell me about your family and how you were disciplined?"

The first response is authoritative and leaves no room for negotiation. The parents' method of discipline has been sent to the jury and given a guilty verdict, complete with a huge dose of guilt. The second response is a reasoned lecture to the parent about alternatives to spanking that provide punishment without spanking. A statement about positive reinforcement as a method to prevent conflict and tantrums is tacked on. However, the clinician has closed the door on negotiation through discussion.

The third response attempts to engage the parent in a dialogue about personal experiences, perceptions and feelings about spanking. This approach provides an opportunity to explore moments when the parent was effective in discipline; it gives the clinician an opportunity to help the parent generalize from these to other situations. Through open-ended or focused questions, the clinician demonstrates respect for the parent's personal history. These simple questions, followed by a pause (the hallmark of active listening), give the parent an opportunity to explore a potentially difficult issue with the child's clinician. Beyond that, it brings about an opportunity for the development of mutual trust, a necessary ingredient for successful education.

For many families, an open and frank discussion about spanking as a form of punishment will require direct, focused questions by the child's clinician. The American Academy of Pediatrics recognizes that corporal punishment in the form of spanking carries significant risks to a child's psychological and physical development. The many effective alternative responses to tantrums and misbehavior have led most child advocates and clinicians to conclude that spanking is an unnecessary form of punishment. After a consensus conference of participating pediatric clinicians and social scientists during which the available research on corporal punishment was reviewed, a policy statement was published to encourage clinicians in their guidance for parents to seek alternative methods for dealing with undesired behavior (Box 15–3).

BOX 15–3   AMERICAN ACADEMY OF PEDIATRICS POLICY STATEMENT: "GUIDANCE FOR EFFECTIVE DISCIPLINE"

Corporal punishment involves the physical application of some form of pain after undesirable behavior. Corporal punishment ranges from slapping the hand of a child about to touch a hot stove to identifiable child abuse, such as beatings, scalding and burns. Because of this range in the severity of punishment and the form of punishment, its use as a disciplinary strategy is controversial. Although significant concern has been raised about the negative effects of physical punishment and its potential escalation into abuse, a form of physical punishment, spanking, remains one of the most commonly used strategies to reduce undesired behavior, with more than 90% of American families reporting having used spanking as a means of discipline at some time. Spanking, as discussed here, refers to striking a child with an open hand on the buttocks or extremities with the intention of modifying behavior without causing physical injury. Other forms of physical punishment, such as striking a child with an object, striking a child on a part of the body other than the buttocks or extremities, striking a child with such intensity that it results in marks lasting more than a few minutes, pulling a child's hair, jerking a child by the arm, shaking a child and physical punishment delivered in anger with intention to cause pain, are unacceptable and may be dangerous to the health and well-being of the child. These types of physical punishment should never be used. Despite its common acceptance and even advocacy for its use, spanking is a less desirable strategy than time-out or removal of privileges for reducing undesired behavior in children. Although spanking may immediately reduce or stop an undesired behavior, its effectiveness decreases with subsequent use. The only way to maintain the initial effect of spanking is to systematically increase the intensity with which it is delivered, which can quickly escalate into abuse. Thus, at best, spanking is effective only when used in selective infrequent situations. A number of consequences of spanking lessen its desirability as a strategy to eliminate undesired behavior:

- For children younger than 18 months, spanking increases the chance of physical injury, and the child is unlikely to understand the connection between the behavior and the punishment.
- Although spanking may result in a reaction of shock by the child and cessation of the undesired behavior, repeated spanking may cause agitated and aggressive behavior by the child that may escalate to a physical altercation between the parent and child.
- Spanking models aggressive behavior as a solution to conflict and has been associated with increased aggression in preschool and school-age children.

Continued

BOX 15–3   AMERICAN ACADEMY OF PEDIATRICS POLICY STATEMENT: "GUIDANCE FOR EFFECTIVE DISCIPLINE"—cont'd

- Use of spanking and threats of spanking lead to altered parent-child relationships and make discipline substantially more difficult when physical punishment is no longer an option, such as with adolescents.
- Spanking is no more effective as a long-term strategy than other approaches, and reliance on spanking as a disciplinary approach makes other disciplinary strategies less effective to use. Time-out and positive reinforcement of other behavior are more difficult to implement and take longer to work when spanking has previously been a primary method of discipline.
- Long-term undesired and unintended consequences of spanking may occur for parents and children. Because spanking a child may provide the parents some relief from anger, the likelihood that the parent will spank the child in the future is increased.

Parents who spank their children are more likely to use other unacceptable forms of corporal punishment. The more children are spanked, the more anger they report feeling as adults, the more likely they are to spank their own children, the more likely they are to approve of hitting and to hit their spouses and the higher their level of marital conflict as adults. Spanking has been associated with higher rates of physical aggression in children, more substance abuse and increased risk of crime and violence when used with older children and adolescents. Because of the negative consequences of spanking and because it has been demonstrated to be no more effective than other approaches for dealing with undesired behavior in children, the American Academy of Pediatrics recommends that parents be encouraged and assisted in the development of alternative methods other than spanking for dealing with undesired behavior.

From American Academy of Pediatrics, Committee on Psychosocial Aspects of Child and Family Health: Policy statement on guidance for effective discipline. *Pediatrics* 101:723, 1998. Used by permission.

Some parents find it difficult to accept or understand the push-pull nature of toddler behavior, even when provided with an explanation of the behavior as a requirement for psychological independence. These parents may have experienced a rigid or strict form of child rearing from their own parents, some may have been physically abused as children and others may have a rigid personality structure with limited capacity to tolerate conflict. Parents may also be struggling with issues of autonomy themselves. Whatever their background, these parents need special guidance in behavior management.

Parents must see how easy it is to be drawn into conflict and that it is always a no-win situation. They must see how the child's needs for control are undercut by a power struggle on the one hand and by lack of control on the other. For some families, cultural imperatives act as a strong influence in shaping parents' approach to discipline. Secure limits that are consistently and kindly presented are what the child needs. It may be helpful to provide parents with guidelines to assist them in clarifying their perception of the child's problem and a strategy for intervention. Box 15–4 gives critical questions for effective interactions by parents.

BOX 15–4   HELPING PARENTS ANTICIPATE DISCIPLINARY PROBLEMS

- What am I trying to teach?
- Why is this important to me?
- How am I trying to teach it?
- What is my child learning?

Anticipating problems, the clinician may use this and subsequent visits to explore various change strategies.

Communication Skills

Teaching parents that toddlers often have a receptive vocabulary that is at least 10 times greater than their expressive vocabulary may encourage some parents to talk to their children more effectively. The use of simple, clear phrases and sentences that express parental emotions and directions can be encouraged. Clear directives that are brief and unequivocal and do not imply a choice when there is none are best (e.g., "It's time to go to bed" versus "Would you like to go to bed?").

Anticipating and Short-Circuiting Excessive Frustration

Many children at this age experience a tantrum when their immediate environment overheats (e.g., a supermarket, a large family gathering, dinner preparations at the end of a busy day). The excessive sensory stimulation may be visual, auditory, tactile or, as is often the case, a combination of sensory inputs. The time of the day may be a contributing factor (e.g., in the morning when parents are busy preparing for work or school, at the end of the day when parents and older siblings return home or at bedtime). Many parents are not aware of the temporal and situational patterns that tantrums follow. It may be helpful to suggest change indirectly by asking, "Do you think that changing some of these situations may help your child by decreasing moments of frustration?" Specific suggestions might include shopping at a different time (when the child is more rested or, if possible, without the child) or providing an alternative activity during dinner preparations (e.g., having the child watch *Sesame Street* or some other child-oriented television program or videotape or arranging for an older sibling to play with the toddler).

Consistency in Discipline

Children at this age require consistency in all aspects of their life. Too many caretakers, too many different activities and too many different people giving different cues confuse the expectations and responses of a toddler. It is not surprising that parents often have inconsistent approaches to child rearing in general and to toddler discipline in particular because they are products of different families and often of conflicting parenting styles. In addition, the inconsistencies in behavior responses may be between a grandparent and parents or between the parents and daycare personnel. When inconsistency in discipline becomes apparent, the clinician should point out the advantages, indeed the necessity, of providing consistency. A conference with both parents is often required to explore and solve this problem. Basic philosophies, as well as very specific issues, must be discussed in a frank, open manner within a family. This process ideally starts in the first year; it becomes a clear necessity in the second.

The link between the action and the response of the parent has to be very close in time at this age for the child to get the linkage. Delayed responses will only confuse the child about what is expected. Toddlers don't operate according to rule-based thinking (a cognitive achievement that emerges several years in the future). They may respond to a parent's direction but not learn the rule behind the direction. Repeated redirection will be needed because the child's memory and rule-based skills are still very immature.

Behavior Modification

Reinforcement of positive behavior and ignoring minor negative behavior form the core of **behavior modification**. Some parents encourage negative behavior unconsciously by either over-reacting to minor outbursts of anger or making frequent demeaning statements when behavior is contrary. Point out that this kind of attention only raises the child's interest in pursuing negative behavior. Conversely, frequent praise for positive behavior teaches the child that parental attention and appreciation are the reward for doing things well, such as drinking from a cup independently, using a potty seat, asking for a toy or milk or making something with toys.

Children younger than 2½ usually need specific help to move to an activity that is not forbidden. Give them the alternative and praise their participation in it. Yelling "No!" across the room only invites a toddler to tease by doing it again.

Dealing with Tantrums

When parents recognize that most tantrums in children at this age are a result of acute frustration, the simple method of *distracting the child from the situation* that appears to be associated with the frustration is usually effective. In fact, distraction as a way of life may be the method of survival for many families at this stage of development! Suggest that the child can be *physically removed from the conflictual or unsafe environment* and placed in a less conflictual or safer place. An alternative toy, a book or an interactive game with a parent or other person usually serves to ameliorate a screaming child if given with a hug or loving touch. Body contact is important.

Other tantrums will require a *verbal dialogue* between the parent and child. Removing the toddler from the conflictual environment and sitting with him in a quiet place are the first step. *Holding the child closely* while talking is settling and reassuring for some children. *Asking a question or making a statement that reflects the child's feelings* at the moment gives the child an opportunity to reflect on the emotional content of the behavior, a feeling or thought that may not be available unless it is articulated by a person the child trusts (Box 15–5). Examples of this form of communication are shown in Box 15–6.

Although the intensity of the tantrum, the child's temperament and the parent's ability to confront the emotional challenges will predict the effect of this method, it is a very powerful tool, not only as a method of response to negative behavior but, more significantly, as a potential foundation for parent-child communication about feelings.

BOX 15–5   EXPRESSING EMOTIONS THROUGH IDEAS

Greenspan's model for child development emphasized the interaction between emerging emotional capacities and thought processes at different ages. He has pointed out that an 18-month-old exhibits **specific behavior to express emotions through ideas:**

- *Dependency and security*—Caring for and holding a doll or stuffed toy.
- *Pleasure*—Showing smiles and excitement to accompany play; indicating fondness for certain food or a special toy.
- *Curiosity*—Hide-and-seek or exploring drawers or closets; search play with dolls or stuffed toys.
- *Assertiveness*—Making needs known verbally; putting a doll or stuffed toy in charge of activities of other toys.
- *Protest and anger*—Using words such as *mad* to express anger; getting mad at an uncooperative toy.
- *Setting self-limits*—Punishing a doll or stuffed toy for being naughty; responding to parental "no."

In this model, "a tantrum is seen as the result of a frustration—an inability to master a task, to communicate a desire, to understand why things are as they are." After a calming-down period, the parent can then re-engage the child in the world of ideas and teach a valuable lesson: closeness between parent and child can occur even after a disruptive emotional experience. By teaching a child to label feelings and learn to make use of pretend play and by using words to discipline, the child's emotional and cognitive skills are blended to encourage growth. Greenspan offers the following example of managing a toddler temper tantrum: "Jimmy enjoys taking care of his stuffed dog in pretend play, but has temper tantrums when frustrated. Today, his mother cannot find his green car just when he wants it. He manages to say, 'Car. Green,' and then when it doesn't instantly appear, he turns red in the face and starts kicking, stomping and throwing things all over the place in a full-fledged tantrum. At moments of rage like this, your teaching about ideas obviously needs to wait until you have calmed the child down. So Jimmy's mother yells a little, threatens a little and physically stops Jimmy from kicking until he quiets down. The two then sulk in mutual annoyance for a few minutes with Jimmy going off by himself and starting to play. At this point, his mother sits next to him, becomes a partner in his play and then gives him a hug to show that everything is all right. While she is giving him a hug, she also says, 'Are you still angry?' This gives the child a chance to learn the word for the emotions he felt, as well as the idea that emotions can be labeled. Gradually, his mother explains about patience and how to look for things he cannot find right away. Later on, when he wants his green car again, his mother might be able to convince him to be patient and look further. She can show him, even in hide-and-seek fashion, how to look. 'Is Mr. Green Car in the closet? No, he's not here. Under the chair?' etc. This use of ideas will probably not work each time, but he may be willing to wait and look rather than throw a tantrum at least some of the time. Your ability to tolerate intense emotion and to reconnect with your child will encourage his use of ideas to express feelings."

Modified from Greenspan SI: *Psychopathology and Adaptation in Infancy and Early Childhood: Principles of Clinical Diagnosis and Preventive Intervention.* New York, International Universities Press, 1981; and Greenspan S, Greenspan NT: *First Feelings: Milestones in the Emotional Development of Your Baby and Child.* New York, Penguin Books, 1985. Used by permission.

BOX 15–6   TANTRUMS: STATEMENTS THAT UNLOCK A CHILD'S FEELINGS

- "Gee, you sure are upset right now!"
- "Sometimes we get real angry and upset inside us when things aren't going well."
- "Isn't it awful when you can't do something you really want to do?"
- "You seem really mad at me now."

Time-out Period for Excessive Tantrums

When a child with a severe tantrum does not respond to verbal communication or to being picked up, it may be helpful to give the toddler a time-out period. The removal of positive parental attention in the form of a time-out increases compliance with parental expectations by 25% to 80%. An explanation is required ("you will stay there until you stop crying; mommy [or daddy] is in the kitchen, and you can come to me after you stop crying"). For some children this technique redirects out-of-control behavior, allows the anger to run its course and provides a time for reinvestment with the parent as the tantrum terminates. When time-out is used consistently for an age-appropriate duration (approximately 1 minute for each year of age), not excessively, and with a planned strategy for escape behavior, it is more likely to be successful.

For some parents, reading a pamphlet or book on the behavior of toddlers during this period may be helpful (see Chapter 28). Other parents benefit from a parent-toddler play group or a parent education class. Having a list of available resources in the community can be extraordinarily helpful. The child's clinician can be helpful as a guide to parents who are going through the experience of a toddler with tantrums. However, it is important to refrain from simply providing parents with a "recipe" for behavior change. Behavior modification techniques are helpful as part of an overall management plan that includes an understanding of the many variables contributing to the child's problems. Listening carefully to parents and children, observing parent-child interactional styles in the office and communicating with them through active listening skills will often provide a sufficient foundation for the parent to understand both the nature and response to various negative behavior. "Prescriptions" for behavior change can give the clinician a false sense of security. Teaching parents about their toddler rather than how to change their toddler's behavior has a bigger payoff in the long run. Having said this, some specific guidelines can often help parents in distress (Boxes 15–7 and 15–8).

A comprehensive approach to the assessment process includes consideration of the parent-child relationship, shaping and teaching desired behavior and reducing undesired behavior; this model will guide the clinician in determining which aspects may require intervention.

Anticipating Parental Distress

The rapid changes in the development of a toddler may be overwhelming for single (especially adolescent) mothers, socially isolated families, families experiencing economic stress and families undergoing a significant life event (e.g., divorce, illness or an unplanned move).

Young children are barometers of the family's emotional life. Although regressions in recently acquired milestones are common in all children at this stage, they are predictable in

BOX 15–7   DISCIPLINE IN EARLY CHILDHOOD MANAGEMENT: CONCEPTS FOR CLINICIAN

- *Achieving a helping relationship*—Parent should perceive the child's clinician as someone available to discuss behavioral outbursts and other negative behavior.
- *Identifying problem areas*—Through a screening checklist or focused questions, developmentally predictable behavioral problems should be queried.
- *Exploring genetic, historical and social predisposing factors*—Include questions on maternal depression, prenatal events, perinatal stress, the health of siblings, the vulnerable child syndrome, substance abuse and the parents' own childhood memories.
- *Viewing parenthood as a developmental process*—Recognize that parenting skills are established through maturation, knowledge, experience and guidance. Development of effective parenting skills takes time.
- *Encouraging parents to take an active role in deciding how to manage the child's behavior*—Explore methods previously used by the parents and provide support for their methods or suggest modifications that might be more effective.
- *Respecting different parenting styles*—Cultural, social class and past experience provide parents with variable responses to child behavior. Variations in child rearing in families can be instructive for the clinician. A "best" way to manage a behavioral problem does not exist.
- *Providing appropriate models*—Increase parental awareness that children imitate and identify with their parents' behavior. While modeling healthy adult behavior, the clinician can be a useful guide to the parent.
- *Consistency*—Rules are essential for discipline. For toddlers, the number of rules should be limited and parents should enforce only the important ones. This should help with consistency.
- *Talking about discipline*—Parents (and other child care providers) should discuss with each other expectations for the child's behavior and agree on management approaches. Discuss acceptable conduct as well as unacceptable behavior.
- *Rewarding appropriate behavior*—Praise, encouragement and rewards increase a child's happiness, security and self-esteem.
- *Punishment to discourage some behavior*—Consistency is important. Design to motivate socially approved behavior and to be specific for a particular offense. Explanation must accompany punishment. Carry out as soon as possible after inappropriate behavior. Administer in the context of a warm parent-child relationship.

Modified from Smith EE, Van Tassel E: Problems of discipline in early childhood. *Pediatr Clin North Am* 29:167, 1982. Used by permission.

children of families experiencing increased stress. Developmental regressions in toddlers include refusal to use the potty seat, throwing food when in the highchair, screaming with seemingly mild frustration and increased periods of night awakening. Although these types of behavior are transient setbacks in development, they are particularly frustrating to the parent in distress. The child's demands may be just too much for the parent to handle. He or she may not be able to see beyond the behavior. Some parents internalize the child's behavior and seem

---

BOX 15–8 **DISCIPLINE IN EARLY CHILDHOOD MANAGEMENT: CONCEPTS FOR PARENTS**

- Provide exemplary models.
- Frequently discuss with each other behavioral expectations and agree on uniform approaches to management.
- Limit the number of rules and talk about appropriate behavior with your child at a calm time.
- Expect your child to need several trials to learn appropriate behavior.
- Compliment your child frequently concerning correct behavior.
- Establish and maintain schedules and routines.
- Give your child choices when appropriate.
- Anticipate and avoid unnecessary conflict situations.
- Use punishment sparingly, but consistently.
- Individualize punishment for particular offenses and provide simple explanations why you are punishing.
- Be mindful of individual and marital needs apart from your child.

Modified from Smith EE, Van Tassel E: Problems of discipline in early childhood. *Pediatr Clin North Am* 29:175, 1982.

---

to see it as a failure in parenting ("She was so good at eating by herself and using the potty seat a few weeks ago. What have I done to cause this new behavior?"). Along with guilt, these parents experience anger and fatigue as the toddler's infantile responses become more difficult to manage in the presence of acute or chronic family distress. An astute clinician will either anticipate or recognize the accompanying anxiety or depression in the parent (or its effect on the child), explore the severity or chronicity of the problems and, when appropriate, offer assistance in the form of referral to a parent group or a counseling resource.

In concluding the office visit, the clinician will find that a summary statement about the child's current stage of development is beneficial when it is then followed by what the parents might anticipate.

QUICK CHECK—15 TO 18 MONTHS

- ✓ Walks and runs
- ✓ Climbs
- ✓ Uses both hands equally
- ✓ Says more than 10 words. Understands one-step commands.
- ✓ Plays game: peek-a-boo
- ✓ Imitates household tasks
- ✓ Takes off some clothing

Continued

QUICK CHECK–15 TO 18 MONTHS–cont'd

- ✓ Uses a spoon
- ✓ Drinks from a cup
- ✓ The emergence of self-regulatory skills (feeding, falling and staying asleep, walking, talking) encourages autonomy
- ✓ Anger outbursts peak between 18 months and 2 years
- ✓ Developmental prerequisites to toilet training include voluntary control of anal and urethral sphincters, ability to sit on the potty quietly with intent to have a bowel movement, desire to please the parent and self as positive reinforcement, ability to sequence the events
- ✓ Self-feeding requires and enhances fine motor skills, hand-eye coordination, autonomy and learning to choose and enjoy different textures and colors of foods
- ✓ Anticipating tantrums and short-circuiting excessive frustration by distraction, talking (expressing to the child her feelings when angry) and time-out periods are effective responses to tantrums

HEADS UP–15 TO 18 MONTHS

- Social interactions should include good eye contact, gesturing with a finger and a desire to show the parent an object.
- An expressive vocabulary of fewer than five words is a significant delay.
- If a child does not point to a body part when asked, consider hearing loss or receptive language delay.
- A toddler who has difficulty learning self-feeding, sleeping alone and limited exploratory play may not be reaching the expected goals for autonomy.
- A parent who spanks a toddler frequently will benefit from a discussion of normal toddler development and behavioral alternatives to corporal punishment.
- Recognize the value of a "teachable moment" when a parent disciplines a child with physical force or harsh language. Modeling alternative methods pays off.
- Take notice if a parent seems embarrassed by a transitional object … another teachable moment.
- Take care to not overinterpret isolated delays in development (e.g., refusal to use a cup, preference for self-play in a temperamentally shy toddler, insistence on sleeping in the parent's bed). A comprehensive developmental history and observations are required to sort out a delay in achieving autonomy.
- Screening for early recognition of autism is part of health supervision visits between 15 and 18 months of age. In addition to a specific screening test, be suspicious if a toddler does not respond to social interactions with you or a parent, speak any words, understand directions or gesture with a finger.

RECOMMENDED READINGS

For Parents

Brazelton TB, Sparrow JD: *Discipline: The Brazelton Way*. Cambridge, MA, Da Capo Press, 2003.

Brazelton TB, Sparrow JD: *Feeding: The Brazelton Way*. Cambridge, MA, Da Capo Press, 2004.

Brazelton TB, Sparrow JD: *Toilet Training: The Brazelton Way*. Cambridge, MA, Da Capo Press, 2004.

Guide to Potty Training: Available at http://www.babycenter.com.

Volkman FR, Wiesner LA: *Health Care for Children on the Autism Spectrum: A Guide to Medical, Nutritional and Behavioral Issues*. Bethesda, MD, Woodbine House, 2004.

For Clinicians

Beers NS, Howard B: Managing temper tantrums. *Pediatr Rev* 24:70-71, 2003.

Brazelton TB, Christophersen ER, Frauman AC, et al: Instruction, timeliness, and medical influences affecting toilet training. *Pediatrics* 103:1353-1358, 1999.

Committee on Psychosocial Aspects of Child and Family Health: Guidance for effective discipline. *Pediatrics* 101:723-728, 1998.

Larsen MA, Tentis E: The art and science of disciplining children. *Pediatr Clin North Am* 50:817-840, 2003.

Rapin I: The autistic spectrum disorders. *N Engl J Med* 347:302-330, 2002.

Siegel B: *The World of the Autistic Child: Understanding and Treating Autism Spectrum Disorders*. New York, Oxford University Press, 1996.

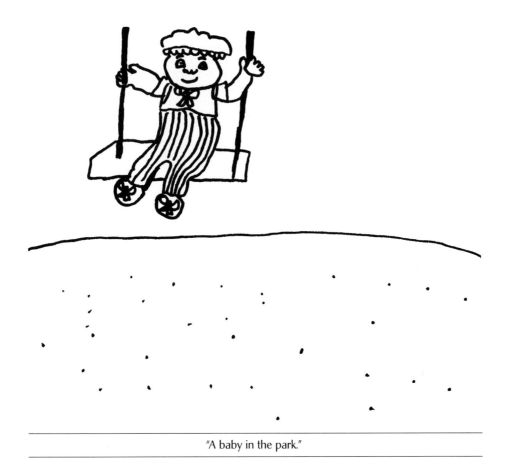

"A baby in the park."

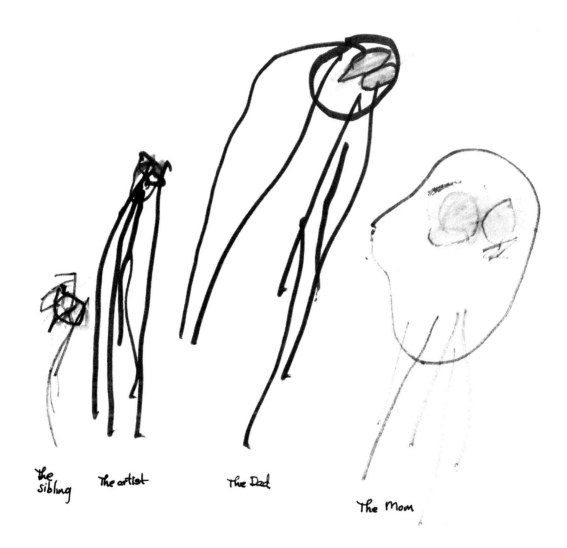

the
sibling   The artist   The Dad

The Mom

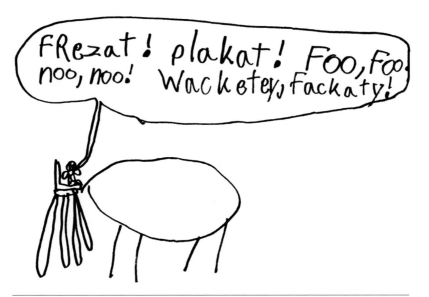

CHAPTER 16

"A baby learning to talk." By Ryan Hennessy.

Two Years: Language Leaps*

SUZANNE D. DIXON

This chapter focuses on the development of language from infancy onward. It provides the cognitive and social context of language development and looks at variations in language. Abnormalities and difficulties with language are discussed.

Key Words

- Language Development
- Language Difficulties
- Language Delays
- Gestures
- Bilingualism
- Hearing
- Speech Difficulties
- Symbolic Function

Cody, age 2, comes in for an ear check after an episode of otitis media. His tympanic membranes now appear nearly normal. On questioning, his mother says that he has about 10 to 20 single words and hasn't put together any words except "gimme." He is the fourth child of this family, born 8 years after his next older sibling, Cody had a mildly difficult birth, but recovered well. He has had six episodes of otitis media since birth. His mom says that he doesn't talk more because all of his sibs do everything for him. "There's no need for him to say anything, or even point, for that matter," she says. She feels he's "younger" than the other kids were at his age, but she says that she's to blame; she really enjoys her baby. Cody doesn't say anything in the office. Note: This case illustrates some of the common misconceptions and pitfalls regarding language assessment. Cody needs another look. An approach to Cody and his mother's concerns will be discussed in this chapter.

The second birthday falls in a period when a whole new set of capabilities emerge, including the core concept of one thing standing for another, called **symbolic function**. Another closely aligned concept is the ability to understand rules and systems that generalize from one situation to another. Language comes out of and further fuels these basic cognitive processes. Major reorganization of brain systems at this time coincides with this behavioral shift. **Language development** and growth in cognitive abilities together allow the child to interact

---

*The chapter is dedicated to Elizabeth Bates, Ph.D. (1947–2003), for her early contribution to this work and for her studies of child language worldwide.

with the world in new ways, and their appearance represents a big transition in development, from infancy to childhood. A new plateau is reached—the era of the talkative, questioning, active 2-year-old.

COGNITIVE ABILITIES

Language assessment in clinical settings should become a prominent part of child health surveillance for several important reasons. Work in developmental psychology has defined more of the links between language and cognitive abilities. A child's "language age" is likely to predict his cognitive abilities and his functional level. A look at language is a look at the mental structures that may be critical to the skills needed now and in the school years and beyond. Language also forecasts later school concern. For example, although a child who has early **language difficulties** may not have continuing **language delays** per se by school entry, he may have verbally based learning disabilities, difficulties in speed and accuracy of verbal processing and social adjustment problems. Early identification and remediation through the provision of appropriate services may prevent school failure and its emotional sequelae.

Second, the chief complaint of language delay may identify youngsters with atypical development, such as the autism spectrum of disorders, a class of disabilities that appears to be on the rise. For these youngsters, early remediation through jump-starting language before the age of 7 gives them a substantially improved outlook. These youngsters are hard to spot early if one does not have strong vigilance about language development beginning even in the first year.

Finally, global developmental delay that has no major motoric component is often manifested in the second year as language delay. *Child health care providers rarely miss disabilities in the motor sphere, but those involving cognition and language are often missed or dismissed in spite of the fact that they are among the most common of developmental disorders.* This won't happen if the clinical milieu is set up to regularly evaluate language and if the clinician has a strong sense of how language develops, including the limits of variability. To dismiss a concern about language without careful appraisal means that many types of problems, now and in the future, will be missed.

LANGUAGE DEVELOPMENT COURSE

Language, of course, begins long before the second birthday and continues beyond it. The specific patterns of early childhood language development have been summarized by many workers. The following represents a synthesis of these works (see Table 16–1).

Prenatal and Infancy

Language development begins before birth as the fetus perceives the sounds transmitted to the womb, quiets or alerts to them and begins to synchronize movements to mother's voice and body sounds. Increasing evidence suggests that the fetus responds to environmental sounds long before birth and begins to develop some memory of these auditory experiences. Specific pieces of music may result in the fetus turning toward the source and showing heart rate changes suggestive of alerting and awareness.

Responsiveness to specific sounds and interactional synchrony between infant movement and parental voices and rhythm are well developed at birth. Discrimination of even similar

TABLE 16–1   **Clinical Evaluation of Language Skills**

Age	Receptive Skills	Expressive Skills	Specific Indication For Referral
0–1 mo	Recognizes sound with startle; turns to sound and looks for source; quiets motor activity to sound; "prefers" human speech with high inflection	Differentiated crying; body language showing positive and negative response	No response to pleasing sound when alert; neonatal sepsis; meningitis; neonatal asphyxia; prematurity; congenital infection; familial deafness; renal abnormalities; aminoglycoside therapy
2–4 mo	Prolonged attention to sounds; responds to familiar voice; watches the speaking mouth; enjoys rattle; attempts to repeat pleasing sounds with objects; shifts gaze back and forth between sounds	"Eh, ih, uh" (hind mouth vowels); cooing, blows bubbles; enjoys using tongue and lips; reciprocal cooing; play dialogues; loudness varies	No response to pleasing sounds; does not attend to voices
5–7 mo	Seeks out speaker; localizes sounds; understands own name, familiar words; associates word with activity (e.g., bath, car)	Initiates sounds; pitch varies; babbles with labial consonants ("ba, ma, ga"); uses sounds to get attention, express feeling; sounds directed at object	Decreased or absence of vocalizations
8–12 mo	Begins word comprehension; responds to simple commands—"point to your nose," "say bye-bye"; knows names of family members; responds to a few words, those associated with specific objects	First words, 5–6—"mama, dada"; inflected vocal play; repeats sounds and words made by others; "oo, ee" (foremouth vowels); intentional gestures	No babbling with consonant sounds; no response to music
13–20 mo	Single-step/element commands; identifies familiar objects	Points to objects with vocalization; vocabulary of 10–50 words; pivot and open class words, rate and content vary	No comprehension of words; does not understand simple requests
18–24 mo	Recognizes many nouns; understands simple questions	Telegraphic speech; vocabulary of 50–75 words; 2-word sentences, phrases; stuttering common	Vowel sounds, but no consonants; no words
24–36 mo	Understands prepositions; can follow story with pictures	Identifies body parts; vocabulary of 200 words; dependent on phrases, 3-word sentences; uses words for expressive needs; pronouns; early grammar	No words; does not follow simple directions; no sentences

TABLE 16-1 **Clinical Evaluation of Language Skills—cont'd**

Age	Receptive Skills	Expressive Skills	Specific Indication For Referral
30–36 mo	Understands some syntax (difference between car hit train and train hit car); understands opposites; understands action in pictures	Sentences of 4 or 5 words, 3 elements; tells stories; uses "what" and "where" questions; uses negation; uses progressive and past tense, all regular form; uses plurals, regular form	Speech largely unintelligible to stranger; dropout of initial consonants; no sentences
3–4 yr	Understands 3-element commands	Talks about what she is doing; uses "I" with grammar by her own rules; vocabulary of 40–1500 words; speech intelligible to strangers; "why" questions; commands; uses past and present tense; passive speech in spontaneous speech; nursery rhymes; says colors, numbers 1–4, full name, sex; articulation of "m, n, p, h and w"; 4-word sentences	Speech not comprehended by strangers; still dependent on gestures; consistently holds hands over ears; speech without modulation
4–5 yr	Understands 4-element commands; links past and present events; decreasing ability for second language acquisition	2700-word vocabulary; defines simple words; auxiliary verbs "has" and "had"; conversation mature with "how" and "why" questions in response to others; articulation of "b, k, g and f"; 5-word sentences; "normalizes" irregular verbs and nouns; increases in accessibility of forms	Stuttering; consistently avoids loud places
5–6 yr	Understands 5-element commands; can follow a story without pictures; enjoys jokes and riddles; can comprehend 2 meanings of a single word	Correct use of all parts of speech; vocabulary of 5000 words; articulation of "y, ng and d"; 6-word sentences; corrects own errors in speech; can use logic in recounting story plots	Word endings dropped; faulty sentence structure; abnormal rate, rhythm or inflection
6–7 yr	Asks for motivation and explanation of events; understands time intervals (months, seasons); right and left differences	Articulation of "l, r, t, sh, ch, dr, cl, bl, gl and cr"; has formal adult speech patterns	Poor voice quality, articulation
7–8 yr	Can use language alone to tell a story sequentially; reasons using language	Articulation of "v, th, j, s, z, tr, st, sl, sw and sp"	
8–9 yr		Articulation of "th, sc and sh"	

sounds (e.g., pa, ba) is present in the first weeks of life, although this ability may be lost later in the first year if a specific sound is not present in that child's language. This is true, for example, with the "r" and "l" sounds, which are not differentiated in Japanese. A selective attention to one's own language, parents' voices and changes in tone or prosody in the surrounding language has been seen in newborns. Infants give selective attention to speech sounds and normal phrasing and recognize violations in their native language by the second half of the first year. Children in the first year acquire a sense of what sounds are words or the units of their language. They pay more attention to real words than to nonsense sounds or sounds that don't occur in their own language. They are building a storehouse of words that will serve them in the second year when they begin to develop an expressive vocabulary of their own.

Expressive language also begins early; cooing, the production of vowel sounds without the formation of syllable units, begins in the first 2 months of life. The loudness of cooing starts to vary at about 1 month of age, and pitch variation develops between 2 and 4 months of age. "Conversations" with 2-month-olds should thus show some variation in tone, as well as sound. Cooing sounds are heard from children who are completely deaf, though with decreased frequency and not in a conversational or interactive setting. Babbling, the production of sounds containing both vowels and consonants, is heard starting at 4 months and continues to increase in quantity and complexity with age. Babbling is heard in a similar manner in all language groups around the world. Babbling requires a marked increase in motor control of all the oropharyngeal musculature; it exercises the coordination of these speech organs and allows the child to discover the ability to talk. The quantity and quality of babble, but not its presence, are less in children who have reduced or no hearing or who are rarely interacted with verbally. Deaf children don't add this tonal variation to their babble. Listening to a child babble is not a waste of time.

> Emma at 6 months seemed to be unusually hyperalert, and her few sounds had a wooden, flat tone. She smiled when Dr. Johnson leaned over her and spoke, but she wouldn't "converse" or respond to what was said to her. She didn't have any babbling dialogues typical of a 4- to 6-month-old infant. Note: This is indicative of an infant with significant hearing loss.

Imitation of adult speech, called jargon or jabber, with the phonetic and intonational features of the child's native language starts at about 7 months and occurs regularly by the ninth month. This always precedes the first words by 4 to 5 months. Jabber is not nonsense, but a real step along the road to real language.

Gestures

Pointing at objects begins between 9 and 12 months and is a very important language milestone. It always precedes the naming of objects and is the gesture language equivalent of naming. Linguistics calls touching, pointing at and holding up objects "proto-declarative," thus emphasizing this linguistic importance.

It also testifies to the child's ability to engage in shared social attention, which in turn tells us that a child has a sense of himself as separate from another. Children with autism have a difficult to impossible challenge in achieving this core mental capacity, beginning in infancy and beyond.

> Dr. Evans looked at Caleb, age 18 months, and then pointed and looked at the picture on the wall. Caleb looked at Dr. Evans' finger briefly and then went back to playing with the wheels on a small car he carried. Note: This child needs screening for the autistic spectrum of disorders because of the absence of "joint attention" with Dr. Evans.

Gestures are part of emerging language abilities. Whereas pointing is the precursor to naming, some gestures may be the precursors to asking. These are called instrumental gestures or "proto-imperatives." For example, a toddler's pointing and grunting at the cookie jar is a request for the contents. Symbolic gestures used in play at 13 months are highly correlated with later language ability (e.g., recognizing a telephone by lifting it toward the ear, categorizing a shoe by touching it to the foot or labeling a toy car by moving it back and forth on the floor). These gestures then expand to be even more elaborate pantomimes, demonstrating a connection between two events, imitating an event and developing themes in play. They are analogous to short descriptions or stories. *Children who can say or wave "bye-bye" or do "pat-a-cake" with a verbal prompt are testifying to emergent cognitive and language skills.* Children with a rich gesture communication system in toddlerhood are likely to develop normal linguistic skills even if they are late bloomers in terms of verbal language production itself. The earlier these gestures occur, the sooner the combining of words will begin. Children without such gestures are likely to have persistent language difficulties. The clinician is well advised to ask about, observe and engage in gesture games with the infant and toddler. These games are not trivial. Always wave "bye, bye" and do "pat-a-cake" or "so big" with small patients.

FIRST WORDS

By the age of 1 year, a child usually has two to eight "words," short utterances that are produced in a specific context or to identify a specific person, event or object. The minimum competency would be **one word** other than "mama" and "dada" and following **one-step commands** and **pointing**.

A toddler both overextends (e.g., using the word "doggy" for all interesting animals) and overly restricts (e.g., using the word "doggy" only for the family dog) the meaning of these early utterances in the struggle to order and understand the world. The child is experimenting with the rules and structure of language and will gradually refine this so that "dogs" are the creatures we identify as such and Fido will get his own proper name. Feedback is absorbed from listening to others' use of language rather than specific teaching about terms or words. The child may point and look for an affirmation of naming. From this feedback and rapt attention to the language around him, the toddler puts the linguistic puzzle together. Being immersed in a rich verbal environment facilitates this process.

The acquisition of expressed new words during the period from about 12 to 18 months tends to be quite slow. These words are likely to be simple, salient and overgeneralized naming that allows the child's needs to be met and permits primitive sharing of simple observations;

these are called the nominative and instrumental functions of these early utterances, and they always come before the sharing of observations or describing of people or events. This is true in both typically developing children and those with language delays. Things that a child can act on ("ba" for ball) or things that change or move ("ca" for car) are usually the first named. The size of the average spoken vocabulary of an 18-month-old is between 50 and 100 words, but this is extremely variable between children and may even fluctuate periodically within a given child, who may use a word only in a special context and not anywhere else. Words will appear and disappear in seemingly random fashion during the first part of the second year.

A child may depend more on others' gestures and visual reinforcers in the context of the family's simplified, overemphasized speech to increase her own language capacities. Families do expand and clarify utterances directed to a child through a process that may help fuel further language development. Talking to children, responding to their utterances as though they had full communicative intent and avoiding overcorrection of word attempts will boost language skills. A parent should be overly dramatic in using gestures, provide emphasis on important words and repeat phrases for clarity. Expansion of the child's utterances to full sentences provides a model and acknowledges the child's communication.

Most parents do this spontaneously because it gets a child's interest and attention.

> Hannah, age 2, said "Soo on" while waiting for her exam. She grabbed her shoe. Her mom said, "Yes, I know you'd like to put your shoes on and go home. But you have to be checked first. No shoes now." Note: Hannah didn't understand all her mother said but she does know that she got a response to her wish and she got the "no" and "shoes" linked. Her mother expanded what Hannah said into a real sentence.

The apparent lag period in early language progress is usually followed by an explosion in either words or phrases. The second half of the second year and the beginning of the third are characterized by rapid increases in vocabulary and the use of verbs, adjectives and even some adverbs. The most significant event in this period is the creation of original linkages of words that express a complete and original thought (e.g., "da da come," "dight hot," "now nigh dark"). These combinations imply, but may not explicitly have a subject, verb and perhaps an object or modifying word, although they are telegraphic or without connecting words over three fourths of the time. They are in contrast to the simple naming of objects or expression of simple demands (e.g., "doggy," "wa-wa") that are characteristic of the "prelanguage" heard earlier. Some prelanguage may have sentence forms (e.g., "I wanna," "ah done"), but because these phrases are always used all together in a single utterance, they are called *holophrases* and are not real sentences. True sentences show original linkages and associations and involve the interchange of word combinations across differing circumstances. They generally emerge when the vocabulary reaches a threshold of at least 50 words, often reported by parents as "too many words to count." Between 2 and 2½, the child starts to add some modifiers (e.g., "big truck"), some possessives (e.g., "my car") and some functional words such as "on" (e.g., "shoes on"). Other prepositions blossom between 2½ and 3. Words expressing time and sequence come in between 3 and 5 (e.g., "I do bath, then do story").

A 2-year-old shows an understanding of the rules of language through the differential ordering of words to alter their meanings, such as "go car" versus "car go." Even with their *telegraphic speech* (i.e., with some parts missing), toddlers knows word order. More than 90% of utterances in a 3-year-old are grammatically correct in terms of word order and sequence. New constructions (e.g., "I like it.") for a child of this age are sometimes learned in their entirety and applied in several contexts as an experiment.

THE BRAIN BASIS OF LANGUAGE

The processes of learning words, word order and the semantic cues of language seem to reside in several areas of the brain, including the right and left parietotemporal and the frontal areas. In contrast to adults, in whom language function is nearly exclusively left sided, children have an evolving brain geography for these functions. As a word or phrase is learned and becomes part of the established language bank, the left temporal area becomes the site for this ongoing use of language. Word retrieval and the rapid recognition of words and utterances, nearly automatic, become available at a time of brain reorganization, at about 18 months to 2½ years old. The laying down of language subsumes bilateral brain systems, whereas the ongoing use of previously learned language is increasingly localized to the left temporal lobe, particularly the essential elements of grammar. This geographical distribution has some flexibility. Preschool children with early brain lesions in the left hemisphere will still acquire and use language, but with an altered time frame and facility. Other areas of the brain seem to pick up these functions in these circumstances. School-age children experiencing left-sided injury will have more struggles with language, particularly grammar.

UNDERSTANDING LANGUAGE

Receptive language is always ahead of expressive language, so a child always understands more than she can say. This usually results in a mild to moderate degree of frustration, which is a source of energy for a child trying to expand linguistic skills. It can also lead to developmental stuttering, the verbal tumbling over words that won't come out fast enough to satisfy a busy preschooler's mind. This is very different from the stuttering that is a block in speech production, usually with an initial sound of a word that emerges in the late preschool and early school-age years. A little help with slowing down, best guesses about what the wanted word really is and the avoidance of pressure or embarrassment will help a young child get mouth in line with mind in learning to speak.

Receptive language is usually more regular in its development than expressive language is because it is more closely linked with cognitive development. It is a better predictor of both long-term language competency and general cognitive abilities in most children. Expressive language is more variable because it is influenced by individual temperament, environmental prompts and constraints and even the interpretive skills of the listener. The clinician should be much more worried about a child who has difficulty understanding age-appropriate utterances that are presented without visual prompts than about a child who has little to say, but does follow verbal input at an age-appropriate level.

For the clinician, the development of receptive language means caution should be used in discussions with a parent in front of a child because understanding will be far ahead of what the child says. Even if vocabulary is not available to the child, the prosody, general idea and some words will be understood. Sensitive subjects and negative behavior or situations should be discussed out of earshot of a child older than 3. Even some younger children may be bothered by such discussions.

PRIVATE SPEECH

Children in the preschool years practice speech in private, as well as with others. "Crib speech" serves linguistic, emotional and cognitive purposes inasmuch as it is used to sort out the day, the experiences, the struggles and the misunderstandings. Crib speech offers a direct view of the child's mind at work, putting language and life in order.

> Ryan, almost 4, was in his room for a nap with a stuffed dog as his companion. His mom heard his conversation. "Go, go go gooooooing, ing ing ing, thing sing a song. We didn't go go sosobad. Stop hitting now wowwow. You go to sleep right now wowwow. Put jacket for the store in the store in the car in the car. I mean it. The red jacket. The red jacket, with Barney."
> Note: Ryan is very busy, working on suffixes, sound, rhyme, the "w" sound, prepositions, pronouns, compound adjectives, adverbs and, it sounds like, some discipline issues about a car trip that may not have occurred because of some behavioral issues. He tells us a lot about his language development, his abilities and how he uses them to manage his day.

The presence of private speech is taken as evidence that language derives from within rather than being just the result of the need to communicate with others. This type of language also appears to support the notion that language fuels cognition; that is, it serves cognitive functions.

LANGUAGE MILESTONES

Because of the variability in expressive language, it is easy to appreciate the tendency to ignore language issues in clinical settings. However, this is not wise because the effectiveness of intervention depends on timing. A clinician should be concerned about the child who fails to reach the minimum competencies shown in Table 16–2. With such a child, the clinician should take a more detailed look at language and evaluate neurological concerns, possible **hearing** problems and other social-interactional issues. These are the limits of acceptable language progress.

The years between age 2 and 5 are characterized by a gradual expansion in sentence complexity (i.e., words or word-like utterances). The length of a child's phrases and sentences increases dramatically during this time from an average of one or two elements at younger than 2 years up to three to five elements by age 4. Linguists use this measure, mean length of utterance (MLU), to evaluate language maturity. Clinicians can evaluate the longest thing a child says to get an approximation of this measure. *It should increase at every visit between the ages of 2 and 5, roughly corresponding to a child's age as a minimum competency.*

> Dr. Moffet asked Mrs. Martin what was the longest thing her daughter says. Samantha, age 3, was reported to say "Me go car now," "Jay Jay hit Max," and "Too many done" when finished with her dinner. Note: She's right on target for her age.

TABLE 16–2 **Backstop Parameters that Call for Referral If Not Met**

Age	Milestone
Newborn	Turns to a soft voice, especially the parents'
By 3 months	Cooing sounds. Looks alert, interactive, smiles
By 6 months	Coos and jabbers and does more every day Turns to a new sound and familiar voices, laughs
By 9 months	Babbles mamamama, babababa Knows name, turns when called
By 12 months	Points at objects Has 1 word in addition to "mama" and "dada" Follows 1-step commands Gives or shows objects to the caretaker
By 18 months	Produces 5 or more words Comprehends more than 50 words
By 2 years	Produces more than 50 words Puts 2 words together Follows 2-step commands Points at pictures in a book Names or attempts to name objects Uses "words" to request things
By 3 years	Talks in sentences most of the time Is understood by strangers at least half the time Says name, age, gender and birthday month Names most objects in her daily life and at least 3 body parts Tells stories in 3-sentence or 3-phrase "paragraphs" Knows 1 color
By 4 years	Sustains a conversation Understood by a stranger Uses pronouns

Rules are overapplied after children start to put words together, so "mistakes" are made that didn't appear earlier. The first sentences are experiments in grammar and syntax. "He has two feets," "The mices are teasing the cat," and "The boy putted the cars away" are all examples of these expected errors. This represents linguistic progress, not regression. A late preschooler is now conscious of rules governing language and is overly fastidious in their application. He will self-correct these irregularities over time without teaching; no didactic instruction is needed here.

Verb tenses are added in orderly sequence; systems of negation and the form of questions also have their own specific developmental course. The "w" words ("what," "when," and the perennial favorite "why") appear in a 3-year-old's talk.

The regularity of these processes is quite striking. A 2-year-old can communicate with family members easily; a 4-year-old should be intelligible to almost anyone who speaks the child's language 100% of the time.

After 5 years of age, all the basic components of language are in place, although these forms become more accessible and usable with time. A vocabulary of 800 to 14,000 words is common by age 6. Poetry, puns and jokes, all subtle turns on language, are enjoyed by early grade school. The study of grammar is appreciated with relish in the early school years, and foreign languages have particular interest for the child at this time. Foreign languages learned early create at least bilingual people and facilitate the later learning of other languages. Vocabulary increases should be a lifelong process, and sentence complexity increases into adult life. Table 16–1 shows the developmental progression of these language milestones.

WHY DO CHILDREN SPEAK?

The question "Why do children speak?" raises considerable controversy among psycholinguists and is not satisfactorily answered by any one school of thought. *Innate theorists*, or nativists, contend that children speak because a predetermined neurosensory capacity (i.e., language acquisition device [LAD]) kicks in at some point in development. These theorists note the regularity in language development across all cultural and language groups and the production of sounds in deaf infants. However, this theory cannot account for the experientially determined disturbances in language in a neglected and emotionally disturbed child or for the interactional variables from child to child that strongly influence language development. Experience is needed, in the nativist's point of view, to trigger this genetically determined capability. Other than that, this theory sees the environment as relatively unimportant to the learning of language.

The *learning theorists* (see Chapter 2) maintain that children speak because they imitate the speech around them and are rewarded for their efforts. Language emerges from the need to name objects, make demands and comply with the verbal environment around them based on the models and reinforcements provided them. Certainly, children in isolation do not learn language, and children learn the language and dialect to which they are exposed. However, these theorists do not account for the unsolicited and private babble and practice done by the infant and young child that serves no communicative intent, even up through the school years. Predictable developmental "mistakes" in grammar and syntax made by children at certain periods have no parallel in adult speech. These detours cannot be accounted for by imitation. Indeed, they are temporarily unavailable to specific adult correction. Adults rarely correct or negatively reinforce these language errors in their children, and yet children correct themselves. Adults respond to the content and factual correctness rather than the form of the child's speech, and that is as it should be. In general, practicing speech with a child does *not* improve the quantity or quality of language, so direct imitation does not explain the bulk of language development. Or as stated by Cazden, "as 'foots' and 'goed' and 'holded' show, children use language they hear as examples of language to learn *from*, not samples of language to learn." Although a model for speech is necessary, children translate adult speech into their own grammar or rule system, thus implying a more complex processing problem than simple imitation.

The *interactionalist school* presents a synthesis of these perspectives, saying that children speak as an outgrowth of their interactions with parents and significant others. These important people in a child's life respond to, elaborate on and clarify early utterances, and these interactions fuel the child's growth in language. Basic cognitive processes must be present to allow children to use that input in the development of their own language skills. The neural basis of language must be present to take in the linguistic experience, order it and reproduce it in original combinations. Children exposed to only mechanical speech (e.g., television) do not speak. Language is an outgrowth of adequate emotional development and serves the emergence of new cognitive skills. The social environment is organized to bring a child into it as a participating member, no matter what the cultural context.

In support of this position, observations of early language suggest that this interaction is vital. The amount and variety of babbling and imitative speech production at 9 to 18 months are, to some extent, a reflection of the amount of the mother's (or significant caretaker's) speech that the child has experienced. However, during that late infancy–early toddler period, subsequent growth in language competency is dependent on the amount and variety of *responsive* speech. The size of a 2-year-old's vocabulary is directly dependent on how much the mother speaks to her. In other words, the development of language is built on early interactions with caregivers and is augmented later by the presence of a rich, conversational environment. The presence of early dialogues with the child, building and expanding on the child's own utterances and the later enriched verbal reinforcements around the child are directly related to early language acquisition.

As clinicians, we can make use of all these perspectives in conceptualizing language development. Children speak for the following reasons:

- They have a basic neurosensory and cognitive readiness.
- Speech around them provides models.
- Speech is fun, both alone and, more importantly, with significant others.

Deficits in any of these areas will be reflected in abnormal or delayed language development. The clinical perspective should be to look for basic neuromaturational competencies, a rich linguistic environment and evidence that the child is loved, talked to responsively and free of other sources of developmental energy drain. An appropriate and responsive environment can support the development of language. Box 16–1 gives ideas on how to provide that environment.

LANGUAGE AND COGNITION

Language development is intricately entangled with cognitive development. Much discussion and research have been devoted to the question of whether language is necessary for cognition (i.e., whether we need words and semantic structure to think) or whether language is merely an outcome or reflection of growth in mental capacity. This chicken-and-egg question aside, the clinician will find that language assessment becomes increasingly enmeshed in other areas of functioning as a child grows because the usual evaluation of language, using standard instruments, is really one of cognitive growth and vice versa. Most often, language and cognitive development *are* linked in an individual child, but not necessarily so. Language development, particularly in a population of disabled children, is highly predictive of overall functioning, and language remains the best predictor of cognition in general. School systems are heavily biased toward verbal skills, so it is not surprising that school performance and

BOX 16–1   SUPPORTING LANGUAGE DEVELOPMENT IN YOUNG CHILDREN

- **Talk to the child.** Beginning in infancy, talk to the baby, naming things in the environment and narrating the events of the day. A rich verbal environment supports language development all the way to college.
- **Speak slowly** and in short phrases to a young child and give emphasis to particular words. Higher pitch gets a young child's attention.
- **Talk in regular language forms**, including complex sentences, to provide good models to imitate. Children with more advanced language forms have families who speak to them in longer utterances. Use pronouns as appropriate; don't substitute proper names.
- **Respond to the child's speech** as though it has meaning. Beginning at 2 months, respond to the baby's sounds with an echo or an enhancement. The baby will learn that her noises create a response.
- **Repeat what a child says** often so that the child experiences being heard.
- **Respond to the meaning** and not the form of the child's speech. Expand on what is said; don't correct the attempts. Help the child get ideas across.
- **Ask questions and wait for an answer.** Language development is enhanced by giving kids a prompt and time to respond. Children who are expected to answer will have enhanced language competency.
- **Look at books together,** name the pictures and talk about the images and the stories. Let the child start to tell the story his way when ready.
- **Never punish or shame** a child for any language effort. Give a new model if needed, but don't overcorrect or drill.
- **Increase interest in language** with exposure to music and rhymes.
- **Encourage gestures** to communicate and to use in games. These will enhance, not detract from the development of speech.

linguistic abilities are linked. Early language disorders are highly predictive of learning difficulties in school, and most studies show that greater than 40% of children with early language difficulties will have learning difficulties in school. The language concern may be the chief complaint, but a comprehensive look at the child and the environment is needed when this problem becomes evident.

Both directions are possible. Emotional and cognitive deficits may be secondary to primary language disorders, particularly in a society that places so much emphasis on verbal competency and formal schooling performance in its children. Conversely, emotional disorders may have language delay symptoms. In any case, a language-delayed child must be carefully and comprehensively assessed for these associated difficulties.

VARIATIONS IN LANGUAGE DEVELOPMENT

Receptive and expressive language in the normal population of children varies significantly. In addition, style differences surface, with some children adopting "frozen" phrases in their entirety (e.g., "I wuv you") and others hesitantly building sentences from a large stock of available words (e.g., "Daddy botta Julia"). Some are late to develop expressive language, whereas some use words or phrases very early. Late talkers who do catch up are more likely to have a rich gesture communication system early on and to have normal comprehension.

Minority groups in the United States may be at a disadvantage in language evaluation and its close relative, cognitive assessment, as measured in the school setting and in standardized tests, for several reasons:

- Vocabulary differences
- Unfamiliarity with verbal interchange with adults in a test situation
- Temperament differences
- Systematic differences in grammatical structures that lead to misunderstandings and assumptions
- Inhibition based on fear of ridicule

A minority child in a majority setting may be inhibited from using advanced language structures. Compounding the problem is the tendency for even well-intentioned teachers to interact verbally with students who are verbal themselves, take verbal initiatives and respond with longer utterances. A reluctant child from any group will get increasingly less verbal encouragement, practice and reinforcement.

Socioeconomic class differences in language development may additionally reflect other differences in the verbal environment. Middle-class children experience a richer verbal environment, have received instructions in a complex verbal form and are required from an early age to use verbal interchanges. Not unexpectedly, language in this group is often more advanced in early childhood. The socioeconomic link with language development is strong.

MYTHS ABOUT LANGUAGE DEVELOPMENT

Parents and clinicians alike may explain away a child's language delay with one of several formulations that have no grounding in science, adherence to which may lead to delay in diagnosis and treatment. Examples of such formulations include the following:

- *His brothers get him everything he wants, so he doesn't have to talk.* Although children lower in the birth order, when compared with firstborn children, show a slight delay in expressive language in terms of the quantity of utterances, they should have no such delay at all in receptive language, gesture language or crib speech. In addition, the type and complexity, if not the quantity, of things said should follow developmental expectations for age. Siblings can prompt language a bit and may provide vocabulary, both good and bad. However, birth order effects do not account for significant delays or an atypical language progress.

- *He's a boy, so what do you expect?* The gender difference in language development is small, with girls being ahead of boys in both quantitative speech measures and complexity after the first birthday. As a group, girls retain the advantage in verbal tasks throughout school. Again, this is a subtle difference of weeks to months, and it applies to groups. There is much individual difference. Significant delays cannot be explained by gender. Many detailed tests of early language have different norms for boys and girls to account for these small differences. If a screening test does show delay, further specialized evaluation should take gender into account. In a pediatric setting, gender issues should be ignored.

- *He's in a bilingual household, so we expect him to be delayed.* **Bilingualism** means a lot of different things, and research is not clear because of the nonexperimental nature of this situation. However, a few conclusions can be drawn from the work that has been done. Children raised in bilingual households do have a slight delay in *expressive* language up to about 2 years of age while they put the components of language together. They mix the syntax and vocabulary of both languages, perhaps using both languages in a single utterance. However, a single object will have a single name in one or the other language until age 2. After that, children are able to switch appropriately from one language to another in context and have a *combined* vocabulary that meets the usual expectations. Bilingualism is not a good explanation for language delay after age 3 and even before if we look at the receptive skills and the ability to form early word combinations. Bilingual exposure facilitates language development rather than hampering it over the long term. If delays are present after age 3 in a bilingually exposed child, an underlying cognitive deficit or ongoing conflict surrounding the child is being played out in the use of one language or another.

- *He's lazy.* Young children have an internal drive to mastery in this area and all others (see Chapter 2), which means that they exercise newly developing skills as they emerge. They don't hold back unless they are fearful, stressed, intimidated or ill. If developmental energy is lacking, it is because the energy is needed for other purposes. If a child is performing below age level, it's because that's the best the child can do at that time. The clinician should consider other intrusions on a child when a delay is appreciated. To say a child is lazy reveals a basic lack of understanding of the nature of child development broadly.

Aiden, age 2, was taken into foster care after experiencing neglect and emotional abuse. On the initial evaluation his foster mother reported that he spoke just a few words and often acted like he didn't understand even the simplest of requests. Three months later she reported that he just started "talking up a storm" at home, although he was shy with strangers. Note: The clinician should have performed a hearing test at the initial intake. If that was normal, this short 3-month time frame is appropriate for a reevaluation. If he hadn't blossomed across that interval, a referral to a speech and language specialist, as well as an appraisal of development, would be appropriate.

- *He'll grow out of it.* This is usually the case experientially. All but a few children learn to speak eventually. However, as we have seen, children with early or continuing delays are at risk in early childhood for emotional difficulties, for behavioral problems and, over the longer term, for subtle or not so subtle language and learning difficulties because of what the lack of language prevents them from doing. It may also index a general developmental delay.

All these viewpoints do not explain a significant language delay or justify significant delays in further evaluation or referral. Beware of such unfounded explanatory models. Further clinical work should be done to investigate the nature of the delay and its etiology.

CLINICAL LANGUAGE ASSESSMENT

Some peculiarities regarding the appraisal of language in the usual clinical settings provide a bit of a challenge, such as the following:

- Most standard language assessments depend on expressive language, which in turn is the most variable aspect of language and one that is difficult to evaluate in a medical office. Gesture language and receptive language are much better indicators of long-term language development, but these areas are rarely the target of appraisal. This requires a careful history or, better, a chronology because as these competencies emerge over time, we get a broader picture of the whole process.

- Language, particularly but not exclusively expressive language, is an "acute phase reactant" that stagnates or even regresses in the face of any stressor, such as illness, separations from primary care providers and family changes. Because these are the times and circumstances during which we often see children, it is even more imperative that a good record be taken at the regular health supervision visits, when stressors are at a minimum. Otherwise it may be unclear whether a language delay is primary or secondary, short or longer term.

- The office visit itself is a stressor, so productive language is difficult to assess because children often do not speak for the clinician. Indeed, in some cultures and subcultures, the very idea of interacting verbally with an unfamiliar adult is very foreign. Direct observation of all you'd like to evaluate is very tough.

- Recall of language milestones, even by sophisticated observers, is notoriously faulty, whereas almost all families remember the exact moment a child walked alone, a gross motor milestone. *Current* language production is the only reliable report. If you miss asking the question, the history taken later becomes so unreliable that it is nearly useless unless language is egregiously delayed. "What can he say (or understand) today?" is the only reliable question. Recall is seriously flawed.

- Parents are so skilled at interpreting the child's intent and providing so many gesture contexts and visual prompts that they and you may overestimate the child's isolated receptive language abilities. Although you want parents to be that way, it can be problematic in assessment. Furthermore, atypical use of language may be thought of as indicating precocity. General parental report may be misleading unless your questions are very specific.

Mrs. King reported to Dr. May, when asked about language development, that her son of 28 months not only said sentences, but that they were several words long. This was a surprise because Dillon had said no words and was not pointing at the 12- and 15-month visits. He had been an irritable, somber baby whose general development had been a bit slow. Saying "ah" and screaming were the only sounds Dr. May heard in the office. When being given his shot by the nurse, the boy was heard to echo very clearly, "Now this won't hurt a bit" and "Hold still." Further investigation suggested that he had no spontaneous speech or gesture language and that his social interaction and toy play were atypical. A diagnosis of autism was confirmed on referral. Note: Echolalia is a specific and common feature in the speech of children with autism. Getting a clinical report of exactly what a child says as his longest spontaneous utterance will help clarify the child's capability. No pointing at a year should have been an earlier clue of trouble in this case.

Setting the Stage

To do a good job with ongoing language assessment of children in a primary care setting, the whole interaction has to be set up with this as a goal. It takes no more time, but it does take a commitment, a focus and a framework to evaluate the child's linguistic skills. *The office staff should listen to the child's utterances at the beginning of the visit, during weighing and measurement procedures and in interaction with the parent or parents.* Instructions that are part of the routine should be given first *without visual supports*, but with a gesture added if needed. Keep your hands in your pockets or at your sides and look at the child while giving instructions. Give one-step instructions (e.g., Take off your shoes) and then lengthen instructions based on expectations or until you get confusion (e.g., Take off your shirt and get up on the table).

Be aware of an interfering parent in this interaction with the child because that interference may be telling you something. The parent may already know that the child can't understand your requests, and that in itself is a clue that you are asking for something beyond the child's linguistic ability. Children may signal their difficulty by ignoring you, looking at you very intently, changing the task, trying to guess what you want or leaving the scene.

Interactions with toys in the room, in the waiting room and in the course of the examination provide a language sample on which to build an appraisal, although such interactions usually represent minimal competency. A variety of toys that include dolls, a toy telephone, books and pictures on the wall may provide prompts that will bring on language. But don't count on it. The best assessment is still the direct recording of what a child is saying at that time by parental report, done at each health supervision visit.

When to Worry

One should not only track normal development but also have a system to make referrals at a particular time (see Table 16–2). Minimal expectations should be met or a referral made. One needs this backstop because it is all too easy to focus on motor development, to explain the lack of language in the clinical setting or to say "We'll check it next time."

The best assessment is the report of the parent on the child's *current language function,* including receptive and expressive language and, for the youngest children, gesture language (Table 16–3). *Parents expressing a concern about speech or language will be justified about three quarters of the time, so ignoring such a complaint is foolhardy.* Further assessment is almost always needed. It can be done quickly with the checklist provided in Table 16–2 or with the language component of several parent questionnaires that should be part of every health supervision visit. Table 16–1 gives an expanded checklist. If these indicate the possible presence of a language delay or atypical use of language, the primary care clinician or a specialist should take a more detailed look. The infant and toddler forms of the MacArthur Communicative Developmental Inventory (CDI) provide this detailed look at a child's language up to the age of 30 months. A few more questions on social development will help address the possibility of a disorder that falls in the autistic spectrum (see Appendix). Also, Table 16–3 presents primary care records that identify the emergence of real language delay.

TABLE 16–3   **Case Study in Emergence of True Language Delay***

Medical Chart	Comments
2 mo: Small child, doing well	The continuing small size of this child may have contributed to the delay in recognition of the language problem. Our expectations of development are lowered in a proportionally small child in general
4 mo: Petite. Happy	
6 mo: Sitting. Pulling up. Cooing. Jabbering. Things in mouth	Cooing should have been present at the 2-mo and surely by the 4-mo visit. Babbling at this age is what we're looking for
8 mo: Petite. Not too verbal	A key observation. Expect lots of "talking" at this age
12 mo: Pulls to stand, cruises, crawls. Da, da. No words, no pointing. Petite	These phonemes are coming in late, should be strung together and one word present. The absence of pointing is suggestive of real delay. Motor development is normal
15 mo: Walking well, running. Jabbers. No words. Will get hearing test. Growth at bottom curve. Mom small. Note: Hearing test OK	Worry is setting in. The first step is always a hearing test
18 mo: Understands a lot. Her own language. No words. Affectionate. Play OK. Does bye-bye, pat-a-cake. No pointing. Mom not concerned; was late talker	Receptive language is considered, but without an assessment, we can't be sure that this child is using spoken language alone with the support of gestures. No words by this time is abnormal. Autism is considered, hence the comments on play, affective development and imitation. However, these imitative games mentioned are first-year-level imitation. As usual, imitative play and language track together, and both are delayed in this child. Family history is important, but not enough to ignore the problem at this point

*Notes on development extracted from a primary care record: child with no health concerns and five entries for minor illnesses, one for otitis media only, not included here.

Differential Diagnosis

The primary care clinician should consider other conditions for which language delay could be a symptom:

- Hearing loss
- Global developmental delay
- Psychosocial deprivation
- Chronic illness
- Acute stressors
- Autism spectrum of disorders

- Selective mutism
- Developmental language disorder

Although these categories are not mutually exclusive (i.e., most autistic children are delayed, and most neglected children have slowed development), they do provide direction for further assessment and intervention. About half the children with language delays have delays, overt or subtle, in other areas. Moreover, behavior problems are very common in the language-delayed population. A developmental language disorder is a focal impairment in language with sparing of other mental functions and abilities.

Even if the final diagnosis is in the category of specific developmental language disorder, the job isn't over. Even with therapeutic and educational intervention, this group is at risk for difficulties at home and with peers, and they may have difficulties in school, both cognitive and social. Specialized intervention that puts language in place before age 7 is imperative here because interventions are most effective before this time. If a child has no language before puberty, it is unlikely that language will emerge thereafter. Behavioral problems may arise from frustrations with communication, or they may come from a neurological foundation in common with the language issues.

SPEECH DIFFICULTIES

Clear articulation of the sounds of speech is distinct from the content and form of these utterances, which is language (Table 16–4). The ability to reproduce the sounds of one's native language has its own developmental course. A child in the first year of life can distinguish all the sounds that exist in his language (losing the ability to hear the sounds that are not in his native tongue before 9 months of age). However, the child may not be able to say all the

TABLE 16–4 **Speech Disorders**

Type	Description
Deficits in resonance	Disorders are characterized by abnormal oronasal sound balance. Deficits most commonly appear as hypernasality (e.g., in cleft palate) or hyponasality (e.g., in adenoid hypertrophy)
Voice	Problems appear as deviation in the quality, pitch or volume of sound production. Such impairments have either psychological or physiological bases. Thyroid disease and laryngeal polyps from overuse are some considerations
Fluency	Disorders reflect disruption in the natural flow of connected speech. The most common type of fluency disorder is stuttering
Articulation	Disorders include a large group of problems often encountered by the clinician. They are characterized by imprecise production of speech sounds. Most articulation "problems" are common at certain ages and are, in fact, normal. However, their persistence often requires intervention

From Levine M, Brooks R, Shonkoff JP: *A Pediatric Approach to Learning Disorders.* New York, John Wiley & Sons, 1980.

complex blends of sounds until school age. Intelligibility by an unfamiliar adult (i.e., the clinician) should increase with the child's age, being about 50% of the time for a 2-year-old, 75% for a 3-year-old and 100% for a 4-year-old. By 2 years of age, beginning consonants should not be omitted ("oy" for "boy"). By 3½ years, the ending consonants should always be present ("did" should not sound like "di"). The "th" sound will not be present until age 3; the "r" and "l" sounds will be mixed until age 5.

If speech in general sounds babyish or immature for the child's age although the form and complexity are at age level, an articulation problem is probable. However, language and **speech difficulties** often overlap.

Some general irregularities in speech require referral or further evaluation, such as the following:

- A decrease in the amount of speech
- Lack of change in speech for 3 to 6 months in a child younger than 5 years
- Explosive or constantly loud speech
- Hoarseness
- Awkward, unusual cadence or lack of prosody (emotionality) in speech
- A child being embarrassed by speech

Some speech irregularities should draw the clinician's attention to oral-motor function and, perhaps, motor function overall. Poor articulation of frontal consonants, which gives the speech a garbled or swallowed character, may provide a clue to hypotonia or mild cerebral palsy, particularly if accompanied by drooling or difficulty swallowing. An overly nasal quality of speech may suggest palatine dysfunction, perhaps a submucosal cleft palate. Hearing loss must be considered with any speech concern.

There is reason to investigate speech if the child is ashamed of it or teased about it or if it is noticeably less mature than that of other children the child's age. Additionally, if the child regularly experiences frustration in trying to get the meaning across, a formal evaluation is needed. Referral should be made to a speech and language specialist experienced in working with young children.

DATA GATHERING

What to Observe

An office visit offers an important opportunity for evaluation of language development. Observing the following will help in such an evaluation:

- What does the child say in amount, clarity, prosody and length?
- How much of what the child says do you understand?
- How much does the parent interact with and speak to the child? What kinds of things are said? Is the child expected to answer?
- What does the child understand? Give one-, two- and three-step commands to see what the child can do.
- What verbal output accompanies play in the waiting or examining rooms?

BOX 16–2   SAMPLE QUESTIONS FOR PARENTAL REPORTING OF SEQUENTIAL ITEMS

- When did your infant smile at you when you talked or stroked his face?
- When did your infant produce long vowel sounds, such as "eeeee" or "aaaaa"?
- When did your baby first give you the "raspberry"?
- When did your child say "dada" or "mama," but inappropriately?
- When did your child begin to use "dada" and "mama" appropriately?
- When did your child say a word other than "dada" and "mama"?
- When did your child first point at objects?
- When did your child begin to follow simple commands, such as "Give me _____" or "Bring me _____," accompanied by a gesture?
- When was your child able to follow simple commands without an accompanying gesture?
- When did your child begin to speak jargon—to run unintelligible words together in an attempt to make a sentence?
- How many body parts can your child point to when named? Which ones?
- When did your child start to put two words together?
- When did your child use three pronouns?

Modified from Capute AJ, Accardo P: Linguistic and auditory milestones during the first two years of life: A language inventory for the practitioner. *Clin Pediatr (Phila)* 17:847-853, 1978.

What to Ask

The following are examples of questions to ask the parents. Box 16–2 gives more examples.

- What can the child say now? Words? Phrases? Sentences?
- What is the longest thing the child says?
- How many words does the child know? (Expect a number up to about 20, "a lot" usually indicates 20 to 50, and "too many to count" generally means more than 50.)
- Can the child follow one-, two- and three-step commands? (Be sure you leave out gestures and visual supports.)
- Does the child know his name? Siblings? Age? Pets?
- Ask the following of the child, using picture books, simple toys and a toy telephone to help:
- What's that? (pointing to a picture)
- Which one is the _____? (in a book)
- Give me the _____ (from among the objects).
- What's your name, etc.? Start a conversation.
- After age 3, ask a child to describe an experience, such as a birthday, an outing.
- Present one- to three-step commands as part of the physical exam.

Assessment

Use Table 16–2 to look at a child's language. If that raises a warning flag, look at Table 16–1 to see whether you should be really concerned at this time. If so, the following are options for the next step:

- Use the Early Language Milestone (ELM) or other instrument to look at the issue in more detail. The MacArthur CDI, the Receptive Expressive Evaluation of Language (REEL), Clinical Language Assessments (CLAMS), CELF and other assessments are available for a more detailed look.

- Evaluate general development, oral-motor function and emotional responsiveness to look for comorbid conditions.

- Ask for more details of the family history and medical risk factors for hearing loss or developmental delay.

- Order a hearing test. Any language delay requires this.

REFERRALS

If data indicate the need for further examination and possibly treatment, consider the following specialists:

- A speech and language pathologist familiar with young children should be involved early for evaluation and treatment.

- For concerns about general development, a developmental specialist, pediatric neurologist or child psychologist should see and evaluate the child. The Denver (II) is a helpful screening tool in these cases and can be used in a primary care setting (see Appendix).

- Any suggestion of hearing loss requires the consultation of an ear, nose and throat physician, as well as a skilled audiologist. It's *never too early* for hearing augmentation.

- Early intervention services, special education or a language enhancement program should be consulted, depending on the specifics and the services available.

- Loss of language skills, severe language difficulties or the presence of seizures requires an electroencephalogram with consideration of Landau-Kleffner syndrome.

ANTICIPATORY GUIDANCE

Offer parents the following guidelines regarding their children's language:

- Parents can support language development by talking *with* their children, engaging them in dialogues, asking questions and encouraging them to narrate experiences. The linkage of tactile and verbal games and the reading of body language cues in the first year begin this process.

- The playful use of language in the second year through rhymes and jingles fuels interest in words.

- Expanding the child's expressions and speaking clearly and simply with correct words and grammar are also important.

- When talking about a present object or event, beginning the description with "look" or another orienting word allows the child to focus attention. Important words should be repeated.
- Narration of parental activities and caretaking events provides a rich verbal environment.
- Encourage the use of words rather than actions to express feelings and wishes.

READING TOGETHER

Reading of stories from infancy onward enhances language, literacy and school performance and should be consciously encouraged by the clinician. Reading together supports language with its own developmental course. Parents who may find it awkward to know what to say to their young children may be supported in their efforts at verbal exchange through the specific use of books together. Offer parents the following types of advice on the progression of reading together:

- Beginning in the first year, parents may point to objects in books and identify them.
- Parental pointing progresses to the child's pointing and naming things in the early second year of life.
- Explanation of a picture with brief descriptions of the immediate action grows into short story telling by 2 to 3 years of age.
- Children who are 3 and 4 years old will expand the action beyond the picture, can follow stories and can anticipate events through the medium of books.
- Children older than 7 years regularly enjoy stories without pictures.
- Jokes and riddles for 5- and 6-year-olds are often based on words with double meanings or vagaries of language. Enjoyment of these by parents and kids reinforces this new plateau of language development.
- Poetry and other interesting uses of language can be introduced at this time, if not earlier. The clinician should have a stock of simple jokes and puns in mind to highlight this new skill in a clinical setting.

SUMMARY

The language of the second year of life is a landmark of change for the child and the family. The child can now share observations of events, recall past events to himself and others and communicate original thoughts and feelings to others. For most children, this is a liberating and exciting event. For parents, this often marks the undeniable end of infancy. Their child becomes more of an individual and an active participant in family life. Much of the work of exposing the child to objects and events, talking to him without obvious response and learning about him through body language and nonverbal response now pays off as the child speaks. The joy, amazement and amusement of toddler speech are tainted by the loss of a totally receptive infant. This step requires developmental work for the whole family. Language acquisition marks another step in individuation for the child and a separation within the family. It may also represent the single most significant developmental process in that it may be unmatched in its complexity and in the fact that it makes the child particularly human.

QUICK CHECK–2 YEARS

- ✓ Is understood about half the time by strangers
- ✓ Uses two-word phrases
- ✓ Follows two-step command
- ✓ Has a vocabulary of 20 to 50 words or more
- ✓ Stacks at least five cubes
- ✓ Makes horizontal lines and circular shapes with paper and marker
- ✓ Can kick a ball
- ✓ Uses a spoon and fork
- ✓ Goes up and down stairs, two feet on each step
- ✓ Names seven body parts
- ✓ Runs easily and often
- ✓ Takes off clothes and helps with dressing
- ✓ Washes hands
- ✓ Points at pictures in a book
- ✓ Imaginary play, combining two or more objects

HEADS UP–2 YEARS

Children with the autistic spectrum of disorders (pervasive developmental disorders) have the following:

- Absent, atypical and/or substantially delayed language that encompasses receptive, expressive and gesture language
- Markedly impaired social interaction, with a failure of reciprocal interaction, shared joint attention
- Failure or marked impairment in the ability to understand the feelings of others or understand that others have different thoughts and perspectives
- Restricted range of interests and/or atypical interests and activities
- Stereotypical movements such as spinning, hand flapping, toe walking
- Interest in the parts of objects such as the wheels on a toy car, the knob of a door, the legs of a toy dog
- Failure to or delay in imaginative play

Despite a wide range of manifestations, impairment in communication and interaction with others is at the core of this class of disorders.

Several screening instruments are available if this group of disorders is suspected: the Modified Childhood Autism Test (MCHAT), the Pervasive Developmental Disorders Screening Test (PDDST) and the Ages & Stages Questionnaires (ASQ). They can be found in the Appendix.

RECOMMENDED READINGS

Agin MC, Geng LF, Nicholl M: *The Late Talker: What To Do If Your Child Isn't Talking Yet.* New York, St. Martin's Press, 2003.

Apel K, Masterson J: *Beyond Baby Talk: From Sounds to Sentences. A Parent's Complete Guide to Language Development.* Roseville, CA, Prima Press, 2001.

Bialystock E: *Bilingualism in Development: Language, Literacy and Cognition.* New York, Cambridge University Press, 2001.

Richardson S: The child with delayed speech. *Contemp Pediatr* 16:55, 1992.

Thal D, Bates E: Language and communication in early childhood. *Pediatr Ann* 18:299, 1989.

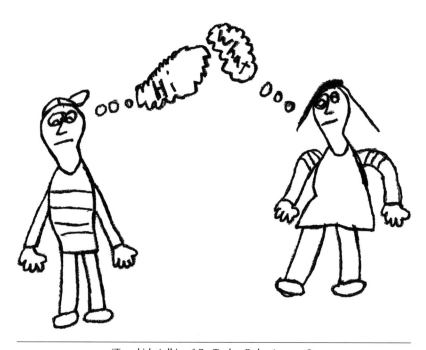

"Two kids talking." By Taylor Roberts, age 9.

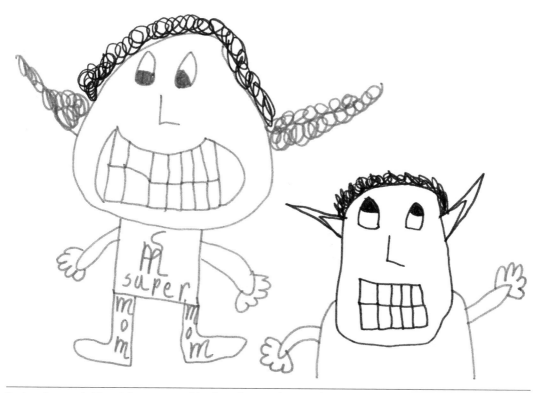

Fantasy has made Mom into some combination of a superhero and a pretty formidable figure. Large teeth, horn-like hair testify to her power. The child below is bit scary himself, with ears that give him a devil-like image and teeth to match Mom's.

CHAPTER 17

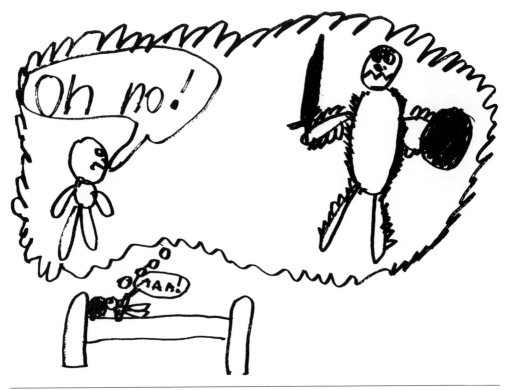

"A scary dream." By Ryan Hennessy.

Three Years: Emergence of Magic

SUZANNE D. DIXON

This chapter looks at the roles played by fantasy and imagination and how they affect behavior day and night. It lays the foundation for counsel regarding support for this aspect of development and the avoidance of inappropriate prompts to fantasy. Sleep disorders of toddlerhood are discussed. The influence of television and computers on children is presented, as well as the expected developmental course of fears across childhood.

Key Words

- Computers
- Imagination
- Fantasy
- Representation
- Imaginary Friends
- Lying
- Fears in Childhood
- Dreams and Nightmares
- Monster
- Night Terrors
- Sleep Disorders
- Stories, Fairy Tales
- Television

Mr. Jackson brings in his 3-year-old son because the boy does not tell the truth about drawing on the wall and spilling milk. He says Jayden has an imaginary friend who is always sitting in his chair at home. Jayden also seems to be afraid to take a walk after dinner with his dad, a thing he used to enjoy. Jayden has nightmares at least twice per week, which he never had before. His dad wonders if he is turning into a "wimp" and needs more discipline. He says nothing frightening has happened to his son to make him so fearful. Note: In this chapter you'll find out not only that Mr. Jackson has nothing to worry about but also why Jayden is having all this "strange" behavior. The case illustrates the phenomenon in development that some behavior appears regressed but is really evidence of growth in the cognitive and emotional domains. This chapter will discuss those gains.

Although the charm and fascination of a child's **imagination** are apparent to all caretakers, we rarely reflect on its significance and the function of this mental facility. The emergence of imagination is both a marker of cognitive growth and a tool for mental and emotional development. It is a probe into the inner life of a child, provided that we ourselves have a mental framework on which to place a child's play, stories, fears and actions. Imagination is in full flower at age 3, so it is the perfect time to examine what this aspect of development can tell us about a child. A 3-year-old floats at a hazy border between reality and **fantasy**. If you let yourself be pulled into his world, you'll learn a lot and be ready to offer informed advice on many areas of preventive mental health. You will also have more fun. Selma Fraiberg's classic book *The Magic Years* should be required reading for all child health care providers so that they can understand and appreciate this special aspect in the development of young children.

REPRESENTATION AS A CORE MENTAL FUNCTION

The young of all higher animals play—with actions, objects and with others—but only human young appear to engage in fantasy play. This uniquely human mental function, along with true language, relies on the child's ability to let one thing stand for something else. This is called **representation** and is the foundation of both language and imaginative play. Although children do simple imitation, even delayed imitation, at a much earlier age, the late second to fifth years of life see the creation of unique play in scenarios, with roles, costumes, voices and sequenced events. Play goes beyond simple mimicry or single roles at this age; it now contains novel components and combinations. Play changes across this time frame in three ways:

- Play becomes more detached from real-life objects, e.g.,

    A 1-year-old pretends to drink from an empty toy cup.

    A 3-year-old makes a cup into a hat or a banana into a telephone.

- Play becomes less self centered, e.g.,

    A 1-year-old dances like his mom.

    A 3-year-old makes his dolls dance and talk and take on roles.

- Play becomes more complex and prolonged, e.g.,

    A 1-year-old runs a car around a track.

    A 4-year-old plays "house" with dolls, his little brother and a friend, changing the drama all afternoon.

The clinician can monitor children progressing along this continuum over time. Children stuck at simple imitation, by themselves, with no reinvention of objects are not progressing in this core cognitive function and need to have their development appraised very thoroughly. It's never a waste of time to ask about and observe a child's play because it is a probe of cognitive development.

Similarly, real language emerges across this same time frame. Words and sounds are learned to stand for objects, actions, relationships and feelings. It's no surprise, then, that language and imaginative play are linked because they are based in the same core function. Delays in one area are often linked to delays in the other.

Tools for Cognitive Growth

This new mental capacity, the ability to use fantasy, emerges in toddlerhood and, like all new abilities, is exercised frequently. The child now uses mental actions to transform events, actions, sounds and meanings beyond the immediate. This is an active mental process attesting to a new level of ability that is used to order experience and learn about the world. The ability to fantasize strengthens the ability to learn and in no way detracts from the skill of understanding "the real world." Quite the contrary, as stated by Fraiberg, "A child's contact with the real world can be strengthened by periodic excursions into fantasy in a world where the deepest wishes can achieve imaginary gratification" (see Fig. 17–1). The ability to use imagination and fantasy opens an entirely new world for a child. Previously, this world was limited to direct experience. Now the child can imagine possibilities, causes and sequences of events that go beyond the immediate or even the possible. He can also fear these mental creations as well.

 Jaime looked at the pattern of bathroom tiles and thought he saw a face. He wondered who was behind the wall. He refused to go to the bathroom by himself.

A child of this age can review, rework and repetitively process the events of daily life through actions, language and "mental movies." Events of the day may be overwhelming and incomprehensible at this age. Through fantasy the child can recall them, process at his own rate and set down memory.

Sidra was heard talking to his stuffed animal in bed at night. "Now, just you stop this. I tol' you never to do it. Bad Barney. OK, you're all right now." Clearly he was reworking a little rough spot in his day.

Overall, fantasy fuels the cognitive functions of attention, memory, reasoning, language and creativity. It is no surprise that the more extensive the make-believe play, the more advanced the child's cognitive abilities are likely to be.

Martin and Esteban were playing firemen with pretend hoses, running around and putting out imagined fires. Kevin said, "Now the firemen go to space. There's a rocket fire." They then sat down and "blasted off".

Interactional play is now a regular event that replaces parallel play and results in more elaborate schemes than children usually come up with on their own. Fantasy is the glue that often holds these interactions together. Children frequently recall and experiment with rules, limits or behavior in their play. Fantasy can serve, as well as define, a new level of cognitive growth throughout the preschool years.

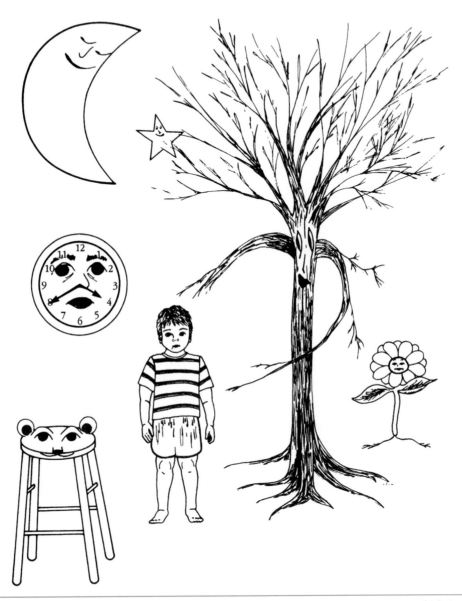

Figure 17–1   The magical quality of a preschool-aged child is illustrated in this picture, in which inanimate objects are assigned human feelings and motives (animism).

Tools for Emotional Growth

Fantasy also serves emotional growth in that it allows children to experiment with strong feelings, work through areas of tension and assume aspects of identification with those around them. They can try out new roles for themselves in a safe, flexible way in imagined forms, such as roles of the opposite sex, their parent, a monster or an animal. Emotions become integrated.

Every time Connor talked to his doctor about visiting his newly remarried Dad on the weekend, he got into the posture of a dog and used his "growl voice." The doctor rightly identified that Connor was having a hard time dealing with the new situation.

Negative feelings can be expressed in creative ways through fantasy that won't draw rejection or punishment, especially when those feelings are directed toward loved ones. Fantasy is the buffer from overwhelming feelings on the child's part and overwhelming response from the adults. Fantasy provides the ability to work through interactive difficulties with siblings, playmates, parents and caregivers. These melodramas allow not just venting but also preservation of self-esteem and practice at resolution. The child has strength and power in fantasy life that cannot be achieved in real life. Aggressive themes may be evident in the play of the mildest mannered child. Costumes, puppet play and doll play are forums and props for this developmental work. In fact, much therapeutic work in the preschool years involves tapping into emotions through the medium of fantasy play by using puppets, dolls, toy animals and drawings.

Expressive language abilities lag behind the child's cognitive capacities, so these nonverbal forms of communication are particularly important for a young child. The child can both work through and communicate feelings, frustrations, anxieties and wishes in safe ways. Adults should pay close attention to play to understand what the child is about. Helping adults see the play of childhood as a valuable indicator of a child's emotional state and as an outlet for emotional release is an important clinical role.

Emma, age 4, went to great lengths to keep her doll Margie with her at all times and became frantic when Margie went missing for even the briefest time. She usually wrapped Margie over and over with a blanket, making it very tight and covering the doll's face. Dr. Anison pointed out that maybe Emma was working out her worries for herself since her military dad was deployed to combat. Her mom had just thought she was being babyish and oppositional.

Tools for Social Growth

The emergence of fantasy allows a child to play with other children in new ways. The assumption of imaginary roles, however brief and ever changing, allows longer and more elaborate play periods, as well as richer solitary play. One child can be caught up in another's imaginative structure, be challenged while having fun and learn from the interaction. Play with older children allows preschoolers to function at a higher level, whereas play with younger playmates allows for the development of nurturance and the ability to successfully guide another.

Olivia, age 3, was playing house with her 5-year-old cousin. She was pouring the "tea" (water) into cups when her cousin told her to "Be careful. Tea makes a big stain." Olivia asked, "What's a stain?" "A big mark you can't get out even if your mom washes it." Olivia was just settling in when her cousin announced that they now had to do the washing. Olivia hadn't done that before. They turned over the step stool for a pretend basin. Note: Olivia is being pulled up by this interaction with her cousin into play that is much more complicated than what she would do on her own.

Cooperative play involves learning about give and take, negotiation skills, assertiveness and demands for communication beyond the circle of family "interpreters." Play with age-mates teaches one to cooperate and resolve conflicts. It teaches compromise and negotiation skills and fuels the development of a sense of justice and fair play. Play with others, or interactional play, should be the norm at this age rather than parallel play, as was seen earlier. Experiences with a variety of playmates offer the best opportunity to learn these important skills. Healthy fantasy play with others, in dramas, stories and long sequences, is associated with enhanced social competency. So a history of rich play periods with others should be reassuring. Children in isolation or those who cannot play with others need a second look.

Devon's preschool teacher reported to mom at the end of the school year that Devon was still "pretty much on his own." He rarely interacts with the other children and usually plays with the trucks by himself. Note: This remark might be made about a shy 3-year-old at the beginning of preschool, but at the end of the year, this description is worrisome. Devon's behavior and development need a second look.

Parent interaction in play can increase the complexity and length of play episodes, provided that the parent doesn't take over, push too hard or ignore signs of disengagement (e.g., the child leaving, playing with something else). Parents, however, cannot provide an exciting enough play experience by themselves. Children in the third year and beyond need other children, such as relatives, neighbors, a play group or a preschool group. Parents should think of peer play at this age as a necessary enhancement for the child, not a substitute for their primary social experiences in the family. Introduction of a group experience is nearly mandatory at age 3 if it hasn't occurred before. Some children will need more time and support than others to embrace this expanded world. Mild stress with group play is inevitable and is a prompt for growth in social competency. Learning to get along, to initiate interaction and to get your own position across to others is an important task at this age. Play interactions are the landscape for these skills to emerge.

Imaginary Friends

Imaginary friends are very useful to young people. They are created by many children, but particularly by girls, firstborns and only children. About 25% to up to 45% of children aged 3 to 7 will invent these companions at some time. These magical creatures serve many functions, such as the missed presence of a parent, an idealized parent, a playmate, the willing slave of a toddler struggling with power and autonomy issues or the victim in a power struggle. These friends can be the scapegoats for misdeeds, a comforter after discipline or even a jolly companion for a long afternoon or a dark night. These valuable creatures come and go, depending on the situation. Too careful a scrutiny of them or even too much attention to them by adults makes them disappear because they don't survive in the hard light of reality. They should be prized and respected as being the product of a creative, adaptive and developing person. No evidence shows them to be harmful, to be indications of pathology or unmet needs or to be cause for concern. In fact, children who have such companions tend, as a group, to have more complex pretend play and more advanced skills of mental representation and are more sociable.

Lies, Thefts and Other Misdemeanors

An active imagination is a healthy asset even if it generates "untruths." Children at this age do not (indeed cannot) intentionally plan to deceive another. However, their reports of events, particularly under pressure, most often reflect how they perceive things to be, how they creatively process these impressions, how they wish things were or how they think things should be to please. These perceptions are real even if the reported events are not. These stories are not formed out of moral lassitude. They should be seen as "creative coping" with a situation that may be stressful for the child. Parents should reflect on the underlying issue rather than struggle with the content of the story. Untruths should not be supported, but it does no good to press a child to retract back a story. Reflect on the obvious and formulate a specific action plan to correct it. The child will know that the story is not correct. Forcing an admission of **lying** will just cause the child stress and greater reliance on the safe fantasy. Generally, children older than 6 to 7 have the ability to purposely lie, separating their own mental creations from objective truths.

Mrs. Curtis looked from the broken vase to her very guilty-looking 3$\frac{1}{2}$-year-old daughter, Alissa. Mrs. Curtis said, "I'm very sad about this vase. You shouldn't be playing in here. Now let's clean it up. I hope you feel sorry for what happened." Note: Mom didn't confront Alissa about something that was obvious. She stated the problem and directed the child to the appropriate feeling and action.

Children also have very fluid concepts of property rights when it comes to things they want. They may "borrow" a sibling's toy or a playmate's three-wheeler if the object is attractive enough. They may then imagine that it is OK, that the owner said it was OK or that they will give it right back. The guilt of a candy heist at the grocery store is easily covered over by such fantasy. Clearly, the rules of society and the rights of others must be taught to young children,

BOX 17–1   RESPONDING TO "CRIMES" OF TODDLERS

Developmentally Appropriate
- "I bet you wish that the crayon marks weren't on the wall. Let's clean it together."
- "You and Jeremy must have had a fight. Tell him you are sorry for hitting, and let's go out to swing."
- "Give Jason's truck back; it's his, not yours. Ask him before you play with it."
- "My pack of gum is in your room. Put it back in my purse. Ask me if you want gum."

Developmentally Inappropriate
- "That's Jason's truck. How would you feel if he took your things?"
- "Play nice."
- "Did you take the gum in my purse? Tell me, did you? You can't just take things that belong to other people. How would it be if everyone did stuff like that?"

so such behavior shouldn't be ignored. Parents must give a message, in very concrete terms, about what is acceptable behavior and how to correct a wrong. Generalities such as "behave" or "act nice" make no sense to a young child. Children this age cannot understand the event from the other child's perspective, nor can they understand the need for a broad social order (Box 17–1). This comes later in the normal progression of moral development, which is linked to the sequence of cognitive abilities. They have a hard time generalizing from one situation to the next, even if adults think the situations are similar. So be specific about what is expected in each instance.

Ms. Washburn said to her son Jared, "Give Clayton's truck back to him now. The rule is: don't take anyone's toys unless you ask them. No borrowing."

FEARS IN CHILDHOOD

Every child, beginning in infancy, has fearful responses to some things, but at this age, fears become more complex. The child can imagine fearful things that *might* happen and can imagine other meanings to the things that have happened in the past or are occurring in the present. Current and future events can be feared not just for their immediate danger but for what is perceived as an anticipated or ongoing threat. The ability to fantasize can enlarge and modify these real or perceived dangers, as well as help the child manage them better.

Fears in childhood have their own expected developmental course and are presented in Table 17–1.

Types of fears seem to be linked to cognitive development (i.e., bright children have precocious fears; delayed children have fears consistent with their mental age). Although subject to both individual and circumstantial flavoring, the objects of fear are remarkably consistent across children. Some emerging fears appear regressed but really have to do with an emerging and expanding imagination. For example, a fearless 5-year-old may become afraid of a monster in the closet after turning 6.

TABLE 17–1 **Fears in Childhood**

Age	Fears
0–7 mo	Change in stimulus level, loss of support; loud, sudden noises
8–18 mo	Separation, strangers, loud events, sudden movements toward, touching, physical restraints, large crowds, water, being bathed
2 yr	Loud sounds, dark colors, large objects, large moving things, hats, mittens, changes in location of physical things, going down the drain or toilet, wind and rain, animals
2½ yr	Movement, familiar objects moved, moving objects, unexpected events linked (e.g., Grandma in mom's hat)
3 yr	Visual fears, masks, old people, people with scars, deformities, the dark, parents going out at night, animals, burglars
4 yr	Auditory fears, the dark, wild animals, mother's departure, imaginary creatures, recalled past events, aggressive actions, threats
5 yr	Decrease in fears; injury, falls, dogs
6 yr	Fearful age; supernatural events, hidden people, being left or lost, small bodily injuries (e.g., splinters, small cuts), being left alone, death of loved ones, the elements, fire, thunder
7 yr	Spaces (cellars), shadows, ideas suggested by television, movies, being late for school, missing answers in school
8–9 yr	School failure, personal failure, ridicule by peers, disease, unanticipated events
10–11 yr	Wild animals, high places, criminals, older kids, loss of possessions, parental anger, remote possibilities of catastrophe (e.g., earthquake), school failure, pollution
12–17 yr	Physical changes in one's own body, isolation, sexual fears, loss of face, world events

Modified from Jersild AT, Holmes FB: *Child Dev Monogr* 20:358, 1935; and Ilg FL, Ames L, Baker SM: *Child Behavior.* New York, Harper & Row, 1981.

No child can be protected from the task of working through these fears. Children's fears, especially in early childhood, seem to cross cultural barriers, although the intensity of the child's response and the *specific* circumstances that intensify fears vary from child to child and across cultural or subcultural groups. In general, girls tend to be more anxious and fearful than boys, starting in the first year of life, but there is much individual variation. The expression of fear is individual and ranges from fleeing or calling for help to shyness or irritability or even to increases in activity and aggression.

David Elkind suggests that as children are exposed to increasingly complex issues and adult developmental issues, we may anticipate that the situations and concerns that evoke fears may also grow in diversity and complexity. For example, fear of pollution, war, car accidents, terror or even direct interpersonal violence may be part of many children's lives because of broad media coverage of world-wide events.

> Luke told Dr. Rogers that he was worried that Osama bin Laden was coming to "get" him and his family by driving a plane into their house. Note: Television coverage of recent events may be changing the fear profiles of young children. Children do not understand causal complexity, so identifying one person or one specific action is the way a child mentally contains and then expresses complex fears.

Management of Fears

Fears cannot be avoided, and they shouldn't be because they serve to keep us safe, restrain our behavior and help us draw what we need from the environment. Support for adaptive coping and protection from unreasonable fears are the goals here, not the elimination of fears completely.

It's healthy for toddlers to be afraid of strangers, dogs, noisy environments and separation from care providers. Stranger anxiety peaks from 8 to 18 months, and separation anxiety is expected. New adults should approach a toddler slowly after talking to a familiar adult and should be prepared to back off if the child resists their approach. Children should not be told to kiss every stranger or pet every dog or be scolded for crying at a stranger's approach. Repetitive patterns of parental leave-taking and return rituals help toddlers cope with necessary separations and the fears they may incite.

Preschoolers' imaginary fears should be respected. Parents should acknowledge the fearful feeling without adding credence to the imaginary creature or events. Reassurance of support and safety and giving a child a sense of control of part of the situation will restore some equanimity. Drawings and pretend play with dolls or with other children can be used to cope. Attempting to argue kids out of fantasy is usually futile. Avoidance of overwhelming images or events will help keep the lid on excessive fearfulness. Giving children time to size up a situation before acting will also help.

School-age children need openings to expose their fears and worries and focused discussions on what might happen. They can use words and reasoning to cope with fears, tools not available to a younger child. At school age, information generally reduces fears, whereas it may overwhelm a preschooler. Unmentionable events become very fearful. Reassurance of the normalcy of fears is usually helpful. Good models also help show children this age how to face fears. Parents can help by sharing some of their own worries and concerns and then talking through how they have coped or will cope. Kids, particularly those older than 5, like to mentally rehearse or talk through their plans about fearful things.

> Jackson's family was moving to a new house. He asked his mom over and over where his bed was going and where would he take his bath. His mom reassured him that his bed would be moved to his new room, which was painted blue, and that his room was right next to the bathroom, which has yellow walls and white tile. He drew a picture of his new house and showed it to everyone in the neighborhood, being careful to show the address. He calmed down considerably after taking a "walk through" with his family.

Most days in a clinical practice offer opportunities to learn of children's fears and their coping styles (Box 17–2). It's also a chance to model support for a child when fearful events come up. Empathy, minimal discussion and providing some aspect of control will help.

The interpersonal environment of children who are chronically or excessively fearful should be examined to see whether it lacks support for resolution of their fears or whether it is too overwhelming for these children to cope. Past events, separations and abandonment leave a scar of chronic fearfulness that may become generalized over time. These children need more extensive evaluations. Children who are too shy or fearful to make age-appropriate relationships with others need a very careful look. (Remember Devon and his teacher's report earlier in this chapter). Their linguistic skills, social awareness or sense of security should be evaluated. Extremely shy and fearful children are at high risk for emotional disorders and should be monitored closely. Anxiety, depression or specific phobias may be present. They may be the victims of teasing, bullying or rejection.

A child's fears should never be dismissed as trivial. The fear is real even if the object of the fear is not. They offer clear testimony to a child's affective, cognitive and social level. Fears are the other side of fantasy, and both are to be respected as sources of and testimony to mental growth.

Nightmares and Night Terrors: Things That Go Bump in the Night

The emergence of representation skills means that **dreams and nightmares**—nighttime fantasies—will also make their appearance. They are another piece of evidence of this new level of cognitive ability. They serve as additional resources for resolution of the dilemmas and tensions of daily life. Nighttime fantasies are a useful outlet for a young child, as well as for older children and adults.

Nightmares and dreams are the product of rapid eye movement (REM) sleep, a mentally active part of the sleep cycle. Not every REM period has dreams; they are more likely to emerge in the early morning, particularly as the child grows. Children may waken from dreams and may or may not be able to tell you about the content of these dreams, depending on their cognitive level and linguistic skills. These children respond to comfort and reassurance. When a child remembers the dream or has specific nighttime fears (e.g., **monster** in the closet), general reassurance is needed, not an exhaustive search of the room for a monster. This "buying in" of the parent just adds confusion (was that monster real?), anxiety (I guess there could be a monster in my closet) and inability to get help (my mom even has to get the monster out). Dream content is a jumble of things and events for mental sorting and cannot be taken too literally. However, dreams increase at the time of stress because they serve as a strong coping mechanism. Kids caught in a recurrent pattern of the same dream need help to look for the stressor, *not* exploration of the dream content itself. Firm, consistent bedtime rituals help all kids cope with nighttime fears and awakenings. Avoidance of overly intense images on television and videos will cut down on some nighttime fears.

Night terrors, on the other hand, are abrupt partial wakenings from deep sleep (non-REM) and are accompanied by dramatic physiological arousal with no wakefulness or responsiveness to comfort. Children appear flushed and wide eyed and may produce screeching cries but are unresponsive to comfort. They will not remember the event later. Though very frightening to parents, they are not harmful and go away without intervention. Parents should keep kids safe while they thrash around but shouldn't expect either responsiveness or memory. They usually

BOX 17–2   IMPENDING INSERTION OF AN INTRAVENOUS LINE: MANAGING FEARFULNESS IN MEDICAL SITUATIONS

Situation

Madison, age 18 months, needed an IV started because of croup. She clung to her mother throughout the whole assessment, really yelled as the nurse approached and was whiny but consolable. On the table she struggled with the restraints and went into a hysterical pitch when her mom left to retrieve a purse left in the waiting room. On mom's return, she stopped screaming, but sobbed inconsolably. She barely flinched with the stick itself. In her room, in the tent, she slept. Her mom was in the bathroom when she awoke, and she immediately screamed and grabbed her blanky.

Helps at this Age:

Presence of mom, loved one

Avoiding eye contact with a stranger

Support of a lovey

Ability to protest

Maintenance of as much of a routine as possible

Situation

Caleb, age 3½, saw the preparations for the IV. The nurse seemed to have pointed teeth like a lion, and her long fingernails were sharp. He thought he'd never get away if she pinched him. The IV looked like it could crush him, and the syringe looked the size of his dog at home. It might just go right through his arm into his heart—Clunk! Move your arm away! He was really sorry he wrote on the walls this morning—this was a pretty bad punishment. He thought the nurse was really dumb to put the needle in one hand when that sore red part was on the other. He wished he had brought his Power Rangers—they'd get 'em. The nurse asked him what color cover he wanted on his IV.

Helps at this Age:

Calm reassurance

Reassurance of lack of blame

Ability to use fantasy to cope

Limiting long explanations

Giving control where possible

Situation

Brandon, age 9, asked the nurse a million questions in the treatment room while they were getting set up: "How big is the needle? Will you die if a bubble gets in? Do you ever slip? How long will it take for the medicine to go in? Can the needle come out? What if you move?" He said he was sure he wouldn't cry. He wanted to hold still. In a small voice he said over and over, "don't cry, don't cry, hold still." His dad asked him if he wanted him to hold his hand. He said, "No thanks," and looked up at the ceiling.

Helps at this Age:

Good, calm explanations

Questions answered concisely

Exact expectations laid out clearly

Provision of a time frame, a plan

Giving a little time for getting ready

Respect for apparent lack of need for support

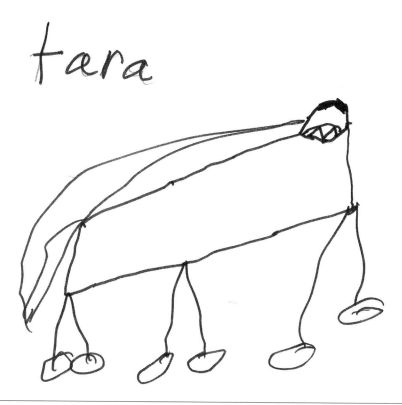

A boy, age 10, draws a bug that attacks him at night. It all started after his dad was killed.

occur in the second sleep cycle (the 11-o'clock news phenomenon), increase at times of fatigue and stress and run in families. Somnambulism (sleep walking) and somniloquy (sleep talking) more typically emerge in the middle grade school years, but they can start in the preschool period, run in families and increase at times of stress, including changes in the environment and when overly tired or under emotional duress. It is a partial awakening or disruption in the sleep cycle. Sleep talking is a product of either REM or non-REM sleep and is rarely a concern. Real secrets are hardly ever revealed. Nearly half of children will do some sleep walking or talking, some of the time. Talking usually emerges before walking as a sleep disturbance, and these children are often described as restless sleepers in general.

The parenting role is to keep the environment safe for a night wanderer by blocking stairs, entrances or any dangerous situations. A door alarm may help alert the parent to an episode, but that depends on the parent awakening. Benzodiazapines have been used in only the most severe, recurrent cases for short periods and possibly work through alteration of the sleep cycles.

Bruxism, or teeth grinding, is also common, being reported in as many as three fourths of children. There are many conditions that result in this behavior, but most cases are termed "simple" and are mild, transient concerns. Interestingly, children with severe temper tantrums at the age of 4 or 5 are more likely to grind their teeth at night. An older child may be willing to use a teeth guard to avoid teeth damage. Self-hypnosis, progressive relaxation and mental imaging have also been used with older children. If this problem is severe, referral to a sleep center for evaluation is recommended.

STORIES AND BOOKS

Stories, including **fairy tales**, are a delight to kids and are useful as well. They assist kids in working through their own fantasies, conflicts and experimentation with roles. Bettelheim, in his classic work, talks about the adaptive significance of fairy tales. He encourages adults to read the stories right through without interpretation. He believes that kids should construct their own explanations of the story based on their own issues. A little less dogmatic approach would be to allow the child to discuss anything about a story with pauses, mild prompts for comment and a brief response from the parent. This approach, along with urging the child to retell a familiar story, has been shown to be effective in improving reading and speaking skills in young children, even in the relatively short term.

Book reading starts early:

- In the first year, children should become familiar, turn pages and learn to look at the pictures.
- Between age 1 and 2, children can name objects or actions of one picture at a time.
- At age 3 to 4, children learn how the pictures are connected in a story and can then tell the story with no book present.
- The ability to guess "what will happen next?" is really evident at age 5 to 6, about the same time that the child appreciates motivations in the book's characters.

Listening to how parents read to their child will tell you not only about the child but also about the interaction between parents and child. Simple books in the exam room allow this observation to be made incidentally. Direct clinician involvement in encouraging reading (e.g., Reach Out and Read Program) seems to be highly effective in improving language skills and parent-child interactions. If children are read to at home, they will do better in school, have more complex vocabularies and ask more complex questions. A clinician who actively encourages reading really does make a difference. Cooperative ventures with local libraries and book stories is good "preventive medicine" for pediatric patients.

TELEVISION AND MOVIES

The average American watches 6 or more hours of **television** per day, and most children older than 2 watch at least 3 hours per day. Because TV is such a pervasive part of children's lives, it is important to look at how and to what degree TV affects children.

The influence of TV on young children has been a matter of concern since the 1960s. These concerns include the form of television (i.e., how it delivers information), the content of the material and what other parts of a child's life TV displaces. These areas will be discussed in turn.

The Child's Perspective: Reality TV

Television delivers many different types of information, some commercial, some pure fantasy and some factual or documentary. A child younger than 5 cannot distinguish between these categories and will remain confused about what's what on TV until at least age 7. As we have seen in this chapter, a preschooler lives with one foot in fantasyland at all times anyway, so TV is always "real" at that age. A preschooler cannot distinguish what is pretend and what is not. Furthermore, the cognitive ability to know that one thing can stand for another (representational ability) is just emerging and remains incompletely developed until age 7 or so. The unreality of TV is only appreciated after that age. Children believe that all the characters act and feel as portrayed and that they somehow live in the TV setting between shows. Children younger than 8 have a hard time connecting scenes and seeing motivation and consequences of action. They assume ongoing relationships and do not understand the concept of acting and rehearsing, even if all this is explained to them. For all these developmental reasons, watching TV is a very different experience for a young child than for an older one or an adult.

The Medium Is the Message

The mode of TV is to present material in short, fast-moving bits of imagery and talk to maintain attention. Children younger than 3 are fascinated by these images but don't have the cognitive skills to understand or link them. Children younger than 8 need a lot more processing time to understand what's going on than adults do, and they do not benefit from close-ups, music or lighting techniques to draw attention to salient features of the story; these techniques are confusing to them. Flashbacks and multiple story threads make no sense to preschoolers or even young grade-schoolers. As in real life, kids need a lot of support to make transitions, and that is not generally available on most programs when transitions are made frequently and fast. Even youngsters in middle school will be challenged to follow the action in a fast-paced program or to remember earlier events that explain motivation or consequences. The *mode of TV*, then, means that kids miss a lot of what they see, often don't make connections and are likely to focus on the most intense, not the most important images and story components. The ideas of sequential events and long-standing motivations are lost in this complex, rapid delivery mode.

New data by Christakis and colleagues suggest that early exposure to television is associated with attention difficulties in middle childhood. This finding adds further imperative to limit early (as well as late) exposure to this media.

Couch Potatoes

Because of these factors and the receptive nature of the media itself, watching TV *requires little active mental work*. At a time when the central nervous system is establishing important connections based on active mental processing, time spent watching TV is time on idle. It is also time taken away from more physical play, family and peer interaction and other activities that are interactive. This is the displacement problem with TV. Moreover, the inactivity, combined with food advertising, sets up the link between TV, obesity and physical inactivity. It's unhealthy to be a couch potato.

Content of Television

The *content of TV* is also of concern in three areas: stereotypes, values and violence. Although much has been done in the past 2 decades to broaden the diversity in TV programming, stereotyped images still show women as dependent and less competent; the elderly as weak, foolish and incompetent; and minorities as comic figures, similar to images from an earlier era. Most families will find some of the situations, solutions and relationships depicted on TV at odds with their own values, including sexual mores, attitudes toward drugs and alcohol, suggestive conversations and innuendos, attitudes toward crime and law enforcement and so forth. Without other models or alternative views on how to handle life's problems, kids quickly pick up TV programs' solutions and assumptions. Consequences of actions are not depicted, and children are left to believe that certain actions have no negative outcomes. As discussed earlier, school-age kids handle fears and stress through adaptation of role models and through mentally practicing how they would handle various situations. TV images fall on fertile ground at this age for models and solutions. "Reality" TV is taken as reflecting real-life possibilities, which older children and adolescents continue to harbor.

Children are highly influenced to seek toys that are advertised, many of which require minimal mental or physical activity.

The area most studied is the effect on children of exposure to *violence*, which more than 80% of TV programs contain. There is no question that children will show more aggressive behavior after being shown aggressive acts on TV, and children who watch more TV are, as a group, more aggressive. Most infectious diseases have weaker proof of causality than the huge body of research now showing links between viewing violence and aggression. Imitation of actions viewed on TV can be seen at the age of 14 months, so it's no surprise that older kids imitate what they see. This has been shown in multiple studies. Reducing TV exposure to violence will reduce aggressive behavior. The vast bulk of evidence would agree that watching violent images is associated with acting more aggressively, or as stated by Cole and Cole after a review of the literature, "The current consensus is that watching violence on television does in fact increase violent behavior in many viewers, whether or not they are otherwise 'predisposed' to it." So-called children's programs on average contain more violence than TV content in general. The link has been made repeatedly in many studies with a diversity of designs in a multitude of settings.

Is TV all bad? NO! Parental involvement can significantly improve the value of TV for children. In addition, a lot of good shows are developed with a young child's needs and interests in mind, such as pre-academic, social and fantasy programs. Children can be exposed to things, good and bad, that wouldn't otherwise be available at home. Without TV, they would miss some of the "language of their own culture"; others would miss exposure to children and families of different cultures. However, it takes parental involvement, vigilance, interaction and discussion to help children link what they see on TV with their lives, reflect, clarify, emphasize the main points and place their own interpretations on the programs (Box 17–3). This means that the TV shouldn't be a baby-sitter, shouldn't be on during meals, shouldn't be in the bedroom and should be limited in time and content. The American Academy of Pediatrics advisory on media education gives very clear support for these restrictions, provisions and recommendations.

Most of the discussion about TV also applies to videos and movies. Parents may be more involved in the choices in these venues, and the beginning of a rating system and published reviews are available to help concerned parents make choices. A word of caution, however— many videos labeled for kids, such as TV cartoons, contain violence without consequences, pacing that exceeds children's ability to follow and stereotypes. All these cautions apply to Internet viewing and video games. Research on these influences is just beginning.

A good clinician will be sure that the waiting room TV and/or videos give the right messages about the place of viewing screens in children's lives.

BOX 17–3 PARENT MANAGEMENT OF TELEVISION AND VIDEOS

Spouses should discuss the TV plan for their child on the first birthday and review it every birthday thereafter.

- Never use TV as a reward.
- Limit watching TV to 1 to 2 hours per day maximum.
- Plan what to watch; don't "surf"!
- Turn off the TV when the program ends.
- No TV during meals.
- Consider channel lockouts or V-chips.
- Specifically suggest and set up another activity.
- Discuss programs with kids, including advertising.
- Check on the policy of the use of videos and spot check its practice in daycare, preschool or school.
- Contact local networks and sponsors for accolades and complaints.
- Watch **with** kids.

YOUNG CHILDREN AND COMPUTERS

Computers are now a regular part of the lives of most of America's children beginning in the preschool period. As discussed by Li and Atkins (2004), even most low-income and rural children have frequent access either at home or elsewhere. Access is more frequent and prolonged with higher socioeconomic status. Although computers in schools are nearly universal, many preschools have some computers available as well. About two thirds of families with children have home computers, and most of them have programs for children. According to some reports, parents spend on average over 2 hours per week working with their young children on computers, with children spending a lot more time on their own.

Studies on the developmental impact of computers have not been thoroughly researched, and there are conflicting results given the complex, changing and varied nature of this phenomenon. Although some reports suggest that computer time does nothing to enhance cognitive skills and may even have a negative impact on social skills, the bulk of the evidence suggests the opposite. Some aspects of cognitive ability and school readiness skills, including visual-motor skills, may be enhanced by this exposure. Furthermore, some data suggest that time spent just cruising the computer, becoming familiar with its use, is more valuable to preschoolers than any specific content. Appropriateness of programming and adult supervision are linked to a positive impact within the usual parameters of use.

The Internet has also made inroads, with even preschools using the web with frequencies approaching 10% and rising. This can be an aid to learning in a school-age child and adolescent, but what role it should play in very young children's lives is unknown. It's likely to be negative for any child if inappropriate content is accessed or if it becomes addictive and takes valuable time away from social interaction and physical activity.

Video game playing is in another category and has not been studied in very young children. The violent and solitary nature of most games, with fantasy not differentiable to young children, is likely to prompt the same concerns as television viewing.

DATA GATHERING

What to Observe

The clinician should observe and make note of the following:

- The child's use of toys in the office. Suggest the use of puppets, small doll figures, blocks, small cars, a blackboard. What does playing with toys reveal about the child's cognitive level?
- Ability to fill in empty times (e.g., time in the waiting room or during mother's interview) with imaginary events.
- Does the child approach and play with other kids? How do these interactions go?
- Interest in books. Does he look at the pictures, point, name or tell a story?
- General response to the office environment and any manifestations of fear, wariness. How does the child cope?
- Is the child wearing a costume, a special shirt or carrying a toy that tells you about an interest in "pretend"?

What to Ask

The clinician should ask the following questions during the examination:

- How does the child use fantasy at home?
- What are the child's favorite toys? How are they used?
- Does the child have imaginary friends or an interest in costumes or role-playing?
- What types of books does the child like? How does he read them?
- Does the child discuss imaginary events, sequences or creatures? What role do they serve?
- How much television does she watch? What programs? Are parents present?
- Does the child sing television jingles, talk about advertised products?
- Is the child assigning new functions to familiar objects (e.g., toothbrush becomes a spaceship, a banana is a gun)?
- Is the child having dreams or nightmares?
- What things make the child fearful?
- What is the parents' response to nightmares and fearful situations?
- Who does the child play with? What activities do they do together and how does she play?
- What about "untruths" and "unlawful borrowing"? How is it handled?
- Does a child have regular social experiences with other children?

ASSESSMENT

The following factors should be assessed during the examination:

- Does the child move into puppet or doll play?
- Can the child accept and use your own fantasy suggestion (e.g., tongue blade becomes a car)?
- Will the child accept a nonsense word for a familiar object?
- What does the child do with some nondescript objects (e.g., several tongue blades, paper clips, paper cup)?
- Is the child fearful? If so, how is fear handled?

ANTICIPATORY GUIDANCE

The following are some guidelines for clinicians to help guide parents of toddlers:

- Explain the importance of handling the TV monster. Encourage limiting television to 2 hours per day maximum. Go through child-oriented programs of value. A parent (or other adult) should participate in viewing for at least half the time the child is watching TV. Reflection on show content should occur during and after the show. In other words, parents should make it a social and active event.
- Encourage play with toys that require at least two thirds of their use to be determined by the child (e.g., blocks, balls, toy buildings, dolls, puppets, crayons and paper and simple vehicles).

- Relate to parents the usefulness of stories, imaginary friends, role-playing and "untruths."
- Reflect on the emergence of dreams and nightmares as markers of this new phase of cognitive and affective development. Welcome them as indicators of healthy mental development. Parents should respond to the child's reaction to the nightmare rather than the content of it. Brief reassurance of the parent's protection should be central to this response. Parents should never dismiss or attempt to explain away this or other frightening experiences.
- Parents should read to the child every day. Hand out books from the office and have a variety of books available.
- Parents should preview books and perhaps develop good library habits or exchanges with friends beginning in the third year of life.
- Old clothes and simple costumes are good props for this phase of development.
- Parents should never ignore a child's fears. They tell of the child's inner life and developmental level. Listen patiently.
- Parents should not stress or elaborate on their own concern about a situation that frightens the child. Assurance of parental protection and support is most important.
- Parents should never force the child to meet the object of fears. The child should not be ridiculed or threatened for being afraid.
- If a child appears excessively fearful or nightmares are very frequent, look at the child's daily experience for evidence of overstimulation and exposure to emotions or situations that are overwhelming.

QUICK CHECK—3 YEARS

- ✓ Tells **3** things about himself: first name, last name and age
- ✓ Imitates **3** figures: line, circle and cross
- ✓ Builds **3** cube structures: tower of 8 to 10 cubes, a train and a bridge
- ✓ Uses **3** types of utensils: spoon, fork and cup/pitcher (i.e., can pour liquids)
- ✓ Speaks in **3**-word (or more) phrases or sentences
- ✓ Carries out **3**-step commands
- ✓ Can be understood **three** fourths of the time by a stranger
- ✓ Understands **3** prepositions (e.g., on, under, next to)
- ✓ Counts **3** objects
- ✓ Rides a **3**-wheel vehicle using the pedals
- ✓ Does simple puzzles of **3** or more pieces
- ✓ Dresses with supervision
- ✓ Alternates feet on stairs, at least going up
- ✓ Walks on tiptoe, a few steps at least, on request
- ✓ Does make-believe play
- ✓ Understands (but may not like) turn taking

⚠ HEADS UP–3 YEARS

- Children who fail to develop fantasy play should be looked at very carefully. These children may be found to be in the autistic spectrum of disorders. Delayed or atypical language adds to this concern. Profoundly affected children will hopefully have been identified earlier, but less severely involved children may not be evident until their play and social interaction are seen to be atypical.
- Most children today are in some kind of out-of-home care even if it is a regular play group, Sunday nursery or a formal preschool. If not, evaluate whether a child is getting enough peer interaction.
- Children asked to leave or are thrown out of one or more daycare or preschool setting are at high risk for having significant behavioral or developmental concerns. Most early childhood providers have the skills and patience to work with a wide range of children. A child who falls outside their coping range needs serious evaluation.
- Children who continue to have severe anxiety about separation from family or fail to engage in a supportive preschool/daycare setting need another look. Either their attachment to their care providers is tenuous/strained, they have suffered traumatic separations in the past or they have primary anxiety disorder or depression.
- Depression at this age is characterized by frequent periods of irritability, whininess, rages or fearfulness. Changes in appetite or sleep may or may not be present. A strong family history of depression heightens concern.
- Video screen addicts make their first appearance at this age. Children should spend no more than 2 hours in front of a TV or computer screen each day, and that should be supervised. A TV in the bedroom is a setup for obesity, lowered physical activity and poor sleep patterns.
- With exposure to television advertising, many children develop unhealthy eating habits at this age. Ask and counsel now before such patterns are set up.
- Resistance to go to bed, awakenings with nightmares and returning to their parents' bed are expected at this age. Good sleep rituals and consistent management are needed here. Most children give up naps before age 4. If they do not, expect diminished nighttime sleep.
- Children at this age should be making strokes with crayons and circular elements. The first people drawings should start to make their appearance. If they do not emerge, evaluate fine motor skills, particularly as part of a general developmental appraisal.

RECOMMENDED READINGS

American Academy of Pediatrics: Media education. *Pediatrics* 104:341-343, 1999.

American Academy of Pediatrics: Children, adolescents and television. *Pediatrics* 107:423-426, 2001.

American Academy of Pediatrics: Media violence. *Pediatrics* 108:1222-1226, 2001.

Anderson CA, Bushman BJ: The effects of media violence on society. *Science* 295:2377-2379, 2002.

Bushman BJ, Hussmann LR: Effects of televised violence on aggression. In Singer DG, Singer JL (eds): *Handbook of Children and the Media.* Thousand Oaks, CA, Sage, 2001, pp 223-254.

Elkind D: *The Hurried Child: Growing Up Too Fast Too Soon.* Reading, MA, Addison-Wesley, 1981.

Fraiberg S: *The Magic Years.* New York, Scribner, 1959.

Healy J M: *Endangered Minds: Why Our Children Don't Think.* New York, Simon & Schuster, 1990.

Li X, Atkins M: Early childhood computer experience and cognitive and motor development. *Pediatrics* 113:1715-1722, 2004.

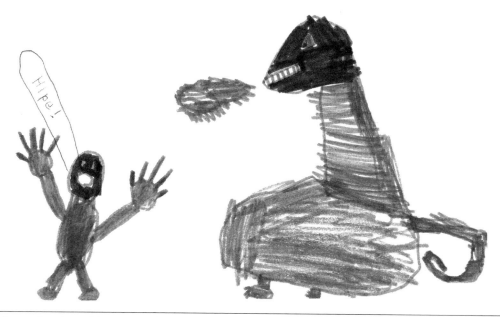

Neil, age 4½, shows his stress in the face of an imaginary dragon attack. His large hands and grounded feet suggest that he feels able to handle this terrifying situation. Aggressive themes are often in the drawings and play of 3- to 6-year-olds and not uncommon later.

CHAPTER 18

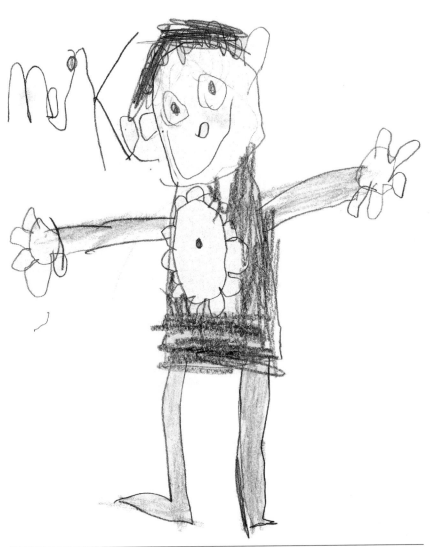

A 5-year-old girl draws a picture of herself. By Meike Messick.

Four Years: Clearer Sense of Self

SUZANNE D. DIXON

This chapter describes the child's central task of establishing an individual identity. The progression of understanding one's gender and sexual self, ethnic identity and how one stands with one's peers is presented. Sexual behavior, typical and worrisome, is discussed. The issues of aggression and the evolution of moral development are placed in a developmental context. These issues are all prominent at this age, but the issues are discussed as they roll out across childhood and adolescence.

Key Words

- **Self-concept**
- **Initiative and Guilt**
- **Gender Identity**
- **Gender Stability**
- **Gender Role**
- **Sexual Exploration**
- **Ethnic Identity**
- **Aggression**
- **Moral Development**

Samuel's mom apologizes as you enter the exam room for a health supervision visit, saying that her son "looks like a mess" today but "he insisted on wearing these clothes." She also apologizes for her delay; the teacher had pulled her aside to say she was worried that Samuel was being "too aggressive on the playground." Mom's concerned about that, as well as that his lying has become frequent. Samuel sits and looks out the window, his Power Ranger in hand, with a Batman T-shirt, a string of beads around his neck and red fingernail polish. A baseball cap tops off his outfit.

The 4-year health supervision visit often brings into sharp focus the important process of development of the self as an individual with definition beyond the immediate family. Exploration of the place, the roles and the identity that one has is the proper work of this age. This is done through observing the modeling of significant others, trying out various persona in looks and actions and experimenting with social roles in the family, the preschool and the neighborhood and with peers. These are the child's laboratories in developing a real sense of self in many dimensions.

The child is beginning to be able to describe himself, whereas before he couldn't even understand the request "Tell me something about yourself." Now this query or a comment

435

TABLE 18–1   **The Emergence of Self-Concept: How Kids Describe Themselves in a Developmental Perspective**

Level	Physical	Activity Based	Social	Psychological
Categorical identification (4–7 yr) Basic descriptive features Concrete, often external	I have green eyes. I'm 5 years old.	I play soccer. I play on the computer.	I'm in Mrs. Smith's class. I'm Jake's friend.	I think about Power Rangers. I'm happy.
Comparative assessments (8–11 yr) The lineup of self with peers Linear, often rigid and rule based	I'm stronger than most kids. I have the longest hair of anyone in my class.	I'm not very good at school. I'm good at math, but I'm not so good at reading. I'm the best kicker on the team.	I'm the second most popular girl in my class. I do well in school because I do more book reports than anyone.	I'm not as smart as most kids. I cry more than the other kids.
Interpersonal implications (12–15 yr) Sense of self based on relationships Personal characteristics as the basis and reasons for relationships Often lack of flexibility	I am soooo ugly; everyone makes fun of me. I have blonde hair, which is good because boys like blondes. No one sits near me because my pimples are so bad.	I play basketball, which is good because girls like athletes. I treat people well so I'll have friends when I need them. I like to join things so I can do things with people.	I can keep a secret, so people trust me. I'm very shy, so I don't have many friends. I can almost always get the rebound, so people pick me for their teams.	I understand people, so they come to me with their problems. I'm the kind of person who loves being with my friends. We can talk about anything.

Modified from Damon W, Hart D: *Self Understanding in Childhood and Adolescence.* New York, 1988, Cambridge University Press.

such as "You look very strong to me" and the follow-up prompts result in a lot of rich information. Damon and Hart have characterized how children from 4 years onward describe themselves along the physical, activity, social and psychological dimensions. These stage shifts testify to how the sense of self emerges over time, in the context of social interactions (Table 18–1). By asking a child to describe himself at health supervision visits through adolescence, first with concrete probes and later with more open-ended questions, we can monitor an increasingly refined **self-concept** along several dimensions. How a child sees himself along these dimensions helps us chronicle this stage-based emergence of a sense of self. A child should be able to define some aspect of himself that is positive and satisfying, even if other dimensions are concerning for himself or others. Home, school, sports and activities are the locations in which a child defines himself. We should ask about activities in these locations in order to tap into how a child sees himself.

A preschool child is faced with the task of gaining enhanced mastery over emotional, sexual and aggressive impulses. He is learning not only who he is, but also how he is expected to behave. More self-control, self-care and self-regulation should be asked of him to support healthy development; the family must be ready to give more over to him at this age. If not, struggles, diminished self-esteem and anger or sadness ensue.

This visit marks the time at which the clinician can really interact in an extended way with the child herself. The child in turn becomes an active and usually cooperative participant in the assessment process. She can converse about past and future events, can ask and answer questions and is often curious about herself. Data are easy to obtain; she'll usually reveal everything by word or action. This should be an efficient and quite entertaining encounter if you focus on what kind of person this child is becoming, how she defines herself and how she gets along in the outside world. Interventions on behavioral regulation, sexual issues and moral development as a foundation for discipline can be very effective at this age. These discussions can now be directed to the child, as well as to the family.

LANGUAGE AND MOTOR DEVELOPMENT: NEW SKILL LEVELS

Enhanced skills in the areas of language and motor development at this late preschool period give the child new ways to figure out who he is (Table 18–2). Language skills blossom during this period, which enables complex social interactions that go beyond the family. They also help the child get more specific information from all aspects of the environment. The child's vocabulary increases, and speech begins to contain all the elements of adult speech with regard to syntax and grammar. The "w" words—who, what, when, etc.—enable him to probe every event in detail. The use of conditional phrases, qualifiers and subordinate clauses means that his narratives, arguments and negotiations are much more complex. Although speech may be slightly imperfect in articulation (e.g., "r's" and "l's" may still be confused), the child is, for the most part, intelligible to strangers (e.g., the health care provider) virtually 100% of the time. He has a whole host of "facts" ready for recitation (Table 18–2). You should be able to have a real, though brief conversation with a 4-year-old. The length, complexity and content will vary by temperament and context. A child of 4 should be able to interface a bit with the outside world without the full interpretive skills of the parent.

Large motor skills have now improved, so more elaborate play and outside activities are available to the 4-year-old (Box 18–1). Fine motor skills have also matured, so work with pencils, scissors and other tools produces more skilled craft creations. Competence in activities that demand greater accuracy or careful timing and sequencing, such as baseball, ballet, soccer, football or a complex project with several steps, is still several years off, although many sports activities are enjoyed and are to be encouraged. The components of these activities that are still to emerge are the following:

- Understanding rule systems and applying them in context
- Advanced motor planning (e.g., running and catching a ball on the run)

TABLE 18–2 **Language and Cognitive Skills in Preschoolers**

Language Area	Ability Level
Vocabulary	Hundreds to thousands of words; parents can't even begin to count
Verbs	Uses suffixes and helper verbs (have, had) to indicate past, ongoing and future
Nouns	Uses plurals, including some but not all irregulars ("mice" but also "feets")
Adjectives and adverbs	Lots
Intelligibility	100% to strangers
Articulation	A few errors ("r" and "l" confusion)
Prosody (emotional expressiveness)	Lots
Content	Asks questions using "w" words Uses clauses and phrases Understands conditionals; e.g., "If it rains tomorrow, we will ..." Can give full name, gender and age of self and siblings; name of the teacher; and the name of at least one friend and can describe that friend Identify colors, perhaps some letters and numbers. May write name or a few letters Can identify composition of object and function ("What's a car made of?"; "What does your heart do?") Can follow a story, anticipate events and ascribe feelings and motivation ("What will happen next?"; "How does he feel?") Copies a "+" Draws a person with two to five parts Sustained cooperative play

- Sustained attention to the actions of others (e.g., anticipating the action on a playing field)
- Memory skills (e.g., football plays; baseball instruction, "if this happens, do that")
- Ability to conceive of the steps of a task leading to completion (e.g., basketball play setup)

Although these activities may be introduced at this age, pressure to succeed at team sports should not be applied. These activities will look very different at this age than they will even 1 to 2 years later. Cooperative group games, excursions around town and craft activities involving more than one step can be anticipated, learned and enjoyed.

Four-year-olds can assume more responsibility for washing and dressing themselves. They should pick their own clothes within the bounds of cleanliness, decency and specific outside rules (e.g., long pants for church). They should be able to do simple, regular household chores, although these should be one- to two-step tasks (e.g., collect the wastebaskets and throw their contents in a bin) and very specific (e.g., "pick up the blocks," not "clean your room"). Practiced, prompted and praised activities always take more time than the adult doing the task, but these

> ## BOX 18–1   MOTOR SKILLS IN PRESCHOOLERS
>
> - Walks up and down stairs, alternating feet
> - Skips on one foot
> - Can broad jump
> - Climbs up jungle gym
> - Throws overhand and catches a large ball
> - Stands on one foot for longer than 10 seconds
> - Holds a crayon well
> - Uses scissors
> - Can use a computer mouse
> - Uses table utensils well except a knife
> - Pours reliably
> - Dresses self (mostly, most of the time)

are ways to build a sense of responsibility on top of the child's new skills. This will build a sense of self that includes being a contributing member of a family.

SOCIAL AND EMOTIONAL DEVELOPMENT

Much of the developmental work of this period has to do with the acquisition of enhanced self-control over sexual, emotional and aggressive impulses through identification with important adults and older children in the child's life. Internalization of norms and expectations for behavior is part of development of the concept of self. Self-regulation is the working task here. Acceptance of the limits of behavior through identification with positive role models is the job.

Freud emphasized the strong attachment that children, beginning at 3 to 5 years old, show for the parent of the opposite sex. This closeness is often associated with a certain amount of anxiety that motivates the child at about 6 years of age to redirect identification to the parent of the same sex. Successful negotiation of this "Oedipal phase" helps instill the beliefs, morals and behavioral manner of the parents, including the societally defined gender-specific behavior.

Lisa told her mom she was going to marry daddy when she grew up. She then marched off in her mother's shoes.

Erik Erikson emphasized the conflict between the feelings of **initiative and guilt** at this age. Taking the lead, standing up for oneself and making needs clear are a big part of the work at this age.

Jared grabbed back the toy crane that Michael had just taken from him and said he had it first and wasn't finished. Then he asked Derek to play with him. They "did cars" in the corner.

Learning to take social initiatives without ever feeling excessively guilty or impinging excessively on the rights and feelings of others is a sign of healthy emotional development during the preschool period. Conversely, a child who is always bullied, is taken advantage of or uses adults as mediators all the time needs some support to take more initiative in social interactions. All kids swing back and forth between the extremes, but a child who is overly shy or clingy all the time or, conversely, overly intrusive to others needs help. The bully, one who knows how to relate only through aggression, domination or disrespect of others, also isn't on track with this developmental work. Children who have no friends at this age or who are always marginalized in the preschool or neighborhood are of concern. The other kids know whether a child is beyond the norms of aggression, guilt or dependence on adults, even if they cannot report why that child is disliked. Other children are generally good barometers of appropriate social adjustment.

DEVELOPMENT OF GENDER CONCEPT

The part of self-concept that includes gender emerges in stages, beginning at birth but becoming prominent in the preschool period. One's *anatomical gender* is obviously determined at conception and during fetal life, and many components of sexual behavior, perceptual and cognitive structures and aspects of emotional life are influenced by genetic and prenatal forces. When the gender of an infant becomes known, the interpersonal environment starts to add to that definition of self. Parents immediately begin a style of interaction that varies by gender in talking, in holding, in expectations and in the application of meanings to appearance and behavior. This *gender attribution* is difficult to change after it is ascribed in the first hours to days after birth.

Doug Martin described his newborn son as "really strong." Eric Johnson told the doctor he was surprised how delicate his newborn daughter's hands were—"like my wife's."

Genital exploration begins in infancy, but a peak of interest occurs in the middle of the second year. By 2 years of age, a child knows that she is a girl and that genital touching is pleasurable. She has a **gender identity** that is nearly impossible to alter thereafter. Furthermore, she is able to classify other people correctly by gender using hair or clothing. The continuity, immutability and permanence of this attribute (**gender stability**), however, will take years to be clearly acquired, so it's not uncommon for a young preschooler to say that he will grow up to be a mommy or that the new baby girl will become a "big boy like me." The exploration of different identities with cross-gender dress-up, fantasy play, stories and statements is the way children learn that gender is a stable part of one's self. In preschool this is an appropriate, normal activity. Children younger than 3, and often older, define gender by external attitudes rather than by differences in genitals, although when asked, they reveal that they know that boys are, in the words of Mr. Rogers, "fancier on the outside" whereas girls are "fancier on the inside." Clothing, hair styles and possessions may actually be more salient, hence the belief that gender may be as changeable as your costume.

The preschool years are ones in which a child acquires a sense of what expected, gender-specific behavior is. This is the beginning of acquisition of the **gender role**, the external behavior that reflects the inner gender identity. Play activities and toy preferences, language, body posture and movement start to become subtly differentiated in the second year but become striking by age 4. Children are more rigid than adults in judging what is gender-appropriate play after age 5, no matter how liberal or how restrictive their environment has been, because they cling to rules and predictability to order their world. As they solidify an understanding of this aspect of themselves without the ability to blend categories of anything, they may go through almost hyper-male or hyper-female role-playing. This stereotyped definition of gender role stays through grade school.

When asked if the girls in his school played baseball, Samuel, age 6, replied that that was silly. "Girls don't play baseball; they do soccer."

Specific interest in the genitals of self, as well as others, reaches another peak at this age, so **sexual exploration** is to be expected. Sexual interest then goes underground at about age 6 with the forces of socialization and with children learning that sexualized interest or behavior, at least that done in public, draws disapproval. Children older than 6 who are still seductive or exhibitionistic or do any sexual exploring publicly are atypical and require further investigation.

Interest in sexual issues bubbles just under the surface across grade school, however, as evidenced by the fascination with jokes, words, gestures or stories that have to do with elimination or implied sexual function. These continue throughout grade school. Peeks at pornographic material, as well as renewed interest in sexual information, are common as middle school approaches. During adolescence, sexual interests are prominent as the child works toward an understanding of the sexual part of himself, his sexual orientation and intimacy (see Chapters 21 to 23).

Boys' Play and Girls' Play

We can learn a lot from the play patterns of kids, so it's not lost time to ask about it at any age. From the preschool period on, play shows marked gender differences. Although scientists note these in the second and third year and some studies even show infancy differences, it's really beyond age 3 that these play pattern differences are obvious. Boys play more physical games and hierarchical and one-upmanship games in which there is a winner and a loser; they are likely to play in larger groups. Their games usually involve a lot more action, even if played on a computer. Boys can be seen building the highest tower or the longest train. They like to say they run the fastest and gladly report successes in competitive play. They may be threatened if someone suggests an alternative activity.

Girls play in smaller groups and have games in which there is no winner or even an endpoint. They enjoy the process of play with a lot of inclusion in role-playing. They are less overtly aggressive, although verbal aggression and some manipulation of people are regularly observed. Girls build enclosures; they change roles frequently so that everyone gets a turn at being the boss, the teacher or the mom. They try to get lots of kids involved with their play and

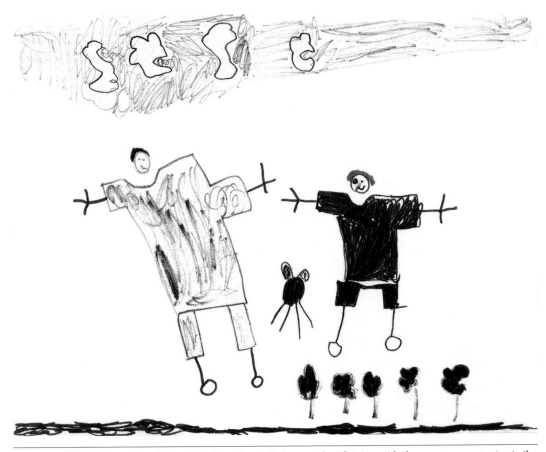

A 6-year-old aligns himself with his dad, with a dog in between. Identification with the same-sex parent sets the stage for defining oneself. By Johnathan Zuidema, age 6. (Note the landscape.)

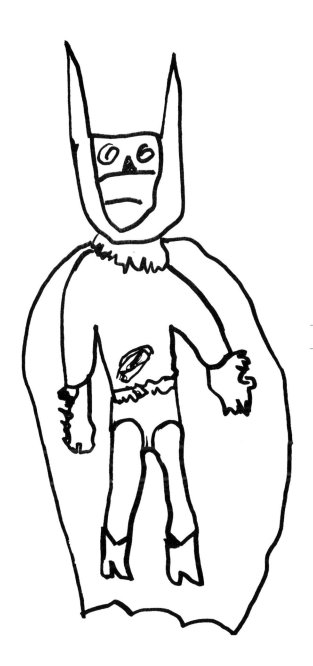

"A picture of me." By T. W.

may make offers to get them to do so (e.g., "you can be the mom if we play house"). They like it when people have other ideas, but they generally try to reshape the proposal, engaging in what is often a prolonged negotiation. Both sexes imitate household activities as they play house at age 3. The girls take over at age 4, and the boys run around with their own, more active games. Standoffs, space violations and mutual raiding of play spaces continue to occur, however. After age 5, children with a clear sexual identity will choose same-sex playmates if they have a choice.

Sexualized Behavior

Young children will often engage in behavior that reflects their interest in these sexual matters; this should be expected. Parental responses should be in concert with a family's own values, but they should include clear, nonhysterical feedback from which the child can learn the expected norms. Shaming a child, punishing without explanation or refusing to discuss this area of behavior sets the stage for sexual problems later. Moral, social and family rules may restrict specific behavior; the clinician should be aware of what's abnormal for children at a given age, developmentally harmful or indicative of inappropriate sexual experience or emotional deprivation. Box 18–2 lists some parameters to apply when confronted with questions about whether some sexualized behavior is within the normal range.

Sexual behavior is likely to emerge and be obvious in the preschool period, whether it is flirtatious behavior with an adult or exploratory behavior with another child, so it's a good

---

BOX 18–2   SEXUAL BEHAVIOR IN CHILDHOOD—WHEN TO BE WORRIED

- Masturbation begins in infancy and is nearly universal from toddlerhood on. There is no evidence that it is problematic unless one of the following is true:
  It is compulsive and takes a child away from other activities
  It is consistently done in public in spite of counsel to do otherwise
  It is done in groups
  It is done with objects
- Exploring of other children's genitals, or "playing doctor," is very common. It is worrisome if one of the following is true:
  It is forceful exposure or touching, not mutual
  The participants are more than 2 years apart in age
  Penetration is attempted
  Behavior is accompanied by aggressive themes or activities
- Infrequent interest in pornography is common, but repeated, chronic interest is a concern
- Simulated intercourse or penetration with objects is abnormal in childhood
- Explicit sexual conversations with significantly older or younger children
- Preoccupation with sexual themes in play or conversation
- Sexual activities or exploration with animals
- Violent sexual ideas, themes in play or actions

time to elicit parents' concerns and to encourage sex education at the level of the child's concerns. Areas of concern should be given developmental context.

"Sex education" begins in infancy with establishment of comfort with physical touching and emotional closeness. It becomes explicit in this preschool period when children begin to connect sex organs with reproduction and sensual pleasure, and it includes the development of the ability to set limits and not be forced to closeness on any level. Children should be given the freedom to ask questions about this area. Parents should provide accurate answers for the questions asked, following the child's lead. At this age, a full explanation of sexual intercourse is not usually needed or wanted. Parents who follow a child's lead generally provide the right level of information and set the stage for coming back for more when the child is ready.

Annie paraded around the living room in her mom's nightie while her dad read the paper. She said she was practicing her dancing.

Sexual Exploration

Preschool children show a great deal of interest in the "private area" (roughly the part of the body covered by a bathing suit) of themselves and others. Games involving undressing or exploration of another child's body are common by age 4. "Toilet talk" becomes particularly interesting as the structure and function of these private areas are verbally explored. Sex play, sometimes played as "mother and father" or "doctor," is common in preschool children. Children of this age often attempt to engage in physical contact with other family members, such as touching their mother's breasts; both "exhibitionistic" and "voyeuristic" activities are common and normal. Such behavior should be seen in the positive sense that it testifies to the child's work on resolution of these important relationships. It does not predict continuance of this behavior, but does demand explicit feedback about what the norms really are in the home and school.

Mrs. Allen found Jessica and her friend Kyle, both 4, under the blankets in Jessica's room. Jessica's panties were down and they both looked guilty. Jessica said they were playing house. Mrs. Allen explained that "clothes off is not good play." She redirected them to some play outside. A similar episode was never repeated.

Such behavior in children can lead to conflict between parent and child and can also create strained relationships between parents with differing views on management. It is helpful for the pediatric clinician to be able to reassure parents that sexual play among preschool children is a natural consequence of growth in the child's cognitive, emotional and social development. The parents' response will reflect their own views, but it should incorporate this developmental framework. Parents can be told that children of this age are intensely interested in learning about themselves and their bodies and that this interest extends to other children and adults as well. In fact, this is the age at which children are most likely to notice differences between individuals, including differences in weight, race and eye color, as well as sex organs. Again, observing and noting these differences help the child obtain a clearer sense of herself as a unique individual with specific traits and characteristics.

At what point parents need to set limits on sexual exploration by preschool children is a matter for each family to decide, consistent with its own values and tolerance for such behavior. Parents may be told, however, that overreacting to sexual play in childhood may only temporarily suppress such behavior, actually heighten sexual curiosity and create unnecessary anxiety in the child. On the other hand, parents who are overly permissive may expose their child to situations that are beyond his ability to handle. This, in turn, may be anxiety provoking for the child. In general, parents should be helped to communicate to their children that an interest in the genital organs is healthy and natural, but that nudity and sex play are not generally acceptable in public, between children and adults or when forced on anyone. Parents should discuss the degree of nudity allowed in a family to ensure consistency. Parents should also tell children of this age that no other person (including friends and family) has permission to touch them on their "private area." Such conversations between parent and child should take place on numerous occasions before adolescence if the child is to incorporate these values as his own level of understanding matures.

ETHNIC IDENTITY

In the preschool years children become increasingly aware of the differences between people and the similarities and differences between themselves and others. With an interest in categorizing and labeling these observed differences, preschoolers come face to face with racial differences and **ethnic identity**. By the age of 4, children can sort dolls and pictures by ethnicity and, even at age 3, will be able to group people about half the time. Skin color is less salient than other features such as dress, behavior and speech. They then can label themselves on this dimension. This is the age to discuss racial differences in appearance as these issues emerge, either by direct questions or through stares by children. Children exposed to a multi-racial environment may notice ethnic differences earlier; those with less exposure may be less aware. Nonetheless, before school age, children clearly notice, label and then begin to develop expectations based on ethnic differences. If parents don't want these concepts guided entirely by outside (particularly media) forces, they have to take opportunities to discuss stereotypes, prejudice and pejorative language directly. If racial issues are dismissed as not appropriate to talk about, children will develop their own ideas. These ideas will be shaped by what they see and hear and will be in line with their cognitive imperatives to label, categorize and make linkages. Children will not be kept "color-blind" by putting this issue underground.

AGGRESSIVE BEHAVIOR

Overly aggressive behavior may become a problem during the preschool years because emotions, a sense of self and identification with powerful figures are developmental themes. A child engages in problematic aggressive behavior when she shows a disregard for the feelings, property, rights or physical safety of other individuals. Aggressive behavior can be distinguished from assertive behavior, in which the child attempts to satisfy her own needs in a direct, energetic, perhaps even willful manner while still respecting the basic rights of other children.

In contemporary Western culture, we want our children to certainly be assertive (and a *little* aggressive), but not *really* aggressive. The child must struggle to keep **aggression** under *her own control* while becoming appropriately assertive. The balance is hard to achieve and is probably a lifelong process; the struggle is prominent at this age. The expanded social world and enhanced interpersonal abilities bring this issue forward at this age.

Some theorists find that aggression is a biological instinct and believe that better child-rearing practices channel this aggressive instinct into socially acceptable behavior. Because our evolutionary past favors successful competition, we are prewired to be aggressive. Other theorists view the development of aggressive behavior as a response to frustration in the early life of a child and positive reinforcement for aggressive behavior, which occurs in some families, and as a result of a child following the model of powerful adults who exhibit aggressive behavior. The former theory of aggression as instinct is supported by the ubiquity of aggressive behavior in preschool children. Films taken of children in preschool settings indicate that all children engage in aggressive acts toward their peers many times each hour. Other evidence shows that girls will engage in frequent aggressive behavior like boys do, provided that they feel relatively ensured of going undetected; girls may also be particularly verbally assaultive.

These aggressive acts are rewarded in early childhood because most of the time the aggressor gets what he wants. On the other hand, theories that view aggression as a learned response are supported by studies showing that many problematically aggressive preschoolers come from homes in which the parent-child relationship is of a hostile, rejecting type or where interpersonal and environmental violence is often present. Such children may merely be imitating their parents' disciplinary behavior or interpersonal style. A child's aggressive behavior may be the only behavior that draws parental attention, thereby embedding such behavior as a habit and style for the child. Television and movies model physical aggression as the way to solve problems, and aggressiveness may be increased by this exposure (see Chapter 15).

Developmental Course

The developmental course of aggression is that aggressive physical acts to get a desired object typically begin early in the second year. By the third year, they are surpassed in frequency by verbal aggression. *Hostile aggression*, an aggressive act designed to hurt another person without any object being involved, may become prominent in the fourth to sixth years and requires support to resolve. Girls particularly exhibit *relational aggression* as they isolate, distance or exclude another person. In preschool, children challenge many other children of different ages, sizes and abilities. By grade school, they have learned to restrict the targets of aggressive challenge to kids with whom they have a chance of winning. These tussles are inevitable and provide an opportunity to learn about self, relationships, negotiation skills and the limits of behavior. Unless conflicts are excessive, adults should stay out of the middle because children need to learn to self-regulate. Significant imbalance in this back-and-forth or escalating pattern between peers or siblings may require some intervention, suggestions for alternatives or exploration for the basis of the excessively combative interaction. Arguments and some fighting are inevitable, however.

Behavior That Calls for Closer Attention

Preschools in general understand these outbursts of aggression and usually help children learn to control themselves, use words to negotiate and redirect their attention. If a preschool says that a child is overly aggressive to the point that staff members cannot handle her or don't see progress, this is a serious concern for the clinician to address. Being thrown out of preschool is highly suggestive of a serious behavioral problem that demands clinical attention.

To understand a particular child's aggressive behavior, the clinician can take an appropriate history from the parent. The following are things that trigger the need for exploration of the chief complaint of aggressive behavior:

- The more serious the aggressive behavior is (i.e., bodily harm)
- The more frequently it occurs
- The more widespread the settings (home, school and community)
- The more frequently that hostile aggression occurs rather than object competition aggression

Isolated instances of aggressive behavior, regardless of the degree of actual physical or property damage incurred, can be part of a normative growth process. A child who appears chronically angry or anxious is more worrisome than a child whose aggressive act comes out of a positive, open approach to life in general. An angry child may not feel good about himself or his place in the family or society or trust that his needs will be met with consistency. Sad (depression) is very close to mad (anger) and bad (misbehavior) in early childhood. Chronic aggressors may be depressed or anxious youngsters. These issues call for further exploration, suggestions for support for a more positive self-image or, occasionally, referral to a mental health professional.

DISGUISED ANGER AND AGGRESSION

The following are examples of behavior that is really disguised aggression:

- Fecal soiling in a child who has previously demonstrated normal bowel control
- Fecal smearing
- Intentional self-destructive, self-injurious behavior
- Intended destruction of objects
- Willful harm to animals

 Jeremy came into the classroom while everyone else was outside. He opened several kids' lunches and stepped on their sandwiches.

Biting behavior beyond the age of 2½ calls for further exploration. It indicates a delay in language, lots of anger or levels of frustration beyond the norm. Such behavior must usually be interpreted as angry, aggressive acts. An "accident- prone" child may likewise be demonstrating aggressive behavior toward self. Girls who are labeled "sneaky" may be covertly aggressive, and this label should not be disregarded. Children labeled by other children as *bullies* generally need at least short-term intervention. Children's drawings with teeth, strong force lines and lots of forceful coloring-in should be looked at carefully and cautiously to see whether aggression is predominant in feeling and thought.

BEGINNINGS OF MORAL DEVELOPMENT

Through a gradual process of identification of parents, the foundation for **moral development** is laid down. A 4-year-old shows increasing reasoning ability and can apply this ability to some moral issues, but the child is still "flawed" in judgment because of thought processes. She can understand rules but still bends them to accommodate immediate circumstances, especially under pressure. The primary goal is to obtain approval and reward (and avoid negative outcomes), so behavior is still shaped by a close link between behavior and consequences. A 4-year-old can understand the idea of promises but can't always keep them herself when time or new circumstances intervene. The child can recognize the difference between truth and fantasy but doesn't always tell the whole and complete truth.

Justin told his mom that he didn't break his brother's truck, in spite of clear physical evidence and the lack of another, plausible suspect. He said he was trying to fix it.

"Inaccurate talk" is a better term than "lies" at this age. Premeditated plans to deceive will be a possibility after the age of 6 to 7 years. At age 4, the child can recognize the rights of others ("It's Johnny's turn now."), but not always respect those rights because his own needs are paramount. Property rights are often a little vague, particularly if the property is attractive. The child may really believe that he's "just borrowing" a toy. He cannot cognitively take the part of the other "dispossessed child," so an appeal to retrospective empathy really has no meaning at this age.

Merrill said that her friend Kristin had said she could borrow her Barbie when it came home with Merrill from preschool. Kristin's mom called later, saying her daughter said Merrill stole it and that she was crying. Merrill and her mother drove over and returned it.

On the other hand, a 4-year-old demonstrates a good sense of justice ("That's not fair; Jason never gets to be first.") and can show unselfish sympathy and concern for others when directly confronted with some unfairness or sadness on the face of another.

Moral judgments must be confined to the immediate instance, so lessons should be structured with the specific (e.g., "Give Sarah's book back. She did not say you could borrow it," *not* "Don't take other people's stuff."). A 4-year-old wants to please, wants approval and may even become a bit self-righteous in this newfound awareness of the rules that govern conduct. The child likes consistency, clear expectations and instances in which the same judgment is applied to every-one. Direct, specific feedback on both correct and incorrect choices, as well as the experience of consequences being closely linked to actions, is the force that begins to infuse a moral code at this age. The child's moral sense is still linked to the specific consequences of her actions rather than any abstract moral code. She is building that sense over time through specific interactions and reactions.

DATA GATHERING

What to Observe

- What is the child wearing? Does this reflect some aspect of who he is trying to become and who he wants to be?
- In the waiting room, what does he do, play with and say? The office staff can really help.
- What is his relationship with his mom or dad? Has it seemed to change since the last health supervision visit? What are his signs of growing independence?
- Does he initiate an interaction with you? Does he carry on a conversation?
- Does his manner or appearance reflect a specific gender identity?
- What toys or activities does he bring with him? What do these tell you about his sense of self?
- What kind of picture does he draw? What does it reveal about him? How does he hold the crayon?
- Does he separate from the parent easily, such as for weighing or another nonstressful event?
- Can he dress and undress himself? Does the parent intervene, expecting a problem?
- Can he follow a three-step command and get up on the exam table without difficulty?
- Is there appropriate shyness about examination of the genitals or even undressing?

What to Ask

The following are examples of questions to ask the child:

- How are you? Why did you come today? Comment on appearance, clothing or possessions that are evident.
- Do you have anything you want checked? Is there anything you want to ask me?
- How are things in school/daycare/home, good or not so good?
- What is your favorite thing to do there? What is bad that you have to do?
- Tell me your friend's name? What do you do together? What do you play?

These questions and conversation should be continued as you explore how this child sees herself in her world and who is important in her world. You are also listening for language, in line with the skills outlined in Table 18–2. Specific questions are presented in Table 18–3. You should be able to understand all of the child's speech. Parents should allow and enjoy this conversation; excessive intrusion at this age means something is of concern.

TABLE 18–3 **Questions to Be Asked during Examination**

Questions for Children	Objective
Does a dog live at your house? Is it a boy or girl dog? How can you tell?	Assess the child's awareness of sexual differences; if the clinical situation suggests any confusion in the child's own gender identity, the clinician may follow with questions such as "How can you tell if you are a boy/girl?"; "What do you like about being a boy/girl?"; "Is there anything you don't like about being a boy/girl?"
What do you do when you want something and mommy/daddy says you can't have it?	Assess the child's perception of his own responses to parental limit setting: does the child admit to throwing tantrums that he later regrets (a good sign)? Does the child relate a number of different levels of responding to frustration (e.g., "sometimes I cry, but sometimes I just go to my room and play.")?
How do you like your preschool/daycare center, etc. (by name if possible)?	Assess the child's reaction to and success in separation from family members.
What kinds of play activity does your child enjoy?	Parental reports can provide much information about the child's actual motor skills (e.g., "Can she ride a three-wheeler?") and social skills.
What does the child's preschool teacher (baby-sitter, grandparent, etc.) say about him/her?	Obtain additional information about the child's personality and behavior while separated from parents, and at the same time assess parents' openness to feedback about their child from outside the home; some parents find it difficult to accept any negative feedback about their child, whereas other parents seem surprised at favorable reports from outsiders about a child with whom they are experiencing difficulty.
What do you like most about your child? What would you say is his/her most troublesome quality?	Determine the parents' capacity to identify and articulate the child's positive and negative qualities; an inability to report some highly positive quality is unusual for parents and should be a sign for further evaluation by the clinician.
How often does he/she misbehave? What kinds of things does your child do? What do you usually do when this happens?	An assessment of discipline practices at this age is absolutely essential; the clinician should be alert to the presence of inappropriately high or low behavioral expectations during this period; disciplinary techniques may be inconsistently applied, too harsh or otherwise ineffective.

TABLE 18–3 Questions to Be Asked during Examination—cont'd

Questions for Children	Objective
Do you take your child out to dinner at a friend's house or a restaurant?	Assesses the parents' comfort with their efforts to help the child meet social expectations outside the home; regardless of the parents' standard of behavior, parents should have a degree of confidence in their child's behavior by age 4 or 5.
How does your child act when angry? What does your child usually do when another child grabs something away from him/her?	Allows the parents to discuss concerns regarding the child's aggressive behavior or lack of aggressive behavior.
How does your child show you that he/she knows he/she is a boy/girl?	Allows the parents to discuss the child's gender identity formation and their own degree of comfort with it.
Has your child expressed an interest in his/her body by asking questions or by examining him/herself or other people?	Allows the parents to discuss evidence of sexual curiosity in the child while defining this as a normative process.
Does your child behave differently around his/her father/mother than around you? In what way are your child's relationships different with each of his/her parents?	Provides an opportunity for the parents to discuss the Oedipal phenomenon at its various stages while allowing the clinician to assess and comment on the age appropriateness of this behavior.

Parental issues should also be elicited. Some exploration of these issues should be done with the child present, but all sensitive or negative concerns should be discussed without the child. The child can be asked to draw with the supervision of office staff, or a return appointment can be set up. Any sign of serious shame or embarrassment calls for a change in the venue of the discussion. Children should not be shamed or embarrassed, although their own views of difficulties should be elicited.

Dr. Gann said to Mark, "Your mom tells me you've had to stay in from the playground many times. Tell me how that happens. What starts these problems?"

Ask parents for several details about the child's life, such as the following:

- Child's favorite type of play
- Child's favorite toys
- Child's preferred playmates
- These all give clues to the child's sense of himself.
- Ask how the child contributes to the household with chores, duties.
- Ask about how much self-care she does.

ANTICIPATORY GUIDANCE

The following guidelines can help the clinician guide parents of 4-year-olds:

- Assess the appropriateness of the child's preschool setting. Does she need more or less structure, more or less self-control? What are her relationships with the other children? Does she have friends and engage in cooperative, sustained play?

- Discuss the normalcy of sexual exploration at this level. Elicit questions and concerns.

- Discuss with the family appropriate limit setting, management and the importance of consistency in family expectations.

- Discuss toys and play vis-à-vis a broad range of interests but with expectations of sex-specific activities. Stress the importance of role-playing.

- Explain the importance of reviewing television and movies that children watch and of limiting exposure to violent and/or sexual themes and sex stereotyping.

- Explain the importance of peer play and help a family orchestrate playmates if this does not occur naturally. A child this age should bring kids home (or participate in parent-initiated get-togethers), or the parents should find out why the child does not.

- Explain the basis for outbursts against the same-sex parent and "over" attachment to the opposite-sex parent. Physical closeness should continue, with parents being alert to the need to limit overly sexualized behavior.

- Children should have regular responsibilities around the house.

- Self-care should be nearly complete, although checks and prompts on cleanliness, as well as finishing touches, will still be needed.

- Discuss stories with social or moral themes. Begin to build a sense of systems, rules and norms.

- Discuss sex education for the preschooler. This usually includes providing names for all genital parts and explaining that touching of genitals should be done only in private and that breasts are for feeding babies. Parents should answer the child's questions but not overload her with too much information at one time.

- Children need to be counseled about their own private parts, that they are for no one to touch except parents and health care providers. Children should be empowered to resist all touches that feel bad. Parents should give them permission to discuss these. All reports of bad touches should be taken seriously.

- Caution parents about the differences between "inaccurate talk" and "lies" and the difficulty with respecting the property rights of others at this age.

- Overly aggressive behavior should be discouraged but *not* answered with aggression because that gives a mixed message and has been shown *not* to be successful. Encourage parents to model appropriate problem solving.

- Differences between people (because of individual, ethnic or disabled characteristics) should be discussed openly, neutrally and positively. Children's curiosity about these issues should be respected.

- Discuss the importance of family rituals and traditions in giving children a sense of self.

- Children enjoy going through baby books and seeing old pictures of themselves as they struggle with a sense of self. Going over a baby book and displaying baby pictures are good ideas. Telling the birth story or a special anecdote helps define one's point.

! HEADS UP—4 YEARS

- Children who adamantly and persistently insist that they are of their opposite gender, particularly if they repudiate their genitalia, need further psychiatric evaluation.
- A child described as a persistent bully or one who is often the target of bullying needs further evaluation and intervention at home, in preschool and beyond.
- At this age, a child should be understood by a stranger (e.g.: the clinician) virtually 100% of the time, with only minor articulation difficulties. If not, a speech and language evaluation and hearing test are needed.
- Vision should be easy to test using a chart. Vision should be better then 20/30 in each eye. If not, opthalmological referral needed.
- Children still biting at this age need a behavioral exam. This degree of uncontrolled anger and its primitive manifestation need a mental health referral. The same holds for fecal smearing.
- Children at this age should be doing the bulk of their self-care: bathing, dressing, eating. If not, there is something concerning in the child, the parent and/or the interaction between them.
- Children not daytime toilet trained at this time need a second look for urological issues and development generally, unusual environmental circumstances or unusual parent/child interaction. Resistance to training after age 4 is likely to be very difficult to manage.

ACKNOWLEDGMENT

This chapter benefits from the earlier contributions of Nicholas Putnam, M.D.

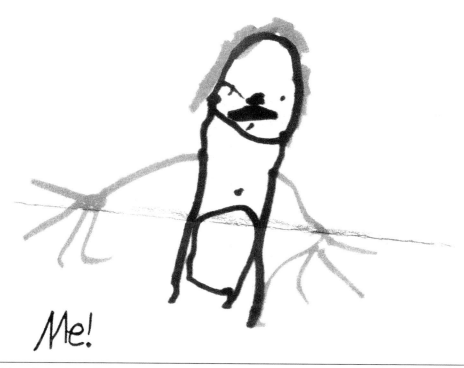

"Me." A boy depicts himself. The sexual themes shown by the form, the lower appendage and the belly button are obvious. These elements show the normal interests of the age. By Logan Henderson, age 5.

CHAPTER 19

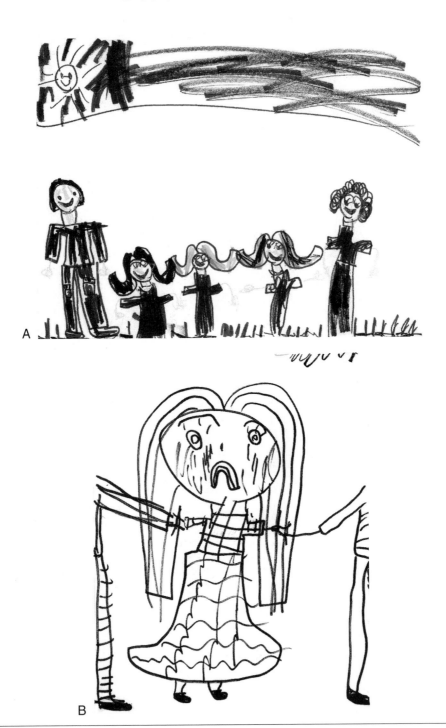

A, A 5-year-old shows her upbeat spirit in this drawing of family and friends (original in bright-colored markers). **B**, The same 5-year-old shows herself clinging to her parents' hands, reluctant to separate for a school event. School entry has its ups and downs (original in dark brown). By Katherine Auerswald.

Five Years: Opening the School Door

MARTIN T. STEIN

Kindergarten represents a significant set of developmental expectations and achievements that come together as a child achieves mastery of specific cognitive, social and motor skills. Neurological maturation, preschool learning and interactions with peers and family members are some of the elements that can be assessed objectively at this visit. Understanding a child's educational and social strengths and vulnerabilities can assist both parents and pediatricians in planning for school entry.

Key Words

- Assessing Strengths and Vulnerabilities
- Individual Variation
- Language
- Communication Skills
- Attentiveness
- Prereading Skills
- Separation and Socialization
- Drawing Interview

FOCUS OF DEVELOPMENTAL WORK

Entry into kindergarten between 5 and 6 years of age is a time of significant developmental expectations and achievements. It is a moment when multiple biological events and psychosocial tasks find a common ground focused on educational and social achievements—sustained attention for classroom learning, prolonged separation from parents, comprehension and expression of language and interactive and cooperative play (Box 19–1). It is a time when children develop a sense of mastery through achievements in cognitive, social and motor skills. For the majority of children who have been in preschool, kindergarten is a natural extension of an earlier learning experience. However, contemporary educational expectations of kindergarten students are similar to those of first and second grade students one or two generations ago! The kindergarten experience may have an enduring influence. Getting off to a good start is of critical importance.

Entering kindergarten is a qualitative change in cognitive and psychosocial tasks compared with preschool experiences. Children are still in the preoperational ("prelogical") stage of cognitive development. Their responses to the environment are guided by egocentric, animistic (giving living status to inanimate objects) and idiosyncratic thinking processes (see Chapter 2). Imagination and fantasy run high. It is also a time when gender identification is explored in interactive games and dress. Simultaneous with these cognitive and psychological growth characteristics is an acceleration of language (both expressive and receptive) and articulation.

> **BOX 19–1   DEVELOPMENTAL TASKS FACING CHILDREN AT SCHOOL ENTRY**
>
> - Separation
> - Increasing individualization
> - Integration of cognitive skills required to learn to read
> - Ability to form relationships with other children and adults
> - Ability to participate in group activities and follow rules and directions
> - Gradual formation of a sense of self or identity, both inside and outside the family environment

A pediatrician who understands the importance of this moment in development is prepared to make the most of the 5-year health supervision visit.

Knowledge about the family's educational expectations, stability and potential to monitor school progress is an important observation that a clinician should make at this time. A primary care provider who has provided longitudinal care for a child about to enter kindergarten is aware of the risk factors (e.g., prematurity, hearing impairment, family disharmony, mental illness) that may have an impact on cognitive skills and social learning. This knowledge can guide a focused school entry evaluation by tailoring observations, questions and screening tests to meet the needs of an individual child and family.

The focus of this visit is to discover a child's **strengths and vulnerabilities** that will have an impact on school function. It is not a "school readiness" examination to determine whether a child has the skills to enter kindergarten. Most children at this age will be in a school experience, ready or not. The goal here is to identify and inform parents about those aspects of development that will either further or hinder success. If not, they will and should enter some modified learning milieu. When clinicians attend to the wide variability in normal development, the 5-year-old office visit will be a useful guide for parents and teachers. When a clinician discovers a significant delay in development (e.g., in language, visual-perceptual or social skills) or an emotional vulnerability, appropriate assessments can be planned, followed by communication with the child's school. Then they can be ready for a particular child, with adaptations geared to ensure success.

THEORETICAL FRAMEWORK

The conceptual framework of cognitive social learning theory is a valuable clinical tool in understanding the reciprocal interactions that shape an individual's sense of competence (see Chapter 2). Bandura's model of social learning emphasizes the important influences of modeled and observed behavior on learning. Mastery of a cognitive or social task brings to the child a developing sense of competence as an individual. Cognitive social learning theory takes into account the mutual influences of the individual, the physical and psychosocial environment and the task or behavior to be learned. All these factors are important in learning.

A skilled clinician approaches the evaluation of a child's school readiness with healthy caution because the **individual variation** in "normal" behavior and cognitive function at this age is substantial. *Readiness at a given age does not necessarily imply either accelerated or retarded development.* The purpose of a school entry evaluation should not be placed in the context of prediction of disease, a condition or dysfunction, but as a clinical opportunity to optimize the chance for a successful early school experience. The limitation of existing tools for assessment and the potential power of a medical pronouncement support the need for proceeding with caution in the evaluation for school readiness.

The time before school entry is an opportunity for the clinician to systematically review a 5-year data base that should be available to critically assess the potential fit or lack of fit between child, family and school factors. It is unlikely that moderate to severe developmental problems, disabilities or illnesses will have gone undetected up to this time when the child has received previous comprehensive pediatric care. The exception is a child who has not received comprehensive medical care in the past—a new immigrant, a child of a homeless family, a foster child or a child who has been outside the mainstream of medical care because of parental mental illness or significant economic stress. In contrast, when health care has been provided, the clinician will have participated in the care plans related to special education interventions for a child with these chronic conditions. The Individuals with Disabilities Act mandates an equal educational opportunity for children and adolescents with chronic disabilities from birth through the 22nd birthday. Knowledge about this law and its application in each community is the first step toward effective pediatric advocacy.

PARENTS' EXPECTATIONS

The parents' expectation for school performance is an important part of the assessment, as well as an opportunity to learn more about the family. Two children may be similar in their temperament characteristics, social behavior, ability to attend and screen out distractions, visual-motor abilities and language development. However, their performance in school may be different, depending on parental views and expectations that are in contrast to the expectations that the school environment places on them. Therefore, determining the attitudes, values and expectations of the parents is important. It is often useful to know about the educational philosophy and individual differences of local schools. For example, parents may describe an "active, inquisitive, independent and creative" 5-year-old who is later described by a teacher as "restless, stubborn, resistant and rebellious." Parental desires and expectations for performance may be reviewed at this visit and compared with the child's preschool experiences. This process is often helpful in forming more realistic expectations of the child. Problems result when underexpectations and overexpectations are placed on the child's school performance.

Despite wide variation in the term "normal," several critical areas within the child deserve special attention at this time. These developmental requisites provide some touchstones in the evaluation process (Box 19–2).

BIOLOGICAL FACTORS

We know that prematurity, maternal illness, poor nutrition and adverse perinatal events can potentially affect brain maturation and subsequent developmental outcomes. We are becoming increasingly aware of the more subtle effects of these factors on learning abilities and specific areas of cognitive function, such as memory, attention and visual/motor skills. These outcomes arise from a number of intrauterine, perinatal events. In addition, early life experiences

BOX 19–2   CRITICAL AREAS DESERVING SPECIAL ATTENTION

- Presence or absence of potential biological insults to the nervous system
- Indicators of language dysfunction
- Indicators of problems in attention and impulsivity
- Successful socialization or separation experience from the parent or parents

influence brain maturation after birth. Dendritic growth, myelination and synaptogenesis are active in the early years of childhood. These neurological changes are influenced by genetic, biological processes that interact with the physical and psychosocially mediated aspects of the environment.

It is increasingly being recognized that early biological factors such as low birthweight are further influenced by potentially modifiable environmental influences, such as poverty, maternal education and the home environment. Minor surgical procedures, hospitalizations, self-limited illnesses and other medical or biological events were previously thought to have little bearing on issues of education and future learning. Now it appears that such events may have a significant influence on *specific* cognitive abilities, emotional factors or motor competencies (see Chapter 26).

Recurrent otitis media, often associated with mild transient conductive hearing loss during each episode, probably does not have an adverse influence on language and learning as once thought. Persistent middle ear effusion in an infant or toddler, in the absence of moderate to severe hearing loss, is not associated with subsequent developmental delays in cognition, speech or language or with psychosocial/behavioral problems. Recurrent otitis media seems to have its greatest effect on early language development in children living in homes with the least amount of language stimulation.

LANGUAGE

An early delay in language development has been shown to be the best single predictor of later learning problems. *Particular attention should be given to a child who has a history of early language delay, even if the current language competency falls within the expected range.* We should also be alert to how the child's language developed. Were there problems in fluency, comprehension and the naming of objects? Expected language milestones leading up to school entry are shown in Table 19–1 and discussed in greater detail in Chapter 16. These language developmental tasks are associated with other areas of cognitive functioning that are important to the tasks of new learning that will be expected in school.

It is now recognized that children with **dyslexia** (a problem in reading associated with normal intelligence, motivation and education) have a neurobiological defect in a specific component of language development (see Chapter 20). These children, who constitute up to 7% of a school population, have a deficit in their ability to break down the smallest segment of speech in a word. This deficit in phonological awareness can be detected during a pediatric evaluation. Focused questions at school entry, including letter identification, letter-sound association, verbal memory and word retrieval, may identify children who have a problem with

TABLE 19–1   **Selected Language Guideposts**

Skill	Age 2 yr	Age 3 yr	Age 4 yr	Age 5 yr
Comprehension	Follows simple commands; identifies body parts; points to common objects	Understands spatial relationships (in, on, under); knows functions of common objects	Follows 2-part commands; understands concepts of same and different	Recalls parts of a story; understands number concepts (3, 4, 5, 6); follows 3-part commands
Expression	Labels common objects; uses 2- or 3-word sentences; uses minimal jargon	Uses 3- to 4-word sentences; uses regular plurals; uses pronouns (I, me, you); can tell age, sex and full name	Speaks 4- to 5-word sentences; can tell story; uses past tense; names one color; can count 4 objects	Speaks sentences of 5 words; uses future tense; names 4 colors; can count 10 or more objects
Speech	Intelligible to strangers 25% of the time	Intelligible to strangers 75% of the time	Normal dysfluency (stuttering)	Dysfluencies resolved

phonological awareness and are at risk for dyslexia. These **prereading skills** are assessable and should be part of the pediatric school entry assessment. Letter recognition, naming (objects, letters, numbers and colors) and visual matching (identifying words that begin with the same letter from a list) are among the best predictors of reading readiness. A family history may be helpful here because classic dyslexia and some other types of learning difficulties do run in families.

Most developmental tests overemphasize verbal skills in estimating intellectual competency. However, when performance in school is considered, these verbal skills and the cognitive functions that underlie them may be of central importance. Bilingual or non–English-speaking families may present special challenges in the assessment of children's language development. The clinician should be wary of ascribing learning and language problems entirely to bilingualism, however. It is often noted that true language delay is present in both English and the natal language By school age, confusion in use of the two languages should be gone, and the child should not have language dysfunction because of bilingualism.

ATTENTION PROBLEMS

At or before the age of 3 to 4 years, a cluster of behaviors that have been associated with a high risk for school learning problems is identifiable; such behavior includes a high degree of motoric activity, lack of ability to sustain attention and impulsivity with limited ability to delay gratification. However, these should be red flags in the preschool history and indicate a need for more vigilance of the child at school entry. The progressive improvement in a child's ability to focus and to differentiate between what is important to a task and what is not is often a key factor in how well the child can master early learning skills in the standard school environment (see Chapter 20). A child of 5 who can sustain attention only when information is given in a certain mode (e.g., a teacher or parent sitting next to a child and mentoring the learning process) or when all distractions are eliminated will have difficulty when faced with the complexities of the usual classroom with multiple forms of stimulation and sensory input.

Belinda's mother remarked to her daughter's clinician that Belinda had a hard time sitting still and completing homework in the second grade. Belinda's mother observed that she was easily distracted when doing work in the classroom. The clinician suggested moving Belinda to a seat near the teacher to encourage keeping her on task and finding a quiet place in the home for homework, free of visual and auditory distractions. These accommodations allowed Belinda to accomplish more work at school and at home.

Attention problems are difficult to evaluate in a pediatric office setting, an environment that usually lacks excessive visual and auditory stimulation. Frequently, problems with attention will become apparent during testing for neurodevelopmental capacities or in the course of more prolonged visits. Information about the preschool experience and activities around the home will also provide useful information about attentiveness.

SOCIALIZATION AND SEPARATION

It is increasingly rare for a child not to have had frequent experiences outside the home and away from parents before entering school. The clinician can obtain information from both the preschool teacher and parent about a child's behavior after separating from a parent and a child's experiences with new adults and other children in a preschool environment. For some kindergarten children, riding a bus to school is a new experience that may challenge social skills and modify the response to separation. Preschool teachers' written observations, when blindly rated on such characteristics as peer relationships, teacher-pupil relationships, independence, participation in group activities, leadership characteristics, task orientation, attention span and persistence, self-confidence and immaturity, were found to be relatively good predictors of school achievement and behavior in later elementary school.

The relationship between a child and a parent is modified by a developmental leap at the time of entering school. Not only is the child learning to successfully negotiate a period of separation from the parents, but parents themselves must also be able to separate from the child. A child with a shy or timid temperament may be challenged when separated from a parent at the start of school. The best predictor of successful separation and entry into school is a previous successful experience. Parental views on their child's vulnerability and the pattern of child rearing up to this time will have an impact on this process. As in other areas of medicine, a focused history will help the clinician identify problems on which to work and strengths to reinforce. Individual components of social-emotional readiness skills at school entry are found in Box 19-3.

BOX 19–3 SOCIAL-EMOTIONAL READINESS SKILLS AT SCHOOL ENTRY

- Self-regulation: ability to control impulses, modulate attention and activity level and regulate emotional reactivity for at least short periods
- Executive function: planning and organizing skills, following directions, ability to demonstrate sequences and to take turns
- Capacity to tolerate separations from parent or primary caretaker; to be responsive to the teacher
- Ability to master new experiences
- Play skills, including taking turns and sharing

Adapted from Sturner R, Howard B: Preschool development 1: Communicative and motor aspects. *Pediatr Rev* 18:291, 1997.

Taylor had a difficult time separating from either parent when she started preschool at 3½ years old. After 3 weeks of refusal to venture out at all and prolonged crying when either parent left her at preschool, she was withdrawn from the class and cared for at home by her grandmother. At 4½ years old, she had the same experience with a preschool. Taylor was described by her parents as shy and fearful of new experiences.

Recognizing that difficulty with separation experiences might affect kindergarten entry, Taylor's clinician counseled her mother about the benefit of arranging multiple brief separations—with other child care persons, while playing at the park and at a friend's home—and said that an early visit to the school, before the start date, might make Taylor more comfortable with the new teacher and classroom. In addition, the clinician recommended that Taylor's mother ask for the names of children who will enter kindergarten with her daughter and arrange for a few to spend time with Taylor before the beginning of school. The clinician also suggested a children's book about starting school that might allay Taylor's fears.

PICKING A SCHOOL

Parents may ask the clinician for advice on what **type of school**—public, private, parochial or specialized—to select if they have a choice. The clinician should ask the parents for a little more information before venturing a suggestion:

- What are the traditions and social expectations of the family?
- What was the parents' experience with the schooling they received?
- Are they under any misconceptions regarding the quality of education that can be obtained?
- What is the profile of the children in a given school?
- Will this child fit in, be able to make friends and succeed?
- Are the parents concerned about ethnic or minority mixing?

In general, quality education is available in most schools and is often highly dependent on the teacher. Research indicates that continued positive effects of preschool and Head Start experiences, especially for low-income children, are dependent on the quality of the subsequent school experience. Therefore, a parental visit to a prospective school should be advised. This is desirable even if no choice is anticipated because all children do better if parents are visible and involved from the start. A classroom environment that is able to adapt to the needs of a wide variety of development levels would be the most ideal. Public schools, for the most part, have access to a greater range of specialized services for children with special needs than do private or parochial schools. In some public school systems, a cluster of schools focus on a specific area of interest (e.g., science, math, drama, music, history) that may be more suitable to a particular child. Parents can also be encouraged to inquire about classroom size, which may vary within schools and between school districts. Smaller class size may enhance learning in children with learning disabilities, inattention or behavioral problems.

"SHOULD WE DELAY KINDERGARTEN FOR A YEAR?"

Frequently parents may ask whether the clinician thinks their child should be kept back at home for another year. Parents who perceive their child as excessively shy and slow to warm up in new situations, clingy, less advanced than others in motor or language skills or shorter than most children of the same age may raise this issue. A child should almost never be kept out of school. Socialization, learning and school readiness activities are often exactly what is needed and should not be delayed. In a study of early reading and mathematics achievement, younger first grade children made as much progress over the school year as did older first graders and made significantly more progress than older kindergarten children did. Preliminary data now suggest that old-for-grade students (even those who have not been retained) have increased rates of behavioral problems, especially as adolescents. Children with special challenges to learning will need this evaluated and addressed, the sooner the better. A year's delay will not make the problem go away; it will just delay the remediation. Beware of a child described as "immature." This label usually masks specific issues with learning, attention or social skills. He needs attention now.

Questions about delaying school entry can serve as a springboard into exploring reasons for the parents' concerns. If it turns out during evaluation that serious, previously undetected developmental problems are present, appropriate diagnostic and remedial efforts should be instituted. However, these efforts often involve school-based resources and special programs. When in doubt, the clinician should encourage attending school, even with a modified program, rather than continuing daycare or remaining at home.

When the child experiences difficulty or when adjustment or advance in learning does not occur, further evaluation and referral are indicated. Psychoeducational testing aimed at formal evaluation of cognition, attention and behavioral factors that could impede progress may be necessary. Waiting 1 year for the child to "mature" only serves to delay necessary remediation. If the educational expectations are found to be excessive and the child is within the range of normal abilities for age, adjustment of the learning environment is required rather than the child being labeled as deviant. Repeating kindergarten as a remedial step without formal evaluation and program restructuring is not indicated and is invariably nonproductive.

DATA GATHERING

The assessment before **kindergarten entry** should include a complete update and review of the child's medical history and the family's medical and social history. Previous daycare or preschool experience should be reviewed. Rocky past experiences may suggest additional considerations. Data should also be obtained on preschool resources, expectations, requirements and educational programs and philosophy.

The examination and formal assessment procedure should include a general physical examination with a growth assessment if one has not recently been completed. It should include a neurological screening and documentation of visual and auditory acuity. Finally, some paper-and-pencil tasks or assessment tools should be administered. At this age the child should be at least moderately comfortable with the examination as long as the parent is present, should be able to answer simple, concrete questions with clear and intelligible speech and should comply with requests. The child should be an active part of the assessment process. Early in the interview, questions should be directed to the child with the message, "You are the patient, I am your doctor and your thoughts and responses to questions are important to me."

What to Observe

The clinician should observe the child carefully during the interview and examination and during even brief separations from her parents to make assessments regarding development. Table 19–2 outlines age-appropriate observations of development, temperament and curiosity.

What to Ask

Table 19–3 presents questions that should be asked during the examination. Questions can be directed to the child, to the parent or to both participants as the clinician engages child and parent during the encounter (see the "therapeutic triangle educational mode" in Chapter 4).

Examination and Assessment

Observing and talking with the child during the process of obtaining a careful history will yield a strong medical data base, as well as insight into language and social skills. Careful attention to the child's social responses, language comprehension and expression, body language, attentiveness to questions and motor skills adds to the data base. Drawing, paper-and-pencil tasks and games of developmental assessment can be accomplished before the physical examination as a way to develop rapport and give the child the message that she will enjoy the office visit. In some situations, information from the physical examination will have priority.

Clinicians find value in the selection of developmental tests they believe they can administer in a reproducible, standardized way. The Denver II developmental screening test (see Appendix), Draw-a-Person and figure copying (see Chapter 5), Pediatric Examination of Educational Readiness (PEER), drawing of geometrical figures and other tests can be used. Office personnel can administer some or all of these tests, and the physician can review the data.

Table 19–4 shows age-appropriate abilities. Familiarity with these behaviors, drawn from the most popular tests for young children, will assist the pediatrician in the assessment process.

TABLE 19–2   **Observations to Be Included in Examination**

Observation	Assessment
Is the child quiet and reserved, outgoing, verbal, inquisitive, at ease or frightened? Does the child initiate questions or comments?	Child's social interaction during the interview and examination. How does the child handle interactions with adults, parents and non–family members?
Is the child active, passive, slow to warm?	Child's language and verbal skills (see Appendix and Table 19–1)
Can the child be completely understood? Is language appropriate for age? Are sentences clear, compound and complex? Is articulation clear? Does the child modulate speech well?	Child's language and verbal skills (see Appendix and Table 19–1)
Does the child show excessive dependence or independence? Observe separation effect(s) if the occasion arises. What does the parent allow the child to do?	Parent-child interactions
Can the child follow 1- to 3-step instructions and assist with the examination by holding still, looking at a specific point, cooperating on the neurological examination? Is the child easily distracted by environmental stimuli?	Ability to attend and cooperate
Does the child show evidence of the ability to solve hypothetical problems, ask questions, draw interesting pictures?	Curiosity, creativity, problem-solving ability

Observation of how the child approaches various tasks, including those to facilitate the physical examination, can be revealing:

- Can the child follow auditory directions with no visual clues? (e.g., "Take off your shoes, get up on the exam table and sit back.")
- Can these be one-, two- or three-step directions?
- How attentive to the task is the child (e.g., can the child complete a drawing)?
- How facile is the child with pencil tasks (e.g., holding a pencil with a mature grasp, steady lines that are connected, clear hand dominance)?
- Is the task easy or slow and pressured (e.g., what does the child's face look like while doing the tasks)?

Children at risk for learning disabilities can and should be identified at school entry. This is especially important because most 5-year-old children with a learning disability have not been recognized at the beginning of kindergarten. A conservative estimate of the prevalence

TABLE 19–3   Questions to Be Asked during Examination*

Question	Objective
Tell me about _____. What words would you use to describe _____?	Determine the parents' views of the child; what characteristics they mention first; it is better to have parents describe behavior rather than make judgments about it ("he gets along well with other children").
What happens when _____ is with friends or playmates? Who in the family is _____ like? How do you expect _____ to do in school? Why?	Follow-up of this line of questioning can open up areas of parental concern, expectations and their own experiences with the education system.
To the child: Do you have any friends? What do you do with your friends? How are you the same/different than your friends? Who in the family are you like? Your mother, father or who? How do you expect to do in school? Why?	
Tell me what you know about the school where _____ will be starting?	Should bring out a real or imagined view of today's school; whether there has been a visit to the school or discussion of the school with neighbors may indicate the degree of parental investment or interest.
Describe how he uses crayons, pencils, scissors.	One child may laboriously use scissors to cut out a doll, whereas another will be engaged in a task, use the scissors, lay them down and proceed with the next task.
What does he like to do? Dislike? **To the child**: What do you like to do?	This may help in determining leisure time use, amount of television viewing, interest in reading or being read to.
If _____ does _____, what do you do?	Helping the parent focus on behavior will give information on discipline methods and parental ability to cope, guide, direct and support the child.

*Some questions are for both child and parent. They can be used when the clinician is interviewing them together or separately.

of learning disabilities is 7% of school-age children. Since the most common learning disability is a specific problem in reading (dyslexia), targeted questions and developmental tasks that assess early reading skills should be a routine part of the examination. Box 19–4 has specific questions about letter identification, verbal memory and letter-sound associations.

For a child in whom problems with attention or learning are suspected from historical data or observations in the office, a brief neuromaturational assessment is indicated. An evaluation

TABLE 19-4   **Appropriate Abilities at Preschool and Kindergarten Entry Ages**

Year	Abilities
3	Picks longer of two lines Can point to chin and teeth on request Cuts with scissors Makes 3-cube pyramid in about 15 seconds Copies a circle Jumps with both feet together
4	Goes upstairs and downstairs one foot per step Copies cross (+) Washes hands Can tell "how many" when shown 2 circles Completes "A hat goes on your head, shoes on your ..."
5	Dresses self (except tying shoelaces) Copies square Can count 6 objects Can answer: "Why do we have houses, books, clocks, eyes, ears?" Can tell: "What is a chair made of? A dress?" Knows (or can be taught): address, phone number, where mother and father work Finger counting (how it is done, pointing to or not) and finger identification Digit span—should be able to repeat 4 digits forward
6	Tells how a crayon and a pencil are the same and different Can tell differences between common objects: dog and bird, milk and water Can complete "A lemon is sour, sugar is. ..." Can tell what a forest is made of

From Hoeckelman R, Blatman S, Brunell PA: *Principles of Pediatrics.* New York, McGraw-Hill, 1978.

BOX 19-4   TESTS USEFUL IN IDENTIFYING CHILDREN AT RISK FOR DYSLEXIA

- Letter identification (naming letters of the alphabet)
- Letter-sound association (e.g., identifying words that begin with the same letter from a list: doll, dog, boat)
- Phonological awareness (e.g., identifying the word that would remain if a particular sound were removed: if the /k/ sound were taken away from "cat")
- Verbal memory (e.g., recalling a sentence or story that was just told)
- Rapid naming (rapidly naming a continuous series of familiar objects, digits, letters or colors)
- Expressive vocabulary or word retrieval (e.g., naming single pictured objects)

From Shaywits SE: Dyslexia. *N Engl J Med* 338:307, 1998.

for digit span (recall of four numbers at 5 years old), memory of serial commands (at least four directions) and right-left discrimination may reveal problems with attention, listening skills, impulsivity and organization. An assessment of coordination, motor and spatial functions is accomplished by an evaluation of motor tasks (e.g., standing on one foot for 5 to 10 seconds, hopping on one foot, climbing up onto an exam table, throwing a ball) and visual-perceptual tasks (e.g., drawing a person with at least six to eight body parts and copying standard geometrical shapes). Previously undetected mild cerebral palsy is diagnosed during a standard neurological examination through the evaluation of muscle tone, strength, gait and reflexes. A clumsy child with a normal motor examination does not have cerebral palsy; a clumsy child with hyper-reflexia, toe walking and limited dorsiflexion of the ankle is likely to have cerebral palsy.

Many health care providers find it valuable to ask a 5-year-old: "Draw a picture of your family doing something" (see Chapter 5). The neuromaturational skills (e.g., visual-motor integration and fine motor coordination) and psychosocial characteristics of the child and family are revealed in often remarkable and surprising ways in these drawings. Clinical interpretation of the drawing should be cautious, however. The drawings also provide an opportunity to enhance the content and quality of communication with children and parents (see Chapter 5 for how to use family drawings in pediatric practice).

An alternative use of drawing skills at this age is through the "drawing interview," as described by Sturner and Howard. In this format, drawing is used as a conversation piece. The child is asked to draw a person while the clinician interviews the parents ("Please draw a picture of a boy or girl."). This is followed by the "drawing interview," which consists of a list of questions from which the clinician can choose to engage the child in conversation. Compliment the child's effort on the picture, if completed, and record any spontaneous comments.

1. "Do you think it is a picture of a boy or a girl?"
2. "Tell me a make-believe story about this boy (or girl)"
3. If no response, restate the above, i.e., "Just tell me something about the boy/girl."
4. "What else is he/she doing?"
5. When the child stops, repeat what was said. Add, "What else happens to the boy/girl?"

No child should enter school without the benefit of formal vision and hearing acuity tests. Many schools have such screening programs in place. Updating of routine immunizations and other health screening tests (e.g., tuberculosis and lead tests in high-risk communities) are now requirements in the United States for a child to enter and remain in school. A screening urinalysis is recommended only once during childhood, usually at the 5-year-old examination.

STANDARDIZED EVALUATIONS FOR SCHOOL READINESS

Because of increasing pressure on schools to ensure academic success of their students, some schools have instituted testing to determine so-called readiness for formal schooling. Such tests are often neither standardized nor evaluated with regard to reliability and predictive validity. The decision to enter public school is always based on legal age of entitlement. No child should be deprived of this right, although the learning environment should be, and by law is required to be, adapted to individual needs. A distinction must be made between tests of

TABLE 19–5   **Neuromotor Accomplishments**

Age (yr)	Gross Motor Skills	Fine Motor Skills
2	Runs well Kicks ball Goes upstairs and downstairs (one step at a time)	Builds tower of 6 cubes Imitates vertical crayon stroke Turns book pages singly
3	Goes upstairs (alternating feet) Jumps from bottom step Pedals tricycle Stands on 1 foot momentarily	Copies circle Copies cross (+)
4	Hops on 1 foot Goes downstairs (alternating feet) Stands on 1 foot (5 seconds) Throws ball overhand	Copies square Draws person with 2 to 4 parts Uses scissors
5	Stands on 1 foot (10 seconds) May be able to skip	Copies triangle Draws person with body Prints some letters

Adapted from Levine MD, Carey WB, Crocker AC: *Developmental and Behavioral Pediatrics*, 3rd ed. Philadelphia, WB Saunders, 1999, p 39.

academic readiness, which evaluate the child's ability to perform basic learning skills, and developmental screening tests, which attempt to evaluate a child's level of gross motor, fine motor, language and personal-social development in comparison to the performance of age-mates. What one has learned at home does not ensure the ability to profit from a specific educational environment. Conversely, lack of academic skills does not predict school failure.

Most clinicians are familiar with the items from the Denver II screening test and with the task of copying geometrical figures—a circle (3 years), a cross (4 years), a square (5 years), a triangle (6 years) and a diamond (7 years). The forms should be presented to the child to copy, and the clinician should not routinely demonstrate drawing the form. A nice tripod grasp of the pencil or marker should be seen at this age. Table 19–5 presents a summary of expected neuromotor accomplishments. Special attention should be paid to these tasks with children who were born prematurely, exposed prenatally to alcohol or other drugs or experienced a difficult perinatal course and with children who have postnatal risk factors that may affect development (e.g., head trauma, meningitis, physical abuse, emotional abuse, witnessing violence). Children from families whose members have experienced school difficulties need careful appraisal because many learning differences run in families.

The PEER test is an expanded neurodevelopmental assessment. It allows the clinician to engage in structured play with a child while deriving information about developmental achievements and learning. Designed for children 4 to 6 years of age, the PEER requires more time than the usual health supervision visit. Although it is not used as a routine screening instrument for all children and has not been standardized against traditional neuropsychological tests, it may be a useful tool to use with a child when there are concerns about development and learning after a screening assessment during a health supervision visit. It is also a useful tool to practice developmental assessment at this age and learn to use selected sections of the PEER for a particular child during a health supervision visit.*

ANTICIPATORY GUIDANCE

The greatest danger in assessment of school readiness is a tendency to overinterpret findings. The clinician should avoid dogmatic pronouncements about prognosis. Strive to describe the child in the most accurate way possible. The 5-year-old health supervision visit should yield significant data to allow the clinician to enumerate educational and behavioral strengths and vulnerabilities. Each child's particular strengths should be brought into focus so that the parents and the school may build on them. Clearly identify areas of concern. For most, it will not be possible to predict the outcomes. Concentrated efforts at support can evolve, and occasionally remediation will be indicated. Examples of two summaries from the 5-year-old health supervision visit follow:

> Ethan, age 5 years, is an only child. He has no serious health or medical problems; he displays the behavior, skills and knowledge of most 5- to 6-year-old children. His ability to handle paper-and-pencil tasks is more like that of a 4-year-old. He holds a pencil with a fist-like grasp very close to the point and perpendicular to the paper. The parents, college graduates, describe him as fun loving, able to concentrate on things and having several good friends. He had a good preschool experience and preferred large motor activities, the sandbox, cars and trucks to drawing and puzzles. The clinician's knowledge of the school's kindergarten program is that attempts are made to take children at the speed they can work, and formal prereading skills are introduced after the first month of school.

Ethan's many assets are described. The observation of immature graphomotor skills suggests the need to monitor fine motor–dependent learning. Some of these children will have difficulty using visual information or listening when writing at the same time.

> Emily, age 5 years, is the third of five children and the only girl. She has a history of recurrent ear infections, but her hearing at this time has been tested as normal. She is slightly overweight for height. She tends to be shy, apprehensive in new situations and quiet in large groups. However, her neurological examination and developmental assessments show her to perform at or above age level. She learns most readily with visually presented material. Her parents describe her as "serious." She has two close friends. Jefferson School's small class size should be ideally suited to bring out the skills of this lovely girl and to encourage gross motor activities.
>
> Medical concerns and a slow-to-warm-up temperament are delineated in the context of a normal examination and development. Emily's strength as a visual learner and the need to encourage physical activity are nicely balanced in this summary.

---

*The PEER can be ordered from Educator's Publishing Service, Inc., 31 Smith Street, Cambridge, MA 02138-1089.

Pediatric clinicians in these situations can be optimistic and encourage the parents to be regularly involved in visits at open houses and to listen to the child's descriptions of the school experience. Ongoing monitoring of each child's progress and fit with the school is indicated.

The clinician's door should always be open to a discussion of how the child is doing in school. With the increased mobility of today's society, the clinician should be aware that children who have moved frequently are more likely to have emotional and behavioral problems and are more likely to repeat a grade than are students who have never moved. If the response to a

HEADS UP—5 YEARS

- "Immature" is not a pediatric diagnosis. A child so labeled requires further evaluation.
- Assess past separation experiences (preschool and child care) and temperament in order to recognize a child who is especially shy and slow to warm up. Use the opportunity to guide parents in ways to modify the transition to kindergarten.
- Developmental assessment at school entry: Start with the neurodevelopmental milestones that include the motor, language and social skills found in the Denver II. Take the next step to evaluate the cognitive neurological processes that either confirm school readiness or may lead to further assessment or close monitoring.

TEST	FUNCTION
Ask the child to tell you about a movie or video seen recently	Oral expression, memory, sequencing
Read the child a paragraph, followed by a few questions	Auditory processing and oral expression
Ask the child to copy a square, a triangle; to draw a person or the child's family	Fine motor and visual-spatial skills
Ask the child to tell you about the picture	Oral expression and affect
Ask the child to repeat a series of random and sequencing numbers (age minus one)	Short-term memory
Ask the child to complete a four- to five-step task in the order given	Auditory processing and motor skills
Ask the child to make up a sentence from three to four words	Expressive fluency and imagination

- The school entry exam is an optimal time to screen for developmental disabilities—visual impairment (refractive error and strabismus), hearing loss, mild cerebral palsy, language or speech delay, dyslexia (see Box 19–4) and visual-spatial dysfunction.
- A child who is a year or more delayed in motor milestones should be assessed for previously unrecognized cerebral palsy (e.g., can't skip, delayed on figure drawing, difficulty holding a pencil or crayon). A neurological assessment for long-tract signs will establish the diagnosis.
- Assess the mental health of the child and family—evidence of depression, anxiety, oppositional behavior.

query of how a child is doing in school is less than a superlative from a parent, it deserves further exploration. Carrying out the school entry assessment sets the stage for ongoing monitoring of family and school behavior and achievement. In this way the clinician can be alert to early signs of a lack of fit between what the child brings to the situation and what the parents and school expect. In addition, the clinician can share in the joy and excitement of a young school-age child's successful social and intellectual growth.

ACKNOWLEDGMENT

Dr. Philip Nader contributed to this chapter in previous editions.

RECOMMENDED READINGS

For Parents

Berenstein S: *Berenstein Bears Go to School.* New York, Random House, 1978.

Berenstein S: *Berenstein Bears Trouble at School.* New York, Random House, 1987.

Comer JP: *Child by Child: The Comer Process for Change in Education.* 1999. New York, Teachers College Press.

Gesell A, Ilg F: *The Child from Five to Ten.* New York, Harper Brothers, 1946.

Schor EL (ed): *Caring for Your School-Age Child: Ages 5 to 12.* New York, Bantam Books, 1995.

Zeifert H: *Harry Gets Ready for School.* New York, Puffin Books, 1991.

For Professionals

Dworkin PH: School readiness. *Curr Opin Pediatr* 3:786.1991.

Halfon N, Regalado M, Taafe K, et al: *Building a Bridge from Birth to School: Improving Developmental and Behavioral Health Services for Young Children.* New York, The Commonwealth Fund, 2003.

National Association for the Education of Young Children: NAEYC Position Statement on School Readiness (1995). Available at http://www.naeyc.org/resources/position_statements/psredy98.htm.

Palfrey JS, Rappaport LR: School placement. *Pediatr Rev* 8:261,1987.

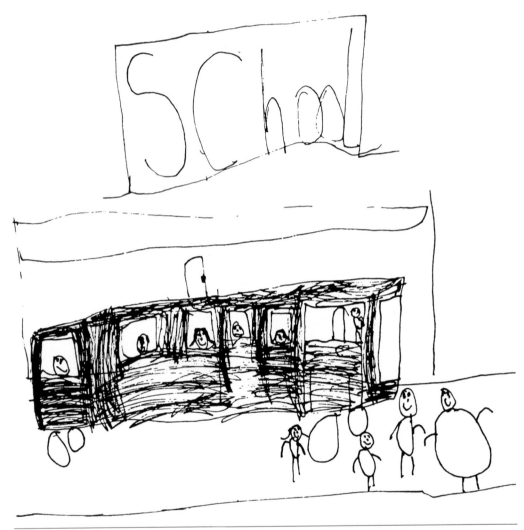

"A girl and a boy get on the bus. Their parents are watching."

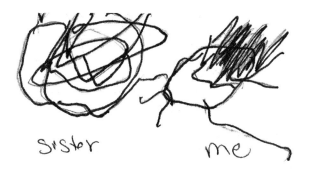

sister

me

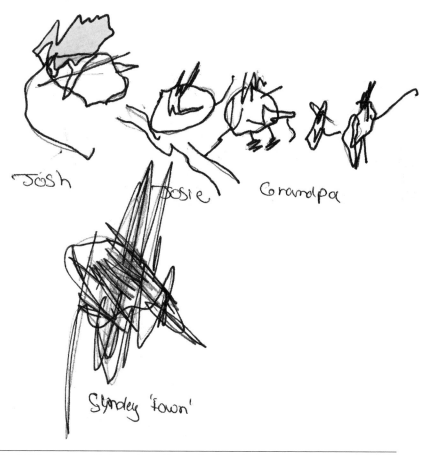

Josh

Josie

Grandpa

Sydney 'town'

Siena and her teacher at school. This six year old shows herself proudly aliened with her teacher. These personal relationships are vital at this age.

CHAPTER 20

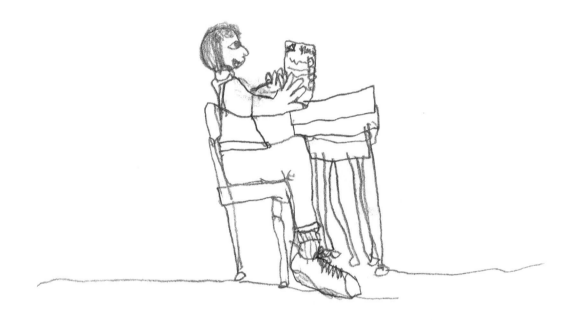

A young lady shows her interest in reading and her considerable skill in drawing in this self-portrait. By a girl, age 8.

Six to Seven Years: Reading, Relationships and Playing By the Rules

MARTIN T. STEIN

The first grade is a time of cognitive challenge coupled with the requirement for sustained attention for learning. Educational strengths and weakness emerge during this time. It is an opportunity for pediatricians to provide early recognition of problems with attention and specific learning disabilities that interfere with classroom learning.

Key Words

- Cognitive Changes
- Concrete Operations
- Attention and Learning
- Learning Disabilities
- School Refusal
- Truancy
- Separation Anxiety

Bryan, age 6 years, was referred at his school's request to see if "something couldn't be done" about his activity level. His first grade teacher thought him much more active than the other boys in her class because he frequently spoke out of turn, moved about the classroom during less structured class periods and invaded his peers' work spaces and private conversations. He was an only child whose parents both worked. He was adored by all four grandparents, who lived nearby and provided much of his daily care. His parents encouraged his outgoing personality and excellent verbal skills and were quite tolerant of his high energy level during their times alone with him. Psychometric evaluation by the school psychologist documented Bryan's academic achievement at above grade level in all academic areas.

His pediatrician found him to be physically healthy with no neurological abnormalities and with a history of excellent language and motor development. He was rather presumptuous in his stance toward the pediatrician, asking the doctor what kind of car he owned and how much the examination would cost. His mother had difficulty concealing her amusement at this inquiry by Bryan.

Psychosocial family stress and a family history of attention deficit/hyperactivity disorder (ADHD) were absent. Bryan's pediatrician requested information from his parents and teachers about specific behavior associated with ADHD (see later in this chapter). When she concluded that criteria for ADHD were exhibited, the pediatrician recommended that Bryan's parents work closely with his teacher in making clear to Bryan their support of classroom behavioral expectations. His parents began to follow through with the teacher's rewards and consequences for unacceptable behavior at school. Improvement in impulse control was not dramatic, but by second grade his teacher commented that Bryan was a "challenging, but gratifying student to have in class."

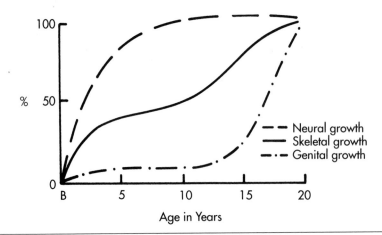

Figure 20–1   Organ growth curves drawn to a common scale by computing values at successive ages in terms of growth. (Modified from Harris JA, et al: *The Measurement of Man.* Minneapolis, University of Minnesota Press, 1930.)

A 6-year-old child stands on a threshold of exciting new cognitive and social experiences. With regular school attendance actually required for the first time, this age marks the beginning of a lifetime of obligations and adherence to schedules and routines imposed outside the familiar family environment. For some children and families, this time of transition may present a crisis. At the same time, it provides an opportunity for rapid cognitive, social and emotional growth.

The accelerated physical growth of preschoolers begins to slow as children enter the years of middle childhood. By the age of 5 years the brain has attained approximately 90% of its adult weight and size, and over the next 2 years, final myelinization of the central nervous system will be completed (Fig. 20–1). Brain maturation, however, continues through the school-age period as new neuronal connections (synaptogenesis) are formed. This process coincides with qualitative advances in cognitive capacities. Simultaneously, the child may participate in activities requiring the integration of fine and gross motor skills, such as dance, sports and, in the classroom, handwriting and arts and crafts projects.

COGNITIVE DEVELOPMENT

A 6-year-old begins to show less evidence of the cognitive stage described by Piaget as "preoperational" thinking—or thinking marked by magical qualities. A sensitive clinician will find most first graders questioning many of their previous assumptions about the world. The typical 6-year-old does not take fantasy for granted and may question magical events to find their logical and "real" explanations. However, she may have difficulty performing mental operations that involve simultaneous changes in more than one variable. Such situations confuse her, so she may adopt a single, simple explanation and continue to focus on one aspect of a situation, a phenomenon known as centration. For example, the child may believe that a tall, narrow bottle of soda contains more soda than a short, wide bottle with an equal volume merely because the former is taller. Likewise, a child may be able to make her way from home to school with great accuracy, but may be unable to mentally reverse the directions to appropriately plan the trip home. She may be able to participate in a multifaceted game, but will have difficulty learning it from verbal directions alone or explaining the rules with clarity. She may resent a sibling whose birthday "comes before hers" without consolation from the sense that soon thereafter the situation will be reversed.

The age at which children demonstrate these changes in cognition varies considerably, often beginning around 6 years of age and gradually evolving over the next 4 to 5 years. Piaget was able to demonstrate preoperational thinking and the transition to concrete operations with simple techniques and the use of readily available materials. For example, an adult can form a ball of clay for a child and ask him to form a similar ball with "as much clay" as the first ball. When the child agrees that both balls have exactly the same amount of clay, the tester can flatten one of the pieces, roll it into a narrow cylinder or break it into two or more chunks. If the child is asked which of the original two balls now has the most clay, his answer and reasoning may reveal his capacity to "conserve mass" cognitively despite the physical manipulations that were carried out before his eyes. However, a child of about 6 years or younger may also give an answer that demonstrates he does not conserve mass cognitively. The child may state that the original ball of clay now contains more clay because it is longer than the other ball or less clay because it is flatter. The child who retains the concept of mass despite these changes in appearance has achieved, in part, a new level of reasoning called "concrete operations" (Fig. 20–2). He can understand that dimensions and weight are two different aspects of an object and that one can change one aspect without changing the other.

By the age of 5 years, most children demonstrate that they understand the concept of conservation of length as well as mass. Many younger children will maintain that a long string and a shorter wooden stick are the same length if they are arranged so that the ends of the string coincide with the ends of the stick. Conservation of mass and weight are accomplished mentally by most children 1 year or more later, and conservation of volume is achieved much later, when children reach the last 2 years of grade school. This orderly progression of mental abilities to understand the real world testifies to the regular pattern of brain maturation that lays the groundwork for the learning experiences school provides. However, some magical thinking still remains.

Six-year-olds continue to demonstrate many of the preconceptual qualities of thinking typical of preschoolers (see Chapter 17). First graders may still believe the sun and moon were made artificially and move because man or God makes them move. They may feel sorry for a car that is heavily loaded with passengers as if the car had feelings. In fact, even adults may think in egocentric, magical ways, depending on many factors, including the context of the cognitive task. The ways in which children think and attain knowledge as they develop into middle childhood are apparently less rigidly tied to specific Piagetian cognitive stages than was once believed. However, the fundamental principles of Piaget's cognitive model of development provide useful insights into the emerging thinking processes of children. Reasoning and understanding are tied to actual situations and objects at this stage, concrete aspects of the world. Hypothetical reasoning and abstract thought will have to await adolescence or later to emerge (see Chapters 22 and 23).

These abilities translate into the typical school-based tasks presented to children. Because this stage is marked by the ability to consider multiple variables concerning objects or situations

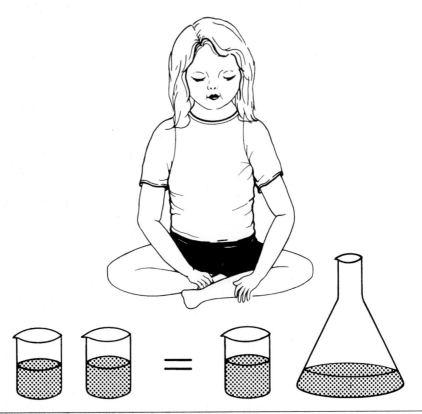

Figure 20–2   This child is proudly able to appreciate that equal volumes of water are maintained when the shape of the container is changed, a demonstration of conservation of mass in a child who has entered the stage of concrete operations.

simultaneously, children can perform mental operations related to concrete objects (e.g., adding or subtracting objects, creating maps), understand serial relationships (e.g., ordering pictures, number concepts) and appreciate classification systems. Classification tasks, common in modern schoolwork, require the identification of a common factor in groups and subgroups.

Although the thinking process of a 6- to 7-year-old is qualitatively different from the thinking of older school-age children, the typical first and second grade child should demonstrate certain qualities that make possible productive classroom participation and learning. In first grade, academic demands are made in addition to the behavioral, social and emotional expectations of kindergarten. Academic failure in the first grade results when children cannot demonstrate in school that they have the capacity to perform the primary decoding tasks of reading, solving simple addition and subtraction problems and writing simple sentences with properly spelled words. *Although these skills are generally taught to all children at about the same age, normal children vary substantially in the age at which they achieve the capacities to read, spell and work with numbers.* Psychologists call this the "5/7 shift," reflecting the range of normal development in this transformation of cognitive abilities. Learning to read, in particular, seems to bloom at varying times, yet it is the cornerstone of achievement in the primary grades. However, a modest delay in the development of these abilities, even if the delay is maturational and not otherwise significant, can create serious psychological and behavioral difficulties for a child whose self-image is tarnished by the experience of academic failure at an early age.

Academic difficulties in the first and second grades may diminish the child's self-esteem, color her future attitude toward school and result in considerable anxiety in parents. It is important that the pediatrician begin to help the parents understand the source of their child's academic difficulty and collaborate with the child, her parents and the school in designing a program to address the child's specific needs while helping her feel successful in one or more areas.

A useful model to evaluate academic success in the first grade curriculum assumes that children have both the cognitive power and the cognitive style to deal effectively with the classroom environment. A child with insufficient cognitive power may be generally dull, with mild or borderline mental retardation that does not become apparent until the child is faced with the academic demands of first or second grade. Selective cognitive deficits (i.e., learning disabilities) may appear in a child who otherwise shows normal intelligence. A child with even a mild form of mental retardation may have a history of delayed attainment of early milestones in language development. Another child with a selective learning disability may seem bright, with a good fund of general knowledge and normal developmental milestones, but has difficulty with specific academic tasks during the first grade in a way that is quite unexpected by parents and teachers, who perceive the child as normal in intelligence and in demonstrating good work habits.

Amrita was premature (28 weeks' gestation) with mild perinatal asphyxia and required oxygen supplementation for only the first week of life. There were no other postnatal complications; a brain ultrasound at 1 month was normal. Motor and social milestones were normal in the first 2 years of life when corrected for gestational age. At 2 years, when she started speech therapy, her vocabulary was limited to 5 words; at $2^1/_2$ years, 15 words; and at 3 years she spoke in short sentences with plurals and pronouns. An audiogram was normal.

Amrita's parents were not aware of any problems in preschool. Her kindergarten teacher commented on Amrita's slow acquisition of letter and number recognition but also noted her "calm and easygoing ways."

Note: The delayed language skills in this child may have been an early sign of a language-based learning disability, a global cognitive deficiency, limited exposure to spoken language at home, psychosocial stress or a maturational delay in language development (see Chapter 16). The pediatrician, aware of an increased risk for learning disabilities associated with prematurity, performed a screening test for dyslexia (see Box 19–4). Significant deficits in achievement of age-appropriate language skills associated with reading were documented. A screening audiogram, visual acuity test and complete physical examination were normal. Amrita's pediatrician concluded that a psychoeducational assessment, including standardized tests for aptitude, achievement and behavior, was the next step to sort out a specific learning disability from mild or borderline mental retardation. Amrita's teacher was notified about the recommendation, and her parents were informed about the Individual Educational Plan (IEP) process.

> **BOX 20–1   ACADEMIC UNDERACHIEVEMENT AND BEHAVIORAL PROBLEMS: CLUES TO ETIOLOGY AND INTERVENTION**
>
> - *Neurologically based* problem with sustained attention
> - *Learning disability* that limits the effective mental manipulations necessary for learning
> - *Psychological disorder*, which may be a primary cause of school failure or a secondary manifestation of a learning disability or chronic inattention
> - *Disorganized home environment*, which may be the result of marital discord, poverty, a major life event change, substance abuse or child/spousal abuse

A child who has difficulty learning in the first 2 or 3 years of formal schooling is often a challenge to pediatric clinicians because of the similarity of behavioral symptoms and academic outcomes for a wide variety of developmental, neurological and psychological conditions. A good clinician appreciates that these many variables may be variations on a normal spectrum of behavior or may reflect problems that are inherent in the child or her environment. This is often a very tough call. Inattention and distractibility in the classroom, poor organization skills, frequent daydreaming during learning exercises and awkward social skills are often found in many first and second grade children who are not achieving academic progress. Some children may have little previous experience with the demands of the typical first grade classroom. In children who display such behavior, with or without poor school performance, the clinician should consider four broad categories that can provide useful clues to etiology and intervention (Box 20–1).

PROBLEMS WITH SUSTAINED ATTENTION AND LEARNING

Perhaps the most common disorder of cognitive style in the differential diagnosis of academic failure is ADHD. A child with a primary attention disorder has a neurologically based intrinsic inefficiency in maintaining selective attention.

- The process of attention in a learning situation has different components that may reach maturation at different chronological ages in an individual child.
- These functions of attention include
  - Planning and reflection
  - Vigilance and awareness of salient information
  - Resistance to distraction
  - A sustained mental effort
  - An ongoing monitoring capability to detect errors and make corrections
- Concepts of attention distinguish between the selectivity and the intensity of attention. Selectivity refers to the process that modulates responsiveness and prioritizes specific stimuli. Intensity describes the ability to activate and maintain attention over time. One or both aspects of attention may be weak in an individual child.
- A history of early temperamental difficulties (e.g., withdrawing from novel situations, slow to adapt, intense emotional responses or negative moods [see Chapter 2]), perinatal

stressful events and sleep disorders are found in some, but by no means all, children with an attention disorder.

- Minor neurological abnormalities (so-called soft neurological signs) may be apparent on physical examination in some children with attention problems These nonlocalizing neurological findings include motor impersistence, synkinesis (moving a body part without intention when focusing on another body movement, also known as "mirroring"), right-left confusion and poor short-term memory.

- Inattention associated with poor listening skills, impaired memory, impulsivity and disorganization may not be seen in a nondistracting, comfortable pediatric office setting, where the clinician provides for containment of focus and eliminates distractions. Signs of inattentiveness will often become apparent only after a child with a significant attention problem is asked to repeat a series of digits, follow a serial command or demonstrate right-left discrimination.

- Although a deficit of attention is the central problem in children with ADHD, many of these children are overactive (hyperactivity) and demonstrate problems with impulse control as well. The diagnosis is made largely on the basis of a medical and behavioral history, including teacher and parent reports. The physical examination is usually unremarkable. Teachers, who have the advantage of classroom observations, identify far more children as inattentive and overactive than parents or clinicians do.

- To succeed in the classroom, a first grader must be capable of focused and sustained attention for periods of 25 minutes to 1 hour. Good students in standard settings are not easily distracted, are selective in what they attend to and must be able to shift the focus of attention rapidly. Parents and teachers are not surprised when a child who lacks these qualities earns low marks in the first grade, often after experiencing a difficult time in kindergarten. Such a child may be seen as so unhappy, so distractible or so preoccupied that academic failure can be predicted early in the school year.

As a guide to clinical assessment, the core symptoms of inattention, hyperactivity and impulsivity have been described with specific clusters of behavior in the hyperactive/impulsive domain and the inattentive domain (Box 20–2). The American Academy of Pediatrics' evidence-based guidelines for primary care clinicians in the evaluation and diagnosis of a child with ADHD include the following specific recommendations:

1. In a child 6 to 12 years old with inattention, hyperactivity, impulsivity, academic under-achievement or behavior problems, primary care clinicians should initiate an evaluation for ADHD. Early recognition of ADHD in primary care pediatric practice is ensured when screening for core symptoms and problems in school and social relationships during health supervision visits. The following screening questions are useful:
   - How is your child doing in school?
   - Are there any problems with learning that you or the teacher has seen?
   - Is your child happy in school?
   - Are you concerned with any behavioral problems in school, at home or when your child is playing with friends?
   - Is your child having problems completing class work or homework?

BOX 20–2 DIAGNOSTIC CRITERIA FOR ATTENTION-DEFICIT/HYPERACTIVITY DISORDER

Categories of ADHD

- **Attention-Deficit/Hyperactivity Disorder, Combined Type**: This subtype should be used if six (or more) symptoms of inattention and six (or more) symptoms of hyperactivity-impulsivity have persisted for at least 6 months. Most children and adolescents with the disorder have the combined type.
- **Attention-Deficit/Hyperactivity Disorder, Predominantly Inattentive Type**: This subtype should be used if six (or more) symptoms of inattention (but fewer than six symptoms of hyperactivity-impulsivity) have persisted for at least 6 months.
- **Attention-Deficit/Hyperactivity Disorder, Predominantly Hyperactive-Impulsive Type**: This subtype should be used if six (or more) symptoms of hyperactivity-impulsivity (but fewer than six symptoms of inattention) have persisted for at least 6 months. Inattention may often still be a significant clinical feature in such cases.

Inattention

- Often fails to give close attention to details or makes careless mistakes in schoolwork, work or other activities
- Often has difficulty sustaining attention in tasks or play activities
- Often does not seem to listen when spoken to directly
- Often does not follow through on instructions and fails to finish schoolwork, chores or duties in the workplace (not because of oppositional behavior or failure to understand instructions)
- Often has difficulty organizing tasks and activities
- Often avoids, dislikes or is reluctant to engage in tasks that require sustained mental effort (such as schoolwork or homework)
- Often loses things necessary for tasks or activities (e.g., toys, school assignments, pencils, books or tools)
- Often distracted easily by extraneous stimuli
- Often forgetful in daily activities

Hyperactivity

- Often fidgets with hands or feet or squirms in seat
- Often leaves seat in classroom or in other situations in which remaining seated is expected
- Often runs about or climbs excessively in situations in which it is inappropriate in adolescents (may be limited to subjective feelings of restlessness)
- Often has difficulty playing or engaging in leisure activities quietly
- Often "on the go" or acts as if "driven by a motor"
- Often talks excessively

Impulsivity

- Often blurts out answers before questions have been completed
- Often has difficulty awaiting turn
- Often interrupts or intrudes on others (e.g., butts into conversations or games)

- Some hyperactive-impulsive or inattentive symptoms that caused impairment were present **before the age of 7 years.**
- Some impairment from the symptoms is **present in two or more settings** (e.g., at school [or work] and at home).
- Clear evidence must exist of **clinically significant impairment** in social, academic or occupational functioning.

From American Psychiatric Association: *Diagnostic and Statistical Manual of Mental Disorders,* 4th ed. Washington, DC, American Psychiatric Association, 1994.

2. The diagnosis of ADHD requires that a child meet the criteria of the *Diagnostic and Statistical Manual of Mental Health Disorders*, fourth edition (DSM-IV), including
   - Documentation of at least six of nine categories of behavior in the hyperactive/impulsive domain and/or in the inattentive domain
   - Presence of such behavior in two or more settings (e.g., home and school) for at least 6 months
   - Presence of some of the behavior before 7 years of age
   - Significant impairment in learning and/or social interaction

3. Assessment of ADHD requires evidence directly obtained from parents or caregivers regarding the core symptoms of ADHD in various settings, the age of onset, the duration of symptoms and the degree of functional impairment.

4. Assessment of ADHD requires evidence directly obtained from the classroom teacher (or other school professional) regarding the core symptoms of ADHD, the duration of symptoms, the degree of functional impairment and coexisting conditions.

5. Evaluation of a child with ADHD should include assessment for coexisting conditions. Common coexisting conditions include mental health problems (e.g., oppositional defiant disorder, anxiety disorder, depression, conduct disorder) and learning disabilities (see later).

6. Other diagnostic tests are not routinely indicated to establish the diagnosis of ADHD. Current evidence does not support the routine use of other diagnostic tests, including hematocrit, blood lead, thyroid hormone levels, brain imaging studies, electro-encephalography and continuous performance tests.

When these criteria are applied, approximately 6% to 9% of school-age children seen in a primary care pediatric setting will have behavior associated with academic and/or social impairment consistent with ADHD.

Similar to most pediatric disorders of behavior, accurate diagnosis of ADHD is complicated by the fact that much of the core behavior can be seen in the course of typical child development. The American Academy of Pediatrics published a diagnostic classification of the broad spectrum of normal and abnormal behavior in infants, children and adolescents seen in primary care medical settings. The classification of child and adolescent mental diagnoses in primary care in the *Diagnostic and Statistical Manual for Primary Care (DSM-PC), Child and Adolescent Version,* can assist clinicians in the process of sorting out a typical developmental variation from a disorder that meets specific diagnostic criteria. For ADHD and other behavioral conditions, DSM-PC is helpful in separating developmentally typical overactivity, inattentiveness and impulsivity from behavior in children who need further evaluation and treatment.

The diagnosis of ADHD should be made with careful deliberation, including assessments of a child's behavior by both a parent and a teacher. It is important that parents and teachers understand that this diagnosis is largely descriptive of the child's behavior and does not reveal the etiology of the problem, dictate treatment or predict an individual child's prognosis. Children with moderate to severe ADHD who are not recognized and treated carry a significant risk for serious maladjustment in adolescence and as adults, including problems with educational underachievement, employment, substance use, relationship difficulties and marital conflicts.

To assist pediatric clinicians in the process of recognition, evaluation and management of school-age children with ADHD in an office practice, the American Academy of Pediatrics has developed a "tool kit" that includes behavioral questionnaires for parents and teachers, samples of letters to communicate with schools and guidelines for medications, behavioral management and classroom/home accommodation. Publications and websites for parents are listed at the end of this chapter.

Measuring the Impact of Intervention

Although longitudinal outcome studies on specific treatments of children with ADHD are limited, specific clinical and educational interventions will have a positive impact. When the treatment plan for a child with ADHD is developed with a chronic disease perspective, there is a better chance for adherence to treatment plans, improved health and disease status measures and higher levels of satisfaction. Treatment begins with providing parents and the child with information about the condition—the biological basis for ADHD and the effects of the school, home and community environments. Guiding and advocating the parents in their work with the child's school, ensuring coordination of health and other services and helping families set specific goals are appropriate pediatric roles.

Initially, three to six target outcomes (improvement in symptoms associated with ADHD), agreed on by the parents, child and teacher, can be of enormous help after the diagnosis of ADHD in a child. Target outcomes bring precision to the setting of treatment goals with the parents and child and direct the follow-up process. Examples of target outcomes include improving written and verbal communication; improving academic performance (e.g., completing homework, greater volume of work; strengthening efficiency and accuracy); decreasing disruptive behavior; improving self-esteem; reducing the degree of supervision needed at school or in the community; and enhanced safety, such as in crossing streets or riding bicycles. Additional goals may address improving the core symptoms of inattention, hyperactivity and impulsivity. The goals should be realistic, attainable and measurable.

Treatment of ADHD

Behavior modification strategies and accommodations in the classroom will diminish many target behaviors and enhance adjustment to school. Behavioral therapy includes programs with specific interventions that have a common goal of modifying the physical and social environments to alter or change behavior. Major components of behavioral therapy are the provision of rewards for demonstrating the desired behavior (e.g., positive reinforcement) and consequences for failure to meet the goals (e.g., punishment). Repetitive application of the rewards and consequences gradually shapes behavior (see Table 20–1). Behavior therapy should be differentiated from other forms of psychological interventions designed to change a child's emotional status—such as cognitive therapy, psychotherapy and play therapy. Although these interventions may be useful for conditions associated with ADHD (e.g., anxiety, oppositional behavior and depression), they are not effective for treating core ADHD behavior. Accommodations in the classroom include front-seat placement to allow for more frequent monitoring by the teacher, assignments in written form, smaller volumes of work and assistance in organization of class work and homework.

TABLE 20–1   **Effective Behavioral Techniques for Children with Attention-Deficit/Hyperactivity Disorder**

Technique	Description	Example
Positive reinforcement	Providing rewards or privileges in response to desired behavior	Child completes an assignment and is permitted to play on the computer
Time-out	Removing access to desired activity because of unwanted behavior	Child hits sibling and, as a result, must sit for 5 minutes in the corner of the room
Response cost	Withdrawing rewards or privileges because of unwanted behavior	Child loses free-time privileges for not completing homework
Token economy	Combining reward and consequence. The child earns rewards and privileges when performing desired behavior. She loses the rewards and privileges as a result of unwanted behavior	Child earns stars for completing assignments and loses stars for getting out of her seat. Child cashes in the sum of her stars at the end of the week for a prize

From Reiff MI: *ADHD: A Complete and Authoritative Guide.* Elk Grove Village, IL, American Academy of Pediatrics, 2004, p 140.

The use of medication improves the inattentiveness, hyperactivity and impulsivity in 70% to 80% of school-age children who have this disorder, often making them more ready to learn. Medication will not improve academic achievement directly. Over 150 randomized controlled clinical trials of school-age children with ADHD support the benefit of stimulant medications (methylphenidate and amphetamine). In addition, a nonstimulant medication, atomoxetine, may be useful for treatment of ADHD behavior. Not only are documented benefits seen in core ADHD symptoms, but in many cases medication also improves a child's ability to follow rules, improves relationships with peers and parents and decreases oppositional behavior and anxiety.

A randomized, controlled multicenter study of school-age children (7 to 9 years old) demonstrated that both medication alone and medication in combination with behavior modification significantly improved core ADHD behavior over a 14-month study period; the beneficial effects were sustained to a lesser extent at 24 months. The combination of medication and behavior management was most effective when ADHD was associated with parent-child conflict, social skills dysfunction or anxiety. Parents and teachers were more satisfied with the combined therapy.

Medication will not by itself turn a student's Ds into As and will not correct a specific learning disability. An unjustified shift to a medical versus an educational diagnosis may lead to unduly high expectations from the medication and the lack of a directed, specific educational program. Whereas a medication is often the most effective intervention for a child with ADHD, it should not be used without equal attention to the learning environment, individual learning style, coexisting conditions and the psychosocial assessment of the child and family.

Evaluation and management of children with chronic inattention involve ongoing contact with the school, as well as referral to educational and mental health specialists when indicated. The pediatrician must therefore develop an alliance with the child, parents and teacher so that long-term collaboration is possible. An environment that supports the child's efforts to maintain focus on tasks and be successful can be created only by this collaborative effort. ADHD should be seen as a chronic illness that calls for close follow-up and timely adjustments in treatments and interventions.

LEARNING DISABILITIES

A learning disability refers to a consistent difficulty in learning basic academic skills related to the acquisition and use of listening, speaking, reading, writing, reasoning or mathematical abilities. Behavioral problems (e.g., ADHD and oppositional behavior) and problems with social interactions may coexist with a learning disability, but they are considered separate conditions. Learning disabilities are neurologically based, a reflection of the "hard-wiring" network of the central nervous system. They are seen in approximately 7% of school-age children with a wide variation in aptitudes—from children with average intelligence to those with superior intellectual abilities. A learning disability is often suspected when the difference between aptitude (intelligence) and achievement (learning output) on standardized tests is wide. In addition, a learning disability should also be considered when a discrepancy of 15 to 20 points is found on the verbal and performance sections of the Wechsler Intelligence Scale for Children–Revised. A learning disability should be seen as a discrepancy or imbalance between one or more cognitive functions. School systems rely on the measurement of this discrepancy to decide which children are labeled as learning disabled and therefore require special services and adaptations. Most learning disabilities do not come to the attention of parents, educators or clinicians until a child is challenged with cognitive work that requires the acquisition and use of reading, spelling or arithmetic skills.

A clinically useful perspective on learning disabilities derives from the recognition that we learn either by visual or by auditory input of information. Assuming that a child has adequate visual acuity and hearing capacity, most learning disabilities can be conceptualized as a developmental variation in the sensory/perceptual-cognitive processing pathways of the brain that follow the sensory input. Visual-dependent learning problems may cause a delay in learning to read and manipulate numbers. Recognition and comprehension of the symbolic language represented by words or numbers are altered in a manner that may affect the development of reading skills (dyslexia) or mathematical abilities (dyscalculia). Children with auditory-dependent learning problems find it difficult to comprehend spoken language when presented with new information. These disabilities are associated with either a visual or an auditory processing disorder that may have a significant impact on the quality and quantity of learning.

Dyslexia, the most common learning disability, is a specific language-based learning disability that affects reading, spelling and written expression. The major neuropsychological deficit is in phonological processing skills. This means difficulty learning the alphabet, lack of alphabet mastery, problems with letter-sound associations and difficulty acquiring decoding skills and sight word vocabulary for reading. Intelligence is normal. The variety of other specific learning disabilities that come to the attention of pediatric clinicians during the early elementary years is presented in Table 20–2.

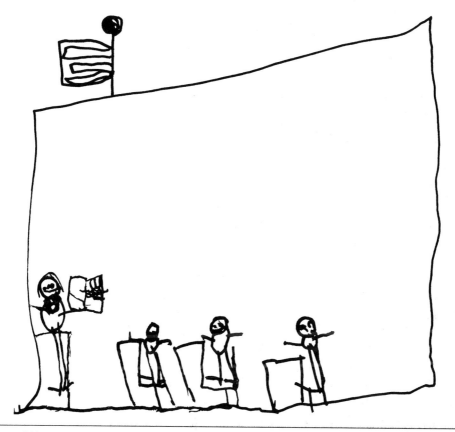

A 6½-year-old boy draws his classroom. The teacher holding the book illustrates the central focus on reading in the first years of school. By Ryan Hennessy.

TABLE 20–2 **Definitions of Learning Disabilities**

Term	Description
Visual perception deficit	Inability to differentiate between similar-looking letters, numbers, shapes, objects, symbols; may habitually skip over lines in text
Auditory discrimination deficit	Inability to distinguish similar sounds ("pig" and "big") or confusing the sequence of heard or spoken sounds ("ephelant")
Dyslexia	Difficulty sounding out letters and confusing words that sound similar resulting in problems acquiring basic reading skills. Dyslexia is a language-based learning disorder associated with difficulty in single-word decoding and phonological awareness (the ability to translate letters and letter patterns into sound with precision and speed). Dyslexia affects reading, spelling and written expression. A core deficit in phonological processing skills leads to difficulty learning the alphabet, lack of alphabet mastery, problems with letter-sound associations and difficulty acquiring decoding skills and sight word vocabulary for reading. Prognosis is best if dyslexia is recognized and treated before grades 4 through 6
Dysgraphia	Difficulty expressing thoughts on paper and with writing associated with unreadable penmanship and problems in gripping and manipulating a pencil. A history of difficulty with drawing (e.g., poorly structured drawings, distorted shapes or missing details) may give a clue to dysgraphia. It is often associated with problems in visual-motor control and fine motor abilities
Dyscalculia	Problems with perception of shapes and confusion of arithmetic symbols leading to poor comprehension of simple mathematical functions. There are three neurological sources for dyscalculia: (1) difficulty with visual-spatial skills; these children often have intact reading and spelling skills; (2) difficulty with arithmetic fact retrieval associated with problems with memorization and retrieval from long-term memory; and (3) difficulties with use of arithmetic procedures such as counting, carrying and borrowing; associated with poor attention and lack of monitoring work when problem solving
Dysnomia	Inability to recall names or words for common objects
Pragmatic language disorder	Difficulty with the use of language in social contexts, including nonverbal aspects of tone, rate of speech and turn taking. Lacking observations skills of nonverbal cues results in impulsive social interchange

The diagnostic assessment of a learning disability is based on more data than the physician can obtain during the interview with the family and examination of the child. It is established by means of standardized educational tests performed by a clinical psychologist or a certified psychomotrist. However, critical clues to a learning disability can be identified by the use of

TABLE 20-3   Screening Questions for Learning Disorders

Reading

What is the hardest thing about reading?

Is it hard to sound out words?

Do you know words by just looking at them (sight word vocabulary)?

Do you forget things that you read at the beginning of a paragraph when you reach the end of the paragraph?

Do you understand what you read?

Mathematics

Do you understand the teacher when he/she is explaining something in math class?

Do you prefer to learn math by having the teacher explain it to you, or would you prefer to see how a math problem is solved correctly?

Do you have trouble remembering things in math? (if yes) What kinds of things do you have trouble remembering?

When you have a word problem, can you figure out what operation you should use (i.e., addition, subtraction)?

Do you make a lot of careless mistakes in math?

From: Lindsay RL: School failure/disorders of learning. In Bergman AB (ed): *20 Common Problems in Pediatrics*. New York, McGraw-Hill, 2001, p 328.

screening questions in a primary care setting (Table 20–3). The "ADHD tool kit," described earlier, also includes specific questions for parents and teacher that screen for learning disabilities. When a learning disability is suspected from the history, several neurodevelopmental procedures often reveal a specific type of disability (Table 20–4). Clinicians will be rewarded by the knowledge that a learning disability was detected early, a time when educational interventions are more likely to be effective.

It is also essential to obtain the results of educational testing from the school or other source or to ask that such tests be performed if necessary. Data on the child's learning patterns and output (grades), attention span and social and behavioral adjustment can be obtained by contacting teachers directly with the parent's permission. Asking a teacher to provide a written response to two questions often yields a rich descriptive profile of a child's learning strengths and weaknesses: "Tell me about ... 's learning style in class; what are his/her strengths and weaknesses; tell me about his/her behavior in class." Teachers are often eager to have an opportunity to discuss with a clinician the children whom they find most challenging. Standardized teacher report questionnaires are available if the pediatrician chooses to obtain a formal profile of school behavior.

Schools are required by federal law to respond to a parent's request to assess learning or behavioral problems that affect school function. Clinicians can play an active role in educating parents about their rights and the referral process, as well as advocating for the child with the school. Two federal laws guarantee the rights of children with learning disabilities to receive timely and comprehensive evaluation and treatment services free of charge: the 1991 addendum to the 1990 Individuals with Disabilities Education Act (IDEA) and Section 504 of the 1973 Vocational Rehabilitation Act. A guide to these service for parents and pediatric clinicians is found in Box 20–3.

TABLE 20–4   **Neurodevelopmental Screening Tests for Learning and Attention Problems**

Pediatric clinicians can include neurodevelopmental tasks as a part of the physical examination. These tasks assess a variety of components of neurological function that are associated with learning and attention. They are helpful in at least two ways. They may give clinicians a clue to a specific learning disability. In addition, as a result of the mild stress induced by the task, often behavior consistent with hyperactivity (fidgetiness, getting up from seat, constant motion, etc.) and inattentiveness (distractibility, off-task, daydreaming) will emerge in the office only during this part of the examination. Examples of neurodevelopmental tests include the following:

Test	Function
Ask child to write a sentence	Written expression and dysgraphia
Ask child to tell you about a movie or video seen recently	Oral expression, memory, sequencing
Ask child to read a paragraph appropriate for age	Reading fluency and comprehension
Ask child to copy a geometrical figure or do a Draw-a-Person test (see Chapter 5)	Fine motor and visual-spatial skills
Ask child to repeat a series of random numbers (at least age minus one from 5–10 years old)	Short-term memory and sequencing
Ask child a multiple-step task to complete in order given (age minus one task from 5–10 years old)	Auditory processing

From: Reiff MI, Stein MT: Attention-deficit/hyperactivity disorder evaluation and diagnosis: A practical approach in office practice. *Pediatr Clin North Am* 50:1020-1048, 2003.

The case of Bryan, at the beginning of this chapter, provides an example of how a child's temperament and experiences in the family can result in disruptive behavior in school. ADHD is only one of a number of disruptive behavior disorders occurring in childhood. Anxiety, depression and oppositional defiant disorder may be associated with similar classroom behavior. In Bryan's case, it would not be appropriate to label his difficulties in school as a disorder because the available information does not include pervasiveness (presence in other settings) or clear evidence that the behavior impairs his educational or social functioning. His hyperactivity and social intrusiveness were, in large part, results of variations in the temperament of Bryan, his parents, grandparents and teacher.

Most specific learning disabilities typically become apparent during first grade, although other subtypes of academic difficulty may emerge initially in the fourth or fifth grade, and still others become apparent for the first time in junior high school with expectations for more planning and organization as learning becomes more complex and challenging (see Chapter 23). This trimodel presentation of these several types will help the clinician be attentive in getting an appropriate evaluation and remediation plan. The family history often provides an additional clue to a learning disability. Patterns of learning disabilities frequently surface during

BOX 20–3   INDIVIDUALS WITH DISABILITIES EDUCATION ACT

The federal law, outlined in the Individuals with Disabilities Education Act (IDEA) and its amendments, states that a "free appropriate public education is available for all children with disabilities between the ages of 3 and 21... ." The difficulties that many parents face in accessing assessment and services for their children within our public education system make it critically important that pediatricians understand how to help parents. Pediatricians can play an important role as advocates for educational services for children with learning, emotional or health conditions.

Information about special education procedures, including the full text of the IDEA amendments, is available from the U.S. Department of Education. Each state's department of education has additional information relevant to your state. The initial assessment consists of procedures to "determine whether a child is a child with a disability and to determine the educational needs of such child." The basic procedures are listed below:

Step 1: Identification

When a child is identified as possibly needing special education and related services, states are required to conduct "Child Find" activities to identify and evaluate all children with disabilities who need special education whether the child is in private, parochial or public school. A request for assessment can be made by the parent, school personnel or other involved persons such as a physician or psychologist. The request can be verbal or in writing (e.g., a dated letter addressed to the principal of the local school and/or the district's Director of Special Education). Parental consent is needed before a child can be evaluated. Parents should keep copies of any correspondence, formal and informal, between themselves and the school; using a notebook format helps keep records in chronological order.

Some schools recommend a Student Study Team (SST) or similar group meeting before considering an assessment for special education. A SST meeting is not a substitute for the special education assessment process. It can be appropriate as a quick look and plan for children with their first school difficulty.

There are some children who are at high risk for persistent and significant problems in school but who have not fallen far enough behind to meet the formal criteria for a disabling condition under IDEA. Children with dyslexia may fall into this category because we can often predict the children who are going to have school difficulties at a young age, yet there may not be a significant discrepancy between achievement and intelligence, which is required to qualify a student as learning disabled. A parent or physician may need to ask for reassessment if school difficulties persist or worsen. Consider also that many of our patients have dual diagnoses and may qualify for and need services because of other health impairments such as ADHD, asthma or anxiety disorders.

Step 2: Evaluation

After a written request is made and received by the school, the school has 15 calendar days to give the parents an assessment or evaluation plan that indicates the areas to be assessed and usually includes specific tests to be administered. Districts vary in the comprehensiveness of their initial assessments. At a minimum, districts will usually assess academic achievement and cognition. It is appropriate for a pediatrician or other specialist to ask for assessments in other areas of probable need, such as language, motor, sensory processing, social/emotional and health.

Continued

BOX 20–3   INDIVIDUALS WITH DISABILITIES EDUCATION ACT—cont'd

The parent reviews, modifies if necessary, signs the Evaluation Plan and returns it to the school as quickly as possible. The school then has 50 calendar days (with extensions for longer school holidays) to complete the testing and hold a team meeting to go over the child's evaluation results and together decide whether the "child is a child with a disability" as defined by IDEA.

Step 3: Eligibility Is Decided

The team meets to determine whether the child is a child with a disability and whether special education services are needed. Parents should not sign special education documents that they do not agree with. Federal and state law outlines procedures to handle disagreements between schools and parents in areas such as eligibility, placement and level of services. Parents or schools can request mediation or due process to challenge team decisions.

Step 4: If Child Is Eligible for Services

If the child is found to be eligible for special education and related services, the Individual Educational Plan (IEP) team must meet again within 30 calendar days to write the IEP. Parents and, when appropriate, the student are part of the IEP team. Services are to be provided "as soon as possible after the meeting." The IEP document must include current levels of performance, annual goals with interim short-term objectives, measurable goals, a list of the specific services provided to the child (e.g., supplementary aids, speech therapy, adaptive physical education, modifications, staff training or supports), extent of participation with nondisabled children, transition service needs and how progress will be measured. An IEP must also state when services begin, where, how often and for how long services will last. Transportation is routinely provided by districts, and many children qualify for extended year programs.

Step 5: IEP Reviews Are Scheduled

The specifics of the IEP are required to be reviewed once a year. Parents or the school can request a review of the IEP at any time, and a meeting must be held within 30 days of a written request for a review. A major review, usually including retesting in the areas of concern, must be held every 3 years but may be done more frequently if needed. Although the criteria for qualifying for special education are fairly specific, there are no specific criteria for exiting special education services. At times, a parent may be told that their child no longer qualifies for special education services; this may not be accurate. Decisions to end special education services need to be carefully examined.

From: Stein MT, Lounsbury B: A child with a learning disability: Navigating school-based services. *J Dev Behav Pediatr* 22:188-191, 191-192, 2001.

a clinical evaluation for school underachievement; specific questions about the educational performance of parents and other relatives are helpful.

It is essential that physicians routinely inquire about the progress of 6-year-olds in the first grade. Any concerns raised should not be dismissed as "adjustment" problems or entirely maturational in origin (i.e., "He will grow out of it" or "He's just immature"). Clinical attention to educational concerns from the start and all along will head off the establishment of a cycle of failures. Children with a primary learning disability can experience academic difficulties without having behavioral or emotional problems if evaluated and addressed early on. However, without diagnosis and intervention, such children may subsequently develop low self-esteem and have disturbances in emotional well-being and conduct as a result of academic frustration. These secondary effects of academic failure will make accurate diagnosis much more difficult later. Because the best medicine is preventive medicine, it is important that learning disabilities be recognized early so that specific remedial measures may be undertaken to lessen the occurrence of secondary psychosocial problems.

PSYCHOSOCIAL PROBLEMS THAT AFFECT LEARNING

A child's emotional life, family environment, school and community are other important factors to consider when problems with learning occur in the first and second grades. Among children with mental health problems (e.g., depression, anxiety, oppositional behavior or conduct disorder), 30% to 80% have problems with academic achievement and classroom behavior. The low self-esteem and poor self-image in these children affect learning, especially in those with an associated learning disability. Chronic family dysfunction or, in a vulnerable child, even a temporary life event change in the family may cause or exacerbate school failure. Separation, divorce, an illness in the child or a family member, substance abuse and child abuse or neglect are seen in many young school-age children with learning problems. Finally, the child's extended environment in the school and community can affect learning. A curriculum that does not fit the learning needs of a child, an unmotivated or overwhelmed teacher, a teacher (or parent) whose expectations for academic success are discordant with a child's abilities or a community where violence is pervasive or where school achievement is not a major goal may have the same effect on learning as a neurologically based learning disability or disorder of attention. Dworkin and colleagues pointed out the following (2004) here.

School processes are more important determinants of students' performance than such features as whether schools are public or private, class size, the age and spaciousness of the school building, and student-teacher ratio. Rather, the school's academic emphasis, expectations for attainment, amount of homework, teachers' actions during lessons, use of group instruction, and use of rewards and praise are major influences on students' performance. Aspects of the school's social environment (such as the amount of praise offered to children) may be particularly important for children from disadvantaged homes in which less emphasis is placed on academic attainment and standards for classroom behavior.

FROM: DWORKIN PH. SCHOOL FAILURE. IN PARKER SJ, ZUCKERMAN BS, AUGUSTYN MC (EDS): *DEVELOPMENTAL BEHAVIORAL PEDIATRICS: A HANDBOOK FOR PRIMARY CARE*, 2ND ED. PHILADELPHIA, LIPPINCOTT WILLIAMS & WILKINS, 2004, PP 281–1284.

SCHOOL AVOIDANCE

All clinicians who work with children sooner or later will evaluate a child who refuses to attend school. Unexcused absences from school follow a bimodal pattern of incidence, with peaks in the early primary grades in about 5% of children, particularly first grade, and a second peak again in junior high school in 2% of youth. The clinician should carefully and systematically determine the reason the child is not attending school. Some children are kept home from school by parents, although most unexcused absences from school are attributable to school refusal by the child.

Most first graders, in contrast to older youth, who refuse to attend school do not roam the community (truancy), but spend the school day at home. These children may have a variety of physical complaints, including stomachaches, headaches, dizziness and fatigue, that often subside as the day progresses. Although a few of these children may be suffering from an actual phobia of school itself or some particular aspect of the school experience such as travel on the bus, most first graders who refuse to attend school appear to be suffering from separation anxiety. When examined in the clinician's office, these children usually appear healthy and have a normal physical examination, although some initially appear pale, sad and emotionally depressed or anxious.

These children are experiencing stress in response to leaving their parents and familiar surroundings for a full day of school. The pediatric clinician may diagnose separation anxiety, which often responds to simple behavioral measures combined with supportive counseling of the parents (e.g., parent stays in class with the child for a short period in the morning and gradually decreases her time in class; takes the child to the school playground on a weekend when other students are not present; arranges a play date with another child after school). Such children may have unusually high levels of anxiety. Some anxiety is normal in all children as they begin their grade school experience. Many children with school-related separation anxiety have a history of difficult separations as toddlers and preschoolers (see Chapter 18). Selective mutism, or refusal to speak to any person outside the home, is a less frequent condition associated with separation anxiety. Some parents may transmit their anxiety about separating to the child and thereby exacerbate the problem. Such families need to be reminded that school attendance in the first grade is compulsory and that separation from family at this time is a healthy and predictable stage of maturation.

The child's clinician must be sympathetic to the physical complaints and initiate a reasonable medical evaluation. Excessive medical attention to the physical complaints, which may occur when a large number of laboratory tests or specialty referrals are ordered, should be avoided when inorganic disease is suspected. The clinician must make it clear to the family that the child is to attend school on a daily basis unless the symptoms are severe enough to require a visit to the physician's office. Returning to school will be both diagnostic and therapeutic. The parents may be reassured that the child will usually settle down in school if he comes to understand that his parents expect and will demand school attendance. Often, the school can support the parent in keeping the child in school. Children with separation anxiety disorder become rapidly asymptomatic as their school attendance becomes more regular. When school refusal does not respond to these measures or when pediatric evaluation of the child or family suggests a serious physical or emotional disorder, a mental health referral may be indicated, as well as perhaps a short course of medication.

School refusal in early adolescence often leads to a more extensive differential diagnostic evaluation. If a junior high school student spends school time in community areas, such as malls, and engages in varying degrees of antisocial behavior, one must suspect a conduct disturbance. Adolescents who remain at home may have physical complaints similar to a 6-year-old's and may be suffering from an anxiety disorder, depression, substance abuse or teenage pregnancy (see Chapters 22 and 23). Some of these youth stay home because they are fearful and have been threatened or mistreated by peers. A small number are experiencing the onset of a serious psychiatric disturbance, such as depression or schizophrenia. School refusal in adolescence that is not clearly truancy should be carefully examined and every effort made to prevent a tragic early withdrawal from school.

DATA GATHERING

Children at the age of 6 may not be as candid in providing information to the physician as they once were. Just as the clinician may observe increasing modesty during physical examination at this age, he may also find the child withholding or distorting her answers to questions about personal, school and family life. Obtaining information with the child and parent present is the most productive technique for 6-year-olds. As with preschool children, it is important to communicate to the child that you value the information she provides about her health and feelings. Asking the child first to describe her physical complaints and beliefs about the reasons for the medical examination may provide an opportunity to deal directly with the 6-year-old's lingering misconceptions about the reasons for the medical encounter. In the course of evaluating the child's physical health, the clinician may gather data about the child's development in the areas shown in Table 20–5.

QUICK CHECK—6 TO 7 YEARS

✓ The brain of a 5-year-old has attained 90% of its adult size. Synaptogenesis persists as a biological marker for cognitive, social and motor maturation.

✓ Six to 7 years begins the shift in cognitive function from preoperational ("magical") thinking to concrete operations (reasoning and understanding connect to actual situations and objects).

✓ The "5/7 shift" refers to the age range of normal development for the acquisition of reading skills.

✓ Academic success in the first grade occurs when decoding letters leads to reading, simple addition and subtraction problems are solved and simple words in short sentences are spelled correctly.

✓ ADHD, a neurologically based disorder in selective attention, occurs in 6% to 9% of school-age children. Diagnostic criteria are specific, including documentation of behavior that reflects hyperactivity, impulsivity and inattention at school and home, persistence of such behavior for at least 6 months (beginning before 7 years old) and an association between ADHD behavior and impairment in either educational output or social functioning.

✓ Coexisting conditions (e.g., oppositional behavior, anxiety, depression and learning disabilities) occur in many children with ADHD.

✓ Medication improves core ADHD behavior in 70% to 80% of school-age children. Behavior management and classroom accommodations are also effective.

✓ A learning disability occurs in at least 7% of school-age children. It may affect the acquisition and use of reading, spelling, mathematical, listening, writing or speaking skills.

✓ Dyslexia, a neurologically based deficit in phonological processing skills, is the most common learning disability. It may impair reading, spelling and written expression.

✓ School avoidance (refusal to attend school) occurs in 5% of elementary school children and 2% of adolescents. It is often associated with separation anxiety in younger children.

TABLE 20–5   Gathering Data

Cognitive Development	
Questions for Children	**Objective**
Where do you go to school? What grade are you in? What are you learning in school? Are there some things you do at school that you really like? Are there things about school that you don't like?	To assess whether a 6-year-old can provide acceptable answers to nearly all these questions. Answers may suggest that the child is having difficulty in particular areas. When the child is reluctant to talk about school or provides very little information, the clinician should then invite the parent to enter the discussion.
What town do you live in? On what street? Do you know your address? Do you know your telephone number?	To assess the child's attention to basic information important to his well-being as he spends increasing amounts of time away from his family; to assess visual or auditory memory skills.
Ask the child to copy a cross (4-year-old), a square (5-year-old), a triangle (6-year-old) and a diamond (7-year-old).	To observe the child's handedness, his ability to grasp and control a writing instrument and his competence in increasingly difficult fine motor and visual-perceptual tasks.
Ask the child to draw a person while you are interviewing the parent.	An estimated mental age may be obtained by using Goodenough's scoring criteria (see Chapter 5). In addition, information may be obtained about the child's attentiveness, tendency to cooperate, compulsivity and even emotional health if the drawing is atypical (see Chapter 5).
What makes the sun come up in the morning? What makes the clouds move in the sky? How can you tell if something is alive?	To assess the child's beliefs regarding causality and to help parents understand that the child remains in a transitional period relative to his cognitive abilities. Most 6-year-olds, regardless of intelligence, will respond to these questions with magical thinking characterized by animism and egocentricity. For example, "The sun comes up in the morning so that I can play."
How do you get to your house from school?	Children at this age continue to be highly egocentric in their ability to give directions and will often leave out important details. This should be interpreted to parents as a normal developmental stage and will help parents understand why it is difficult for children to reverse directions or see the world from another person's perspective.
Have you seen a recent movie or video? Tell me about the story.	To assess the child's capacity for sequencing events, memory and content of a story.
Do you ever have dreams? Do the dreams ever really happen? Where do the dreams take place? What really happens to the people on television who fly or get hurt?	To assess the child's capacity for distinguishing between reality and fantasy, which should be well developed at this age.

TABLE 20–5 Gathering Data—cont'd

Cognitive Development	
Questions for Parents	**Objective**
Does (name) have a problem concentrating or paying attention? Do you think that (name) is more active, less attentive than other children his age?	To assess the parent's perception of the child's ability to attend to a classroom learning environment.
Do you frequently find yourself repeating directions or instructions?	To assess auditory processing maturation.
How is school going? Have you had a conference with the teacher? How does (name) fit in with the classroom? What are the teacher's expectations for (name)?	To assess the parent's understanding and involvement with the school; to model the expected close interaction between parents and school personnel.

Social and Emotional Development	
Questions for Children	**Objective**
Do you know the name of the team that plays baseball or football for your city? What is your favorite movie? What is your favorite television show? Where did you go on your vacation?	To assess the child's general fund of information and the child's interest in and retention of information about events that occur outside the home.
Who are your good friends?	To assess the child's relationships outside the home. By this time a child should have formed several close relationships outside the home. The child should name one and preferably more friends close to his age. A child who does not name anybody or who names an adult, a family member or a much younger child requires further evaluation. The parent may be asked to comment on the child's response.
What games do you like to play?	To assess the child's preferences for solitary versus peer activities. Is he comfortable with the give and take of peer group activities? Does he understand the necessity for and the nature of rules? Is he involved in organized community-wide activities, such as team sports or a religion-based peer group?
Who lives at your house? What do you think about your brother/sister/the new baby?	To assess the child's capacity to express both positive and negative feelings relating to family members and the degree of sibling rivalry that may be present.
Questions for Parents	**Objective**
How long is (name) in school? What does (name) do after school? What jobs does (name) do around the house? How much television does (name) watch each day? What programs?	To assess the demands on the child's and family's circumstances and arrangements. To assess family responsibilities that the child shares.

> ## ! HEADS UP–6 TO 7 YEARS
>
> - Not all school-age children who are wiggly, fidgety and inattentive have ADHD. An assessment of social development, family structure and function and learning strengths and weakness and consideration of physical causes for the behavior are required before making a diagnosis of ADHD.
> - Specific learning disabilities are common in cognitively competent children. Early recognition is critical to a good outcome. Focused questions about learning progress during a health supervision visit will generate clues to a learning disability. Use of the American Academy of Pediatrics evidence-based guidelines for the diagnosis of ADHD will prevent both overdiagnosis and underdiagnosis.
> - Behavior modification for ADHD and oppositional and disruptive behavior is extra-ordinarily powerful when applied appropriately. Knowing the principles of behavior management, having handouts for parents in the office and, in more severe cases, knowing about the referral sources in your community should be a part of every pediatric practice.
> - School refusal in early elementary school is usually due to separation anxiety. It is often associated with physical symptoms in the morning, such as abdominal pain, headache or sore throat. Go further with each case by exploring symptoms of generalized anxiety, depression, an emerging and undetected learning disability or a history of persistent bullying. Primary depression and/or anxiety disorder must be considered.

ACKNOWLEDGMENT

Nicholas Putnam, M.D., contributed to this chapter in previous editions.

RECOMMENDED READINGS

For Parents

Barkley RA: *Your Defiant Child: Eight Steps to Better Behavior.* New York, Guilford Press, 1998.

Levine M: *A Mind at a Time.* New York, Simon & Schuster, 2002.

Levine M: *Educational Care: A System for Understanding and Helping Children with Learning Disabilities at Home and in School,* 2nd ed. Cambridge, MA, Educator's Publishing Service, 2002.

Office of Special Education and Rehabilitation Services, U.S. Department of Education: *A Guide to the Individualized Education Program,* July 2000. Available at http://www.ed.gov/offices/OSERS/OSEP/IEP_Guide.

Reiff MI: *ADHD: A Complete and Authoritative Guide.* Elk Grove Village, IL, American Academy of Pediatrics, 2004.

For Pediatricians

American Academy of Pediatrics/National Initiative for Children's Healthcare Quality (NICHQ): *ADHD: Caring for Children with ADHD: A Resource Toolkit for Clinicians.* Chicago, American Academy of Pediatrics. Available at http://www.aap.org/bookstore. Dworkin PH: School failure. In Parker SJ, Zuckerman BS, Augustyn MC (eds):: *Developmental and Behavioral Pediatrics: A Handbook for Primary Care,* 2nd ed. Philadelphia, Lippincott Williams & Wilkins, 2004, pp 281-1284.

eQuipp ADHD Module: American Academy of Pediatrics: *On-line Seminars and Office-Based Activities on the Etiology, Diagnosis and Management of ADHD.* Available at http://www.eqipp.org/global/module_overview_prel.

Websites

Children and Adults with Attention-Deficit/Hyperactivity Disorder (CHADD). Available at http://www.chadd.org.

Federal Resource Center for Special Education. Available at http://www.dssc.org/frc.

International Dyslexia Society. Available at http://www.interdys.org. Tel: 800-ABCD123.
Learning Disabilities Association of America. Available at http://www.ldanatl.org, tel: 412-341-1515.
National Center for Learning Disabilities. Available at http://www.ncld.org, tel: 212-545-7510.
National Institute of Neurological Disorders and Strokes, NIH. Available at http://www.ninds.nih.gov.
San Diego ADHD Project. Available at http://www.sandiegoadhd.com.

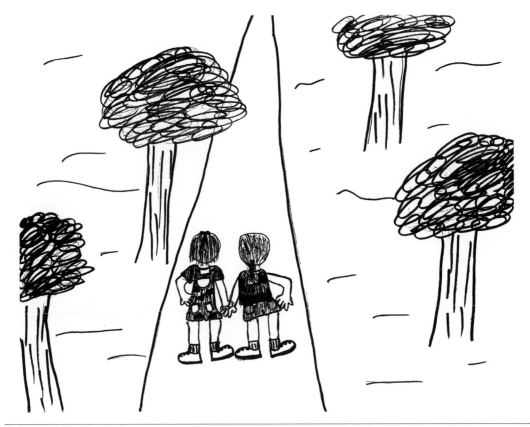

"Friends Forever." A precocious 10-year-old shows herself walking with a friend. Clear distance perspective usually emerges at an older age. By Kaitlin Thomas, age 10.

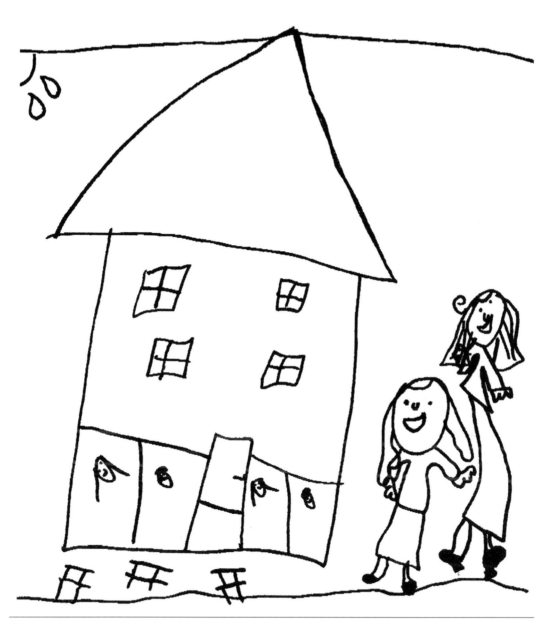

This school age child with William's syndrome demonstrates with her drawing the significant visual/spacial difficulties that track with that disorder. Her verbal skills are good, causing one to expect more of her than she can do.

CHAPTER 21

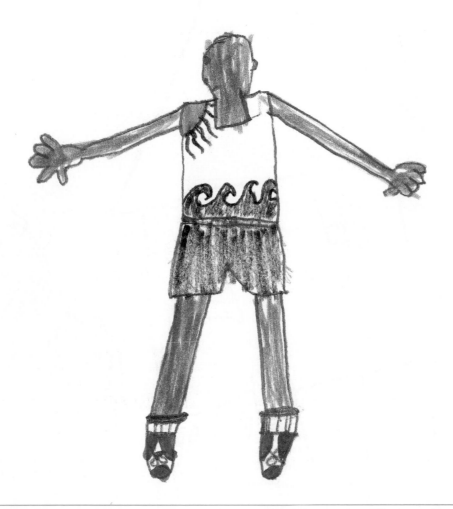

A 9-year-old shows himself ready to take on the world. Details of his clothes and the profile show advanced skills.

Seven to Ten Years: World of Middle Childhood

ROBERT D. WELLS and MARTIN T. STEIN

This chapter describes the cognitive, social and motor skills that are necessary for learning in school and during play. Developmental growth in emotional regulation and thinking brings new opportunities and vulnerabilities.

Key Words

- Mastery of Cognitive Skills
- Moral Development
- Conscience
- Separation
- Learning Disabilities
- Coping Skills
- Friendships
- Stress
- School Performance
- Sports
- Computers

Middle childhood is a period of significant changes in cognitive, social and motor development. Skills, emotional regulation and thinking all grow substantially through this period. Developmental tasks include expansion of a child's intellectual, moral and social reasoning, the development of a conscience and social activities guided by rules of conduct. The ability to access previously gained knowledge, organize it and express it verbally and in writing reflects maturation of the central nervous system in areas of perception, memory, reasoning, reflection and insight. The quest for social involvement and social acceptance highlights middle childhood. Biological and environmental influences act as both risk and protective factors during this period of growth. Understanding a child in this period requires consideration of all of these complex threads of developmental change.

Aaron, age 9 years, was brought to you after a 1-week history of headaches. He is a fourth grader in a school for gifted children and has been earning excellent grades. You know the family well because he has two younger siblings (ages 3 and 6 years) and because his

Continued

mother often calls and visits the office with acute concerns. Aaron was born after 5 years of infertility in his parents. His father, an attorney, is even-tempered and serious. His mother is a part-time teacher in computer sciences and has always been intense. She is concerned that Aaron's headaches are the result of a brain tumor because he has also had a major change in his behavior. His paternal grandfather died of an astrocytoma when Aaron was 2 years old. Although Aaron was always an intense, but sociable child, he is now withdrawn, irritable and demanding. He has been out of school for 1 week. His mother is unaware of any specific changes or stressful events, but did note that Aaron has recently had problems with friends in the neighborhood. You decide to speak with Aaron alone to assess his developmental and behavioral functioning and determine its potential significance in creating or maintaining his symptoms.

On physical examination, Aaron is a depressed-appearing child with dramatic complaints of headaches that are not well localized. A complete examination, including neurological assessment, blood pressure, screening audiogram and visual acuity, is normal. The child is afebrile and appears physically well.

When Aaron is interviewed alone, he initially denies with irritation any specific concerns. He easily discusses his baseball card collection. When asked about his strengths, Aaron is unable to tell you what he does well.

He says his headache keeps him from doing his schoolwork and admits hating school despite his success. He admits feeling lonely at times and wishes he had more friends. This is his first year out of the neighborhood school. To attend the gifted program, he must travel to the other side of town and thus far has not met any of his fellow students out of school. Note: Aaron's story will be used to highlight many of the important themes of the middle years of childhood. By the end of the chapter, his problems will be solved.

The middle childhood years are, for most children, a time of robust physical health filled with surges of competencies and vulnerabilities in behavioral and developmental areas. This places the primary care physician in a challenging position because visits become less frequent during a time when many behavior and learning problems may appear. Self-awareness, control over new feelings and desires and making a wider net of friendships deepen and evolve. This is not really a "latent" period at all, but one of consolidating and building skills. A lot is going on, but the clinician usually has to probe these normal developmental gains during visits for acute illnesses or minor injuries.

A significant number of school-age children face additional obstacles to developing these competencies. Approximately 30% of all children must cope with a chronic illness, of which asthma, obesity, attention deficit/hyperactivity disorder (ADHD) and learning disabilities are the most common. About 5.5% (3.5 million) of U.S. children have a chronic condition that limits usual activities, and they require additional care during a period of growing independence and self-responsibility. For these children, life is pulling them in two different directions. In the past decade childhood obesity rates have accelerated, thus creating additional concerns about the long-term health of children who have increasingly sedentary lifestyles and access to high-fat/high-calorie diets. A recent study found that only 12.8% of children between the ages of 7 and 12 had a good diet, 79% had a diet needing improvement and 13% had a poor diet. Growth charts published by the Centers for Disease Control and Prevention include gender-specific graphs to chart body mass index (BMI) from 2 to 20 years old. BMI levels between the 85th and 95th percentiles indicate children at risk for obesity, and levels equal to or greater than the 95th percentile indicate children who are overweight (Figs. 21–1 and 21–2). With an understanding that obesity affects self-image, self-esteem and interpersonal relationships, as well as physiological well-being, clinicians should assess and monitor this chronic condition throughout school-age and adolescent development.

In addition, learning problems, exposure to traumatic events and social and family dysfunction all pose significant risks for the development of a wide range of behavioral, academic and psychosomatic disorders. Of school-age children, 15% have an identified behavior problem severe enough to benefit from a formal pediatric evaluation and treatment.

Many more children have hurdles to overcome on a regular basis, and the health care provider may not be aware of all of these. Specific outreach to this group of youngsters through some planned assessments, some acute illness visits and even encounters after injuries all are opportunities to touch the lives of these children. Expanded visit agendas attached to these chance encounters may identify conditions and concerns that would otherwise be hidden.

DEVELOPMENTAL TASKS OF THE MIDDLE YEARS OF CHILDHOOD

New Cognitive Skills

Mastery, in a developmental context, refers to an internalized awareness of achievement. Although it is a part of each developmental stage, mastery takes on special meaning during the school-age years as a result of the child's increased capacity for making many kinds of determinations. New cognitive skills form the basis of these. At this age, a school-age child is able to consider two or more aspects of a situation simultaneously. In making comparisons, he takes into account more than one variable. He appreciates that a tall, narrow lump of clay can be made short and wide without any net gain or loss of clay (see Chapter 2). Such reasoning extends to the child's capacity for making a variety of judgments. He may appreciate for the first time another child who is clumsy but bright, a teacher who is strict but fair or medicine that is difficult to swallow but brings down a fever. For the first time the child has the mental capacity to appreciate that a surgical procedure will cause discomfort yet will produce a desired result.

Children begin to understand that rules in games and in life are the product of mutual consent and respect and that rules may be changed under certain circumstances. Piaget explained how children of elementary school age increasingly take context and motivation into account in making moral judgments. Kohlberg found that school-age children have varying levels of **moral development**. Whereas many behave well in order to earn some tangible reward or to avoid punishment, some are beginning to conform to gain approval from peers and adults. They also see the universality and value of a rule system. Many children at this age focus on clearly defined rules and have difficulty understanding why some people do not behave appropriately. This moral rigidity is developmentally normal, the outgrowth of new cognitive skills to see broad systems, such as rules, that work together.

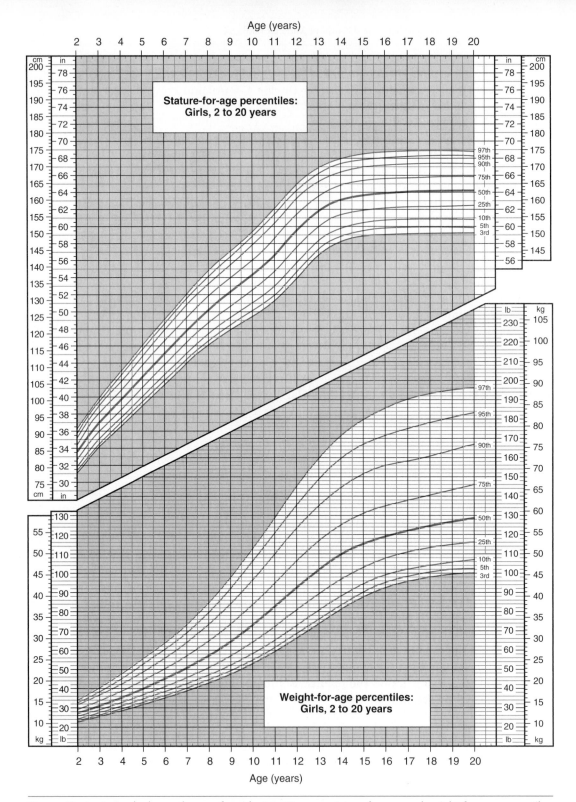

Figure 21-1 A standard growth curve for girls, 2 to 20 years: stature-for-age and weight-for-age percentiles. (From the National Center for Health Statistics in collaboration with the National Center for Chronic Diseases Prevention and Health Promotion, 2000.)

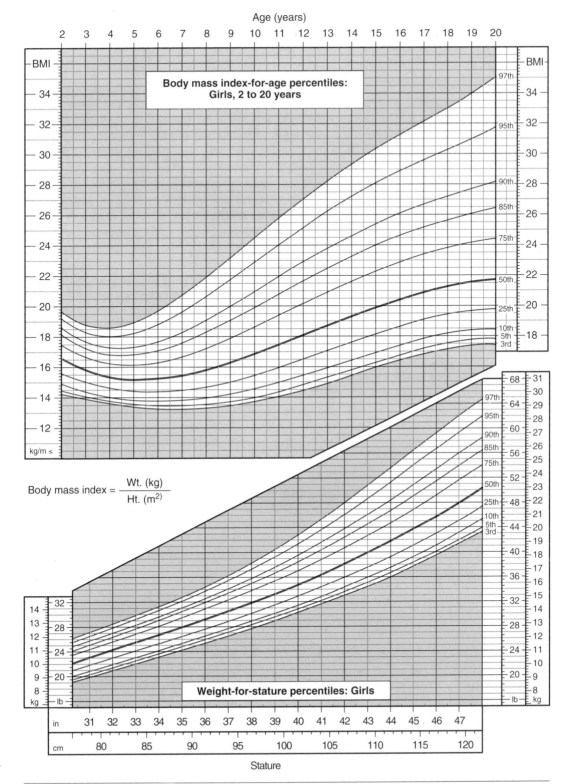

Figure 21–2 Body mass index and weight-for-stature percentiles. (From the National Center for Health Statistics in collaboration with the National Center for Chronic Diseases Prevention and Health Promotion, 2000.)

Identification and Socialization

During this time the child continues to consolidate her identification with important adults in her life. In this process the same-sex parent is an important role model. Other adults inside and outside the child's family also serve as examples for the child and thereby augment the primary organizing force of the immediate family. Freud pointed out the continuing growth during these years of that part of the child's mental life that represents internalized parental values—the superego or internalized **conscience**. Emotional growth and cognitive growth interact and result in the early development of a more personal conscience with less emphasis placed by the child on adult authority or conventional rules. This growth in conscience is found universally and crosses cultural and religious boundaries. The specific belief systems and norms of behavior are developed within the context of the family and, increasingly, that of society as a whole. The basis for understanding these rules is neurodevelopmentally based.

According to Erikson, children this age are negotiating a stage of *contrasting industry and inferiority* in which achievement is linked with self-concept. The ability to compete productively in academic, extracurricular, social and family realms in large part determines the child's sense of self-efficacy at this age. Highly self-efficacious individuals believe in their relative ability to master and control the situation to achieve goals and rewards. In the face of failure and disappointment, children with moderate to high self-efficacy will reapply themselves in an industrious fashion and develop a range of skills for overcoming obstacles. In contrast, low self-efficacy may be both the result and the cause of personal failure in developing social and academic skills. Children of this age are always measuring themselves and their achievements against others. This is part of the normal process but may be exaggerated in families or schools that push competition and competitiveness. Children must experience some success some-where in order to build a strong sense of themselves and a feeling of control over their world.

Although earlier explorations into separation have already been experienced, the school-age years are filled with a need to separate from parents for more prolonged periods. The ability to master these outings (e.g., sleepovers, camp) and to use independent **coping skills** when away from home appear critical for healthy development in this culture. While the separation process progresses during these times of independent activity, the child must still manage to function in the home in a manner that allows for new responsibilities. Children must become part of the family's maintenance system. Chores and homework become frequent testing grounds for these new demands. Conflicts are inevitable as parents teach children responsibility and participation, but these conflicts are really about psychological separation and control. With the child's increased cognitive and verbal sophistication, arguments between parent and child can take on the appearance of a courtroom as each side argues with righteousness over the obvious logic and illogic of the case. Stepping back from the particulars allows parents and the clinician to see the basic issues here. That sets the stage for less contentious interactions.

Fantasy and Identification

The psychological work of school-age children involves the *active use of fantasy and identification* with real and imagined characters who do what the child can only wish to do. This allows an emotionally healthy school-age child to express feelings without losing self-control. A boy who identifies with a professional athletic team may find expression for aggressive feelings by loudly denouncing a rival team (e.g., "I hate the Raiders!"). Although the child may have only recently outgrown a variety of fears, he may boast of his prowess in the face of the unknown by wearing a superheroes T-shirt. He may communicate to others and to himself his capacity for aggression by wearing military clothing and engaging in mock, but fierce battles with real or imaginary opponents. The widespread interest in video and computer games provides a popular avenue for exploring newfound capacities for achieving mastery in fantasized environments. Although this may not be universally healthy, it's nearly universally a part of kids' lives. A school-age girl may identify strongly with the sensuality of a popular actress or singer or with the controlled aggression of a female tennis champion or ballerina. These alignments and affiliations are testimonies to this healthy developmental process.

The physical, aesthetic and aggressive actions of these heroes provide outlets for normal, age-appropriate sexual feelings and drives. Their presence in a child's life can be demonstrated in the clinician's office by asking specific questions ("Who would you most like to be?"), by observing and commenting on the child's clothing and favorite possessions and by reviewing a child's artwork.

It is essential that a child this age be able to spend some of her energy in such fantasy. With emerging maturity, free-form fantasy is typically replaced with more rule-based activities (e.g., games rather than fantasy play). In view of the great appeal of video and computer games, it is also important that the child express herself through active participation in the *real* world, and parents may need help and advice in limiting time spent on solitary recreational activities. Emotional problems may occur when a child becomes lost in fantasy and fails to gain a sense of competence in dealing with the actual world. The boundary between fantasy and reality should be clear at this age. Behavior problems may occur if a child fails to learn to use fantasy as a means of expressing feelings and instead acts out many of her impulses in real situations or isn't clear about the effect of fantasy on herself and others.

Academic Skills

Achievement at school becomes more demanding and complex at this time. Tests, grades and special classes exert significant effects on school-age children. Repeating a grade level is one of the most stressful events for an elementary school child; it outranks the death of a close friend and is just below having a visible congenital deformity. Lesser degrees of academic failure also cause major distress in children. The expectations placed on students by their parents, teachers and ultimately themselves have significant impacts on learning rate, academic ranking and the child's sense of self-worth. Children with exaggeratedly optimistic or pessimistic expectations will demonstrate significant problems in work motivation and frustration tolerance now and in the longer term. Academic failure should be seen as a major trauma to a developing child's sense of self.

Distinct *learning disabilities and learning styles* may become most obvious during this time as the cognitive operations required in class become increasingly complex, sequential and reading based. For mastery to occur, it is important for the child to recognize her capacity to meet the expectations of teachers and parents by assuming responsibility and developing the skills to complete assigned tasks in the assigned time, manner and form that is expected.

By age 7 most children have become proficient in *decoding* basic symbols; they can read, sound out words and understand what a number means. Academic demands change qualitatively midway through grade school and require another set of skills, *encoding*. A child without any previous difficulty decoding may develop a "working disability" manifested by low productivity and difficulty encoding information or using these symbols to learn, understand concepts and pull information together.

In the early grades you learn to read; beginning in third grade you must read to learn. Moreover, once you learn something, you have to show that you've got it, through reports, essays, oral responses or other projects. During the *encoding* process, the child may be asked to access previously gained knowledge, organize it and express it verbally or in writing. Writing an essay and solving a numerical word problem are examples of encoding tasks. Levine and colleagues have termed disability in such tasks "developmental output failure," which can appear for the first time in some children as late as middle school or junior high. Such children form an extremely heterogeneous group with respect to the underlying disorders responsible for their generally poor productivity . Expressive language deficits, attentional deficits, fine motor problems and emotional problems may interact to produce the same clinical picture. These children may be seen as "lazy." Although a few students put little energy into their work because of individual temperamental style, most of these students are handicapped by real neurologically based learning disabilities that can and should be addressed. For example, some children with fine motor difficulties benefit from being given the opportunity to present their work orally, use a computer or present less work of better quality. The clinician serves such children by helping families, teachers and the children themselves see the problem in terms of underlying neurodevelopmental disabilities rather than look at it simply as "work refusal." Through effective advocacy, the clinician can identify these children for further evaluation and educational remediation. There is no diagnosis of "lazy." A child labeled "lazy" or described as "he doesn't apply himself" is a very likely candidate for this class of learning disabilities.

As demand for the volume of output increases, so does the complexity of the academic tasks that face the child in grades 2 through 4. Mussen and colleagues have pointed to five additional aspects of learning abilities that are a result of a higher level of central nervous system maturation that occur at this time:

- Perception—detection, organization and interpretation of information from both the outside world and the internal environment. A child notices more: more details, more similarities and more differences.

- Memory—storage and later retrieval of information. A child can recall more and more and bring information of greater diversity to solving a problem or understanding a situation.

- Reasoning—use of information to make inferences and draw conclusions. The child learns to assemble facts to explain things in increasingly complex ways.

- Reflection—evaluation of the quality of ideas and solutions. The child can compare ideas or consider a proposal before accepting or rejecting it.

- Insight—recognition of new relationships between two or more bits of information.

Successful learning requires an ability to be in a place where one is presented with challenges and to use these cognitive and perceptual abilities. The clinician can examine the child's capacity for such thinking by asking him to tell a story about something that happened to him or about a movie he saw. Alternatively, he can be asked a series of questions that assess increasingly sophisticated educational skills, such as the following:

- Memory—"Where did you go on your vacation?"
- Reasoning—"Why did your family decide to go there?"
- Reflection and analysis—"What did you like best and least about the trip? Why?
- Insight and creativity—"Where would you like to go if you could go anywhere? Why?"

The nature of the child's answers may reveal the capacity to make use of and communicate the knowledge he has, a task that is increasingly important as the child progresses through school. At this stage single words or nonspecific responses may signal a problem.

Expansion of Activities with Peers

School-age children immerse themselves in sports, clubs, crafts, organizations, music, baseball cards, current fads and a variety of other activities. These pursuits reflect a drive to master specific motor, social and artistic skills that are fashioned out of individual experiences, skills and cultural expectations. Some children spend hours drawing, whereas others shoot basketball, write poetry or build remote control cars. Doing the "in thing" becomes extremely important at this age, and most school-age children pursue sex-stereotyped activities with same-gender friendship groupings. Every child should have at least one such area of activity to which she, not just her parents, is committed.

Participation in organized athletic and artistic **activities** becomes an important part of the life of most school-age children. By the age of 6 years, children become aware of their abilities in various areas and in comparison with other children. At this age they may participate in team sports competitively although they rely on adults to structure the activity. At times they may have difficulty maintaining interest throughout the game. They may even be unclear about the outcome of a game in which they were involved. Nevertheless, by 10 years of age, most children have participated in sports and other performance activities in school or outside of it. These activities involve intense training, commitment, physical risk and physical contact. A child involved in such activities gradually learns basic skills, rules and the meaning of teamwork and discipline. She also has fun and develops **friendships**, and this may be reason enough to participate. For a child who is resistant to participation in a team sport, an individual sport (e.g., tennis or swimming), a martial arts program or other structured artistic activity may be an important outlet. Every child needs something beyond school work and family at this age.

Perhaps most central to the school-age years is the *quest for social involvement and social acceptance*. Most children seek to find a place for themselves among a cohesive group of same-sex friends. Their success in maintaining a positive sense of self during the vicissitudes of making and breaking friendships is in part dependent on the resilience of their coping and social skills. Children with positive peer relationships tend to give and receive positive attention, conform to classroom rules and perform well academically. They are also able to initiate social contact in a positive manner and tend to develop pleasant social interchanges with others.

Social skills may include a good sense of humor, an ability to make others feel wanted, a willingness to share, a positive mood, creativity, leadership and negotiation skills. These abilities are developed typically through observation of others (e.g., peers, parents, siblings, teachers and even television). For most children, friendships develop naturally as social involvement is pursued. The child's temperament (see Chapter 2) appears to be an important contributor in a school-age child's ability to develop competency at play and in making and losing friendships.

Challenges to Social Success. Social interactions with peers and teachers in school settings depend not only on the characteristics of the school and the child's abilities and background but also on the child's temperament. A slow-to-warm-up child may resist social assimilation into the school community. He may appear at first as "anxious" or "insecure." Temperamentally difficult children may appear "immature" as a result of impulsive, disruptive behavior in class and on the playground. A child with low persistence, a short attention span, high distractibility and a high activity level is at risk for early unfavorable judgments by peers. Highly impulsive children with ADHD may experience significant problems in initiating and sustaining desirable social interactions because of their underlying temperament. Children who do not make friendships should be evaluated for behavioral problems, special stressors or other conditions.

Bullies. Scapegoating, teasing, bullying and self-isolation become social dynamics that can seriously hinder children, especially those with poor social skills. Approximately 20% of school-age children are involved in bullying—as perpetrator, victim or both. Direct bullying (physical aggression) is more common with boys, increases in elementary school, peaks in middle school and declines in high school; verbal abuse remains constant. Indirect abuse (social isolation such as ignoring, excluding and backstabbing) is more frequent in girls. A recent report observed that 25% of teachers did not see anything wrong with most bullying situations and intervened in only 4% of bullying incidents. Female bullies have a high incident of depression. Delinquent behavior is found more frequently in both boys and girls who bully. As they approach adolescence, a child with a persistent lack of regard for others can be at significant risk for more serious problems, such as bringing a weapon to school, fighting and membership in a gang. Bully victims are typically socially isolated and may lack the social skills to distract bullies. Children with physical and emotional disabilities are bullied more frequently. Children on *both* sides of the bullying equation are at serious risk for long-term problems. Bullying is not all right; it requires prompt adult intervention.

Unusual Children. Social awareness and skill may be impaired in children who have a neurologically based social-cognitive dysfunction, such as a nonverbal learning disability or *Asperger's syndrome.* Essential features of Asperger's syndrome are severe and sustained impairment in social interaction with restricted, repetitive patterns of behavior, interests and activities, but without clinically significant delays in cognitive development or language. Basic language skills are intact (although there may be a history of early delays) in Asperger's syndrome, but there are delays in nonverbal communication skills and the social use of language (pragmatics). Motoric awkwardness, proprioceptor disabilities and poor performance scores on IQ testing make it difficult for such children to engage in the physical aspects of sports, scouting activities or artistic pursuits. A *nonverbal learning disability* is a neurological syndrome involving right hemisphere dysfunction that may also impair social awareness and interactions. There is considerable disagreement about whether these two conditions are the same or are distinct. Such children have relative strengths in verbal/auditory skills, rote memory and early literacy skills, but deficits in visual-spatial organization, tactile perception, motor functions, social skills and executive functions such as self-regulation, planning and problem solving. Deficits in

TABLE 21–1   **Essential Features of Asperger's Syndrome and Nonverbal Learning Disability**

Asperger's syndrome	Sustained impairment in social interaction with restricted, repetitive patterns of behavior, interests and activities but without clinically significant delays in cognitive development or language
	A pedantic style of communication (both in choice of words and in tone of voice)
	Reliance on language-mediated interaction
	Limited use of facial and bodily gestures to communicate
	Restricted social skills (e.g., reciprocal play)
	Speaking loudly, often about unusual, adult-like topics; one-sided descriptions of facts
	Difficulty understanding other people's feelings, intentions and motivations
	Lack of mutual friendships despite an apparent motivation to engage others
	Self-absorption (e.g., talking to self or smiling to self)
	Verbal associations without maintaining a coherent message
	Not adjusting speech to the conversational partner's needs
	Circumscribed interests sometimes involving unusual topics
	Unusual interest in normal topics pursued in an unusual manner (e.g., learning of serial numbers, listing of models)
	Circumscribed interests have an impact on learning and interfere with the child's capacity to maintain reciprocal conversations
Nonverbal learning disability	A neurological syndrome involving right hemisphere dysfunction with strengths in basic verbal/auditory skills, rote memory and early literacy skills
	Deficits in visual-spatial organization, tactile perception, motor functions and social skills
	Problems with executive functions, such as self-regulation, planning and problem solving
	Significant discrepancy on aptitude tests with higher scores on verbal than nonverbal abilities
	Socially engaging with adults but overwhelmed by the complexities of peer interactions
	Difficulty processing nonverbal social cues and integrating sensory-motor information
	Problem in organizing language in a conversation
	Difficulty adapting to novel or complex situations
	Social anxiety and isolation

proprioceptive abilities have been shown to be the basis for some of the motoric awkwardness seen in this group of youngsters. Anxiety and difficulty adapting to novel or complex situations are common in both Asperger's syndrome and nonlearning verbal disabilities.

Distinguishing features of Asperger's syndrome and nonverbal learning disability are outlined in Table 21–1. An assessment of the components of social cognition can help the

TABLE 21–2   **Social Cognitive Dysfunction: Troubled Subcomponents**

Subcomponent	Trouble
Weak greeting skills	Initiating social contact with a peer skillfully
Poor social predicting	Estimating peer reactions before acting or talking
Deficient self-marketing	Projecting an image acceptable to peers
Problematic conflict resolution	Settling social disputes without aggression
Reduced affective matching	Sensing and fitting in with others' moods
Social self-monitoring failure	Knowing when one is in social trouble
Low reciprocity	Sharing and supporting, reinforcing others
Misguided timing or staging	Knowing how to nurture a relationship over time
Poor verbalization of feelings	Using language to communicate true feelings
Inaccurate inference of feelings	Reading others' feelings through language
Failure of code switching	Matching language style to current audience
Lingo dysfluency	Using the parlance of peers credibly
Poorly regulated humor	Using humor effectively for current context and audience
Inappropriate topic choice and maintenance	Knowing what to talk about and for how long
Weak requesting skill	Knowing how to ask for something tactfully
Poor social memory	Learning from previous social experience
Assertiveness gaps	Exerting the right level of influence over group actions
Social discomfort	Feeling relaxed while relating to peers

Modified from Levine MD, Unpopular child. In Parker S, Zuckerman B (eds): *Behavioral and Developmental Pediatrics: A Handbook for Primary Care*, 2nd ed. Philadelphia, Lippincott Williams and Wilkins, p 359.

clinician focus on the child's specific problems (Table 21–2). A clearer definition of the social deficits may guide management in a primary care setting (Box 21–1). A child labeled "odd," "a loner," "a geek," "wired" or other such terms may have one of these disorders. He may need a specific component in his school experience to teach the social skills he will not acquire on his own. He may also need assistance in finding a place in the social life of school, such as being the record keeper at sporting events, the "helper" in the computer lab or the money counter for a fund raiser. Providing a structure for such a child will assist in helping him feel valued in the complex world of the school.

Children with difficult, *high-strung temperaments* generally show greater mood intensity and lability and have a greater tendency to develop behavioral and psychosomatic symptoms. Children who tolerate frustration poorly, have difficulties with sharing or stand out as different

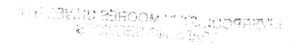

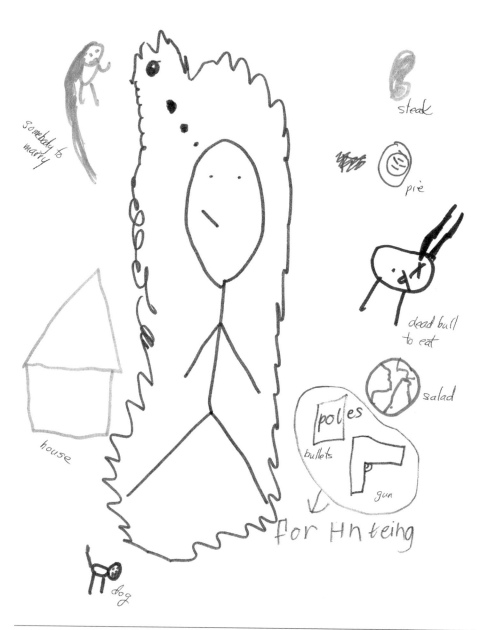

A rural boy of 9 shows himself in the center of all he thinks is important, now and in the future.

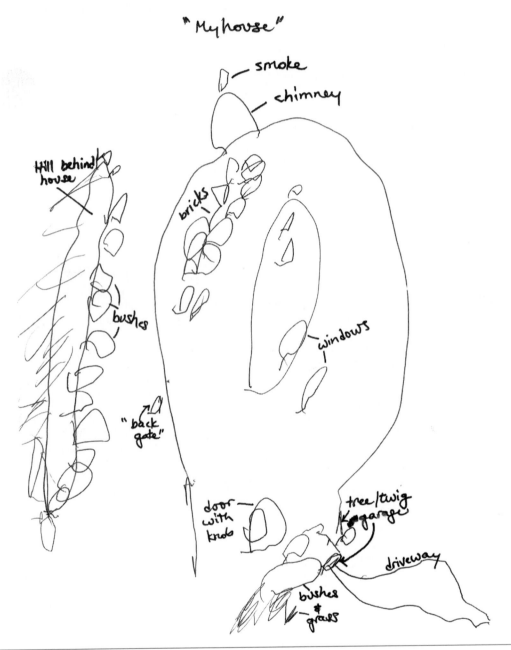

A 7-year-old with Tourette's syndrome and a nonverbal learning disability draws his house. The ideas are far ahead of the actual execution of the drawing. By Ryan, age 7.

BOX 21–1 SOCIAL COGNITIVE DYSFUNCTION–MANAGEMENT STRATEGIES

- **Explain the social skill problems carefully to the child.** This may require multiple sessions; not all affected children can process such information readily.

- **Have the parent of a child who needs social improvement accompany the child to an activity with other children.** Then, during a calm and private interlude, the parent can discuss the social interactions (especially any *faux pas* and transgressions that occurred).

- **Help the child locate one or two companions with whom to relate and begin to build skills.** It can be helpful if such peers share interests and perhaps some traits with the unpopular child.

- **Inform the classroom teacher or building principal if a child is victimized by peer abuse in school.** It is the school's responsibility to make every effort to contain this activity. A strongly worded note from a primary health care provider may be vital in such cases.

- **Help a rejected child develop skills, hobbies or areas of expertise that can enhance self-esteem and be impressive to other children.** Management of such a child should always include a diligent quest for and development of such specialties. Ideally, such pursuits should have the potential for generating collaborative activities with other children.

- **Never force these children into potentially embarrassing situations before their peers.** For example, an unpopular child with poor gross motor skills needs some protection from humiliation in physical education classes.

- **Manage any family problems or medical conditions** through counseling, specific therapies (e.g., language intervention or help with motor skills) and/or medication (e.g., for attention deficits or depression).

- **Identify social skills training programs within schools and in clinical settings.** Clinicians should be aware of local resources that offer social skills training to youngsters with social cognitive deficits. Most commonly this training makes use of specific curricula that are used in small group settings in a school or in the community.

- **Reassure these children that it is appropriate for them to be themselves, that they need not act and talk like everyone else in school and that there is true heroism in individuality.** Clinicians, teachers and parents must tread a fine line between helping with social skills and coercing a child into blind conformity with peer pressures, expectations and models.

From Levine MD, Unpopular child. In Parker S, Zuckerman B (eds): *Behavioral and Developmental Pediatrics: A Handbook for Primary Care.* (2nd Edition) Philadelphia: Lippincott Williams and Wilkins, p 359–60.

---

because of cultural, psychosocial or physical conditions are at high risk for an array of behavioral, somatic and developmental conditions. One study found that being labeled by a teacher as a school-age child who "failed to get along" was a more predictive factor of adolescent and adult criminality than any other single factor. Pay attention to these comments by teachers.

RISK AND PROTECTIVE FACTORS

Adjustment disorder, a condition that describes changes in behavior, mood or academic performance for the first 6 months after a stressful life event, are common in school-age children. Divorce, domestic violence, child abuse, natural disasters or a serious accident or illness

TABLE 21–3   **Internalizing and Externalizing Disorders**

Internalizing Disorders	Externalizing Disorders
Psychosomatic complaints	Disruptive behavior
Depression	Negativism
Withdrawal	Hyperactivity
Anxiety	Conduct disorders

of a family member can all have significant emotional effects on the developmental work of school-age children. The impact of any loss is experienced by school-age children with a growing awareness of its permanence and a feeling of being responsible for events around them.

When **stress** exceeds coping resources, maladaptation results. Some children will respond to stress overload by becoming depressed, anxious or preoccupied with body functions, whereas others may become provocative, angry and demanding. The array of psychological dysfunctions has been conceptualized as fitting into two broad groupings of disorders—internalizing and externalizing (Table 21–3).

Recurrent symptoms of pain, especially head, abdominal and limb pain, are frequent during the school-age years and in some cases may lead to difficulties in functioning in several areas. Although most of these recurrent pains are idiopathic with negative physical examination findings, many parents of these children have higher rates of depression and somatic pre-occupation, thus suggesting a familial pattern of underlying stress.

Habit problems and persistent problems with elimination are also prevalent in school-age children. Affected children and their parents become increasingly concerned about thumb sucking, nail biting, hair pulling and nocturnal enuresis and encopresis as social ostracism becomes more fervent. Recurrent idiopathic pain in school-age children may be a clue to inappropriate anxiety in the child or family and is often triggered by a significant stressful life event.

Differential Diagnosis of Poor Performance in School

Poor **school performance** may be the result of stress overload, sensory-perceptual limitations, learning disabilities, attentional problems, behavioral disorders, retardation or a host of other potential factors. Three percent of elementary-age children have a hearing impairment, almost 25% have visual defects and 1% have a major articulation disorder of speech. In addition, 10% to 20% have a definable learning disability in reading, arithmetic, attention, visual-spatial skills or other areas of neuropsychological functioning. Children with disabilities that limit their capacity for learning are at twice the risk for school avoidance, disruptive behavior problems, depression and psychosomatic reactions. Concern about poor academic performance may bring a child to the clinician; at other times it is the child's emotional or psychosomatic response to the disability that raises parental concern. Behavioral symptoms and somatic functioning that appear during school days but either lessen or resolve during holidays and weekends may be important clues to discovering developmental disorders and behavioral concerns.

Matthew is a 7-year-old white boy who has experienced crampy, periumbilical, abdominal pain almost daily for 2 months. Matthew has been successful in school and sports and has several close friends; the belly aches have not altered any of these activities. He denies constipation, diarrhea, nausea, vomiting, dysuria, urinary frequency, trauma or headaches.

Matthew's birth history and developmental course are uneventful. A comment in the chart at his 5-year health supervision visit was noted: "Bright and verbal child, inquisitive, enjoys drawing and playing with friends, new sibling past year/appears to have adjusted well." The family history is negative for gastrointestinal disorders and food intolerance. The parents both work and are successful in their jobs, and no financial stress or marital discord is evident.

When asked to describe the pain, he points to the periumbilical region and says it is "like the cramps—achy." It lasts from 5 to 30 minutes, occasionally several hours. The pain never radiates, never awakens him at night and is not accompanied by other symptoms. Lying down or sitting quietly usually resolves the pain.

Physical examination (including blood pressure determination, growth measurements and a digital rectal examination), a mental status test and a neurodevelopmental screening test are normal. Matthew's family drawing (completed while waiting in the office) reveals age-appropriate visual-motor skills and an active imagination, appropriate for his age and gender. Signs of anxiety or depression are not observed. Screening laboratory studies (complete blood count, erythrocyte sedimentation rate, urinalysis and stool examination for ova and parasites and occult blood) are normal.

At the initial visit, the pediatrician emphasizes the normal physical examination findings and the absence of associated symptoms that might suggest a specific cause for his pain. A brief discussion about the connection between "feelings and tummy aches" is initiated. A drawing of a transverse section of the intestinal tract is used to show Matthew how the smooth muscle lining constricts and dilates in response to signals from the brain. Strong feelings, such as anger or sadness, can "change the tightness" of these muscles and cause pain. It is suggested that sometimes kids with belly aches may feel pain when they are really feeling a strong emotion. Matthew listens attentively and asks a few questions about the illustration of the intestinal tract. Empirical dietary recommendations are written down: limit dairy products and increase fiber and fresh fruits. A follow-up appointment is made for 2 weeks.

At the next visit, the pattern and frequency of abdominal pain have not changed. A brief interview with the mother alone does not reveal any new information. Matthew is then interviewed alone. When asked why he thinks he experiences the pain, he says, "I guess some kids just get it. I don't know why." Matthew's affect and interpersonal interactions do not suggest either anxiety or depression. Note: This case is representative of the 15% of school-age children described by John Apply who have recurrent abdominal pain without an organic etiology. At the fourth office visit, a referral is made and the psychosocial cause of the pain is revealed (see end of the chapter).

Children with chronic medical diseases carry an additional burden for behavioral and developmental adjustment disorders. Children with central nervous system dysfunction, such as seizure disorders or mild mental retardation, are at three to four times greater risk for behavioral, emotional and learning problems than the general population of children. Differences in adjustment capacities do not correlate with the type of chronic illness; they are most affected by family functioning. The quality of the parent-child relationship, emotional disorder in the parents and marital discord are the strongest predictors of maladjustment for chronically ill and healthy children. In addition, the extent of functional limitation imposed by the illness and its treatment contributes to the risk for maladaptation.

Things That Help—Protective Factors

School-age children with greater intelligence, those with easier temperaments and those from more organized families are at reduced risks for significant behavioral and developmental problems. Flexible coping skills, an internal sense that one can have a positive effect on events and people and good physical health are also important moderators of stress.

Family functioning appears to be both the strongest risk and the strongest protective factor. A genetic predisposition to depression, alcoholism, obesity, learning disabilities, ADHD, conduct problems and psychosomatic preoccupations will raise the level of concern. Often, these factors will become apparent only through a focused family history interview. Of equal importance is the extent to which a family is successful in helping the child develop the necessary skills for social and academic success. Studies of resilience emphasize parental modeling of coping skills and the need to maintain predictable rules and expectations at home.

Social support from friends, family and others exerts significant influence in moderating the range of acute and chronic stress. Although peer friendships are important in helping children become socialized, studies of resilient children who reside in very dysfunctional families suggest that having one healthy, interested, caring and predictable adult can do a great deal for children facing numerous barriers to their development. So even in the most fragmented families, a child can develop in a strong healthy manner if even one adult is passionately committed to him and provides structure and support.

Individual temperament is also a protective factor. Children who are liked by adults and other children are more likely to succeed and have a positive self-image. For clinicians, your own response to an individual child may be a predictor of how others respond. Children who elicit positive feelings from others are likely to do well in life.

ASSESSMENT

Interviewing a school-age child can be a challenge, but certain approaches will help. In recognition of the child's concerns about competency, the first rule is to focus on abilities and strengths. Such an approach will allow the child to present herself in a controlled fashion, thereby furthering the development of trust. Early questions about stressful events or feelings should be avoided until the child settles down and appears comfortable in the interview. Consequently, questions about the three arenas (family, school and social functioning) can be ordered such that the least stressful area is discussed first and the most worrisome is left for last. Predictions about this order can be made from the information gained from parents, your own observations and the current problem.

Developmental and behavioral assessments of a school-age child should broadly assess the child's functioning at home, in school, with friends and in the community. The child and parents can be interviewed together, but some time with the child alone will be important to communicate your sense of her as an independent and competent individual.

OBSERVATIONS

While the clinician is engaged in developing rapport and expanding her data base, her observations of the child and family will be helpful.

- What are the child's and parent's general mood and level of interaction?
- Is the child's behavior appropriate for age, pseudomature or delayed?
- How well does the parent allow the child to speak for himself?
- Are there indications of underlying anger, distrust or worry?
- How age appropriate are the child's basic skills of speech, concentration, attention and compliance?
- How close do the parents seem with each other, and how close are they with this child?
- How do the parents respond when their child seems anxious, angry or embarrassed?
- How much do the parents control the child's behavior during the visit?
- How easy or difficult is it to relate to this child and family?

Questions regarding the child's functioning should focus on strengths and successes, as well as concerns and weaknesses. Such terms as *problems* and *failures* should be avoided. It may be more helpful to inquire about difficult or challenging situations they have had to cope with. Helping the family keep a balanced perspective while discussing the child is extremely important to avoid belittling the child in a disrespectful and potentially harmful fashion. To spend some time with the child alone, explain that this is part of your standard practice with children who are on their way to being teenagers. Showing an interest in getting to know the child and wanting to give him a chance to discuss things in a more private way are also important goals to convey. Clarifying that you will treat him like any competent patient by keeping his communications confidential is also helpful.

DATA GATHERING

The clinician should gather information from the child about all aspects of his life—family, school and social.

The Child Interview

Family Functioning

Tell me about what the family enjoys doing together.

What are you allowed to do now that you couldn't do when you were younger?

What chores do you have at home? How easy is it to do them? What happens if you forget?

If you have a problem at school or with a friend, whom do you talk to about it?

How much fighting goes on between you and your brother or sister?

What are the most important rules at home? What type of punishment do your parents use?

How important is it to your parents that you succeed in school, sports or chores?

What new freedoms do you expect to get over the next few years?

What parts of your parents do you wish to be like when you have children?

Tell me about a usual Sunday. What happens? Who does what with whom?

What do your parents worry about with you?

What are your parents most proud of about you?

What do you worry about at home?

What would you change about your family if you could?

School Functioning

What do you like about school the most?

What do you dislike about school?

What would you change about school if you could?

What subjects are easy? Which ones are hard?

What kind of grades are you getting this year? How about last year? Are you happy with them?

What is your teacher like this year?

Do you ever worry that it is extra hard for you to do something the teacher asks?

Have you ever gotten into trouble for the way you behave at school? What happened?

How much school have you missed recently?

Do you ever visit the nurse's office or feel sick in school?

How do you get along with the other children at school? Do you have friends? Do you have enemies or people who pick on you?

If you were the principal or teacher, what rules would you change?

What jobs or careers do you think you would enjoy?

Do you like to read? Do you read for fun?

What's your favorite subject? Which do you dislike?

Social Functioning

What kinds of things do you like to do after school and on weekends?

What are you good at? What types of things do you enjoy and do well?

Who is your best friend? How long have you known him or her? How often do you get together?

What do you like about him or her? What are some of the things that your best friend likes to do?

Whom did you eat lunch with yesterday (at school)?

Can you talk about worries and problems with your friends?

Have you ever lost a friend? What happened? How did you cope?

Do you and your friends ever fight or have problems sharing? How do you settle it?

Do your friends have special problems in their homes? Do they worry about their parents?

Have you slept over at friends' homes? Have they stayed with you?

What types of things do you wish you could do or learn?

Have your friends become interested in boys or girls? What kind of grades do they get? Are they experimenting with cigarettes, alcohol or drugs? What are they good at?

Do you belong to any teams, groups or clubs?

How well do you behave when you are out in the neighborhood? Do you get in any fights?

Has anyone ever hurt you or made you do something you didn't want to do?

What are some of the harder things you have had to deal with?

Projection/Insight

If you could have three wishes, any wishes, what would they be?

If you were the captain of a space ship, which three people would you take along?

What would you change about yourself if you could make any change?

What are you best at doing?

What is your biggest problem?

Describe yourself like someone else would.

If you could be any age, what age would you pick?

Is this year going better, worse or about the same as last year? How come?

ANTICIPATORY GUIDANCE

The child's clinician can offer specific guidance to the child and family directed toward the development of responsible, competent behavior.

- Counseling about *accident prevention* recognizes the school-age child's cognitive ability to connect an event with an outcome and focuses on the innate interest in controlling one's environment. Thus the need for seat belts and responsible helmet use during bike riding, skating, rollerblading, skiing and snowboarding should be mentioned because these activities continue to be the leading causes of death and injury in children.

- When family risk factors for *obesity* are determined, a balanced diet (low in saturated fats, refined carbohydrates and salt) and regular exercise for all family members should be encouraged.

- Counseling children about *smoking and drinking alcohol* should begin at this age. By encouraging the child's active involvement in these discussions, responsibility and self-control are promoted at an early age . Parents who smoke are more likely to stop when the impact of their smoking on the health of their children is emphasized (e.g., ear infections, allergies, asthma, other respiratory infections and behavior problems). Questions directed to parents about alcohol and other substance abuse in family members can be revealing but are most productive if the child is not present at the time (see Chapter 24). Introducing these risks in the context of understanding children's desires to act more grown-up may encourage a discussion about smoking, drugs and alcohol with children in the home.

BOX 21-2   READINESS FACTORS INFLUENCING SPORTS PARTICIPATION

Cognitive Development (Piaget)—Stages of Understanding Game Rules
- Egocentric play using personal rules
- Cooperative play
- Perception of rules as human productions that can be changed when participants agree

Moral Development (Kohlberg)—Stages of Moral Reasoning
- Self-gratification and avoiding punishment
- Desire to win approval
- Internal sense of ethics (i.e., internalization of a sense of fair play and sportsmanship)

Motor Readiness
- Basic prerequisites: running, throwing, hand-eye coordination
- Minor prerequisites: height, weight, skeletal age
- Specific skills for different sports (e.g., soccer vs. swimming vs. gymnastics vs. baseball)

Psychological Readiness—Achievement Motivation and Desire to Perform Successfully
- Capacity to evaluate own competence
- Capacity to compare own performance with that of others
- Integration of self and comparison evaluations

Modified from Livingood AB, Goldwater C, Kurz RB: Psychological aspects of sports participation in young children. In Camp BW (ed): *Advances in Behavioral Pediatrics*, vol 2. Greenwich, CT, Jai Press, 1981, pp 141-169.

- Parents can enhance the child's feeling of *responsibility* by having clear expectations of the child for initiating and completing chores and homework.
- Gradual increases in *independent activities* can be an encouragement for child behavior that demonstrates trustworthiness and competence.

Extracurricular Activities

Extracurricular activities should be supported, but care should be taken to avoid the "hurried child syndrome," in which the pressures to excel far outweigh the pleasures to explore and experience. This may be particularly true with a school-age child's participation in competitive sports, whether as an individual or on a team. Parents should be encouraged to carefully balance the amount of attention placed on performance and the degree to which the activity is enjoyable and helpful for social maturation. Clearly, some children are very comfortable and ready to participate in competitive sports, whereas others may lack interest, skill or confidence. Box 21-2 lists the developmental skills required for sports participation.

Boundaries and Expectations

Parents may be encouraged to maintain reasonable, predictable and observable boundaries and rules so that the child can accurately predict the parents' positive and negative responses to behavior. Children need to learn a variety of skills, including delay of gratification and tolerance of frustration, which can be developed only when negative events are experienced. Parents may consult with the child about their concerns, but they are wise to avoid premature suggestions or advice in favor of supporting the child's own problem-solving efforts. The clinician can identify areas of stress for the child and invite family-initiated solutions. Changes in the school and social environments that will support positive growth should be encouraged. Parents must get involved in these environments and understand their impact on the child to effect such positive change.

Managing the Media

Clinicians may also anticipate with parents the conflicts that arise in children as they are increasingly exposed to the world outside the family. Children today are aware of violence on a global scale through the media and will almost certainly need help from their parents to deal with the news of events that produce anxiety even in adults and adolescents. Many of today's children are exposed to sexual material that may be perverse or bizarre through television, movies (including videos) and the Internet.

The availability of computers at home and school has had an impact on all school-age children. Cognitive research suggests a link between playing computer games and computer literacy mediated by enhancement of reading ability, visualizing images in three-dimensional space and tracking multiple images simultaneously. Some studies suggest an association between home computer use and improved academic performance. On the negative side, other studies link increased use of the Internet with increases in loneliness and depression. Playing violent computer games may increase aggression and desensitize a child to suffering.

Society supports parental guidance in managing exposure to the media in a number of ways, from the existence of community groups such as the Parent-Teacher Association and the Violence Intervention Project for Children and Families to the movie, television, music and video game rating systems that provide parents with improved information about the type of violence and sexual content involved. Parents should also be encouraged to be mindful of their child's Internet use and may find that Internet-blocking software can help limit the child's ability to enter potentially dangerous sites. Some parents have found it useful to place the home computer in a central area of the home (e.g., the family room) to ensure continuous monitoring. As a children's advocate who is aware of the potential danger of exposure to excessive amounts of television (as well as other forms of passive entertainment), the pediatrician has a responsibility to raise the issue of television viewing and video and computer gaming with parents. Parents must understand the confusion and anxiety such material can engender in a child 7 to 10 years old. Parents can be encouraged to limit the child's exposure and provide an atmosphere in which the child feels free to share concerns and clear up misconceptions.

Finally, for children who experience a major life stress such as a divorce, death or school failure, the clinician should be an advocate for the child by keeping the child's developmental needs in focus and coping strategies intact. At least one domain should remain a positive area of success for the child as struggles continue in other domains. At the close of each visit, the child and parent should be complimented on their particular strengths. Families will come to anticipate these office visits as an opportunity to share their child's achievements, as well as a place to explore current behavioral and developmental concerns.

The case of Aaron, who had experienced a recent onset of headaches, may be evaluated in the context of the developmental issues of a school-age child. Aaron's headaches may stem from stress overload after the loss of a friendship. His social skills appear somewhat limited by his intense preoccupations. His coping style has always been to withdraw and distract by occupying himself with more pleasant stimuli. His parents' responses have often heightened concern and further reinforced his symptomatic behavior. His social skills in developing and maintaining friendships appear lacking.

After ruling out serious physical illness, his parents were reassured. They were encouraged to decrease the secondary gains (i.e., increased attention, new baseball cards, no chores, no homework) and to return him to school. He was allowed to use acetaminophen for pain analgesia but was also forced to be out of his room and out of his house for approximately 1 hour per day. His father was encouraged to involve Aaron in league baseball and to practice regularly with his son to build up his stamina and sense of resilience. The family was also encouraged to have Aaron arrange to bring friends over to the house. Within 2 weeks Aaron's headaches were gone and his social and academic functioning returned to normal. He continues to be a child of somewhat increased risk as a result of a family history of emotional problems and his own difficult temperament and problematic social skills. On the other hand, his intelligence, his organized and concerned family and his general competence may serve as important moderators in helping him maintain a positive adjustment.

Matthew's recurrent abdominal pain persisted after four office visits, at which time he was referred to a child psychiatrist. On the fifth visit with the psychiatrist, during a play therapy session, the patient revealed that he feared his mother's death. Matthew's mother underwent a surgical procedure for a benign condition during a 3-day hospitalization 2 weeks before the onset of his abdominal pain. His mother returned home with a visible vertical sternal scar. Without an explanation for the hospitalization, Matthew interpreted the scar to mean that his mother's death was imminent. When he was told that the scar was from a medical procedure and that his mother was well and would not die, the recurrent abdominal pain resolved.

QUICK CHECK—7 TO 10 YEARS

✓ Approximately one third of all school-age children have some form of chronic illness. About 5% have a chronic condition that limits usual academic or extra-curricular activities.

✓ Fifteen percent of school-age children have a behavior problem severe enough to benefit from a pediatric evaluation and treatment.

✓ The most frequent stress-related physical symptoms at this age are recurrent abdominal pain (prevalence, 15%), headaches and limb pain.

✓ About 20% of school-age children are involved in bullying—as a perpetrator, victim or both.

✓ A 7- to 10-year-old child with normal cognitive development can
Consider two or more aspects of a situation simultaneously.
Take into account more than one variable when making comparisons.
Understand that rules come from mutual consent and respect and can be changed under certain circumstances.
Focus on clearly defined roles.

✓ The superego develops as an internalized conscience representing parental and cultural values.

✓ Sports, hobbies and music reflect the drive to mastery of motor, social and artistic skills. Team sports enhance learning rules, the meaning of teamwork and discipline.

✓ Asperger's syndrome and a nonverbal learning disability are both forms of social-cognitive dysfunction.

✓ Family functioning is the strongest risk factor and protective factor for behavior and learning problems.

HEADS UP—7 TO 10 YEARS

• A quiet, reserved school-age child may reflect an individual temperament, depression or psychosocial stress. A focused history usually provides the needed information.

• Consider the degree to which a child has emotionally separated from her family through success in school, sports and other activities.

• Atypical, disruptive behavior during social interactions with peers may reflect an incomplete development of conscience, a process that internalizes parental and societal values.

• Fantasy at this age promotes identification with real and imagined heroes. Monitor for excessive time in fantasy play with videos, computer games and movies when a child seems lost in fantasies, and fantasy is no longer used as a means of expressing feelings.

Continued

! HEADS UP—7 TO 10 YEARS—cont'd

- Learning problems at this age may reflect a problem with "encoding"—the retrieval of previously learned knowledge, difficulty with organization and either verbal or written expression. A formal learning disability educational evaluation should be initiated. "He's lazy" is not a diagnosis.
- A school-age child who lacks a best friend, is not invited to birthday parties or does not participate in any social play activities with peers is at risk for social isolation. Look for individual strengths that can be encouraged and provide positive comments during office visits that serve to enhance social competency. Make proactive suggestions to the parent.
- Frequently encountered chronic conditions at this age include asthma, obesity, ADHD and learning disabilities. During office encounters, assess each child with these conditions for the acquisition of normal cognitive, social and motor milestones. Recognize increased risks for behavior problems and academic underachievement.
- Physical complaints without an apparent organic cause may be associated with emotional and social stresses in the child's immediate environment—family, school, peers, neighborhood. A focused history, often interviewing the child and parent separately, frequently provides clues to the etiology of the physical symptom. The interview process itself is often therapeutic.
- Ask about bullying—either being bullied or acting as the bully. A pediatric encounter may be the only opportunity for early recognition and intervention to enhance social competency and prevent isolation.
- Family functioning is the strongest risk factor and protective factor for behavior and learning problems.

ACKNOWLEDGMENT

Nicholas Putnam, M.D., contributed to portions of this chapter in previous editions.

RECOMMENDED READINGS

For Parents

Elkind D: *The Hurried Child: Growing Up Too Fast, Too Soon.* Reading, MA, Addison-Wesley, 1988.
Frankel F, Wetmore B: *Good Friends Are Hard to Find: Help Your Child Find, Make and Keep Friends.* Glendale, CA, Perspective Publishing, 1996.
Levine MD: *A Mind at a Time.* New York, Simon & Schuster, 2002.
Levine MD: *The Myth of Laziness.* New York, Simon & Schuster, 2003.

For Clinicians

American Academy of Pediatrics: *Sports Medicine: Health Care for Young Athletes,* 2nd ed. Elk Grove Village, IL, American Academy of Pediatrics, 1991.
Frankel F, Wetmore B: *Good Friends Are Hard to Find: Help Your Child Find, Make and Keep Friends.* Glendale, CA, Perspective Publishing, 1996.
Klin A, Volkmar FR, Sparrow SS (eds): *Asperger Syndrome.* New York, Guilford Press, 2000.
Levine MD: *Developmental Variation and Learning Disorders.* Cambridge, MA, Educators Publishing Service, 1993.

Levine MD, Oberklaid F, Meltzer L: Developmental output failure: A study of low productivity in school age children. *Pediatrics* 67:18, 1981.

Levine S: *Against Terrible Odds: Lessons in Resilience from Our Children.* Palo Alto, CA, Bull Publishing, 2001.

Stein MT, Klin A, Miller K, et al: When Asperger syndrome and a nonverbal learning disability look alike. *J Dev Behav Pediatr* 25:190-195, 2004.

Subrahmanyam K, Kraut RE, Greenfield PM, Gross EF: The impact of home computer use on children's activities and development. *Future Child* 10:123-144, 2000.

For Children

Janover CD: *Josh: A Boy with Dyslexia.* Lincoln, NE, 2004. Available at http://Backinprint.com.

Roby C: *When Learning Is Tough: Kids Talk about Their Learning Disabilities.* Concept Books, 1994. Available at http:// (www.microsoft.com/education.conceptbooks.aspx).

Root A, Gladden L: *Charlie's Challenge.* Linda Gladden, 1995.

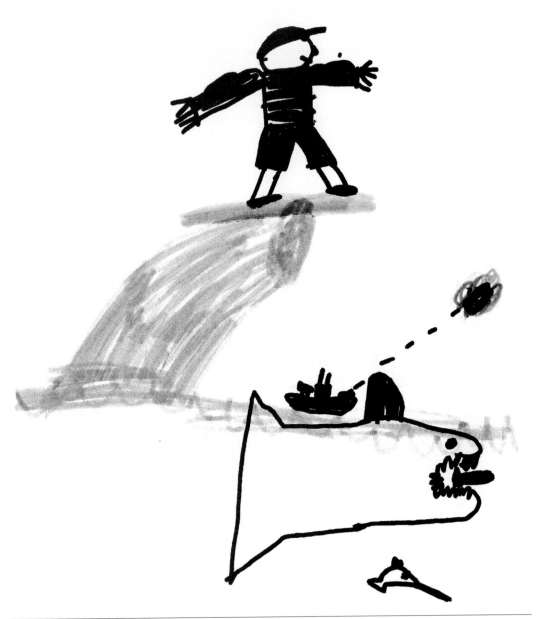

Neil, age 9, shows himself on top of the world, riding a wave above the monster whale, missile-launching ships and swordfish. A good sense of confidence is conveyed.

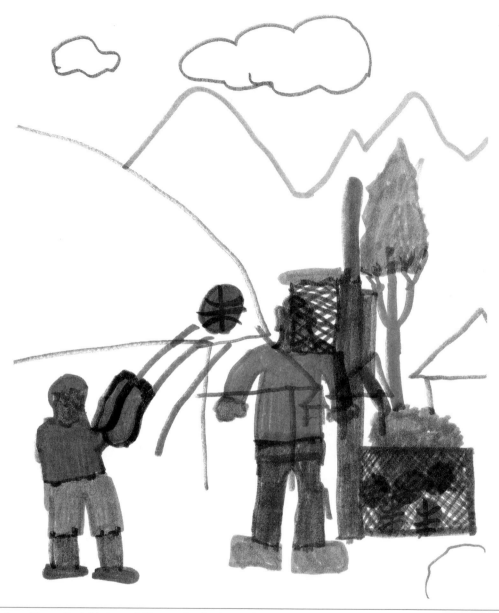

Playing with my Dad. Motor activities can be the forum for rich family interactions if coaching is sensitive to the child's ability to learn complex tasks, understand directions and alter his actions from the instruction. By HH, a boy age 8.

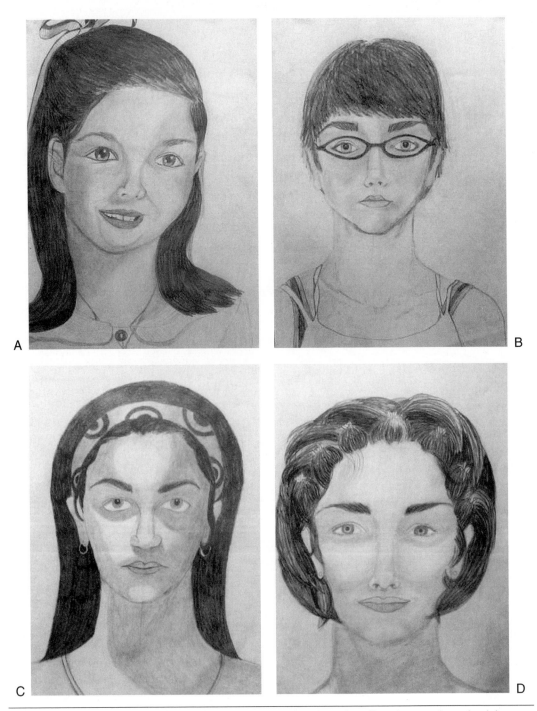

A–D, A series of four self portraits "Myself at Different Ages." She draws herself as she goes through adolescence and beyond. By Shala Abdi, age 16.

Eleven to Fourteen Years: Early Adolescence–Age of Rapid Changes

JENNIFER MAEHR and MARIANNE E. FELICE

This chapter explores the behavioral and physical changes characteristic of early adolescence. The significance of emerging sexual development, importance of peer relationships and limits in conceptualization is explored.

Key Words

- Adolescence
- Puberty
- Thelarche
- Adrenarche
- Menarche
- Sexual Maturation
- Internet
- Independence
- Substance Abuse
- Gangs
- School Transition
- Confidentiality
- Tobacco/Alcohol
- Exercise

OVERVIEW OF ADOLESCENCE

Adolescence is the developmental phase between childhood and adulthood and is marked by rapid changes in physical, psychosocial, sexual, moral and cognitive growth. This developmental phase consists of three substages: early, middle and late adolescence. Early adolescence generally occurs between the ages of 11 and 14 years and midadolescence, between 15 and 17 years. Youth 18 years or older are typically in late adolescence, a substage that extends into the third decade of life. These age ranges are simply guidelines; many other factors contribute to the adolescent's placement in early, middle or late adolescence, including gender, health, cultural background and socioeconomic status. To address the pertinent needs

535

BOX 22–1   DEVELOPMENTAL GROWTH TASKS OF ADOLESCENCE

- Gradual development as an independent individual
- Mental evolution of a satisfying realistic body image
- Harnessing appropriate control and expression of sexual drives
- Expansion of relationships outside the home
- Implementation of a realistic plan to achieve social and economic stability
- Transition from concrete to abstract conceptualization
- Integration of a value system applicable to life events

From Felice M: Adolescence. In Levine MD, Carey WB, Crocker AC (eds): *Developmental-Behavioral Pediatrics,* 2nd ed. Philadelphia, WB Saunders, 1992.

---

of a particular adolescent, it is helpful to first determine in which developmental substage the youngster belongs. This model allows clinicians to tailor their approach to each teen patient.

Certain psychosocial growth tasks are specific to adolescence in general and to each substage of adolescence, as summarized in Box 22–1 and Table 22–1. *The key issues are separation and independence, sexual identity, cognitive expansion, moral maturation and preparation for an adult role in society.* In other words, during adolescence, the individual must ask himself, "Who am I, where am I going and how am I getting there?" For healthy adulthood and personal maturity, mastery of all of the growth tasks is necessary. Like all psychological growth, however, progression through the substages does not occur in a straight line, but is marked by peaks, valleys and plateaus. Progress in one area may influence progress in another area. For example, failure to develop a healthy body image may affect the development of intimacy in relationships.

Despite the persistent myth that adolescence is tumultuous, most youth will complete adolescence without delinquency, school failure, parenthood or drug addiction. Rather, it is a developmental period that may baffle parents, frustrate health care providers and even cause confusion for adolescents themselves. The industrious school-age child who was hard working, compliant and quiet is suddenly seen as rebellious or unpredictable. The wide-eyed, shy child who was previously in adoration of his parents, teachers and pediatrician is now viewed as insolent and outspoken. Without trying, adolescents may evoke uncomfortable feelings in adults who harbor unpleasant memories from their own adolescence. Interaction with teens, however, can be an uplifting experience and a fresh reminder of the idealism of youth. The outspoken young person is actually in the midst of an age of wonderment and is someone who is searching to find herself while learning to make a contribution to society. Caring for a cohort of teens, as they make the journey toward adulthood, can be a marvelous and rewarding experience for a clinician, particularly if those same teens were followed since early childhood.

EARLY ADOLESCENCE AND PHYSICAL DEVELOPMENT

Early adolescence, sometimes called preadolescence, is characterized by the onset of both **puberty** and gradual emergence of independence from the family. As physical changes occur in the body, early adolescents develop sexual curiosity and heightened body consciousness. It

TABLE 22–1 **Growth Tasks by Developmental Phase**

Task	Early: 11–14 yr	Mid: 15–17 yr	Late: 18 yr +
Independence	Emotional break from parents; prefers friends to family	Ambivalence about separation	Integration of independence issues
Body image	Adjustment to pubescent changes	"Trying on" different images to find real self	Integration of satisfying body image
Sexual drives	Sexual curiosity; occasional masturbation	Sexual experimentation; opposite sex viewed as sex object	Beginning of intimacy/caring
Relationships	Unisex peer group; adult crushes	Both males and females in the peer group; multiple adult role models	Individual relationships more important than peer group
Career plans	Vague and unrealistic plans	Vague and unrealistic plans	Specific goals/specific steps to implement them
Conceptualization	Concrete thinking	Concrete thinking and developing introspection and abstract thought	Abstract thinking
Value system	Drop in superego; testing of moral system of parents	Self-centered	Self-centered idealism; rigid concepts of right and wrong; other orientated, asceticism

Adapted from Felice ME: Adolescence. In Levine MD, Carey WB, Crocker AC (eds): *Developmental-Behavioral Pediatrics*, 2nd ed. Philadelphia, WB Saunders, 1992.

is an important transition time that calls for developmental work by both parents and their growing youngsters. With anticipatory guidance, the health care provider can prepare and support the parent and adolescent for these changes.

Puberty

To understand the behavior of early adolescents, one must become familiar with the normal pattern of puberty and appreciate the dramatic physical changes that are a part of it. In the United States, puberty begins for most girls between the ages of 8 and 13 years with the development of breast buds (**thelarche**). It is normal, however, for some adolescents, particularly African American girls, to have the onset of pubic hair development (**adrenarche**) before breast development. Pubescence starts later for boys and begins with testicular enlargement followed by lengthening of the penis and pubic hair development. The majority of boys

TABLE 22–2 **Maturational Staging Criteria for Secondary Sexual Characteristics**

Breast Stage	Female
B1	No visible breast mound
B2	Breast buds: a small amount of subareolar breast tissue
B3	Amount of breast tissue increases
B4	Nipple is distinct from areola; areola forms a mound above breast tissue
B5	Areola recedes to the contour of the breast

Genitalia	Male
G1	Infantile genitalia
G2	Scrotal skin reddens and thins; testes increase in size; minimal or no enlargement of phallus
G3	Continued enlargement of testes; phallus lengthens
G4	Continued enlargement of testes; increased length and circumference of phallus and glans penis
G5	Adult-sized testes (>20 cc) and adult-sized phallus; deeply pigmented scrotum

Pubic Hair	Female	Male
PH1	No pubic hair	No pubic hair
PH2	Long, downy hair on labia majora	Long, downy hair at base of phallus
PH3	Coarse, curly hair in small amount on labia majora and mons pubis	Coarse, curly hair in small amount at base of phallus
PH4	Increased amount, but not on median aspect of thighs	Increased amount, but not on median aspect of thighs
PH5	Triangular-shaped escutcheon; hair extends to median aspect of thighs	Triangular-shaped escutcheon; hair extends to median aspect of thighs

From Long TJ, Fitzpatrick SB, Reese JM, Felice ME: Basic issues in adolescent medicine. *Curr Probl Pediatr* 14:1, 1984.

have entered puberty, by evidence of increased testicular volume, by or before age 14; some boys start puberty as early as 8 or 9 years. The progress of puberty can be followed on physical examination by assigning a Tanner stage, or sexual maturation rating, from 1 to 5 for breast maturation and pubic hair development in girls and genital maturation and pubic hair development in boys (see Table 22–2). Puberty is typically completed within 4 to 5 years and follows a well-described pattern that is summarized in Figure 22–1 and Table 22–2. For instance, **menarche** occurs about 2 years after thelarche: normally between the ages of 10 to 16 years with an average age of onset at 12.5 years.

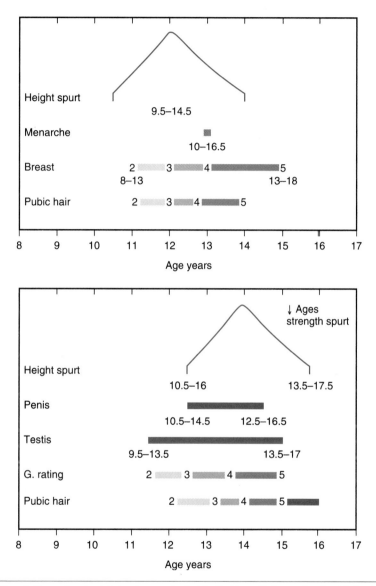

Figure 22–1 **Top**, Pattern of pubertal development of girls. **Bottom**, Pattern of pubertal development of boys. (From Marshall WA, Tanner JM: Variations in the pattern of pubertal changes in boys. *Arch Dis Child* 45:13, 1970.)

Several factors affect the timing of pubertal events and menarche, such as health, nutrition, body mass index, ethnicity and environmental conditions. As a group, African American girls enter puberty first, followed by Mexican American and then non-Hispanic white girls. Similarly, African American boys have been shown to enter adrenarche and complete genital development before Mexican American and white American boys. Because of these ethnic differences, standards for normal **sexual maturation** are being developed for various ethnic groups. In general, however, there has been a "secular" trend over the past century toward earlier puberty and larger growth. This trend is largely attributed to better health and nutrition, although some specialists hypothesize that environmental chemicals as well as hormones in animal and beauty products may be contributing to an earlier onset of pubertal development in some populations. As more studies demonstrate that boys and girls are developing earlier than the commonly used reference norms of Marshall and Tanner, the age cutoffs for precocious puberty are being debated and may be lowered.

WORRIES ABOUT PHYSICAL DEVELOPMENT

Before puberty, the normal bodily changes youngsters experience are quantitative, steady and predictable increases in height and weight each year. With puberty, however, physical changes are much more dramatic and rapid. For instance, height increases suddenly. Girls are growing most rapidly at a mean age of 11.5 years with a **peak height velocity** averaging 8.3 cm per year; boys enter their peak height velocity later, at a mean age of 13.5 years with a peak height velocity of 9.5 cm per year. The physical changes are also qualitatively different from previous years. Hair becomes coarse and appears to grow where it never grew before, major changes occur in the distribution of body fat and musculature, the skin becomes oily, apocrine glands begin to secrete, genitals enlarge, hips widen and breasts develop. It is no wonder that with adolescence, appearance becomes more critical and may be imagined as much worse than it really is.

Early adolescence is a time for agonizing self-consciousness and painful sensitivity to one's own physical changes. Acne may develop, and braces often become necessary. Young adolescents may be unaware or acutely sensitive of the development of body odor and the need for deodorants and more frequent bathing. Furthermore, the physical changes that occur may be asynchronous; that is, body organs and subsystems may appear to grow at different rates, so the arms, legs, nose or chin may seem to enlarge with no apparent respect for overall body harmony. The youngster may not know what to anticipate and may become very anxious about the seemingly out-of-control maturation that he is experiencing. It is not unusual for adolescents to spend hours in front of a mirror or in the bathroom becoming acquainted with the physical changes that appear to take place on a daily basis. Consistent with the healthy self-absorption or egocentrism expected at this age, they imagine that the world is as focused on these changes as they are.

Sometimes the physical changes that are observed are worrisome to young teens, who may harbor their own "explanatory models" for these events. For example, a pubertal boy who has gynecomastia (a normal occurrence in many boys during puberty) may be alarmed that he is developing breasts like a girl or may fear that he has breast cancer; a girl who has been inadequately prepared for menstruation may believe that her first period is a result of internal injury or serious illness. All young adolescents are concerned about their bodily changes, whether they easily reveal their worries or not. It is important for the clinician to uncover and allay these concerns.

Not all youngsters grow at the same time or at the same rate. A seventh grade class picture may show 12-year-olds in all sizes and shapes. Youngsters are acutely aware of how their physical changes compare with those of their friends, and they harbor some anxiety about the comparison. Many youngsters feel that they are growing too quickly or too slowly, too soon or too late. These apprehensions are most often revealed by nonverbal or obtuse patterns of communication. A girl whose breasts are developing more quickly than those of her peers may adopt a hunched posture. A boy whose genitals are not quite as big as those of his friends may find excuses to avoid undressing or showering in the locker room.

The timing of puberty can affect the overall well-being of an adolescent, especially for one who develops early or late. Boys who develop later tend to have poorer self-image and lower educational goals and tend to do more poorly in school than boys who progress through puberty earlier. It is not difficult to imagine a former little league star whose body fails to keep pace with the development of his peers. If he is unable to compete on an athletic team because of delayed physical development, he may have to shed his current identity as an athlete and reevaluate his own sense of who he is and where he is going. Some girls who develop early, but still within the range of normal, tend to have a poorer self-image than girls who develop later. Even a youngster whose maturation keeps pace with peers may feel out of step.

ADOLESCENT IN THE OFFICE

Jeremy, 12, and his father are at the doctor's office for his annual examination. When the nurse calls Jeremy, his father stays behind in the waiting area. Jeremy follows the nurse, has his vital signs recorded and is told to undress and change into a gown. Jeremy then waits alone in the examination room; this visit is the first time that Jeremy has seen the doctor alone.

Before entering the room, the physician reviews Jeremy's chart and notices that he has grown 5 inches since the last visit. Jeremy has always been tall, but now he is far taller than most boys his age. The physician enters the examination room and greets Jeremy with a friendly hello. Jeremy meekly replies, "Hi," and looks down at the floor while fumbling with the ties on his gown. When the doctor asks, "What brings you to the clinic today?" Jeremy shrugs and says, "I don't know." Further questioning about school and home brings similar answers—shrugs, nods of the head or a short "yes" or "no" answer. At a loss to proceed further, the clinician calls Jeremy's father back to the examination room. Jeremy appears relieved at the sight of his dad.

Note: Despite Jeremy's mature appearance, he was feeling awkward while alone in the examination room with the physician. Jeremy wasn't sure how to answer the physician's questions and was feeling especially self-conscious because he was wearing nothing but an examination gown. It became clear to the physician that Jeremy was feeling uncomfortable. Many young teens like Jeremy have difficulty with the interview process because of their limitations with conceptualization and abstraction; clinicians quickly discover this during the examination process and have to adjust their interview questions to accommodate the developmental stage of the youngster. As with most younger adolescents, it may have been more helpful to have both Jeremy and his parent together

Continued

initially to obtain a more complete history. Waiting to have Jeremy change into the gown until after the history may also have reduced Jeremy's discomfort.

While the physician talks with Jeremy and his father, it becomes apparent that as Jeremy has grown, more expectations have been placed on him by his family, coaches and teachers. Most people who meet Jeremy think that he is 14 or 15 years old. Even though he feels more comfortable with his boyhood friends, he often finds himself hanging out with older teenagers who are closer in size to him. Jeremy reveals that he feels under pressure to be the best player in sports. Some teachers look to him to be a leader, and when a disruption occurs, Jeremy feels singled out. At home, Jeremy finds himself doing more chores, such as putting away groceries, doing lawn work and watching his younger siblings. His father confesses that sometimes they forget that he is only 12. They have given Jeremy more autonomy to set his own schedule and social and school activities.

People's expectations of adolescents are usually based on their size and appearance rather than their age. Pointing this out to Jeremy can help validate some of his feelings. His parents may need to talk with teachers and coaches to discuss Jeremy's concerns and to see whether any other issues are at play. It appears that Jeremy may appreciate more limit setting and guidance from his parents at this particular point in his life. Parents may need assistance from the physician in deciding how to make these changes. Jeremy needs to know, however, that as youngsters get older, parents usually do expect more household help from them than in the past. Before Jeremy leaves, the physician takes additional time to discuss the further pubertal changes, both physical and emotional, that he can expect. The clinician also takes time with the father to provide him with a developmental perspective of early adolescence; the clinician discusses issues relating to body image adjustment, separation from parents, appropriate limitations in the ability to project cognitively and the importance of supportive friends.

SEXUAL DEVELOPMENT

As a young adolescent ponders the various changes taking place in his body, he begins to have an acute interest in sexual matters, but is not usually sexually active. An 8-year-old child may scorn romantic movies as "mush" and be embarrassed or even disgusted to see a couple kissing or embracing. The same child as a 12-year-old may now be fascinated by such matters and may even spy on older adolescent couples to learn from them. Early adolescence is the age when parents may find "adult entertainment" magazines hidden under their adolescent's bed. Parents are usually caught off guard by this "early" interest in sexual matters and may believe that the child is already sexually active. As a result, parents may act more restrictively or punitively than in the past. It may be more helpful, however, for parents to turn this discovery into a teachable moment about issues of sexuality.

Many young teens do not know what the term "sexually active" means. For instance, they may not consider having oral sex as being sexually active. Some early adolescents do experiment with sexual practices such as oral sex and seem to approach sex as though it were all a game, with little or no importance or emotional context attached. To realize which sexual practices, if any, are actually occurring, it is often necessary to ask teens specific questions regarding their sexual practices and the sexual practices of their friends.

"Janet, have any of your friends started to have sex, like, are they having oral sex, or sexual intercourse, or just kissing? (pause) … What about you?"

Some adolescents formulate concepts regarding sexuality from what they can glean from **television**, movies and the Internet. For the most part, sexual relationships are portrayed in a nonrealistic fashion in these venues. Women may be sexually exploited; information on issues of safe sex and sexually transmitted infections may be lacking; and extramarital affairs, multiple partners and premarital sex may be seen as the norm. On a positive note, television, movies and the media can sometimes serve as an opportunity for conversation between parents and their children on topics such as sex, violence and safety. In fact, children and adolescents are exposed to numerous and various forms of sexual and physical **violence** through both audio and visual entertainment, including video, computer and arcade games. It is helpful for parents to keep track of what their teens are watching on the screen and listening to on the radio or CD player. In this way, parents can help interpret for teens and put into context what they are seeing and hearing. Some parents may realize the need to limit exposure to certain entertainment venues for their teen and curtail the amount of time spent in these activities. This same vigilance applies to the Internet because teens, who often are more experienced in "surfing the net" than adults are, may find themselves with access to sexually explicit material or in potentially vulnerable situations in which they may be exploited.

Michael, a freshman in high school, was seen at his school wellness center for a sports physical. During the visit, Michael expressed concerns that he was "oversexed." On further explanation, Michael relates that he feels like he is always thinking about sex with girls. He has never been sexually active and has never been in any romantic or sexual relationship. To deal with his feelings, he masturbates "a lot," several times per week, when in his room by himself. He states that he is not sure if there is something wrong with him. He goes to church every Sunday and has not discussed the masturbation with his father, who happens to be a minister. Michael is worried that there is something wrong with his strong sexual feelings and the fact that he is masturbating.

The clinician lets Michael know that it is normal at his age to be thinking "a lot" about sex and that many adults and teens his age masturbate for pleasure or to relieve feelings of sexual tension. Michael is reassured that masturbating is a safe practice that won't harm him as long as it doesn't interfere with his day-to-day activities and is done in private. The clinician explains that although masturbating is very common, some cultures and individuals don't like to talk about it and may discourage it.

In early adolescence masturbation is a common occurrence. Many myths concerning **masturbation** (e.g., masturbation causes blindness, acne or hairy hands) exist, and young adolescents need reassurance that in fact, they are untrue. If the subject of masturbation does come up, religious and cultural beliefs by either the clinician, parent or teen may make the discussion challenging and difficult. Sharing factual information such as "many teens masturbate and it does not cause any physical ailment" can be helpful to an inquisitive parent or adolescent.

Male adolescents typically have **nocturnal emissions**, or "wet dreams." An early adolescent boy may be frightened by the occurrence of these emissions because the event happens beyond his control or because he believes the emission to be the result of an infectious disease. Similarly, a female adolescent may note a clear, mucoid discharge in her underpants starting about 6 months before menarche. This discharge is normal and is called vaginal leukorrhea, but both she and her parents may be alarmed and erroneously think that she has a vaginal infection.

DECLARATIONS OF INDEPENDENCE

Anxiety concerning sexuality may prevent parents from supporting the developmental tasks of early adolescence, such as the emergence of **independence** from the family. During the school-age stage of development, youngsters generally identify strongly with their own families and model their actions after their own parents. In adolescence, youngsters have an appropriate psychological need to separate from their parents and establish their own identities as individuals. It is important to be known as Bobby Jones rather than "Mr. Jones' son." In most young adolescents, this task is generally accomplished quietly, without open rebellion, through the choice of clothes, hair, jewelry, music and the increased importance of close friends. In some families, especially those that are close-knit, this process may still pose difficulties.

Erin, 13, prefers being with her friends to joining in family activities. In the past Erin and her mother enjoyed shopping outings together. Weekend picnics and field trips with her parents and little brothers were frequent. Instead of going out with her family, Erin now tries to stay home where she can talk on the phone or "chat" on the Internet with friends, watch television or listen to music. Erin also refuses to shop with her mother; she prefers going to the mall with her girlfriends. When she comes home, she and her mother argue over the clothes and jewelry that Erin has purchased. Now Erin is talking about getting a tattoo or nose ring. Her parents are hurt, and they often find themselves entrapped in futile and potentially harmful arguments with Erin about clothes, cosmetics and other superficial matters. They know that Erin is doing well in school and is responsible for her age, but cannot risk letting go for fear of loss of their control and potential harm to Erin.

This struggle recalls that of an earlier era, the second year of life. Then the bids for independence heralded the transition from infancy to childhood; now these bids are renewed as the child begins the journey from childhood to adulthood. Most parents need that perspective clearly laid out. In this case, Erin's choice in clothing is a concrete way for her to express her individuality and **peer group** identification. She is appropriately identifying more with peers than with family members. Symbols of that identification take on new importance. The more dramatic those symbols, the greater the tensions between parent and child. **Limit setting** is still necessary, such as the amount of time allowed on the phone, computer and television. Compromises can often be found. Instead of a tattoo and nose ring, Erin and her parents may reach a middle ground allowing her to have a temporary rub-on tattoo, clip-on jewelry or pierced ears.

As adolescents separate from parents, they must have the support of a peer group for a safe psychological shelter in which to grow outside the family. The peer group provides a sounding board against which a young teen can test ideas, and it serves as a barometer of her own physical and psychological growth. In other words, the peer group provides an important supportive structure to an adolescent's psychosocial development. An adolescent must often juggle the differences between what friends want and what family rules dictate. Even though the teen must psychologically distance himself from his family, most adolescents do not hate their parents or view their home as an unpleasant place. In fact, adolescents still need reassurance, support and physical affection from their parents. This comforting may be in the form of frequent hugs, compliments, help with homework, attendance at important events or simply taking the time to play a game of cards or to talk. It is essential to reserve time for the family and to create special family traditions in which all family members participate.

SOCIAL DEVELOPMENT AND THE ROLE OF PEERS

In early adolescence the peer group generally consists of same-gender members who share similar interests and spend a considerable amount of time together. An adolescent may belong to several different groups of friends whose members may or may not overlap, for example, one group of friends at school, another from the home neighborhood or extended family and potentially others from various social activities (e.g., church, sports and clubs). Membership in particular peer groups or crowds can be very important to the teen and a means by which to define or label himself and others. An adolescent may not always be able to "get into" the group that he desires and may be forced to accept a peer group of lower social rank. A few teens may not be accepted by any peer group, a condition that can eventually contribute to poor self-esteem, loneliness and depression. Social isolation or alienation, however, is *not* the norm in adolescence and may be a sign of coexisting psychosocial problems.

Rachel is a straight A student, shy and self-conscious. She wears glasses and has braces. She often feels like a nerd and has very few social interactions while at school. Rachel is active in a local choir and takes violin lessons. She has a best friend and enjoys going to the movies with friends from choir. Her parents are proud of her. Her primary care provider is impressed with Rachel's accomplishments and takes additional time with Rachel to talk about issues relating to her self-esteem and self-image.

Comment: This girl's individuality, her temperament, is being played out during adolescence. She has a friend, acquaintances and positive family interactions.

Ann is a straight A student, shy and self conscious. She feels anxious around other kids her age, especially at school. She sometimes gets bouts of shortness of breath accompanied by palpitations and sweating. On weekends and evenings, she stays home to study or just sleeps. She cannot identify a best friend. Her primary care provider is concerned about Ann and performs a thorough psychosocial history, including questions about suicidal ideation. She is referred to a mental health specialist for evaluation of anxiety and depression.

Once in a particular peer group or crowd, the individual members must conform to the norms of the group. Members of the peer group often dress alike. Girls may spend a considerable amount of time together planning outfits and hairstyles. Boys often wear similar clothing, jackets of the same make and color or T-shirts with the same inscription or insignia. Haircuts are alike. To verify these statements, visit a shopping mall for the afternoon and observe a group of youngsters walking by. The tendency to dress alike continues through all of adolescence, but it is most exaggerated in early adolescence. It signals the important work of separation from parents and peer group identification and in that sense is an indicator of developmental progress.

Depending on the particular peer group, conformity pressures can be either beneficial or counterproductive to family values, school performance and overall well-being of the adolescent. Many peer groups encourage individual achievement, for example, in sports and academics, but some may encourage delinquent behavior, such as **substance abuse** or criminal acts. Teens with the lowest self-esteem are the most vulnerable to peer group pressure and may knowingly do things against their better judgment and their parents' wishes. These conformity pressures are felt most strongly during early adolescence.

Gangs are an extreme example of this type of peer pressure. In general, gangs become appealing when other, healthier peer group options are not available. The setting for gangs is most commonly a poor inner-city area, where gangs offer perceived protection from outside threats or a means to social and economic advancement. Once in a gang where violence is part of the culture, the individual members feel compelled to acquiesce and perform as expected, often imposing threats, physical harm and injury to others and their belongings.

SCHOOL MILIEU

Early adolescents are usually in middle school (grades 6, 7 and 8) or just starting high school. For most teens, this is a new social experience with a completely different milieu from elementary school. The youngster must adapt to changing classes, multiple teachers and teaching styles, varying homework loads and testing schedules and a larger student population. Middle school may be the first time that a young person is exposed to youngsters outside his neighborhood. He may meet others of different races, religions and socioeconomic status. These new experiences may make him uncomfortable. Most young people make this transition with minimal anxiety, tempered by the comfort of knowing that their grade school companions are in the same predicament. Youngsters who must attend a new school with all new classmates may be more anxious and frightened. This anxiety may be manifested as psychosomatic complaints (e.g., headaches, stomach cramps, chest pain, shortness of breath),

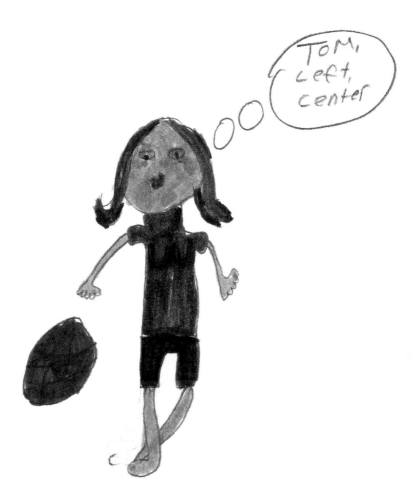

A middle-schooler shows her sports competence but clearly also shows her emerging figure. Her partner on the court is a boy. By a girl, age 12.

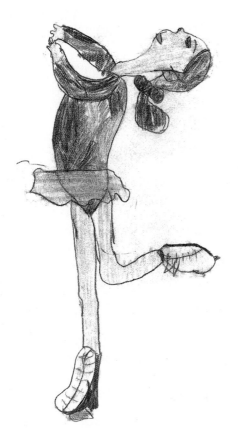

A romantic pose. She is working on profiles, three dimensions, body movement and a changing image of the age. By MD, age 11.

school avoidance (e.g., unexcused absences, tardiness, skipped classes) and academic problems such as declining grade point average.

Youth with an underlying attention deficit disorder who were previously functioning well in elementary school may suddenly experience academic difficulties in this more challenging school environment. These students may require alterations in their medication, additional supervision or strategies with homework completion, as well as meetings between their parents and school staff to develop an individual education plan to meet their needs. All adolescents with prolonged school dysfunction must have a psychosocial as well as physical, neurological and educational assessments. A good start is a visit to the youth's primary care clinician, who can suggest specific areas for further evaluation. **School transition** should last weeks, not months. Continuing school difficulty must be taken seriously and evaluated broadly.

COGNITIVE DEVELOPMENT: IMPLICATIONS FOR THE CLINICAL INTERVIEW

Because of a young adolescent's assumption of pseudo-adult mannerisms or the emulation of older models, it is easy for both parents and clinicians to overestimate their cognitive abilities. When evaluating a child in early adolescence, one must realize that 11-year-olds think concretely; that is, they do not yet have the cognitive abilities to think abstractly, to develop contingency plans or to conceptualize. Piaget classified this stage of cognitive development as *concrete operational thinking*; teens in this stage may experience difficulty organizing large bodies of data or inferential tasks. They may not relate present actions with future consequences. This inability has important implications for health counseling and the management and treatment of illnesses. Explicit linkages and short-term consequences must be spelled out clearly for a young adolescent.

Physicians who care for young adolescents frequently proclaim that they are difficult to interview. Teens may answer questions with only monosyllabic answers. In these instances, the physician is probably not being specific enough for a concrete-thinking youngster. For example, instead of saying, "Tell me about yourself," the clinician may be more successful in saying, "Tell me, what do you do after school?" Because of limitations in conceptualization, young adolescents may be unable to sustain lengthy verbal interviews. Other youngsters may view a physician's questions as a test and interpret the medical interview like an examination at school, with right or wrong answers. In those instances, the physician may glean more information by interacting with the young patient through talking about current events or by asking the teen to draw a picture of himself. This approach may be more successful in getting to the core issues than more "standardized" interviews. Some children of age 11 or 12 may talk more freely in a relaxed, nonformal environment. In addition, a young adolescent may be more able to describe specific behaviors, beliefs and attitudes in her peer group than in herself. The clinician will do well to respect these distancing maneuvers and may even use these approaches in data gathering. For instance, " Some young people your age try cigarettes. Tell me, are any of your friends smoking cigarettes?"

DATA GATHERING

Although experts disagree on the frequency of the adolescent physical examination, all agree that adolescents should be seen annually for **risk assessment**, health education and anticipatory guidance. Obtaining a thorough risk assessment or psychosocial history from an adolescent can take a significant amount of time and expertise on the part of the clinician. Several tools have been developed specifically for adolescent risk assessment, and their use can facilitate obtaining a complete, yet efficient risk assessment. Guidelines for Adolescent Preventive Services (GAPS) from the American Medical Association is a thorough step-by-step guide to the adolescent preventive visit. The GAPS includes several useful questionnaires for adolescent risk assessment, including an Early Adolescent Questionnaire specifically for 10- to 14-year-olds. A Parent/Guardian Questionnaire, as well as useful parent fact sheets, are also included. These questionnaires and parent anticipatory guidance information are available in several languages, including Spanish.

For clinicians who prefer not to use questionnaires, the HEADSS inventory is an excellent tool for ensuring a thorough psychosocial interview. Although several variations exist, the HEADSS acronym typically stands for home, education/employment, activities, drugs, sexuality and suicide/depression. When using the HEADSS inventory to interview a teen, a clinician starts with questions that a teen is used to answering, those about home and school, and then proceeds to more sensitive questions about substance use, sex, abuse and suicide. The idea is that over the course of the HEADSS interview, teens will develop some level of trust that enables them to share more personal information with the clinician. The GAPS questionnaires are developed in a similar fashion: one moves from more mundane questions to those that are more personal and involve some level of risk or trust on the part of the adolescent.

Bright Futures provides useful chart forms for pediatric health maintenance visits, including the early, middle and late adolescent visit. These forms include suggested questions to ask the teen, a history section, physical examination section and an anticipatory guidance checklist. Bright Futures also supplies anticipatory guidance handouts for parents and teens.

If possible, the adolescent physical examination should be performed yearly as recommended by the American Academy of Pediatrics. The annual physical examination presents an opportunity to update immunizations and to screen as appropriate for medical conditions that may affect this age group, such as vision problems, hypertension, weight-related problems, scoliosis, anemia, hyperlipidemia, tuberculosis and sexually transmitted infections. The physical examination is also an ideal time to talk to teens about their bodies and to answer any questions that they may have. Some clinicians may find it useful to perform components of the risk assessment or anticipatory guidance while completing the physical examination, for example, discussing cigarette smoking after listening to the lungs or asking about exercise after examining the heart. The components of the early adolescent health maintenance visit are reviewed in Table 22–3.

GENERAL GUIDELINES

Matters of Confidentiality

Clinicians seeing adolescent patients must develop policies and procedures regarding **confidentiality** and the delivery of adolescent care. These policies should address when an adolescent can give informed consent and receive confidential care for the counseling and treatment of family planning and reproductive health issues, sexually transmitted infections, substance use/abuse and mental health problems. They must also outline situations in which confidentiality will be broken, for example, when a teenager discloses a history of abuse or if

TABLE 22–3 **Components of the Early Adolescent Health Maintenance Visit**

What to Observe	Objective
Interactions between adolescent and parent	To assess whether they communicate well or whether the mother/father answers all the questions for the adolescent or allows the youngster to answer for himself; these interactions may reveal the status of the separation process
The adolescent's willingness to be interviewed and/or examined alone without parental presence	To determine the adolescent's willingness to begin to act independently from his parents

What to Ask (HEADSS Format)	Objective
Home: With whom do you live? How many brothers and sisters do you have? To whom are you closest in your family? How does everyone get along? Do you have any chores around the house? Do you ever get in trouble at home? Do you feel safe at home? What happens in your family when someone gets angry with you?	To assess the teen's family and home situation, patterns of interaction within the family and his/her role within the family
Education: What do you like best/worst about school? What are your favorite and least favorite subjects? Do you have a favorite teacher? Why? Do you do any after-school activities? Who are your friends at school? What are your actual grades? Are you in any special education classes? Have you ever had to repeat grades? Have you ever been suspended/expelled? Do you feel safe at school? Have you ever brought a weapon to school?	To assess the teen's functioning within the school environment
Activities: Do you have a best friend? What do you like to do with your friend(s)? What do like to do on the weekends? Do you play any sports or exercise? How often? Do you belong to any clubs or do any activities besides sports? How many hours of TV do you watch every day? What about computer or video games? How many meals do you eat a day? What are your favorite snacks? Are you happy with your weight? Have you ever tried to lose weight?	To assess the adolescent's function within a peer group and interactions outside the family; to determine whether the adolescent is developing independence from the family; to assess whether activities are healthy ones and within normal for the adolescent's age, including eating habits and exercise

Continued

TABLE 22–3   **Components of the Early Adolescent Health Maintenance Visit—cont'd**

What to Observe	Objective
Drugs: Are any of your friends smoking cigarettes or using tobacco? Does anyone in your family smoke? What about you? Do you or your friends ever drink alcohol? Use marijuana or other drugs? What about sniffing or using inhalants? Have you ever worried about someone in your family who used alcohol or drugs?	To screen for drug, alcohol and tobacco use in the teen, peers and family
Sex/Sexuality: Are any of your friends dating or going out with someone? What about you? Have any of your friends started to have any sexual experiences, including kissing, oral sex or sexual intercourse? What about you? Have you started to have an interest in boys or girls in a sexual way?	To assess teen's interest and participation in sexual activities, as well as those of his/her friends
Suicide/Depression: Do you consider yourself to be happy or sad most of the time? Are you happy with the way you look and feel? Do you wish that you could change something about yourself or your life? What would that be? Are you sleeping OK? How often do you cry? Have you ever thought about hurting yourself or someone else? Have you ever tried to kill yourself? Have you ever been abused, physically hurt or sexually touched in a way that you did not want?	To screen for mental health issues such as mood, depression, concerns over appearance, suicidal ideation and abuse

Physical Assessment	Objective
Appearance/observe styles of dress and hair	To assess importance of peer group identification
Height, weight, body mass index*	To plot the adolescent's growth on a growth chart and screen for obesity, excessive weight loss or weight gain and underweight
Blood pressure	To assess for hypertension
Vision screening	To determine whether there is a vision problem such as myopia
Dental examination	To assess for dental hygiene, caries

Continued

TABLE 22–3 **Components of the Early Adolescent Health Maintenance Visit—cont'd**

What to Observe	Objective
Careful palpation of thyroid gland	To check for a goiter because thyroid disease can occur in adolescence
Note the presence of gynecomastia in boys	Gynecomastia is common in pubertal boys and is generally a source of concern to them
Tanner maturational staging (see Table 22–2 and Fig. 22–1)	To access entry into and progression through puberty
Check carefully for scoliosis	Scoliosis is most apparent during the adolescent growth spurt and should be carefully assessed as early as possible in this phase of development
Examination of the skin	To evaluate for acne or other common adolescent dermatological conditions
Affect/mood	To assess teen's current psychological state and feelings about the visit
Immunizations	**Objective**
May include vaccinations for tetanus, diphtheria, pertussis, hepatitis A and B, varicella, influenza, measles, mumps rubella, and meningococcus	To update or catch up on required and recommended immunizations as per CDC and AAP guidelines
Screening Tests	**Objective**
May include hemoglobin, cholesterol or lipid panel, tuberculosis skin testing, urinalysis, gonorrhea and *Chlamydia* testing	To assess as deemed necessary for anemia, lipid disorders, tuberculosis and genitourinary problems such as sexually transmitted infections
Anticipatory Guidance and Health Education	**Objective**
See further discussion in text	To prepare the teen and parent for what lies ahead and to give information that the teen/parent can use to change behavior and possibly reduce risk

*Body mass index (BMI) = (weight in kilograms)/(height in meters)^2.
AAP, American Academy of Pediatrics; CDC, Centers for Disease Control and Prevention; HEADSS, home, education/employment, activities, drugs, sexuality and suicide/depression.

the teen is at risk of harming herself or someone else (e.g., suicidal or homicidal ideation or personal neglect of a serious medical condition). Organizations and individual clinicians can draw on their state **minor consent laws** when drafting these policies. Clinicians must be cognizant of the minor consent laws for the state in which they practice because these laws do vary from state to state. Hospital and academic centers typically have legal counsel to advise staff on these matters; independent practitioners may obtain information regarding the care of minors from their state government offices or the National Center for Youth Law (see "Resources").

It is helpful to review these policies with both the teen patient and the parent some time around the 11- to 12-year visit for established patients and at the first visit for an adolescent patient new to the practice. Let them know that the teenager will be interviewed separately from the parent for at least a portion of the visit. Some parents also benefit from an opportunity to discuss their concerns privately with the clinician. Separate interviews not only enable the clinician to obtain sensitive information from the adolescent and parents in private but also emphasize the emerging independence of the youngster and help establish rapport. Some pediatric practices send letters to the teen and his parent or parents informing them about confidentiality and separate interviews so that they will not be surprised when they come for the adolescent visit.

> "Sam, I wanted to explain to you and your parents that my role here is as your physician. Now that you are a teen, I will spend a part of the visit just with you to talk about some sensitive issues that many teens your age face. Because I follow the minor consent laws of our state, our discussions about drugs, alcohol and sexual matters will remain confidential; that is, I will not share the information you tell me with your parents or teachers, although I do encourage you to share our discussions with your parents whenever possible. Now there are a few exceptions to the confidentiality rule. I will break our confidentiality in the following situations: (1) if you are at risk of seriously hurting yourself, (2) if you are at risk of hurting someone else and (3) if you have been abused or if your health is in serious jeopardy. I hope knowing our conversations are confidential will make you feel more at ease about talking to me and hopefully make your parents rest easy knowing that you have someone to talk to who can give you factual information on these topics."

Setting the Stage

It is important to try to make the teenager feel comfortable. Adolescent clinics and school-based health centers are particularly adept at customizing the setting to the adolescent patient. If the setting is in a general pediatric practice, it's helpful to have a separate room that is age appropriate in which to interview and examine the teen patient. Reading materials, such as pamphlets, magazines and posters geared toward adolescent issues, should be provided. In this way the teen may be more inclined to bring up sensitive issues or may even find answers to questions that were not addressed during the visit.

Questionnaires

The clinician may want to make use of health survey questionnaires such as GAPS as an adjunct to the patient-physician interview. The use of questionnaires or computerized risk assessments can be reassuring to a teen because it implies that other adolescents have similar problems and concerns. If questionnaires are used for the psychosocial assessment of teens, they must be reviewed before the patient leaves the clinic and cannot replace a face-to-face interview. In practice settings where there are high rates of illiteracy and for individual patients with reading difficulties or low levels of educational achievement, the use of questionnaires may not be warranted.

Choice of Clinician

It is not unusual at this age for a teenage patient to develop a preference for a male or female health care provider. Some teens choose to remain with the clinician who has cared for them since early childhood. Others request a clinician of the same gender. Both situations should be respected and, when possible, accommodated.

Sensitivity in Examination

The examination must be done with sensitivity and awareness of the young adolescent's exquisite self-consciousness and perhaps exaggerated embarrassment. For example, the clinician should give clear directions concerning disrobing and gowning in preparation for a physical examination. If the underwear should be removed, the clinician must say so. The examination should be performed behind a drape or in a closed room to protect the adolescent's privacy. If the teen wishes, a parent or support person may be present during the examination. When a chaperone is not required, the teen may prefer to be examined alone. When a male clinician is performing a breast or pelvic examination, it is recommended that a female chaperone be present. The chaperone can be supportive and reassuring to an anxious youngster, as well as negate any fantasy about the intimacy of the examination.

Narrating the Examination

During the examination itself, it is important to affirm normal physical findings, especially of sensitive areas such as the genitals. The clinician's narration during the physical examination demystifies the clinical encounter and involves the patient while providing valuable information. Concomitantly, the health care provider must use active listening skills to pick up on the patient's underlying concerns. Showing interest along with giving nonjudgmental counseling also lets the teenage patient know that she is taken seriously.

ANTICIPATORY GUIDANCE FOR THE EARLY ADOLESCENT

Physical Development

Young teenagers need reassurance and education about their bodies. Explain the patterns of physical and sexual maturation to each youngster. For example, if a girl has not begun to menstruate but has breast development, the clinician can outline for her the expected pattern of growth, including the approximate time of menarche. The physician may say,

"Mary, I notice that you have begun to develop as a young woman. It will be about 2 years now before you get your first period. Would you like to know more about this?" or "Jack, when I did your physical examination, I noticed that you are starting to have pubic hair. Have you wondered what will happen next?" … "These recent changes in your body tell me that you have started puberty. It's normal to have questions about puberty. Would you like to hear more about it?"

Menstruation

All girls should receive an explanation of menstruation. It is usually helpful to ask the teenager what she already knows about menstrual periods and the menstrual cycle and then build on her knowledge. Teens often appreciate being told that it is normal for their periods to be irregular for some time after menses start. They also need to know that once menarche occurs, it is possible to become pregnant, a natural lead into a first discussion about sex, abstinence and contraception. It is important that young women be exposed to a positive rather than a negative attitude toward menstruation. Pamphlets do not substitute for personal counseling by the health provider.

Masturbation and Nocturnal Emissions

Adolescents may need reassurance concerning masturbation, and adolescent boys may need education about erections and nocturnal emissions. It is often very embarrassing for a teen to be asked about these issues directly. When necessary, it is usually more helpful to say,

"Many boys your age start to have more sexual urges than before. Erections or hard-ons may occur any time of day and sometimes when you are least expecting them. Some boys around your age start having wet dreams; that is, they ejaculate while sleeping, which leaves a sticky, white discharge in their underwear. Boys may also have an ejaculation from rubbing or stimulating their penis; this is called masturbation. I don't know if this has happened to you yet, but I want you to know that this is normal."

Pubertal Development of the Opposite Sex

Adolescents may be ignorant of the development of the opposite sex. Some teens may be too embarrassed to ask questions concerning this topic. It is usually helpful to say,

"What have you learned at school about the changes that boys (or girls) experience at your age? Is this something you'd like to learn more about?"

A brief explanation accompanied by pamphlets is usually sufficient.

Tobacco, Alcohol and Drugs

It is never too early to begin counseling about the health risks of **tobacco, alcohol** and illicit drugs. In fact, a 2002 survey of 12- to 17-year-olds showed that the average age at initiation of cigarette use was 12 years, 12.5 years for alcohol use and 13.5 years for marijuana use. Alcohol is the substance most frequently tried by eighth graders (47%), followed in descending order by cigarettes (31%), marijuana (19.2%), inhalants (15%), smokeless tobacco (11%) and amphetamines (9%). Five percent of eighth graders smoke cigarettes daily; otherwise, daily use of these substances by eighth graders is extremely rare. Almost 20% of eighth graders, however, have used alcohol in the past 30 days and almost 7% have been drunk.

Although these figures may seem alarming, many teens who try drugs, including tobacco and alcohol, will not continue to use them on a regular basis. It is the health care provider's job to provide information on these substances so that the teen will understand the risks involved. Young teens may not care about health risks that will occur decades from now, such as cancer, heart disease and emphysema, and they often don't appreciate the addiction potential. Stressing the short-term effects on health and appearance may be more beneficial. For example, the clinician may say, "Did you know that smoking tobacco affects your physical performance in sports so that you may not be able to run, bike or swim as fast or as long as you might otherwise be able; it also yellows teeth and fingernails, causes bad breath and increases the risks of getting sick with coughs, colds and lung infections, not to mention the increased risks of getting cancer and heart disease." For marijuana, the practitioner may say, "marijuana, like cigarettes, has bad effects on the heart and lungs, including an increased risk of cancer, but it can also slow your reaction time, for example, when driving a car and trying to stop suddenly or playing sports and having to catch, kick or hit a ball; it may also make it harder for you to organize your thoughts and solve problems, so it may become more difficult to get good grades or to say "no" to things that you would normally not want to do, like having sex or using other drugs; it may possibly cause unwanted growth of breast tissue and lower sperm counts in some boys and abnormal periods in girls." Some teens need reminding that most of these substances are illegal or against the law for minors. In addition, they face the financial cost of using and the risk of parental reprimand. With the support of the clinician, school, parent or all three, the teen may be better equipped to resist peer pressure to engage in drug or tobacco use and therefore be less likely to become a regular user.

Exercise and Television

Although some adolescents **exercise**, many do not. For those who do, the exercise may be infrequent and may not involve sustained aerobic activity but rather spurts of running or weight lifting. In addition, many teens no longer receive routine physical education in school. To make matters worse, television and recreational computer use often replace physical activity, and driving and commuting have made walking an inconvenience. Safety concerns, cost, transportation issues, lack of motivation, embarrassment and time restraints may deter the adolescent further from exercising. With the growing problem of obesity, it is imperative to talk about exercise and nutrition with teens (see Chapter 21 for further discussion on nutrition in adolescence). Explore ways that they can add daily exercise to their lives and address any barriers to exercise. Advise the teen and parent to limit television and recreational computer use to less than 2 hours per day. Strongly recommend that televisions do not belong in the teenager's bedroom. If a teen establishes healthy patterns during adolescence, it is more likely that these patterns will be maintained into adulthood.

Safety

Many teens ride bicycles, scooters or skateboards and yet do not wear protective padding or helmets. Most teens travel in cars, and many may not wear seat belts consistently or at all. The clinician can make an impact on the teen by explaining that serious head injuries with permanent disabilities can result from not wearing a helmet and that unrestrained passengers in a car accident may be ejected from the vehicle and die. It is not helpful to preach to an adolescent, but equipping him with information with which he can make his own decision is.

Safety may also be an issue at school, ranging from bullying to gang warfare. It may be necessary to review strategies on dealing with bullying and hostile threats.

If a teen has access to a gun or other deadly weapon, safety measures need to be discussed with the teen as well as the parent. Preferably there should be no guns in the home, but at a minimum, guns should be locked, unloaded and stored separately from the ammunition. Access to guns in the home is a risk factor for both homicide and suicide.

ANTICIPATORY GUIDANCE FOR PARENTS

Pubertal Development

Parents should be informed when a youngster has begun the process of puberty, a fact that may not be obvious to the parent. A simple explanation concerning the expected progression of pubertal development is usually appreciated by most parents, with specific emphasis on matters that will be most noticeable to parents rather than someone outside the family. For example, let parents know that when doing the laundry, they may notice a discharge in a girl's underpants for 4 to 6 months before the onset of menarche. This knowledge will prevent misconceptions about the discharge and will enable the parent to be prepared for menarche to occur so that sanitary pads or tampons will be available. In addition, point out that sexual interest is appropriate at this age and does not necessarily indicate sexual activity. Assumptions of inappropriate behavior may become a self-fulfilling prophecy.

Need for Privacy

Parents should be informed that with the onset of puberty, young adolescents must have privacy. This is best accomplished by allowing the teen to have his own room; if not possible, he should have his own section of a room where he can go and be by himself and not be bothered by siblings or by parents.

Sensitivity to Teasing

Parents should be advised that it is not appropriate to tease youngsters about their pubertal development. Most teenagers are exquisitely self-conscious about their development and may be acutely embarrassed by this teasing. This advice is best given in two ways: (1) by asking the parent if anyone is teasing the youngster about pubertal changes and (2) by asking the parent about his or her own early adolescence. In that context, most parents will recall their own self-consciousness from adolescence and will be more likely to show increased sensitivity to their child's needs. Parents may also need to restrain siblings from making comments.

Quest for Independence

Parents must be reassured that their teenager's quest for independence is normal and should not be interpreted as rejection of the family by the child. Give examples of this situation. For instance, young teenagers may not want to join the family on every family outing or may not want the parents at school or social functions in a chaperone capacity. If possible, another authority figure may do better. Young teens may begin to confide in an adult outside the family rather than their parents, possibly a change from previous years.

It is difficult at times to avoid arguing about trivial things, but it is best to concentrate on physical safety, basic hygiene and school attendance when deciding which specific behavior to address. Parents of a teenager must maintain a delicate balance of providing parental monitoring while allowing the teen to stride toward independence.

HEADS UP–11 TO 14 YEARS

Endocrine Issues

Boys and girls who do not follow the normal pattern of pubertal development (e.g., advanced breast development with little pubic hair growth) warrant an endocrine evaluation. In addition, adolescent boys who have not begun pubertal development by the age of 14 and adolescent girls who have not begun breast development by the age of 13 or had menarche by the age of 16 should be evaluated for pubertal delay.

Chronic Illness

A teenager who has a chronic illness, such as immune deficiency, cystic fibrosis, diabetes or sickle cell anemia, may have delayed or atypical psychosocial development because of dependence on parental support, medical personnel and therapeutic regimens. Physical development, including puberty, may also be delayed secondary to the disease process. With the limitations imposed by the illness, either physically or mentally, adolescence can be an excruciatingly difficult time for a child with a chronic disease. Independence, a positive body image and a supportive peer group may be difficult to obtain. As a result, some adolescents with a chronic illness may become depressed, angry with parents and medical staff and noncompliant with medical therapy. Teens with a mental health condition may experience similar problems with obtaining independence and healthy self-esteem. Adolescents with a serious, chronic health condition often require mental health counseling for support and assistance with adjustment.

Poor School Adjustment

Children who are adjusting poorly to middle school after 6 weeks often benefit from a psychological and/or educational assessment. Such assessment may lead to an individual education plan, tutoring or counseling. Declining school performance should never be attributed to benign causes or be played down with a "let's just watch how things go" statement.

Continued

HEADS UP–11 TO 14 YEARS–cont'd

Friendless Youth

Youngsters who do not have a peer group of friends need psychological or psychiatric evaluation. This signals significant social isolation, often depression, and is a serious matter.

Family Conflict

Families that have persistent conflict may need additional sessions to identify areas of disagreement and to develop strategies to improve mutual respect and functioning. Family counseling may be indicated and may bring significant insight and improvement in family function. Some turbulence is expected in all families, but a decline in functioning or prolonged conflict is not to be expected.

Early Onset of Sexual Debut

Most early adolescents are not yet sexually active. In the Youth Risk Behavior Surveillance of 2001, 6.6% of students nationwide reported sexual intercourse before the age of 13. By the ninth grade, the percentage of teens reporting ever having had sexual intercourse jumps to 34%. Factors associated with **early sexual debut**, usually considered to be sexual intercourse before the age of 15, include being male; African American ethnicity; use of cigarettes, alcohol or other drugs; lack of school attendance; poor school performance; and a boyfriend or girlfriend who is older by 2 years or more. Timing of sexual debut, for girls in particular, has been shown to be greatly influenced by their close friends; that is, if their friends are having sex, they too will be more likely to have sex. The influence of friends is not surprising given the importance of peers in early adolescence. Other reasons cited by adolescent girls for having sex before the age of 15 include a partner pressuring them, curiosity and the desire to feel grown-up.

Fortunately, certain protective factors are associated with a delay in sexual debut, including teen satisfaction with parental relationships, teen perception of maternal opposition to early sexual intercourse, peer group norms to refrain from sex and athletic participation. It appears that a healthy home, peer and school environment can temper sexual drives and protect young teens from coercive or unhealthy sexual relationships. Given the protective and adverse factors for early sexual activity, it is important to ask all teens about their relationship with parents, school grades/attendance/suspensions, use of tobacco/alcohol/drugs and the sexual activities of friends.

Young teens who are sexually active deserve a closer look for problems contributing to or stemming from their sexual activity. It is imperative to ask them about the age of their sexual partner or partners and any history of nonconsensual sex, sexual assault or abuse. The teen, in fact, may be a victim of statutory rape or past sexual abuse. Early onset of sexual intercourse is a risk factor for teen pregnancy and sexually transmitted infections. A frank discussion about sexually transmitted infections and contraception is warranted because young teens usually have no previous knowledge of these topics. In addition, all teens who are having sex deserve thorough and periodic screening for sexually transmitted infections, including an inspection of the external genitalia. Some teens, particularly younger adolescents paired with older partners, experience difficulty saying "no" to sexual advances. Others are unable to assert themselves enough to demand condom use. It is therefore helpful to role-play these scenarios and to remind teens that they do have the right to say no to sex.

RECOMMENDED READINGS

For Clinicians

American Academy of Pediatrics, Committee on Practice and Ambulatory Medicine: Recommendations for preventive pediatric health care. *Pediatrics* 105:645, 2000.

American Medical Association: *Guidelines for Adolescent Preventive Services (GAPS). Recommendations Monograph*, 1997, http://www.ama-assn.org/ama/pub/category/1980.html.

Bright Futures: Guidelines for Health Supervision for Infants, Children, and Adolescents, 2nd ed, revised. Washington, DC, Georgetown University Press, 2002.

Elkind D: Understanding the young adolescent. *Adolescence* 13:127, 1978.

English A, Kenney K: *State Minor Consent Laws: A Summary*, 2nd ed. Chapel Hill, NC, Center for Adolescent Health and the Law, 2003.

Erikson EH: *Identity, Youth and Crisis*. New York, WW Norton, 1968.

Goldenring JM, Rosen DS: Getting into adolescent heads: An essential update. *Contemp Pediatr* 21:64, 2004.

Joffe A, Blythe MJ (eds): *Handbook of Adolescent Medicine, State of the Art Reviews*, vol 14, No 2. Philadelphia, Hanley & Belfus, 2003.

Marshall WA, Tanner JM: Variations in the pattern of pubertal changes in boys. *Arch Dis Child* 45:13, 1970.

Neinstein LS (ed): *Adolescent Health Care: A Practical Guide*, 4th ed. Philadelphia, Lippincott Williams & Wilkins, 2002.

Tanner JM: *Growth at Adolescence*, 2nd ed. Boston, Blackwell Scientific, 1962.

Weiner IB: Distinguishing healthy from disturbed adolescent development. *J Dev Behav Pediatr* 11:151, 1990.

For Parents and Teens

Basso MJ: *The Underground Guide to Teenage Sexuality*, 2nd ed. Minneapolis, Fairview Press, 2003.

Bourgeois P, Wolfish M: *Changes in You and Me: A Book about Puberty Mostly for Boys*. Kansas City, Andrews & McMeel, 1994.

Faber A, Mazlish E: *How to Talk So Your Kids Will Listen and Listen So Your Kids Will Talk*. New York, Avon Books, 1980.

Greydanus DE (editor-in-chief), Bashe P: *Caring for Your Teenager*. Elk Grove Village, IL, American Academy of Pediatrics, 2003.

Haffner DW: *Beyond the Big Talk: Every Parent's Guide to Raising Sexually Healthy Teens—From Middle School to High School and Beyond*. New York, New Market Press, 2002.

Harris RH: *It's Perfectly Normal: Changing Bodies, Growing Up, Sex and Sexual Health*. Cambridge, MA, Candlewick Press, 1996.

Madaras L, Madaras A: *My Body, My Self for Boys*, 2nd ed. New York, New Market Press, 2000.

Madaras L, Madaras A: *My Body, My Self for Girls*, 2nd ed. New York, New Market Press, 2000.

Madaras L, Madaras A: *The "What's Happening to My Body?" Book for Boys: A Growing-Up Guide for Parents and Sons*, 3rd ed. New York, New Market Press, 2000.

Madaras L, Madaras A: *The "What's Happening to My Body?" Book for Girls: A Growing-Up Guide for Parents and Daughters*, 3rd ed. New York, New Market Press, 2000.

Madaras L, Madaras A: *My Feelings, My Self: A Growing-Up Journal for Girls*, 2nd ed. New York, New Market Press, 2002.

McCoy K, Wibbelsman C: *The Teenage Body Book*. New York, Perigee, 1999.

Panzarine S: *A Parent's Guide to the Teen Years: Raising Your 11- to 14-Year-Old in the Age of Chat Rooms and Naval Rings*. New York, Checkmark Books, 2000.

Pruitt DB: *Your Adolescent: Emotional, Behavioral and Cognitive Development from Early Adolescence through the Teen Years*. New York, American Academy of Child and Adolescent Psychiatry, Harper Collins, 2000.

Wolf AE: *Get out of My Life, but First Could You Drive Me and Cheryl to the Mall? A Parent's Guide to the New Teenager*. New York, Farrar, Straus & Giroux, 2002.

Websites

For Parents

http://www.aacap.org/publications/factsfam/index.htm—Excellent site that provides fact sheets on adolescent and mental health issues from the American Academy of Child and Adolescent Psychiatry. English/Spanish.

http://www.advocatesforyouth.org/parents/—An excellent site providing anticipatory guidance for parents on adolescents.

http://www.4girls.gov—Resources on caring for adolescent girls.

http://www.pflag.org—Parents, Families and Friends of Lesbians and Gays.

http://www.talkingwithkids.org—Talk with Kids about Tough Issues—a project of Children Now and Kaiser Family Foundation.

http://www.tnpc.com/parentalk/adoles.html—From the National Parenting Center.

For Teens

http://www.advocatesforyouth.org/glbtq.htm—Great site that includes fact sheets and links on issues for gay, lesbian, bisexual and questioning youth. English/Spanish.

http://www.advocatesforyouth.org/teens—Information on teen health, sexual health and other links.

http://www.freevibe.com—Excellent site to get information on drugs, alcohol, and tobacco that is teen friendly.

http://www.4girls.gov—Information geared toward younger female teens.

http://www.iemily.com—Site for teenage girls about health-related matters.

http://www.iwannaknow.org—Information from the American Social Health Association for teens on sexuality, sexual transmitted infections and related topics with a parent's guide and great links.

http://www.kidshealth.org/teen—A great site for teens on health with separate sections geared toward boys and girls. From the Nemours Foundation.

http://mysistahs.org—A site for and by young women of color.

http://sxetc.org

http://www.teengrowth.com—Interactive website for teens on health and development. Board-certified physicians give advice on topics such as obesity, diet, emotions, alcohol, drugs, family, friends, school, sex and sports.

http://www.teenpregnancy.org/teen/default.asp—Website from the National Campaign to Prevent Teen Pregnancy. A good site for anyone (teen, parent, professional) wanting information on teen pregnancy.

http://www.youngwomenshealth.org—Site from the Center for Young Women's Health, Children's Hospital of Boston. English/Spanish.

For Professionals

The National Center for Youth Law. Available at *http://www.youthlaw.org/*.

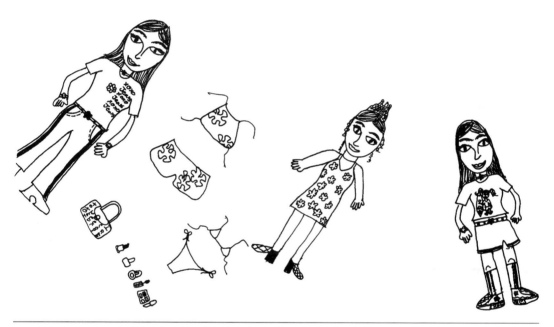

"Dressing for school, party and beach." By Sarah Stein, age 11.

CHAPTER 23

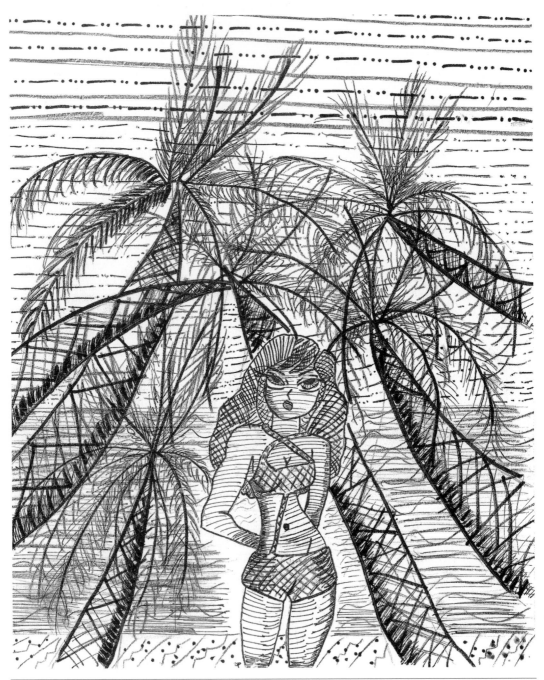

"Girl on the beach." Sexualized images represent the preoccupation of the age. By Kristen Hamilton.

Fifteen to Seventeen Years: Mid-Adolescence–Redefining Self

JENNIFER MAEHR and MARIANNE E. FELICE

This chapter describes the emotional and social challenges facing young people in the heart of adolescence. Sexual issues, independence and self-image are prominent themes during these years.

Key Words

- Eating Disorders
- Obesity
- Employment
- Sexual Activity
- Sexual Minority Youth
- Sexual Abuse/Assault
- Adolescent Pregnancy
- Contraception
- Sexually Transmitted Infections
- Abstract Thinking
- Risk-Taking Behavior
- Substance Use
- Promiscuity
- Depression
- Suicide
- Immigrant Youth
- Out-of-Home Youth
- Sports

Mid-adolescence typically spans the ages of 15 to 17 years. The major developmental task of mid-adolescence is the achievement of a sexual sense of self. This means becoming comfortable with one's sexuality, as well as learning to express sexual feelings in an appropriate manner and to receive sexual advances from another in a comfortable way. For most teens, it means the assumption of culturally defined sexual roles, behaviors and activities.

REFINEMENT OF THE SELF-IMAGE

For an adolescent to become comfortable with her sexuality, she must be comfortable with her body. Most mid-adolescents have already experienced puberty, but they may not yet be comfortable with the results. Hence, mid-adolescent girls and boys spend much time, money and energy on their appearance. Teens may experiment with clothing, hair, jewelry, makeup, tattoos, body piercing and speech in an effort to "try on" different looks and find the real self (see Chapter 18 for the preschooler's similar developmental work). It would not be surprising to observe a 15-year-old girl in pigtails at one medical visit and see her with a sophisticated hairstyle or dramatically changed hair color 2 weeks later at another visit. This experimentation is evidence of developmental work.

The emphasis on appearance is one aspect of the pervasive self-centeredness of many mid-adolescent teenagers. Because they are spending so much time thinking and looking at themselves, they presume that others are thinking about them and looking at them as well. This preoccupation with self may seem to border on paranoia, hysteria or frank narcissism, but it is completely normal. An example of this self-absorption can be observed by watching a group of heterosexual adolescent girls as they are approached by a group of adolescent boys. Each teenager will act and feel as though all attention is focused solely on himself or herself, that everybody is looking directly and completely just at him or her. No wonder, then, that so much effort is spent on the development of an image. This self-centeredness and heightened self-awareness may account for the continual hair grooming, clothes straightening, body posturing and makeup activities that take place in any gathering of mid-adolescents.

GROWING UP IN A PERFECT WORLD—FROM EATING DISORDERS TO OBESITY

Unfortunately, society's preoccupation with physical perfection of the human body can derail adolescents from attaining a positive sense of self and acceptance of their recent physical changes. Youth are bombarded by images of slim, attractive, muscular people and advertisements for quick fixes such as plastic surgery, cosmetic procedures, fad diets and weight-loss wonder drugs. Children and teens today grow up watching television shows in which individuals compete for surgical "makeovers." Not surprisingly, it is becoming increasingly common for adolescent girls to undergo plastic surgery procedures such as rhinoplasty, breast implants and "tummy tucks" just before the start of college or as a birthday gift from parents. Today's emphasis on veneer-thin beauty discourages teens from accepting themselves as they are.

Large numbers of teens, both male and female and even those with no weight problems, have dieted and consider themselves overweight. To lose weight, teens may exercise, restrict dietary intake, use medications and herbal remedies or purge. Teens commonly skip breakfast and avoid lunch while at school. Instead, they will buy snack foods and soda from vending machines and typically eat one large meal at the end of the day. These dietary practices and attempts to lose weight can result in substandard intakes of the calories and nutrients required during adolescence and can even lead to paradoxical weight gain. Adolescent girls struggle most with dieting as they attempt to stay thin despite the physiological changes occurring in them as a result of puberty, such as an increased percentage of body fat and changing body dimensions. An adolescent's normal interest in physical appearance can become obsessive and lead to potentially harmful behavior and **eating disorders**.

Tiffany is 16 years old. Her parents have recently become concerned because they have noticed that Tiffany's clothes are fitting loosely. Tiffany avoids eating with the family and has eliminated sweets, dairy products and meat from her diet. She wakes up at six in the morning every day to run. Although Tiffany continues to do well in school and in her extracurricular activities, her parents have decided to bring her to the family doctor. Tiffany weighs 15 pounds less than she did a year ago at her last visit. Her heart rate is 50 at rest, and her body temperature is subnormal. She has not had a period in the past 3 months and is not sexually active. Tiffany denies using any laxatives or diet pills and states that she does not make herself throw up because it hurts too much. Tiffany likes to weigh herself before each meal to know how much food she can eat. Although Tiffany is concerned about some recent hair loss, she does not think that she has an eating disorder and would actually like to lose 10 more pounds. Tiffany's doctor appropriately diagnoses anorexia nervosa and discusses the referral and treatment options with Tiffany and her parents.

Approximately 0.5% of adolescent girls in the United States have anorexia nervosa and 1% to 5% fit the *Diagnostic and Statistical Manual of Mental Disorders* (DSM-IV) criteria for bulimia nervosa. Not all teens with an eating disorder, however, meet the full criteria for anorexia or bulimia but can be classified as having an eating disorder not otherwise specified. All told, up to 10% of postpubertal females have some form of an eating disorder that presents a threat to their growth and development. Adolescent boys are also affected: 5% to 10% of all cases of eating disorders occur in males. Factors and characteristics associated with eating disorders in adolescents include female gender, puberty, early pubertal development, especially if also mildly overweight, a drive to excel in sports, perfectionism, low self-esteem and difficulties with communication, conflict resolution and separation issues. Certain sports are associated with eating disorders, including dance, gymnastics, figure skating, swimming, diving, running, cycling and those with weight requirements such as wrestling, crew and weightlifting. Teens with eating disorders commonly have other coexisting mental health problems such as depression, anxiety and obsessive-compulsive disorder. If an adolescent meets the criteria for an eating disorder, that youngster should be referred to an interdisciplinary team experienced and skilled in working with this special group of adolescents.

Though not as dramatic or acutely life threatening as anorexia nervosa, **obesity** affects more adolescents and often has negative effects on health and development. In the 1999-2000 National Health and Nutrition Examination Survey (NHANES), over 15% of adolescents 12 to 19 years of age were overweight (body mass index at or above the 95% percentile), a threefold increase in overweight adolescents since the 1976-1980 NHANES II. The escalation in adolescent obesity has resulted in more youth with weight-associated medical and psychosocial problems. Obesity in adolescence negatively affects self-esteem and overall mental health; for this reason, it is important to screen all obese teens for depression. The majority of obese adolescents remain obese as adults, thus stressing the importance of combating obesity as soon as it is recognized.

Regina is a 15-year-old freshman in high school. She weighs 350 pounds and has a body mass index that is off the chart. She makes an appointment with her primary care provider for back pain. A thorough history reveals that she is carrying a 30-pound book bag from class to class. She explains that her school has four levels and her locker is on the fourth floor. To use her locker between classes, she has to walk the stairs several times per day and she gets short of breath after climbing one flight. She feels embarrassed when she can't keep up, is late for class or blocks other students trying to get up the stairs behind her. So she chooses to carry all her books with her everywhere she goes. Her eating habits are likewise affected at school. She feels too embarrassed to eat in the cafeteria where her fellow students will stare at her and joke. So she skips lunch or slips into the art room where she can snack on food from vending machines. She doesn't understand why she is overweight. A risk assessment reveals family issues at home, and a self-reported depression inventory screen scores her in a range requiring further evaluation for possible depression. Her provider schedules several follow-up visits with Regina and her parent to create a diet and exercise plan. A note is written to the school nurse requesting assistance with the book bag problem. She agrees to be referred for counseling. She eventually requires referral to a comprehensive hospital-based program for obese adolescents and may attend a specialized summer camp program for overweight children.

SOCIAL DEVELOPMENT: THE ENLARGING WORLD OUTSIDE HOME

The supportive approval and combined efforts of the peer group fuel self-confidence under the presumed scrutiny of the opposite sex. Even when not "going out" with someone, adolescents benefit from interactions with members of the opposite sex as they learn to expand the peer group from a primarily one-gender group to a group of both boys and girls, from a local neighborhood clique to select groups with individuals of similar interests or talents. Frequently these interactions are initiated through school-based activities such as team sports, clubs, theater, academic societies or elected positions. In these organizations a mid-adolescent has the opportunity to socialize when not actually dating. For many teens this is a safer, more comfortable environment than a formal dating situation.

In addition to developing relationships with peers of the opposite sex, mid-adolescents form other relationships outside the family. They usually make some new friends of the same sex, frequently develop a strong attachment to one or two adults outside the family and begin to care about and for younger children. These are important interactions and expose mid-adolescents to lifestyles and philosophies different from those of their own families.

Most mid-adolescents attend school, typically in a high school setting spanning the 9th to 12th grades. During this time, adolescents may discover new or heightened interests and talents in varying disciplines such as the arts, creative writing or sports; these interests often support the development of a positive self-image and provide an outlet for personal expression. They also provide a means by which a teen can transfer her internal feelings and struggles into something concrete and positive. Teachers and coaches can provide valuable insight into the important developmental work being done by teens as they participate in these activities and are often among the first adults to notice when a teen is troubled and in need of help. Mid-adolescents typically find a particular teacher or coach to serve as an important mentor in their lives.

Many teens will obtain **employment** or volunteer for the first time during mid-adolescence. Some do so out of financial necessity, others as part of their education and some by their own choice. The positive effects of employment during adolescence are numerous and include a sense of accomplishment and responsibility, job experience that enhances the probability of future employment and social skills that come from working with others. Employment allows teens greater independence from parents, which fosters important developmental growth, but it may also result in less parental supervision. Excessive work hours during adolescence can have a negative impact that affects school performance and sleep and possibly increases opportunities for risk-taking behavior. A healthy adolescence requires supportive parental monitoring, as well as a balance between school, work and social activities.

During mid-adolescence, teens may begin to try on various personas by altering dress, manner of speech and political viewpoints, often to the chagrin of their parents. However, these excursions are normal developmental explorations, and by young adulthood, their political and philosophical opinions are usually similar to those of their parents. In fact, for most adolescents, constant conflict and recurrent turmoil are the exceptions rather than the rules, and most adolescents love and respect their parents in spite of disagreements about everyday issues.

SEXUAL DEVELOPMENT

Some say that sexual and aggressive drives are stronger during adolescence than at any other time of life. Learning to appropriately express and control these drives is a major and formidable task of the teenage years, and the need to master these drives is felt most acutely during mid-adolescence, a time when the individual may seem least equipped to control them. Responding to strong sexual drives as well as to peer and cultural age-appropriate expectations, most mid-adolescents will begin to date or "hook up" if given parental permission to do so. Though attracted to their dating partner, most mid-adolescents see their romantic relationships as an opportunity for social gain. The degrees of attractiveness and popularity of one's partner provides are important measures of one's own self-worth and status. During mid-adolescence, romantic relationships tend to be short lived, lasting on average less than 9 months, but become increasingly more important and intimate during late adolescence. Conflict with close friends, especially same-gender friends, may erupt as romantic relationships evolve and sometimes eclipse childhood friendships.

Most mid-adolescents engage in some aspect of **sexual activity** or play, the extent of which varies from adolescent to adolescent and from one socioeconomic group or subcultural group to another. By the 11th grade, over 50% of adolescents have had sexual intercourse and 15% have had four or more sexual partners. Of all sexually active high school students, approximately 63% used condoms the last time they had sex, an improvement over previous decades. As many as 25%, however, used drugs or alcohol before last having sexual intercourse. Some mid-adolescents engage in oral sex and fewer in anal intercourse. Many teens will avoid intercourse or oral sex altogether and engage in foreplay or "outercourse," a slang term used to describe mutual sexual stimulation by pressing up against or feeling each other. Although one cannot presume that all mid-adolescents are having sexual intercourse, one can assume that all mid-adolescents are interested in sexual issues and may be engaging in other types of sexual activities.

> Amber, 16 years old, comes alone and on time for her appointment at the doctor's office. She tells the nurse that she is here for birth control. With family planning forms in hand, Dr. Smith walks into the examining room to see Amber. Although Dr. Smith has been her physician for several years, Amber suddenly seems more mature and independent. Sitting at the small table in the examination room, Amber works diligently on her school assignments. Her nails are long and painted with intricate designs. Dressed in a purple suit with matching shoes, Amber seems like a young adult. After Dr. Smith compliments her for working on her homework, Amber replies that she has auditions for the choir after this and is worried that she won't finish all her work by tomorrow.
>
> At past visits, Amber had not disclosed a history of having had sex. Because she came for birth control, Dr. Smith assumes that she has probably become sexually active. During the interview Dr. Smith asks Amber, "Are you sexually active now?" Amber hesitates in thought for a few moments and then answers, "No." Slightly surprised by this response, Dr. Smith adds, "Are you thinking that you might start having sex soon?" to which Amber answers, "Well, yeah, I already am." With further questioning it becomes clear that Amber has indeed been sexually active for several months and wants birth control pills because she doesn't want to get pregnant. When Dr. Smith asked her about being "sexually active," Amber thought the doctor was asking her whether she is really active, physically, when she has sex.

A health care provider can be easily fooled by the appearance of a teenager. Amber seemed very mature and was indeed taking responsibility for herself and her body. However, she did not understand what Dr. Smith meant by "sexually active." Many teens don't. To some, being sexually active means having multiple sexual partners; having sex recently, for example, in the past month; or having sex frequently, for example, multiple times per week or per day. Being "sexually active" may imply to the teen a heightened sexuality, such as engaging in risqué sexual acts or sex that demands a great deal of physical activity. The term "sexual intercourse" may also be confusing to adolescents—most know what this term means but some teens, especially sexually inexperienced ones, may not.

One can never assume that a teenager understands what is being said or implied when it comes to sex. A health care provider needs to use easy-to-understand language in a non-threatening manner and may need to give examples of what is meant:

- Many teens your age are starting to have romantic relationships. Have you ever been romantically involved with anyone?

- Have you done any kind of sexual activity with this person, like kissing, touching or having sexual intercourse?

- Do you know what I mean when I say sexual intercourse? (Then follow-up with a brief explanation of what sexual intercourse is.)

- Are you using anything to protect yourself from pregnancy or sexually transmitted diseases, like condoms?

• Some teens think that they may be gay or homosexual, that is, some boys (or girls) are sexually attracted to other boys (or girls). Are you interested in being involved in a sexual way with boys, girls or both?

Questions should be open ended so that teens don't feel compelled to answer questions in a certain way. Broaching and discussing the subject of sex with a teenage patient can be challenging for the practitioner. If done well, however, the teenager will feel supported by the health care provider, who has now become a valuable and trusted source of information on confidential and sensitive matters.

SEXUAL MINORITY YOUTH

Similar to adults, some adolescents identify themselves as gay, lesbian or bisexual. Many teens are unsure of their sexual orientation. Others may not yet realize or are not able to admit that they are not heterosexual; this realization may not be faced until late adolescence or early adulthood. Information from adult homosexual men and women shows that most perceived themselves as being different from their same-sex peers as early as childhood but did not develop feelings of being *sexually* different until sometime during adolescence.

In the process of establishing a sexual sense of themselves, many adolescents may wonder whether they are homosexual. Adolescent girls commonly develop crushes on girlfriends or female teachers, and it is certainly not unusual for adolescent boys to experience an erection in the company of other males. Same-sex arousal or experimentation with same-sex sexual activity does not necessarily indicate that an adolescent is homosexual, nor does it predict future sexual orientation. With time, a teenager's sexual preference will become clear.

Teens who are nonheterosexual, however, are at increased risks for psychosocial problems, such as deteriorating school performance, mental illness, substance abuse, homelessness, delinquency, suicide attempts (most notably among males) and prostitution. **Sexual minority youth** may feel isolated and hate themselves. They may be rejected by their families, and they often face peer ridicule and physical violence. Sexual minority youth are more likely to have a satisfying adolescence if they feel supported by their family and friends. Nonheterosexual youth and their families can benefit from interactions with gay and lesbian peer support groups and knowledgeable health care providers.

Unfortunately, many sexual minority youth may be afraid to trust their health care provider because of fears about judgment, rejection and breach of confidentiality. Teens may get signals directly from the clinician or indirectly from the atmosphere in the office that rightly or erroneously tell them that the provider would not be receptive to their sexual behavior or choices. It is critical to create an environment in the office that positively supports and fosters discussion about topics relating to homosexuality. Posters on the wall, visible brochures and the availability of referral resources that support sexual minority youth are examples of ways to accomplish this. Clinicians also need to ask questions regarding sexual orientation because the topic is rarely broached by mid-adolescents themselves. The clinician must be ready to discuss sexual issues with the adolescent patient in a nonjudgmental fashion. This means that the clinician must be comfortable with his own sexuality, as well as comfortable with and knowledgeable about the subject of sex. Clinicians must be aware of their own limitations and biases in this area and must not impose their viewpoints on an adolescent patient.

Dr. Lee had known Lauren since she was 14 years old, treated her asthma, started her on birth control when she became sexually active at the age of 16 and performed Lauren's first Pap smear when she turned 19. It was not until a clinic visit when Lauren was 20 that she disclosed to Dr. Lee that she had been involved with a female girlfriend for the past 5 years. She explained to Dr. Lee that she was just not sure how he would take her having a sexual relationship with another woman.

The physician reacted supportively to Lauren's disclosure but inwardly was quite surprised because she had not shared this information with him sooner. Dr. Lee reflected on his past office visits with her and wondered whether he had ever asked her questions about the gender of her partners.

Note: Sometimes it is difficult for clinicians to take a thorough sexual history on patients whom they have known for years. This case points out, however, that it is equally difficult for adolescents to volunteer this type of information. It is important for clinicians to give teens, even those well known to the practice, the opportunity to discuss their sexual orientation and practices by directly asking them questions on these matters.

James had developed a trusting relationship with his mental health counselor at his school-based clinic. He was being seen for depression and had a history of several psychiatric hospitalizations. During a comprehensive risk assessment, he disclosed to her that he was gay and had been involved in several sexual relationships with men. His counselor advised him that it would be a good idea to see the medical provider at the school-based clinic for further information about safe sex practices and testing for sexually transmitted infections. James adamantly refused. He did not want to meet another provider and trust that person with private information about himself. He did not want to risk being judged. He already felt rejected by his parents and had very little self-esteem left for himself. James eventually agreed to meet the medical provider with his counselor present and did receive testing. The medical provider was accepting of James, and James now felt comfortable enough to return to the medical provider by himself to receive his test results.

Note: This case reflects how some teens are resistant to entrusting personal information with more than one provider. James may never have received testing if it had required him to go to another clinic or if his mental health provider had not been able to introduce him to the medical provider.

SEXUAL ABUSE AND ASSAULT

Not all sexual activity in adolescence is consensual. Teens may be victims or perpetrators of **sexual abuse** and **sexual assault**. The health care provider is mandated by law to report cases of suspected or actual sexual abuse, defined as any contact or conduct of a sexual nature between a minor and a person responsible for the child's welfare, such as a relative, caregiver, teacher or coach. Sexual assault differs from sexual abuse in that the assailant is not responsible for the child's or adolescent's welfare, and in most cases, the decision to report is left to the family or the victim. Sexual assault occurs when a sexual act is committed without a person's consent or with a person who is legally unable to consent, such as a mentally or physically impaired person, intoxicated or drugged person or a child/adolescent under the age of consent as specified by state law.

Acquaintance or date rape is one type of sexual assault and refers to situations of rape in which the assailant and victim know each other, typically in a social way. The illegal availability of flunitrazepam (Rohypnol), the so-called date rape drug, has been associated with an increase in adolescent acquaintance rape. Gamma-hydroxybutyrate (GHB) may also be used in date rape and, like flunitrazepam, can be easily slipped into a drink. Another form of sexual assault is statutory rape, which is based solely on an age discrepancy between two sexual partners, typically when an adult has sex with an adolescent who is younger than a specified age as set by state law or who is more than a predetermined number of years younger than the older partner. The notion behind statutory rape laws is that until a certain age, adolescents are unable to legally consent to sexual intercourse and need to be protected from predatory adults. In some states, health care providers must report statutory rape; this requirement may lead some teens to avoid seeking medical care or to omit parts of the medical history in an attempt to protect their older partners.

Unfortunately, adolescents have the highest rates of sexual assault of any age group. When compared with their adult counterparts, adolescent rape victims are more likely to have used alcohol or drugs before the assault and are more likely to delay seeking medical care after the assault. Sexually abused and/or assaulted teens are at higher risk for teen pregnancy, younger age at first voluntary sex, multiple sexual partners, substance use, depression and eating disorders. Teens may not disclose a history of abuse or assault that occurred in childhood or adolescence until weeks, months or even years later. Parents and victims need to be reassured that this delay in disclosure is normal. Like adult women, post-traumatic stress or rape trauma syndrome can result.

It is important to assess all teens periodically for a history of abuse and assault. An ideal time to ask is during the annual adolescent health maintenance visit. The pre-participation physical examination is also an opportune time to perform a risk assessment and screen for past abuse and assault, especially in those teens who seek medical care only when they need clearance for sports-related activities. Teens receiving care for mental health problems, eating disorders, substance use, early sexual debut and high-risk sexual behavior should also be asked about past or current abuse/assault. Counseling teens about date rape drugs and ways to stay safe (e.g., avoiding drug and alcohol use, not walking alone at night) may help reduce their risk of being sexually assaulted. Teens who have been abused or assaulted benefit from ongoing counseling with a health professional experienced in working with adolescent abuse and assault victims.

ADOLESCENT PREGNANCY

In the United States, approximately 20% of sexually active adolescent girls become pregnant each year, accounting for an estimated 900,000 teen pregnancies per year. More than three quarters of these pregnancies are reported as unintended. When looking specifically at pregnancies in mid-adolescent girls (15 to 17 years of age), 56% result in a birth, 30% are terminated by abortion, and an estimated 14% end in miscarriage. The pregnancy and birth rates for

TABLE 23–1   **Factors Associated with Increased Risk of Teen Pregnancy in Adolescent Girls**

Teen Characteristics	Family/Parent Characteristics	Community Characteristics
Lower expectations for the future	Poverty	High poverty rates
Poor school performance	Low parental educational level	Low levels of education
Ambivalence about or desire for having a baby during adolescence	Parents divorced/separated/ never married	High divorce rate
Negative attitudes toward birth control/condoms	Mother or sister gave birth as an adolescent	High residential turnover
History of multiple sexual partners or older male partners	Less parental support and supervision	
History of sexual/physical abuse or forced sex/sexual assault		
Drug and alcohol abuse		
Earlier age of puberty		

Adapted from the AAP Committee on Adolescence: Adolescent pregnancy—current trends and issues: 1998. *Pediatrics* 103:516, 1999; and Kirby D: *No Easy Answers—Research Findings on Programs to Reduce Teen Pregnancy.* Washington, DC, National Campaign to Prevent Teen Pregnancy, 1997.

adolescents in the United States have been steadily decreasing over the past decade. The decline in the pregnancy rate among high school–age teens has been attributed to both a delay in their initiation of sexual intercourse and improvements in their contraceptive practices. Despite this improvement, the United States still has the highest adolescent birth rate of all developed countries. Some blame this high rate on the fact that American teens have less access to contraceptive services and sex education than teens in European countries do.

The underlying issues and consequences of teen pregnancy are numerous and complex. As shown in Table 23–1, various factors have been identified that place individual adolescents at increased risk of becoming pregnant. Adolescents as a group are also developmentally more at risk for unintended pregnancy than adults are. Cognitively, younger teens have a limited ability to project themselves into a realistic scenario in which they are pregnant or a parent. Therefore, they do not appreciate the need for birth control or emergency contraception. The response of "this couldn't be happening to me" is an all-too-familiar reaction from a teen who has just received the news that she is pregnant or that he is going to be a father. Even for mature teens who have the ability to think abstractly, the overriding drive for pleasure may supersede caution to abstain from sex or to use a condom. Being "caught up in the moment" may take the teen by surprise before initiating birth control or getting condoms. Others may be intoxicated and unable to make sound decisions. Unfortunately, many teens do not know enough about reproductive health and their contraceptive options.

Victoria came to the clinic requesting a pregnancy test because her period was late. She states that she will just die if she is pregnant. Her parents would be disappointed, and she wants to go to college and is just not ready to have a baby. She doesn't know why she and her partner aren't using any protection. She just wasn't thinking that she would actually get pregnant.

Once pregnant, teens are less likely to receive timely prenatal care than their adult counterparts and more often delay care until the third trimester. Adverse health behavior by pregnant teens occurs for a variety of reasons that may include delayed diagnosis of the pregnancy, denial of the pregnancy, desire to hide the pregnancy from parents or partners, conflicting feelings about the pregnancy, barriers to prenatal care, lack of knowledge and/or a developmental inability to focus on the needs of the baby over their own desires and fears.

When compared with pregnant adult women, pregnant teens have a higher incidence of medical complications in both the mother and child, including a higher risk for low birthweight, prematurity and neonatal and maternal death. Children born to adolescent mothers are at increased risk for developmental delay, academic difficulties, behavior disorders, substance abuse and adolescent parenthood themselves. Adolescent mothers are at risk for school interruption, poverty, limited employment opportunities, separation from the baby's father, divorce, single parenting and repeat teen pregnancy. Fathers of babies born to teen mothers struggle as well. Most young men have little idea how to be a father or supportive partner. Like teen mothers, they are more likely to have poor academic performance, higher school dropout rates, limited financial resources and reduced earning potential as compared with their male peers who are not fathers. These multiple medical and socioeconomic sequelae of teen pregnancy are at great cost to society at large. In spite of these risks, some teen mothers do very well as parents, particularly if they receive comprehensive, age-appropriate care before and after the birth of the child, as well as positive social support from the baby's father and/or their own mother.

CONTRACEPTIVE USE

Teen girls typically seek medical services for **contraception** approximately 12 months *after* initiating sexual intercourse. Given this statistic, it is not surprising that about half of all adolescent pregnancies occur within the first 6 months after coitarche and that as many as one fifth occur within the first month of initiating sexual intercourse. In addition to financial restraints, transportation issues and the developmental issues discussed previously, there are numerous reasons why adolescents delay, refuse or avoid obtaining birth control.

In the ideal situation, a teen has a conversation with a parent or health professional about starting birth control and initiates a method before becoming sexually active. Many teens, however, do not want to have this conversation and worry about the repercussions of a parent or clinician knowing that they are sexually active. Some teens think that their primary care provider or health plan may breach confidentiality and inform a parent directly or inadvertently via a bill or health insurance statement. Others may be too embarrassed to buy contraceptive supplies or too shy to discuss issues of sexuality with their health care provider.

Clinicians must be sensitive to these concerns and automatically spend at least a few minutes with every adolescent patient without a parent being present. Posting practice policies on confidentiality and discussing how the practice handles matters under the minor consent law of the state can reassure a teen on what can be expected.

> During a high school health education class, the instructor was generating an open discussion about condom use. One of the students verbalized, " If a guy uses a condom, his girl may wonder what's up. Like she may think that maybe he is sleeping around with other people or that she isn't his main girl. Or maybe she's thinking that the guy doesn't think that she is clean. It's all about trust. If you use a condom, you're not trusting your partner."

Teens who choose not to use birth control may baffle or elude the health care provider. They (or their partner) may actually want a baby or may be testing to see whether they can get pregnant (or get someone pregnant). Some teen couples feel that using condoms equates to a lack of trust or faith in the relationship with their partner. Teenagers who believe they are infertile because of irregular periods, a past sexually transmitted infection (STI) or failure to conceive in the past may see no need for birth control. Fear of the pelvic examination may deter some young women from asking for hormonal birth control, but in most cases, a pelvic examination and Papanicolaou (Pap) smear are not required before starting hormonal contraception. Adolescents may have other fears and misconceptions about birth control, especially hormonal contraception, that keep them from starting a method. Adolescent girls tend to worry about weight gain, infertility, hair loss and changes in menstrual bleeding. Some of these concerns may stem from comments made by friends or family members.

> Michael asked his doctor if there was some way he could be tested to see if he could have kids. He had been with several different sexual partners over the past year, often without using condoms, and none of them got pregnant. He has now stopped using condoms altogether. Michael wants to know if there is something wrong with him.

For adolescents choosing birth control, oral contraceptives and the male condom are the most popular methods. Use of birth control, however, is sporadic, with 32% to 75% of sexually active teenagers reporting current use of any contraceptive method. Girls choosing a contraceptive method with their clinician may use it incorrectly, never start it or quickly discontinue it. Some girls are more successful with their chosen method and will often continue using it during periods when they are abstinent. The sexual partner is influential in whether contraception will be used. In some subcultures, condom use or hormonal contraception is not looked on favorably. Fortunately, hormonal contraception and condom use have been increasing among sexually active adolescents.

After several discussions with her clinician, Maria decides to start taking birth control pills as her contraceptive method. She is dispensed four packs with verbal and written instructions. Maria is also given advice by her girlfriend on how to take the pills. When Maria develops spotting (mild midcycle bleeding from the pills), she stops taking the pills and does not start a new pack until the Sunday after her bleeding stops. Maria returns to the clinic in 3 months. Her urine pregnancy test is positive.

Note: Maria should have been told by her clinician that spotting is a common side effect of the " pill," particularly in the early months, and that she should continue the "pill" as directed if spotting occurs. For this reason, some clinicians ask new contraceptive users to return for a visit in 1 month to check on problems and misperceptions.

Kelsey refuses any form of hormonal contraception. She is afraid of needles and therefore does not want Depo-Provera. She does not want to gain weight like her sister did on the pill and worries that Ortho Evra (a transdermal contraceptive patch) will do the same thing. The thought of putting something in her vagina is "freaky," so using a vaginal ring or diaphragm is out. She is consistently given condoms and a backup dose of emergency contraception by the clinic. Several months later, Kelsey is pregnant. She hadn't been using the condoms and did not want to take the emergency contraception. She shrugs, "I just didn't care one way or the other if I got pregnant."

Note: Despite our best attempts to educate teens about contraceptive options and safe sex practices, clinicians are not able to prevent all contraceptive errors, nor are we able to convince all sexually active teens to consistently use or even start birth control. Short of being with the adolescent at all times, we cannot control what they are going to do or what decisions they are going to make. We can, however, remain accessible and nonjudgmental to them as questions arise and problems develop. We can engage them in discussions about birth control, pregnancy and parenting and what the consequences of a pregnancy would be for them. We can kindly confront them if we identify discrepancies between their actual behavior and their verbal statements about wanting to avoid pregnancies or STIs. It is important to uncover whether their statements accurately reflect what they are feeling—they may simply be telling us what we want to hear. Clinicians caring for mid-adolescents benefit from training on the behavior change model and on strategies to support positive behavior changes.

SEXUALLY TRANSMITTED INFECTIONS

Approximately one in four sexually active teenagers will become infected with a **sexually transmitted infection** every year, and one quarter of all new STIs occur in teenagers. Adolescents have a greater risk of acquiring STIs than do people of other ages because of various biological (e.g., cervical ectropion) and behavioral reasons. As a group, adolescent girls, especially African American girls, seem to be at greatest risk; girls have higher rates of chlamydia, gonorrhea and human immunodeficiency virus (HIV) infection than same-aged adolescent boys do. Excluding HIV, the most common STIs seen in adolescents are chlamydia, human papillomavirus and trichomoniasis.

Receiving a diagnosis of an STI can be devastating to a teen. An adolescent given an STI diagnosis may actually decompensate in front of the medical provider. Giving a positive test result by telephone can be especially challenging because the clinician cannot predict how the teen may react. Similar to receiving a diagnosis of pregnancy, the teen wonders "how could this be happening to me," but often with the additional feeling of being violated by the partner, "cheated on" and possibly permanently damaged or "dirtied." Teens appreciate receiving results without placement of blame on them, as well as factual information about the infection and prompt, on-site treatment. It may take several visits before the teen totally understands her diagnosis and how to prevent future infections in herself and her partner or partners. Even with this knowledge, a teen may not change her sexual behavior and may instead continue to put herself at risk. For adolescents who display repetitive, risky sexual behavior, it is worth performing a thorough screen for underlying, contributing psychosocial issues such as depression, past/current child abuse, family problems, substance use or limits in comprehension because of mental retardation or other disabilities.

Jessica, a junior in high school, has a new sexual partner. She comes to the woman's clinic to "be checked" to make sure that she doesn't "have anything." She admits that her partner has not been using a condom every time they have had sex. She denies any oral or anal sex. She is taking Depo-Provera and recently had a normal Pap smear and negative HIV test. She has no symptoms of an STI, no vaginal discharge, no vaginal odor, no dysuria and no pelvic or abdominal pain. The patient and clinician decide that a pelvic examination is not necessary, and instead a vaginal swab is obtained by the patient herself for microscopic inspection by the clinician. The patient also gives a urine sample for a gonorrhea and chlamydia test. The wet prep is normal except for a very mild elevation in white blood cells. The patient is sent home with condoms after a discussion about ways to reduce her risk for STIs.

The patient is called back to the clinic the following week when her urine test returns positive for chlamydia. She is treated at the clinic and counseled about chlamydia and the importance of remaining abstinent until her partner is treated. The clinician gives Jessica a list of places where her partner can be treated for free and another bag of condoms.

Jessica returns 1 month later with severe lower abdominal pain. When specifically asked, Jessica relates that her partner never got treated. He didn't believe that he had an infection. They started having sex without using condoms several days after she was treated. After a thorough examination, she is diagnosed with pelvic inflammatory disease and started on a 14-day outpatient treatment. Her clinician again stresses that her partner must be treated and the importance of abstinence until everyone completes treatment. The clinician schedules a follow-up visit in 3 days and invites Jessica to bring her partner to that visit if he has not been able to get treatment.

Three days later, Jessica returns with the partner. She is better, but he has not been treated. The clinician takes the opportunity to talk to both of them together about STIs and risk reduction. The partner is tested and treated at the clinic. Both Jessica and her partner also receive HIV testing and counseling. Condoms are given and a follow-up visit is scheduled in 2 weeks.

Note: The clinician here did everything right and could not be faulted with her evaluation, treatment and counseling. Chlamydia is often a "silent STI" with no symptoms in males or females. Time permitting, it may have been helpful for the clinician to role-play with Jessica on how Jessica would inform her partner of the positive chlamydia test. It can be very daunting even for adults to disclose such information to partners. Equipping Jessica with the knowledge that her partner may be asymptomatic with chlamydia may have aided her in convincing him that he needed treatment and may have helped her say "no" to sex until he was treated.

COGNITIVE AND MORAL DEVELOPMENT

Mid-adolescence is usually characterized by a shift in cognitive abilities. Most mid-adolescents have developed the capacity for **abstract thinking** and are usually capable of introspection. In other words, they are capable of coherent, logical thinking, deduction and conjecture and are able to reflect on their own thought processes in an "objective" manner. This stage of cognitive development is known as formal operational thinking in the framework of Piaget (see Chapter 2) and is a giant step in mental development. A mid-adolescent may become fascinated with his newfound intellectual tool, and this aspect of growth may be another factor contributing to the self-centeredness or egocentrism of mid-adolescence: they can now think about themselves thinking. A marvelous sense of self-cleverness may contribute to a positive self-image or a slight disdain for the archaic thought processes of adults.

With the development of abstract thinking, adolescents have new capacities for moral decision making. In younger years, children are in a stage of moral growth in which good behavior results in reward and misbehavior results in punishment (see Chapter 18). Hence, good or bad is determined solely by the consequences. A second level of morality is marked by the need to meet the expectations or follow the rules of one's family, peer group or nation. In fact, maintaining the rules of the group becomes a value in itself for a youngster in mid-childhood. The third stage of moral development consists of a major thrust toward autonomous moral principles that have validity apart from the authority of the group and are based on the individual's own beliefs and conclusions concerning what is right or wrong. This is called adult morality. This last stage of morality usually begins in mid-adolescence, but it is not completed until young adulthood. Some individuals never make this shift.

A mid-adolescent may be capable of making moral judgments based on the principles of a moral code, but unfortunately, the self-centered behavior of mid-adolescents also results in a narcissistic value system, "what is right is what makes me feel good," and "what is right is what I want." This self-centered attitude partially explains the high-risk sexual behavior and exploitation that can occur. Indeed, many activities during the mid-adolescent years may be impulsive, with little thought about consequences. Hence, other psychosocial processes may supersede cognitive capacities.

The prefrontal cortex, which is responsible for executive functioning such as prioritizing tasks, planning, analyzing options and consequences and controlling urges, is the last part of the brain to fully mature and continues to undergo modification into young adulthood. Scientists speculate that teens often resort to emotional decision making because of relatively increased reliance on other areas of the brain. As teens mature and approach adulthood, they rely more on the prefrontal cortex for decision-making processes. Until then, teens are in the midst of developing their abilities to make judgments based on sound reasoning rather than on emotion or on what makes them feel better. Often what feels better during adolescence is what gets the most attention and support of peers. An adolescent may make a logical, well-thought out decision when alone but a more impulsive, risky decision when surrounded by friends or other teens. Understanding brain maturation during adolescence helps explain some adolescent behavior and the lack of consistent good judgment and self-control. More research is unfolding in this area.

> John was out with his friends. His parents insisted that he be home by 10 PM. John was having a great time and did not realize it was past 10 PM until it was already 11. "I gotta go—I'm late!" His friends retort, "What's the point—you're already in trouble? Why go home now? Might as well stay." John is about to call home on his cell phone to let his parents know that he is late, but then decides his friends are right. He'd rather stay here with his friends for now than have to deal with his parents' reprimand.

RISK-TAKING BEHAVIOR AND ADOLESCENT MORTALITY

Despite their better judgment, many mid-adolescents engage in **risk-taking behavior** such as truancy, substance use, unsafe sex, breaking parental curfews or rules, violent or criminal acts or irresponsible driving. Such behavior may lead to school failure, unintended pregnancy, STIs, addiction, juvenile delinquency and personal harm. This risk-taking behavior may ultimately lead to death. It has been estimated that over 70% of all adolescent mortality could be prevented if risk-taking behavior could be minimized. Although there are variations by race and gender, the leading causes of death in adolescents 15 to 19 years of age are (1) unintentional injuries, primarily from motor vehicle accidents; (2) homicides, primarily from firearms; and (3) suicides. Factors contributing to these deaths are numerous and include drug and alcohol use, fighting, possession of weapons, mental health issues, inexperienced teen drivers and lack of seat belt use. Even though not all teens engage in risky behavior, most teens are directly or indirectly affected by violence, alcohol and drugs sometime during their adolescence.

> David was being seen in the emergency room for chest pain. A thorough examination, chest x-ray and electrocardiogram revealed a healthy 16-year-old male. His history was more significant. During the episodes of chest pain over the past 2 weeks, it was difficult for him to breathe, he felt anxious and his heart would beat fast. These episodes usually happened when he was alone and would resolve in about 5 to 10 minutes. With further questioning, the clinician discovered that one of David's close friends was killed in a drive-by shooting exactly 2 weeks ago. David was having panic attacks. The clinician recommended counseling and reassured David that he was going to be alright. The clinician explained to David what panic attacks were and that it was not surprising that he was having them given the recent traumatic death of his friend.

Substance Use

Although younger children are exposed to drugs as early as grade school, the pressure to use them becomes more intense in mid-adolescence. Teens may use drugs for a variety of reasons. Substance use may make it easier for a teen to get accepted into a desirable peer group. For more serious users, drugs may be a coping mechanism to feel better about themselves, to reduce stress or, in some situations, to self-medicate mental health conditions. Many teens will try a drug simply to discover what it feels like to be high or intoxicated.

Overall, alcohol is the most commonly used substance by adolescents: 70% of 12th graders reported using alcohol and almost one half of them reported having been drunk at least once in the past year. More than one half of 12th graders have at some point in their lives used illicit drugs, most commonly marijuana, followed by amphetamines, inhalants and hallucinogens. A significant number of teens are using cigarettes and marijuana on a regular basis: the 30-day prevalence use for 12th graders is about 27% for cigarettes and about 22% for marijuana. Because both marijuana and cigarettes often precede the use of other illicit substances and hard alcohol, their use should not be taken lightly.

Although it is common for adolescents to experiment with alcohol and marijuana, it is not normal for adolescents to be habitually drunk or "stoned," and it is not normal for adolescents to use "hard drugs," such as crack, phencyclidine (PCP) or heroin. Some signs of drug abuse are a drop in school performance, accidents, family stress, legal problems and noticeable changes in behavior, dress or peer group. These substance-using teens need special help. Adolescents who abuse drugs should be referred for drug counseling with mental health workers experienced in drug counseling of youth. Frequently, this requires residential treatment, and clinicians should become familiar with drug rehabilitation agencies in their area of practice. Drug use that alters a youngster's functioning cannot be dealt with in an ordinary pediatric office setting.

Dying to Drive

A mid-adolescent is usually a newly licensed or about to be licensed driver and, as such, is inexperienced in the skill of driving. Often seen as a rite of passage for adolescence, teens and parents may view the teen's driver's license with both anticipation and dread: it allows the teen increased independence from parents and vice versa, but at potential cost. The leading cause of death for all adolescents is motor vehicle accidents. The motor vehicle fatality rate is higher for adolescents, most notably male adolescents, than for any other age group. Teens are most at risk for fatal accidents in their first 6 months of driving and when driving with others. In addition, motor vehicle accidents cause head and spinal cord injuries, which are a major cause of disability for adolescents.

José and Zachary were both leaving in their separate cars from an evening band practice. Because they were neighbors, they decided to race home to see who could get there first. Often ignoring stop signs and traffic light signals, they sped off down the road. José could see that Zachary was close behind him, so he accelerated. In the darkness and at excess speeds, José could not see the people crossing the street until it was too late. José attempted to swerve and slammed his car into a tree. In the process, one pedestrian was struck and killed. José required helicopter transport to the nearest trauma facility and would face criminal charges.

The combination of high-risk–taking behavior and lack of driving experience accounts for an adolescent's increased risk for motor vehicle accidents. Teenagers tend to drive more at night and have a much higher nighttime crash fatality rate. Alcohol use has been tied to about one third of all fatal crashes involving teens. In addition, adolescents use seat belts only 35% of the time. Many states have adopted graduated licensing systems to combat these statistics. Graduated licensure requires the teen to progress successfully through an additional stage called provisional licensing that allows for a more monitored and lower risk environment in which to practice driving before getting full licensure. Although graduated licensing varies by state, the ideal system would require (1) supervision by a responsible adult for the first 6 months of driving, (2) a limit on the nighttime hours during which teens could drive, (3) zero alcohol tolerance, (4) proper restraint of all occupants, (5) a limit to the number of nonadult passengers and (6) penalties such as remedial driving education and prolongation of provisional licensing for violations of any of the above.

COUNSELING PARENTS

During the child's mid-adolescent years, the physician may begin to see the adolescent patient regularly without a parent present, but this does not mean that the role of the parent is unimportant. Indeed, the mid-adolescent years are considered the "heart" of adolescence and may be the most difficult period for parents to face. As mid-adolescents struggle with self-identity, they are characteristically ambivalent about their relationship with parents. Having already progressed through *early* adolescence, they have declared their need for independence in one way or another. But being wiser than their younger selves, they realize that complete independence from parents may be frightening. So, typically, a mid-adolescent "flirts" with a close relationship with his parents, sometimes asking for help and at other times rejecting all offers of assistance for fear that the parent will engulf him and suffocate his independence. This back-and-forth relationship is normal but can be confusing and disheartening for parents.

Some parents have difficulty accepting the fact that they may not be informed about the diagnosis, treatment and counseling of a health condition or behavior in their adolescent. These situations are also difficult for the clinician. At some point, however, teens must take responsibility for their own health as they make the transition to adulthood. Parents may find it helpful to know that their adolescent is acting appropriately for his developmental stage by attempting to individuate or separate from parents in seeking health care on his own. It is also helpful for parents to hear that their teen is behaving maturely by taking responsibility for his well-being and that this health-seeking behavior should be commended.

Nonetheless, the clinician should attempt to work with an adolescent to help him communicate with his parents. Clinicians need to carefully assess the parent-teen landscape and, when possible, urge the teen to disclose information to the parent, perhaps with the assistance of the clinician. It is equally important to gain the trust of the parent as it is the trust of the teen patient. This trust is earned by listening to the concerns of parents and by providing compassionate, high-quality care to their adolescent. In situations in which parents know that their adolescent is receiving confidential care, the clinician can reassure them that they will be immediately informed if the teen's health is ever in serious jeopardy. Once the patient turns 18, however, the adolescent is no longer a minor, and the clinician is usually required to obtain permission from the older adolescent patient before informing parents of any health concerns.

Heather, who is 16 years old, comes with a friend to the clinic for a pregnancy test and STI testing. Her mother calls later that day to talk to the clinician. She wants to know if her daughter is pregnant. The clinician thanks the mother for calling and asks what information Heather has shared with her so far. Heather had told her mother that she went to the clinic because her period was late and that a pregnancy test was negative. The mother is worried that Heather really is pregnant, that she may not have told her the truth. The mother knows that Heather has been sexually active in the past, but Heather told her that she was not involved with anyone now. The mother is not so sure given the late period. The clinician relates that she can understand the mother's concern and explains that although she would like to, she cannot discuss with her any matters that fall under the state's minor consent law, such as testing for pregnancy, until Heather gives her permission to do so. The clinician explains that these laws were created so that teens would feel comfortable seeking out care and counseling about pregnancy, STIs and drug use from trained professionals. The alternative is that many teens would otherwise rely on advice from friends or receive no care at all. So whether a test was done or not or whether it was positive or negative could not be shared at this point. The clinician quickly adds that this confidentiality ends if a teen is at risk of seriously harming herself or someone else or if she discloses a history of abuse. Although frustrated, the mother understands. The clinician says that she will talk with Heather at the follow-up visit to see whether Heather will give permission to allow her to discuss these matters with her mother. She suggests that Heather and her mother come to the clinic together so that they can discuss these issues further in person. The clinician ends on a positive note by sharing her observation that Heather and her mother must have a close and caring relationship as demonstrated by their openness to talk to each other about sexual matters.

Parents must realize that to be of most benefit to a teenager, they must remain a constant and consistent figure, willing to be a sounding board for the youngster's ideas without overtaking and dominating the teen. Mid-adolescents must learn to think through problems to evolve solutions, and parents are a valuable resource to assist in that task. Supportive parental communication, supervision and availability seem to be protective factors toward the development of a healthy and successful adolescent. In fact, recent surveys of adolescents indicate that most teens trust their parents more than other individuals in their lives and want more open, honest conversations with their parents about topics such as sexuality.

DATA GATHERING

Some Guiding Principles

At a minimum, a mid-adolescent should be seen on an annual basis for health maintenance. Table 23–2 outlines components to be included in the annual history and physical examination. The following are additional principles to keep in mind:

- As part of the annual adolescent health visit, it is essential to take a sexual history from every teen patient. Before asking questions about sexual activity, it may be helpful to inquire about sexual development, such as menstruation or testicular changes. These questions can lead to more sensitive areas, such as sexual activity, contraceptive use and symptoms of STIs.

TABLE 23–2   Components of the Mid-Adolescent Health Maintenance Visit

What to Observe	Objective
See Table 22–3 and add the following: Who made the appointment? Does the teen come to the appointment alone? If not, does the parent/guardian accompany the teen to the examination room?	See Table 22–3 and add the following: To assess the teen's level of independence; to determine the nature of the relationship and interactions between the mid-adolescent and the parent/guardian; and to gain insight into the behavior and attitude of the adolescent during the visit
Dress and clothing style of the teen	To understand how the teen sees himself at the present time

What to Ask (HEADSS Format)	Objective
Home: See Table 22–3 and add the following: Ask about the adolescent's function in the family—Are you involved in many activities with your family? Do you accompany the family on many outings? What are your responsibilities around the house? Most adolescents have curfews, do you? Do you feel that your parents are fair in their treatment of you concerning dating and outside events? Most adolescents and their parents disagree on certain issues. What issues do you and your parents disagree on? What do you do if you disagree with your father or mother on a certain issue?	To determine relationships within the family and the degree of parental supervision/limit setting
Education/Employment: See Table 22–3 and add: Have you recently changed schools? How are your grades? Have they dropped from last year? Are you working? Where do you work? How many hours per week? Do you have plans or goals for the future?	To assess the teen's functioning within the school and work environment and progress toward formulating plans for the future
Activities: See Table 22–3	See Table 22–3
Drugs: See Table 22–3	See Table 22–3
Sex/Sexuality: See Table 22–3 and add these additional questions for a sexually experienced teen: How old were you when you first had sexual intercourse? With how many partners have you had sexual intercourse? Were they	To assess the teen's level of sexual risk and need for STI testing, PAP smear screening, pregnancy testing and health education on birth control, STIs and safe sex practices; to screen for sexual assault/abuse; to understand the degree to which the adolescent is sharing this information

Continued

TABLE 23–2 **Components of the Mid-Adolescent Health Maintenance Visit—cont'd**

What to Observe	Objective
boys, girls or both? Have you ever been tested for sexually transmitted infections such as chlamydia, gonorrhea or HIV? Have you ever had an infection from sex? Do you do anything to protect yourself from sexual infections? Have you ever used a condom? How often? Have you (or your partner) ever used any other birth control, such as birth control pills or the patch? Have you ever been pregnant (or have you ever gotten someone pregnant)? What happened with that pregnancy? Have you ever felt forced to have sex? Have you ever been raped? Does your parent/guardian know that you are having sex?	with a parent or guardian
Suicide/Depression: See Table 22–3 and add: Ask about the adolescent's feelings about himself—Most young people your age have experienced a lot of changes in their bodies. Are you satisfied with the way your body has turned out? Is there anything about yourself you wish you could change?	To screen for mental health issues such as depression, concerns over appearance, suicidal ideation and abuse; to determine adolescent's comfort with himself
Physical Assessment	**Objective**
See Table 22–3	See Table 22–3
Immunizations	**Objective**
See Table 22–3	See Table 22–3
Screening Tests	**Objective**
See Table 22–3	See Table 22–3
Anticipatory Guidance And Health Education	**Objective**
See further discussion in text	To prepare the teen and parent for what lies ahead and to give information with which the teen/parent can use to change behavior and reduce risk

HEADSS, home, education/employment, activities, drugs, sexuality and suicide/depression; HIV, human immunodeficiency virus; PAP, Papanicolaou; STI, sexually transmitted infection.

- Adolescents should be asked questions about sexuality, abuse/assault, suicidal thoughts and substance use in private, not in the presence of parents. All adolescents should be assured of confidentiality on matters covered by that state's minor consent law. Clinicians must be aware of their state laws governing informed consent and treatment of minors (see Chapter 22 for further discussion on confidentiality and minor consent laws).

- Teens, like adults, appreciate a clinical environment that is nonjudgmental, supportive and responsive to their concerns. If a teen patient has specific health concerns, these issues must be addressed. If the issues presented are too numerous or complex to resolve at one visit, determine with the teen which issues are most pressing to address at that time. Acknowledge to the teen that his other concerns are also important but will require a follow-up visit to more thoroughly address them. Teens can sense when their concerns are not taken seriously or when the clinician has an agenda that is not congruent with the teen's own interests or reasons for coming to the clinic.

- When interviewing a teen, it is helpful to periodically and verbally paraphrase the teen's concerns and summarize the key points addressed up to that point. In this way, the clinician can be sure that he is understanding what the teen is trying to convey, the teen can be reassured that the clinician is listening and the clinician can reinforce with the teen all the key points discussed. Teens appreciate a health care provider who actively attends to them with frequent eye contact, verbal cues and body language that signal the clinician is listening and interested in what they are saying. At the end of the visit, the clinician should review the plan and ask if there are any further questions. Teens who initially may be hesitant to share certain information with their health care provider may divulge their most pressing concerns at the very end of the visit if given a chance to do so.

! HEADS UP—15 TO 17 YEARS

Teenager with Multiple Sexual Partners

Although many mid-adolescents are sexually active, this activity is usually confined to one partner at a time, so-called serial monogamy, and is an expression of affection. Adolescents who have multiple partners at the same time are outside normal behavior. **Promiscuity** may be a sign of difficulties in the adolescent's life and may be the means by which an adolescent signals that he or she is having difficulties. For example, an adolescent girl with very poor self-esteem and self-image may seek many sexual partners to affirm that she is worthwhile, or a young woman who is not getting along well at home may deliberately flaunt her newfound sexual prowess in an effort to antagonize her parents.

Sex may be used for nonromantic reasons, including rebellion, self-destruction, hostility, acceptance or out of a need for comfort and love. Homeless youth or teens in desperate situations such as gang involvement or severe poverty may depend on sex for their own survival, so-called survival sex, in which they may have sex in exchange for drugs, money or gang initiation. Any mid-adolescent, male or female, who has multiple sexual partners concurrently or within a short period deserves a thorough

HEADS UP—15 TO 17 YEARS—cont'd

psychosocial history to explore the family dynamics, the teen's financial situation and risk factors for depression, suicide or drug abuse. In addition, promiscuous teens should be asked about their past history of sexual or physical abuse.

Adolescent Who Is a Loner

Adolescents should have several close friends and engage in multiple social activities. Those who do not belong to a peer group are defined as loners and are worrisome. Adolescents who are loners may be depressed and at risk for suicide; they may be involved in truancy and drugs; or they may be in the early stages of psychosis, such as schizophrenia, which may begin to manifest in mid-to late adolescence.

Depression and Suicide

A significant proportion of adolescents will meet the criteria for **depression** at some point during high school. In the most recent Youth Risk Surveillance Survey, about 29% of students in high school reported experiencing symptoms consistent with depression in the 12 months preceding the survey. The survey also showed that 17% of high school students had seriously considered **suicide** and 8.5% had actually attempted suicide at least once in the past 12 months. These statistics show that many young people grapple with feelings of sadness and despair.

It can be very difficult in the clinical setting to determine whether an adolescent with suicidal ideation is a harm to himself. Many teens think about it but have no intentions to actually commit suicide. Most of these teens can be evaluated for depression and referred if needed to a mental health specialist. Several self-reported inventory screening tools have been developed for depression and can be used with adolescents. These tools include the Beck Depression Inventory II (BDI-II), the Center for Epidemiologic Studies Depression (CES-D) Scale, the Children's Depression Inventory (CDI) for children 7 to 17 years and Reynold's Adolescent Depression Scale. Caution must be used when interpreting the results of self-reported inventories; a positive screen does not necessarily mean a diagnosis of depression but indicates a need for further assessment and possible referral to a mental health provider.

If, however, a teen says that he is intent on killing himself or can't guarantee that he won't kill himself, a parent or guardian must be informed, and he must be evaluated emergently by a mental health professional for possible admission. Teens who have a plan for suicide and the means to make it happen must be taken seriously. Teens with past suicide attempts, severe depression and/or a destabilizing environment should be monitored very carefully for the development of suicidal intentions. Any adolescent who is depressed should be urged to obtain mental health counseling and evaluation, and the clinician should help the adolescent and parent in obtaining these services.

Decline in School Performance

Deterioration of an adolescent's grades should not be viewed lightly; it may be the result of one of the following:

Continued

HEADS UP—15 TO 17 YEARS—cont'd

- Learning disability
- Inappropriate school, grade or class setting
- Drug use or abuse
- Mental health disorder such as depression, anxiety, post-traumatic stress disorder, psychosis
- Attention deficit disorder
- Family dysfunction or crisis
- Work commitment/excessive work hours
- Family commitment (such as caring for a younger sibling, sick or dying relative)
- Excessive stress or pressure
- School absences because of a health problem or truancy
- Child abuse

Rapidly declining grades in high school may be the first clue to an emotional disturbance because neurobehavioral disorders characterized by disturbances in thoughts or emotions may be first identified by a marked change in school performance. These maladaptive thought processes may interfere with cognitive function to such an extent that a young person is unable to sustain his usual grades.

Immigrant Youth and Acculturation Issues

With the growing immigrant population in the United States, it is becoming increasingly commonplace for clinicians caring for youth to see adolescents who have recently immigrated. Many of these adolescents face acculturation issues in addition to the normal developmental issues of their age. They are at increased risks for psychosocial problems such as depression, anxiety, school failure, involvement with gangs and drug use. They may also bring with them issues that preceded or may have motivated their immigration, such as poverty, medical problems and mental health issues, including post-traumatic stress disorder.

On immigrating, they leave behind friends and a familiar culture, language, environment and, for some, parents or other family members who could not make the journey with them. Now in their new country, they are forced to adapt to their new surroundings, which may include learning a new language, making new friends, adjusting to a different school system and navigating a new set of cultural norms. Some immigrant youth must also work to help support the family and may not be able to attend school. Overall, most immigrant youth adapt more quickly to their new surroundings than their parents. Their adaptation can spark parent-child conflict above and beyond the expected parent-teen disagreements typical of this developmental stage. In response, immigrant parents may become excessively restrictive and protective, especially of their daughters, or some may become emotionally detached from their acculturated adolescent.

Clinicians need to be culturally sensitive and aware of the challenges facing immigrant youth and their families. It is critical to perform a thorough risk assessment for psychosocial problems. Whenever possible, appropriate translator services should be

HEADS UP–15 TO 17 YEARS–cont'd

available that are confidential and professional. Telephone language lines are now readily available and give clinicians quick access to interpreters. In addition, clinicians must be resourceful in providing needed care to immigrant youth because they are frequently uninsured or have very limited access to medical and mental health care services.

Serious Delinquent Behavior

Adolescents who are in trouble with the law need careful evaluation. Although many adolescents are arrested each year, most offenses are minor and are not repeated. Minor offenses (e.g., shoplifting) by young adolescents may not signify a major psychosocial problem and may reflect the young adolescent's struggle with independence and peer group approval. Nonetheless, this behavior should not be ignored. Young people who commit major crimes against people or property or commit minor crimes repeatedly may be having severe difficulties, including sociopathic tendencies or gang affiliations.

Out-of-Home Youth

Out-of-home youth refers to adolescents who are in foster care, runaway, homeless or incarcerated. They are at higher risks for health and psychosocial problems than the general adolescent population. Many of these problems existed before they were out of the home. Although their problems will vary, these teens are more likely to have chronic medical problems, including mental illness; a history of being abused or neglected; school problems, including learning disabilities, truancy and higher drop-out rates; and higher rates of emergency room use, substance abuse, unsafe sex and pregnancy. When an out-of-home teen seeks medical care, the health care provider will probably have to set aside additional time to deal with all the issues presented. The clinician may not have the luxury of follow-up visits for these teens, and referrals to specialists may not be kept. The clinician must therefore attempt to cover all the most pertinent problems and treat any suspected illness before the teen leaves the clinic. This can be quite a challenge!

Min has been living in the United States for 2 years since moving from Korea with her father and younger brother. Her mother died 5 years ago. She self-reports depression since her mother's death. It has become worse since moving here to the point where she shuns her family, instead preferring to stay alone in her room. She is overweight and binges. She is unhappy with her body and eating habits, but does not feel like she has any control over it. To make matters worse, her father is not permitting her to talk on the telephone to her "boyfriend" since he discovered their "relationship." She met her friend at the public library; they traded phone numbers and had been communicating ever since then, but only by telephone. He is the same age and also from Korea. Min does not understand why her father is forbidding her from talking to him. The physician and mental health provider at her school are able to help Min with her depression and eating disorder and assist in the relationship issues between Min and her father.

Mohammed left his country in Africa years ago. His father had been violently killed there, and he emigrated to the United States with his mother and sisters. Mohammed has been going to school and working every day. His mother has a health condition and he feels responsible for supporting the family. He is being seen for palpitations and shortness of breath, is experiencing difficulty sleeping and has frequent nightmares. He is diagnosed as having anxiety and post-traumatic stress disorder. Mohammed agrees to counseling, and his provider is able to refer his mother to a free medical care clinic in the area for women without health care.

Katrina has recently run away from home and is now living with various friends and relatives. She is seeking medical attention today because of painful lumps in her genital area. The clinician seeing Katrina has never met her before but can tell from her unkempt and tired appearance that issues besides medical concerns should be addressed. During the history, Katrina reveals that she has had many sexual partners and wonders if she has an infection; the clinician wonders if she has been prostituting. In the course of the examination, it is clear that Katrina has enlarged, tender inguinal lymph nodes and a purulent vaginal discharge. Cervical testing for gonorrhea and chlamydia is performed, and blood is drawn for syphilis and HIV testing. A urine pregnancy test is negative.

The clinician is concerned that Katrina has cervicitis and syphilis. Rather than wait for test results, the physician gives Katrina medication to complete treatment for gonorrhea, chlamydia and syphilis before she leaves the office. She also receives the first vaccination for hepatitis B and free condoms. Katrina is urged to return to the clinic in 1 week for results and contraceptive counseling. She refuses all offers for psychosocial counseling. On the way out the door, she remembers that she is out of her asthma medicine and is given an inhaler.

The clinician calls child protective services (CPS) to see whether a case has been opened on Katrina. No name matches her name, and the address and phone number that Katrina has given are false. Katrina does not show up for her follow-up appointment. She is positive for gonorrhea and syphilis, and the health department is notified. Her HIV test is negative.

Note: This clinician was very astute to treat Katrina with antibiotics before laboratory confirmation of the suspected infections. Likewise, she may have benefited from the clinician calling CPS before her departure from the clinic. CPS may have been helpful in connecting her to support services or may have recommended that CPS or the police pick up the child directly from the clinic. However, in many cases, the clinician is not equipped or able to prevent a patient from leaving before CPS evaluation. Although Katrina did not return for her follow-up appointment, it would not be unusual for her to return at a later date if she felt that the clinician had cared about her. Although frustrating for the clinician, this case vignette exemplifies some of the challenges of caring for high-risk youth.

ANTICIPATORY GUIDANCE FOR THE MID-ADOLESCENT

Issues Relating to Sexual Activity

Sexual Intercourse. It is not unusual for adolescents to have questions about sexual intercourse, although they may be embarrassed to ask about it and may not know what terminology to use. Young people who are unskilled in lovemaking do not know whether their experiences are normal. They may simply need information about anatomy or physiology, or they may actually require counseling concerning sexual dysfunction. To discuss sexual intercourse with adolescents, the clinician must be comfortable and knowledgeable about the topic of sex and with his/her own sexuality. If this isn't the case, the clinician must be aware of referral resources in the community.

Kimberly's chief complaint at her clinic appointment is pain with sex. She has one sexual partner who is also a mid-adolescent. By report, neither of them have had any other sexual partners. They have been together for 6 months and have used condoms consistently. There is no history of sexual abuse or assault. She denies any type of sexual activity that is "rough" or coerced. Both sets of parents are aware of their sexual activity. The pelvic examination is normal and STI testing is performed. On further questioning, it becomes apparent that she and her partner are not adequately lubricated when they have sex and that this is the most likely cause of the pain. The nurse practitioner recommends a lubricating liquid. Kimberly is embarrassed, but relieved that nothing is wrong with her. The practitioner spends several more minutes with Kimberly to make sure that Kimberly wants to be in this sexual relationship and reminds her that she always has the option of saying "no" to sex. At the follow-up visit, Kimberly reports that the lubricating liquid is working—no more pain. Her STI tests are all negative.

Sexually Transmitted Infections. Adolescents need information about the most common STIs, the disease processes associated with them and ways to reduce risk. Because the quantity of information is so large, STI education should occur in a classroom setting such as at school with reinforcement or review in the clinical setting. Many teens, however, may not receive comprehensive sex education, so it is often up to the clinician to inform teen patients about STIs. Perhaps one of the most important facts to relay to teens is that many people with STIs have no signs or symptoms of infection. In this way, teens will appreciate the need for consistent condom use and periodic STI screening. STI educators, whether a clinician or teacher, must be careful of what they say to the teen. For example, it is more productive to stress the risk of ectopic pregnancy rather than infertility as a result of gonorrhea or chlamydia. Otherwise, some teens may erroneously conclude that if they have ever had an STI, they don't need to use contraception because they are infertile and unlikely to get pregnant.

Although abstinence is the best method to avoid an STI, adolescents who are sexually active and attempting to reduce risk should be commended for any risk-reducing behavior. All sexually active male and female adolescents should be encouraged to receive at a minimum annual screening for gonorrhea and chlamydia and should be offered HIV testing. It is helpful to have pamphlets on STIs and condoms readily available for adolescents to take home and read. However, these do not substitute for the clinician's direct discussion and invitation for questions on STIs and how to reduce risk.

Contraception. Terms such as *birth control* and *contraception* have different connotations for different adolescents. To some it simply means the birth control pill rather than all the various options available, including condoms. A contraceptive kit containing the various forms of contraception can be extremely useful in discussions with teenage girls and boys. In addition, it is very helpful to show adolescents, both males and females, how to properly use a condom. The more confident they are at putting condoms on, the more likely that they will use them. They can practice putting a condom on by placing it over a plastic model or over their own fingers. The clinician should clearly present the pros and cons of each contraceptive method, including the positive health benefits, while attempting to dispel any contraceptive myths that the teen may have. Verbal information should be backed up with informational pamphlets.

When an adolescent girl requests birth control, it may signify that she has already been sexually active for many months. Any inquiry should be met with a positive response. After a discussion with the clinician about the available methods and their associated risks and benefits, some teenagers know immediately what they want to use and should be started as soon as possible. Some teens are more indecisive and may need to talk it over with a parent, boyfriend or girlfriend. If the teen allows, it is helpful to involve the parent to improve compliance and follow-up.

Regardless of the contraceptive method chosen, adolescent boys and girls should know about emergency hormonal contraception so that they can use this option as a backup for contraceptive failure or sexual assault. It is always inappropriate to push a teenager into accepting one form of contraception over another or to demand that a teenager use contraception or become abstinent; the decision must be her own or she will not adhere to it. Although abstinence should be highly recommended, abstinence-*only* education has not been shown to be effective in reducing rates of teen pregnancy or STIs. It is important to teach teens about contraceptive options, as well as the option to say "no" to sex. The discussion of birth control should be seen in the broader context of individual decision making, taking responsibility for one's actions and planning for the future. These developmental skills have obvious applications in many areas.

Teenage Pregnancy. The clinician may meet an adolescent patient for the first time at an office visit for a pregnancy test. The physician should be prepared to make the diagnosis of pregnancy and to discuss the adolescent's options with her face to face. Ideally, pregnancy test results should not be given over the telephone. Once a teen is told that she is pregnant, she may be so upset that she is incapable of rationally thinking through what she would like to do about the pregnancy. It is therefore helpful to sit down with the adolescent before obtaining the test result to think through a possible pregnancy scenario with her:

- Does she want to be pregnant?
- Will she be disappointed if the test comes back negative?
- Would she keep the baby?
- How does she feel about abortion? What about adoption?
- What would her partner want her to do?
- What would her parent or parents say? Will she be able to tell them if she is pregnant?
- If she wants to keep the baby, who would help her take care of the baby, and who would financially support her? Would she be able to go back to school?
- If she is not pregnant, does she want to start or change a birth control method?

If she is pregnant, all options should be presented to her and she should be encouraged to make her own decision. How to handle the pregnancy is always the *adolescent's* decision, not the physician's. She should be encouraged to discuss the pregnancy with her parents, and this can be done with the help of the clinician, who may play an important mediator role in this setting. The teenager should also be encouraged to involve the father of the baby in the decision process, to explore his wishes and capacity for emotional or financial support. A pregnant teen will need a follow-up visit in 1 to 2 weeks to ensure that she is formulating a plan and making steps toward her decision. It is important to transition pregnant teens to prenatal care as soon as possible or, if they desire an abortion, to ensure that the teen does not delay to the point that she requires a more complex procedure or is ineligible for the termination.

Other Health Issues

The Annual Gynecological Examination. It is critical for the clinician to inquire about the age of first sexual intercourse so that adolescent girls can be told when they will be due for their first Pap smear. The American College of Obstetricians and Gynecologists recommends that healthy young women receive their first Pap smear approximately 3 years after first sexual intercourse or no later than the age of 21, whichever occurs first. It is also important to educate adolescent girls about the difference between a Pap smear and a pelvic examination because most of them think they are one and the same. Even though a teen may not need a Pap smear until several years after coitarche, she may need a pelvic examination before then to be fully evaluated for STIs.

The first pelvic examination can be anxiety provoking, even for a sexually experienced teen. Every woman should be educated about the pelvic examination and female genital anatomy before the examination, and if a Pap smear is required, its purpose should be explained in simple language, not to scare a teenager but to educate her about her body and to encourage her to take responsibility for it.

Breast and Testicular Self-Examinations. Most mid-adolescent girls have reached Tanner stage IV breast development and are ready to be taught to perform a breast self-examination. Even though breast cancer is uncommon in teenage girls, this practice instills good health habits at an early age and supports the process of being comfortable with one's own body.

Although testicular cancer is rare, it is the most common cancer in young men between the ages of 15 and 35. The American Cancer Society estimates that approximately 7600 new cases of testicular cancer will be diagnosed each year in the United States and that 400 men can be expected to die each year as a result. Hence, boys should be taught how to perform a testicular self-examination and instructed that if they find lumps or bumps on the testis or in the scrotal sac, they should have an immediate checkup by a physician. This discussion itself acknowledges and verifies a new attitude toward the genitalia.

Nutrition and Exercise. During adolescence, it is important to develop healthy habits, such as eating right and staying fit. Many teens have concerns about their diet, weight and level of exercise as they are faced with the dichotomy of society's overwhelming emphasis on appearance and thinness juxtaposed to escalating **obesity** rates and a fast-food culture. The health care provider can assist adolescents in making sense of these often mixed messages that they receive.

Teens rarely have the knowledge of how to meet their nutritional needs and typically require some guidance on how to improve their nutritional intake. Some mid-adolescents may choose their diet as a mechanism to gain control and independence from their parents. In some cases, these dietary maneuvers to gain control will result in eating disorders, but more often they are short lived and less serious. For example, some teens will opt to become vegetarians or will place themselves intermittently on controversial diets despite the protests of their parents. It is important to identify teens who are actively dieting, skipping meals, restricting certain foods, purging, using medications to lose weight or exercising excessively. It is equally important to identify teens who are eating excess amounts of fast foods or fried foods, binging or not engaging in any form of physical activity. Clinicians should ask the adolescent patient about his/her dietary practices and must ascertain whether the teen has body image or weight concerns. It may be helpful to ask the following:

- Does the teen like the way her/his body looks?
- Is there anything the teen would like to change about herself/himself?
- Does he/she want to gain or lose weight?
- Would the teen like to weigh a particular amount?
- Has the teen ever tried to lose weight (or gain weight)? If so, how?
- How often and how long does the teen exercise?

Clinicians should share their concerns with the teen who has a weight, diet or exercise problem, and together an individual wellness plan can be developed. It is usually helpful to involve parents in this discussion so that their assistance can be given in menu preparation, shopping or planning an exercise program. Parents often share similar problems and may benefit from the discussion.

Overall, adolescent patients need reassurance about their bodies, especially those who are not overweight but think that they are fat. Even teens who are doing well may have questions about their dietary intake and may appreciate information on how to follow a healthy, realistic and sustainable diet that meets their nutritional needs and tastes. Recommending multiple changes to the teen's lifestyle and diet at one time is usually a sure recipe for disaster; teens are more successful if asked to address no more than three changes at a time. Families should be encouraged to eat together as often as possible for nutritional reasons, as well as for benefits to family communication and cohesion. The practitioner may want to remind parents that they are their children's role models in lifestyle choices, such as how they eat and exercise and in how positively or negatively they view their own bodies. Teens benefit from parents who boost their self-esteem and who serve as moderators to society's often one-sided message to be satisfied with nothing less than perfection.

Athletics. Many teens participate in organized **sports**. Most adolescent athletes can successfully combine sports, schoolwork and a social life and reap benefits in health and morale from the experience. For a few adolescent athletes, they may push themselves or be driven by coaches and parents to perform beyond their own limits or to the exclusion of other activities. These teens may not realize to what extent their sports involvement has become all-consuming. They may need someone to provide this perspective. Frequent injuries, stress fractures and chronic pain may be signs of overuse injuries and a signal to the clinician that the teen needs to cut back. Amenorrhea or extreme dietary measures to gain or lose weight for a sport is a red flag that the teen may be jeopardizing his/her own health.

Some adolescents may try performance-enhancing substances in attempts to improve athletic performance. Teens most frequently use protein, mineral and carbohydrate supplements available in health and nutrition stores. Although usually benign, these dietary supplements (e.g., creatine) can increase the risk for dehydration and heat-related illnesses. Teens, parents and coaches need to understand the potential risks associated with the use of certain ergogenic aids, most notably the anabolic steroids (e.g., androstenedione, dehydroepiandrosterone), stimulants (e.g., caffeine, ephedra and methamphetamine) and blood-doping agents (e.g., erythropoietin). For teens who do try these substances, it is usually for a brief period. In 2003, the annual prevalence rates for steroid use was 3.2% for all 12th-grade boys and 1.1% for all 12th-grade girls.

Given that most, if not all teens require clearance by a clinician before participating in an organized sport, the preparticipation physical evaluation is a perfect opportunity to review the importance of proper nutrition, hydration and stretching, as well as to ask about the use of ergogenic aids, tobacco, alcohol and other drugs. Most adolescent athletes welcome a discussion on these topics. The sports physical may be one of the only times that a male adolescent seeks medical attention, so the clinician may want to take advantage of this visit to perform a thorough risk assessment and educate the male teen on testicular self-examination and other pertinent health topics. Some clinicians will also take the opportunity during the sports physical to offer urine STI screening to athletes who are sexually active.

Drugs, Alcohol and Tobacco. Even though many adolescents use drugs and alcohol, they may be reluctant to admit using substances if an authority figure asks them directly. It is often productive to ask first about peer group use of substances rather than about the individual teen's use and then to provide factual information on the possible effects of these substances on health. Similar to taking a sexual history, the rules of confidentiality should be reviewed with teen patients, and they should be interviewed alone to obtain the most accurate history on their drug and alcohol habits.

"Tom, I know that some teens your age are using drugs. What about in your school or in your neighborhood—what are the drugs that are being used? Are your friends using drugs or drinking on a regular basis? Has anyone ever offered you drugs or alcohol? What about at home—are you concerned about someone in your family who is using drugs or alcohol or is smoking?"

When adolescents do admit using alcohol or other drugs, it is appropriate to ask where and when they are using, with whom, how often and how much. For example, have they ever been "stoned" at school? Do they ever use alone? If they are using, how many times per week? An experienced clinician will usually double or quadruple the figure given by the adolescent. Many teens don't appreciate that even if infrequent, ingestion of large quantities of drugs or alcohol can be toxic.

For teens who choose not to use, positive reinforcement is a must. Compliment the teen on his decision to abstain from the use of cigarettes, alcohol or other drugs. "That's great! I realize that it may be difficult at times to not smoke, drink or use drugs, especially if others around you are. You are definitely doing the best thing for yourself and your health by avoiding their use." Leave the door open for future discussions if the need arises. "I'll be here if you ever do need to talk to someone about drugs, tobacco or alcohol or if you are worried about someone you know who is using them."

Teenage Driver. It is unclear whether a discussion on automobile safety between an adolescent patient and health care provider is helpful in preventing motor vehicle accidents. Most adolescents, however, will give at least transient thought to the clinician's observation that more teenagers die as a result of accidents than from any other cause. The clinician should encourage the adolescent to not drive while under the influence of alcohol or other drugs and to not ride in a car driven by someone who is intoxicated. Parents and teens may want to discuss the availability of a nonjudgmental, safe adult from whom the teen may request a ride home if she finds herself in an unsafe situation. Teens should be reminded to always wear a seat belt and to use a helmet if on a bicycle or motorcycle. In states with no graduated licensing system, the clinician may want to review with the parent and teen that it may take some time for the teen to develop mastery over the skills required to drive safely; during this period, it is in the best interest of the teen to drive while supervised by an adult, during daylight hours and without distractions such as loud music, friends or younger siblings in the car.

ANTICIPATORY GUIDANCE FOR PARENTS

Limit Setting versus Power Struggle

It is not unusual for mid-teens to "test" all authority figures, including parents, but this doesn't mean that they do not need or want rules or regulations. Indeed, most mid-adolescents appreciate reasonable limit setting by parents as evidence of parental concern and as safe, boundaries in which to function. However, there is a difference between limit setting and power struggles. Limit setting refers to rules and regulations concerning behavior; power struggles occur when authority itself is at stake, regardless of the issue being discussed. Limit setting is necessary; power struggles should be avoided because someone always loses and that person is inevitably resentful and bitter. One example of limit setting is the curfew. Teens and their parents should decide together on a reasonable curfew; the parent and teen should discuss in advance the consequences that will follow if the curfew is broken. In contrast, a power struggle may involve an argument over one person being "right" and the other person being "wrong." Usually, the subject matter is unimportant; being "right" or winning is all that counts. Because limit setting consists of rules, they may need to be modified as the adolescent matures or the situation changes. Adolescents and parents should be encouraged to communicate as these changing needs arise.

Cross-Gender Parent Attachments

As adolescents cope with sexual issues, it is common for them to experience renewed attraction for the opposite-gender parent. This is the reemergence of the "Oedipal complex" (see Chapter 18). In healthy families, this attraction may be used to bolster the adolescent's self-esteem and provide reassurance to the young person that he is developing into an attractive, normal adult. In most families, this phenomenon is expressed as normal parental-filial affection and pride. In other families, the cross-gender parent attachment is a threatening experience or a source of conflict or pain. In such instances, the conflict is almost always the result of a parental problem. Some parents become frightened by their child's attentions, particularly because it occurs at a time when the youngster is sexually blossoming. A parent may become aloof and distant from a youngster, who in turn finds such action confusing. For example, a father may tell his daughter that she's "too big to be hugged anymore," even though he continues to hug the younger children. Another father may inappropriately respond to his daughter's attentions by taking sexual liberties in the form of incest. It is normal for parents to find their adolescent children attractive. In fact, the son or daughter usually resembles a parent at a younger age or looks like the spouse looked when the parents married. Given this similarity, it is not unusual that the teenage youngster is also seen as attractive. It is *not* normal to act on that attractiveness or to take advantage of the teen's stage of development for personal sexual gratification. All cases of suspected incest should be referred to the appropriate authorities for investigation.

Vicarious Satisfaction in Adolescent Activities

Sometimes the parents of adolescents unconsciously encourage adolescents to misbehave so that the teenager will act out the parent's own fantasies. For example, a mother may warn a daughter to remain a virgin until marriage, yet buy her revealing or provocative clothing. If so, this area should be explored and brought to the parent's attention.

Alyssa was being seen for a follow-up appointment 1 month after receiving a therapeutic abortion. Her mother had insisted that she receive the abortion; Alyssa still had mixed feelings about it. Ms. Right, her nurse practitioner, couldn't help noticing the vivid red velour warm-up jacket and matching pants that Alyssa was wearing. The word "SEXY" was written in large cursive letters across the chest and buttocks of the clothes. Ms. Right commented on her outfit and Alyssa responded that her mother had just bought her the warm-up suit yesterday. Realizing that Alyssa had just come from school, Ms. Right asked her if anyone had said anything to her about her outfit at school today. Alyssa said that she did notice some of the guys staring at her and one of them had slapped her on the bottom when she was walking to class. Ms. Right asked Alyssa how she felt about the reaction she received and what message her clothes may be sending. Alyssa responded that she was not sure. She felt kind of uncomfortable with the attention, but her mother said that she looked so cute in it. Together they came to the conclusion that it would be best to not wear the outfit to school. Ms. Right was able to speak with the mother privately and conveyed her concerns that this type of clothing could be seen as an invitation to boys even when Alyssa did not want the attention. Ms. Right informed the mother that given Alyssa's recent abortion, buying her this type of provocative clothing was sending Alyssa mixed messages. Ms. Right had worried that the mother would not take too kindly to her comments, but to her surprise the mother was very receptive and had not realized that she may have inadvertently been encouraging Alyssa to act out sexually.

Effective Parenting of the Adolescent

It is not easy to be a parent, and the mid-adolescent years may be the most difficult for some parents. They should be prepared for the commonly experienced conflicts involved in raising adolescents. For example, for the first time, parents may face unresolved issues from the adolescent's childhood and unresolved issues from their own adolescence, and they may find their authority as parents repeatedly challenged. Parents should be reassured that the best approach to their teenagers (and to themselves) is to keep the lines of communication open. Parental connectedness—that is, the adolescent's perception of warmth, love and caring from parents—and parental availability to the adolescent are keys to the successful development and health of every adolescent. In most families, parents find themselves growing in wisdom as they struggle with the issues that teenage children force them to face.

RECOMMENDED READINGS FOR CLINICIANS

Dietz WH: Health consequences of obesity in youth: Childhood predictors of adult disease. *Pediatrics* 101:518S, 1998.

Elkind D: Egocentrism in adolescence. *Child Dev* 38:1025, 1967.

Frankowski BL, American Academy of Pediatrics Committee on Adolescence: Sexual orientation and adolescents. *Pediatrics* 113:1827, 2004.

Knight JR: Adolescent substance use: Screening, assessment, and intervention. *Contemp Pediatr* 14(4):45, 1997.

Resnick MD, Bearman PS, Blum RW, et al: Protecting adolescents from harm. Findings from the National Longitudinal Study on Adolescent Health. *JAMA* 278:823, 1997.

Santelli JS, Abma J, Ventura S, et al: Can changes in sexual behaviors among high school students explain the decline in teen pregnancy rates in the 1990s? *J Adolesc Health* 35(2):80, 2004.

Stashwick C: When you suspect an eating disorder. *Contemp Pediatr* 13(11):124, 1996.

Troiden R: Homosexual identity development. *J Adolesc Health Care* 9:105, 1988.

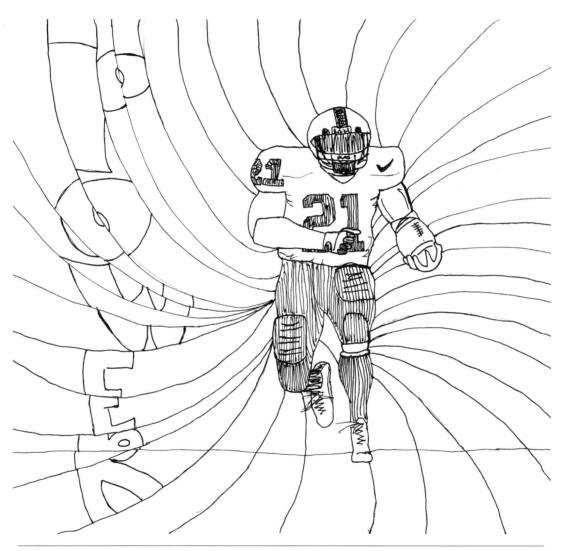

The masculine hero, muscles bulging, is shown in this football player. By Nasir Austin, age 15.

CHAPTER 24

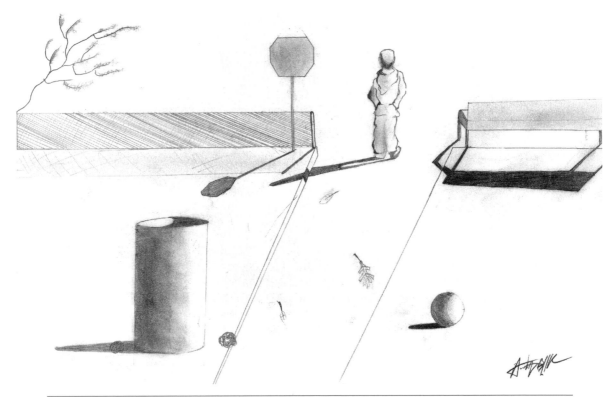

"Still Life." A young person is shown at a boundary, a transition. The landscape looks a bit bleak and scary. By Andre Bullock.

Seventeen to Twenty-one Years: Transition To Adulthood

LAWRENCE S. FRIEDMAN

This chapter will familiarize the reader with some key behavioral and developmental issues of adolescents during their transition to adulthood. Topics include education and vocational transition, intimate interpersonal relationships, and performance of a behavior-focused interview to assess health risk behavior and readiness for independence and to provide anticipatory health guidance.

Key Words
- **Vocation Planning**
- **Critical Life Transitions**
- **Intimate Relationships**
- **Homosexuality**
- **Substance Abuse**
- **HIV/AIDS**

Julie, an 18-year-old high school senior with below-average grades but above-average performance on college entry examinations, has decided to forego application to college and apply for a job selling clothes at a retail store. In spite of pressure from her mother to attend a local community college, Julie wants to be financially independent and live with her boyfriend.

Three years earlier, Julie's parents divorced. She currently lives with her mother and her mother's boyfriend. Gradually, since her parents' divorce, Julie has become moody, has withdrawn from family activities, and has developed a new set of friends who are older and no longer in school. Several months ago her mother discovered a small amount of marijuana and an empty vodka bottle in Julie's bedroom. Julie's father, who now lives in a neighboring town, thinks that his daughter may have a drinking problem, but her mother thinks that she is just behaving like a lot of other teenagers.

Late adolescence is the final stage in transition from childhood to adulthood. The defining issue of this developmental period is realistic awareness of "who I am." The integration of family, peer, educational, social, cultural, and community experiences comes into clearer focus and is grounded in enhanced behavioral, emotional, and cognitive maturity. Many adolescents are now less dependent on peers and are able to develop realistic vocational goals, pursue monogamous interpersonal relationships, and define individual ethical and moral standards. Although the independent "self," defined by vocation, relationships, and values, becomes clearer during late adolescence, realistically these are processes that evolve over a lifetime.

Similarly, by late adolescence, almost all teenagers have accommodated themselves to adult physical stature but continue adjusting to an evolving physical appearance throughout adulthood.

As with earlier stages of adolescence, not all teenagers progress at similar physical or emotional rates. For example, although an 18-year-old boy is physically capable of fathering a child, he may not be emotionally capable of responsible fatherhood. In addition, many factors interfere with normal development. For instance, teenagers who heavily abuse alcohol or other mind-altering substances frequently have delayed emotional, behavioral, and cognitive development. Likewise, the psychopathology of anorexia nervosa, which commonly afflicts girls during mid-adolescence, often involves fear of sexual and emotional maturity and delays transition to adulthood. In general, teenagers given progressive independence and responsibility by supportive family, peers, school, and community are the teens most likely to achieve timely developmental hallmarks. Conversely, individuals who do not appropriately address the issues of early, middle, and late adolescence will probably grapple with these issues into adulthood.

VOCATION PLANNING

As teenagers prepare to enter the adult world, **vocation planning** becomes a preoccupation. Vocational options usually depend on a combination of cognitive ability, educational achievement, financial resources, social environment, and career goals. Superimposed on these factors may be other responsibilities, such as marriage or parenthood. As they enter late adolescence, most teenagers will be in the final stages of completing secondary education. However, some will be attending alternative schools, be school dropouts, or be incarcerated.

Under the best of circumstances, vocational decisions are made after consideration of competing options and when individual abilities and aspirations are satisfied. However, it is common for teenagers to make choices under the considerable influence of friends, family and counselors. Although vocational choices made under such circumstances may work out, they could lead to regret later in life. Delaying a decision for a year or two may in the long run be the best choice.

Julie, who has the intellectual capacity to attend college, has for now decided on other plans. With questions about a drinking problem and perhaps depression, the decision to put off higher education may be correct. With those issues unresolved, the likelihood of Julie failing in college is greater. A timely medical and psychosocial evaluation, possibly followed by intervention and treatment for substance abuse and mental health issues, will give Julie the best opportunity to make the proper decision about what is best for her.

For clinicians, discussion with a patient about future vocational plans may be useful as a catalyst to assess health risk behavior and provide health education and anticipatory guidance. Almost all teenagers will be eager to have such a discussion if it occurs in a nonthreatening, nonjudgmental, and confidential manner. Common transition options are discussed in the following sections, along with vocation-oriented suggestions for health-related discussions.

CRITICAL LIFE TRANSITIONS

Transition to College

Approximately 12 million American teenagers or young adults are currently enrolled in post-secondary school education. Of Americans between the ages of 18 and 24, about half are enrolled in some sort of educational program or have already attended college. Although some believe that college may delay confronting issues of adulthood, the significant variability in post-secondary educational experiences makes generalization difficult. Social and psychological adjustment may be more difficult for those attending college because of parental or social pressure and may predispose to greater degrees of substance abuse and depression. For some teenagers, college may represent the first extended time away from home. In some instances, heavy drinking and drug use, as well as suicidal thought, are related to stress associated with the difficulty of reproducing high school performance in a more competitive college environment. Some teenagers combine postsecondary education with work. This is becoming more common, especially with the growth of organizations that offer degree-granting programs over the Internet.

Transition to Work or Unemployment

Teenagers enter the workforce under a variety of circumstances. Those who have dropped out of school before completing high school generally have greater difficulty entering the workforce and have lower-paying unskilled jobs. A chronic illness or parenthood interrupts the education of a significant number of American teenagers. For some intelligent and capable teenagers, work may be an appropriate choice because on-the-job training may offer sufficient career preparation. Many successful individuals in business, professional sports, entertainment, and the arts never went beyond high school.

Transition to the Military

The military offers structure, discipline, excitement, education, and travel. Traditionally it has been a route of upward mobility for lower socioeconomic populations. The military may be a stepping stone, offering vocational training before entering the workforce, or it may be a long-term career choice.

Transition from Incarceration

A growing number of teenagers spend their adolescence (and often childhood) under social service or juvenile justice authority. In 1997, 368 juveniles were in custody for every 100,000 in the population. Nearly 90% are male and over 60% are members of a minority population. Juvenile delinquency is a complicated subject but is receiving increased study and community awareness. Teenagers who have been in the juvenile system for prolonged periods usually face daunting social, psychological, family, and career obstacles. These obstacles become magnified as teenagers transition from the juvenile to the adult justice system. Because the criminal justice system generally treats minors more leniently than it treats adults, incarcerated adolescents should be made aware that their changing legal status will change their legal consequences. Theoretically, the juvenile justice system places greater emphasis on counseling, rehabilitation and "second chances," whereas the adult system tends to be more punitive. Although the health services provided to incarcerated youth are often superior to those they might receive elsewhere, their health risk behavior is generally greater than that of their peers. Compounding the problem is that many of these teenagers are neglected and disenfranchised and have no health insurance. Most, but not all, are from lower socioeconomic strata. Health problems in this population often include substance abuse, family and interpersonal violence, sexually transmitted disease, poor dentition, and a variety of mental health problems. Transition from incarceration back to society should be guided by the probation system. However, this system is often seriously overburdened, and health issues frequently receive low priority. It should not be assumed that probation officers have the knowledge to anticipate health issues or are aware of health care options. Minors should be informed about the adult legal and incarceration systems.

Transition from Homelessness

The problems of homeless and runaway youth are often similar to those who are incarcerated. A subgroup of homeless youth, but not all, have been incarcerated or involved with legal authorities. Some teenagers are homeless along with their families; some are homeless for short periods and may live with friends or relatives; and others are homeless because they have run away from home and do not plan to return. In the last group, almost all have been victims of physical, severe psychological or sexual abuse. Two thirds to three quarters of all runaways have experienced sexual or physical abuse, with such abuse reported more commonly in girls. The needs of these teenagers may seem daunting but can be managed effectively when they are prioritized. A stable housing situation is most important because it is difficult to address issues of substance abuse or even a medical problem as simple as a respiratory infection if the teenager is constantly uncertain about shelter, food and a place to keep medications.

DEVELOPING INTIMATE INTERPERSONAL RELATIONSHIPS

A well-balanced transition from adolescence to adulthood includes the ability to develop **intimate relationships** with members of both genders. Some of these relationships will be emotional and others will be emotional and sexual. The ability to develop both emotional and sexual interpersonal relationships is inextricably intertwined with the definition of "who I am." By late adolescence, the security found in activities that are group centered gives way to activities that are individual centered. Like other developmental tasks, past collective experience with family, peers, teachers, and community often defines the degree to which intimate relationships develop. Individuals with poor self-esteem, inadequate or inappropriate role models, poor peer group acceptance, depression, or thought disorders may have difficulty developing mature intimate relationships.

Julie has developed an "intimate" relationship with her boyfriend, but her seemingly unresolved issues about her parents' divorce, substance use, and depression put her at risk for unstable interpersonal relationships.

Historical trends redefine interpersonal relationships within a constantly changing cultural context. Over the past half century the nature of marriage and family has changed dramatically in American culture (see Chapter 25). Early in the 20th century, for instance, it was common for American teenagers to marry and begin raising families, often before finishing high school. Those living in rural farming communities were encouraged to have large families to help with household and farm chores. At the same time, out-of-wedlock pregnancy was a personal and family embarrassment and usually resulted in adoption or marriage.

Today, marriage is often delayed because cohabitation is culturally acceptable and both individuals want to continue their education so that each can obtain full-time employment. Concurrently, improvements in family planning and economic necessity have prevented many unwanted pregnancies and have decreased the size of the average American family. Moreover, unmarried teenagers who are pregnant or are parents are no longer ostracized. Although new strategies are constantly being developed to decrease unwanted teenage pregnancy, the status of these adolescents is discussed openly, and they are often accommodated with special schools and parenting programs.

The nature of marriage, as well as the permanency and definition of interpersonal relationships, continues to change. Over half of marriages in the United States currently end in divorce. Many teenagers today are raised in households of divorced parents, and research indicates that they are at risk for repeating this pattern of marital behavior (see Chapter 25). The long-term effects of these changes in social patterns are not clear. However, the next 50 years will probably see continued remodeling of the American family and new roles for religion and other social institutions. Evidence of social change is probably no better demonstrated than in the current dialogue about the characteristics and legitimacy of homosexual relationships, marriage, and families in American society.

GAY AND LESBIAN YOUTH

Only 2 decades ago, **homosexuality** was defined within the context of psychopathology by national mental health and medical organizations. It was rarely a subject of public discussion. Since the 1980s, when the American Psychological Association and psychiatric and other medical societies redefined homosexuality as a normal psychological variant, a greater national dialogue and gradual acceptance of this alternative lifestyle have taken place. The last few years have found major corporations offering health insurance and other benefits to homosexual partners, national figures disclosing their sexual orientation, and a variety of governmental and religious organizations actively debating the legitimacy of homosexual adoption, partner rights, civil union, and marriage.

The etiology of homosexuality is the subject of ongoing research, but it probably involves some blend of environmental and genetic factors. It is estimated that between 5% and 10% of adults identify themselves as exclusively homosexual, and a greater percentage have had periodic homosexual thoughts or experiences. Some studies indicate that up to 20% to 30% of the male population has had at least one same-sex sexual experience, usually sometime during adolescence. These experiences may lead to anxiety, shame, and guilt and do not alone indicate a homosexual orientation. Although homosexual teenagers' acknowledgment of their sexuality is still fraught with the risk of social isolation and physical violence, greater social tolerance in recent years has made many feel more safe about doing so. Like other teenagers, however, homosexual teens become aware of their sexual feelings during early or middle adolescence and often have a variety of sexual experiences before making a definitive lifestyle choice.

Gay and lesbian teenagers can benefit from informed, supportive and nonjudgmental health care providers. Although many positive role models and institutions now exist that can help homosexual youth build self-esteem, in many cases, tremendously negative pressure still comes from family, peer community and society. The social isolation and poor self-esteem many of these teenagers experience may lead to depression, suicide or increased rates of alcohol and drug use. Health care providers should assess the level of self-acceptance in homosexual teens and also assess potential external stressors, such as parents, church, school and peers.

It is important to become aware of peer support groups for teenagers and their families so that referral can be made when appropriate. Most regions have support groups for gay and lesbian youth, and they are usually listed in telephone books or on the Internet or are affiliated with colleges or universities. Parents frequently find support in the local Parents and Friends of Lesbian and Gay Youth (PFLAG), which has a chapter in most urban areas. For social and emotional support, teenagers and young adults who so desire should be referred to a gay and lesbian youth group in their area. If no such group exists, a local college or university may have or know of an appropriate group.

CHRONIC DISEASE

Approximately 2 million teenagers in the United States have a chronic illness or disability. This is a diverse group that is entering adulthood with a variety of medical expectations, needs and concerns. Like other teenagers, their concerns usually center around physical, social and sexual development. Ideally, these concerns have been honestly addressed during earlier adolescence while, at the same time, parents and care providers have allowed the teenager a progressively greater role in making medical decisions. Additionally, realistic identification of academic, vocational and social capabilities is important to enhance self-esteem and peer relationships.

As this vulnerable population enters adulthood, it is especially important for health care providers to assess the capability to navigate a complicated health care system. Probably the most important task is assessing whether health insurance benefits will continue after leaving adolescence. Most teenagers who have relied on parents or the government for health insurance will need guidance about these issues and possible referral to knowledgeable experts. Teenagers who discontinue their education, move out of their parents' house and work at low-wage jobs are most at risk for losing all health insurance coverage.

> Unless health insurance is an employment benefit, Julie's decision to enter the workforce may jeopardize her health benefits if she has been getting them under either parent's policy. Staying in school frequently allows continuation under a parent's policy.

One of the greatest challenges may be the transition to a new set of health care providers for adults. In many cases, patients and parents will have grown up with and become dependent on the same team of pediatric nurses, social workers and physicians. Separation may be difficult for patients, parents and providers, and the process can be managed most successfully over a period of time that allows for several office visits. Ease of transition will depend on parental trust and the patient's ability to assume and demonstrate responsibility for self-care and sensible decision making.

ALCOHOL AND OTHER SUBSTANCE ABUSE PROBLEMS

Natural history studies indicate that most adolescents who use alcohol and other drugs will, as they assume adult roles and responsibilities, spontaneously quit using drugs and develop controlled patterns of alcohol consumption. However, a small proportion will be seriously affected by use during adolescence. Motor vehicle and pedestrian accidents, interpersonal violence, date rape, suicide and decreased use of condoms are all associated with alcohol or substance use. In addition, approximately 20% of adults become dependent on substances, and with few exceptions, harmful patterns of use begin to appear during adolescence. The interviewing section in this chapter should assist in identifying those who need special attention and intervention.

Working with substance-abusing patients frequently frustrates health care providers. Frustration arises because treatment often seems futile, treatment resources are limited, patients and their families are in denial, and patients often do not ask for help. These issues can be addressed partially by learning about appropriate community referral sources, treatment programs, and counselors, including Alcoholics and Narcotics Anonymous groups specifically for teenagers and young adults. The local telephone directory and Internet are usually the best sources for local self-help groups such as Alcoholics Anonymous, Cocaine Anonymous, Narcotics Anonymous and Alanon (for individuals and families living with someone with a drinking problem). Inquiry should be made about local groups specifically for teenagers and young adults. If age-appropriate groups don't seem to exist, local college or university health centers can often provide referral assistance. Denial frequently interferes with patients' and families' abilities to recognize the connection between alcohol or substance use and adverse consequences. Denial is a recognized adaptive mechanism often used by patients and their families to avoid the discomfort associated with admitting a substance abuse problem. It is predictable and can be addressed through multiple visits. In time, denial can be overcome by a respectful, empathic, and supportive clinician. Patients will not change their behavior until they are ready. Although a drinking or drug problem may be obvious, advice to change will be futile if the patient is not ready. Assessing the stage of change (Table 24–1) and working with patients at their current "level" make the process easier and more assessable for the provider and patient.

Chemical dependency is a chronic medical condition with lifelong implications. Like other chronic medical conditions, it has periods in which symptoms are well controlled and periods of relapse. Consequently, successfully intervening with an adolescent does not preclude periods of relapse in adulthood.

Drug Testing

Bioethical principles about patients' rights apply to drug testing. Testing should be performed only for the benefit of the patient and only with the patient's consent. This is often a point of contention between parents of minors and providers. For patients who are no longer minors, it is less of an issue. To begin with, it is important to know what is included in the drug test performed at an individual laboratory or facility. Urine drug testing never includes the most

TABLE 24–1   **Stages of Change: Preparing Adolescents to Change Addictive Behavior**

Stage	Description	Motivational Task
Precontemplation	No acknowledgment of a problem or a need for change	Clinician should present "evidence" of a problem and raise a patient's awareness. Do not expect a patient to agree with a diagnosis or plan Create doubt, increase awareness of risks and problems with current patterns of substance use
Contemplation	Patients are ambivalent about having a problem or needing to change	Clinician should help patients become aware of their ambivalence. Help patients reflect on their comments, such as "You said at times you feel like you should stop drinking. Tell me why you feel that way." Help weigh the relative risks and benefits of changing substance use, evoke reasons to change and risks of not changing, strengthen self-efficacy for changing current substance use
Determination	Accepts problem and willing to attempt treatment	Treatment options (day program, evening program, Alcoholics Anonymous or other 12-step programs) should be provided, and the patient must participate in choosing the most appropriate Help determine the best course of action to change substance use from available alternatives
Action	Attends treatment program and attempts to change behavior	Help establish a clear plan of action toward changing substance use
Maintenance	Requires skills to maintain sobriety and is usually dependent on positive experience and on treatment and its effects	Positive reinforcement by the health care provider, family and social and work environment is important Help identify and use strategies to prevent relapse
Relapse	Recurrence of substance abuse. Some may slip back into contemplative stages	The possibility of relapse should be discussed with patients and, as with other chronic disorders, should not be unexpected Help renew the process of change starting at contemplation

Modified from Samet JH, Rollnick S, Barnes H: A brief clinical approach after detection of substance abuse. *Arch Intern Med* 156:2287, 1996.

commonly abused substance, alcohol. Many laboratories do not include tetrahydrocannabinol (THC—the active ingredient in marijuana) in their screening drug panel. Moreover, the ability to detect drugs depends on the dose and frequency of drug use in question.

Many parents request drug testing as a substitute for teenager-parent communication. Because of this, it is important to explore reasons for the test request. Before a test is performed, parents should be asked the following questions:

- "Why and what do you suspect your teenager is using?" If the answer is something obvious, such as drugs or empty bottles discovered in the teen's bedroom, testing is rarely helpful.

- "What do you plan to do if the test is positive?" It is important that a plan be in place beforehand and that both parents agree on the plan. If the drug in question is used infrequently or in relatively low doses, it is quite possible that the test will be negative.

- "What will you do if the test is negative?" This is not a trivial issue because it becomes more difficult to change the behavior of a substance-using teenager who receives a negative test result.

Testing is always justified if the teenager consents. It can also be helpful to satisfy parental concern before the teen is allowed to get a driver's license or to continue use of the family car. In addition, it can be a way for those in recovery to prove and maintain abstinence.

 Julie should be evaluated to assess her "stage" of substance use or abuse and to determine what type of intervention, if any, is appropriate. At the same time, she should be assessed for depression. Because substances themselves or the effects of withdrawal can mimic mental health problems, coexisting mental health problems are best evaluated when the patient is known to be substance free for several weeks.

TAKING A MEDICAL HISTORY

As with all teenagers, the clinician must ensure confidentiality before beginning the interview. Because the questions may seem embarrassing, intrusive, or trivial from the patient's perspective, it is important to reassure patients that all questions are asked to provide advice about maintaining health and avoiding disease. Patients 18 years or older are legally adults.

Julie is 18. Legal statutes require that all decisions about health care be her own. This is the case even though her parents may be "paying the bills."

For those who recently became adults, it is important to reaffirm the legal provisions of consent and disclosure, especially if the patient is accompanied to appointments by a parent. Most teenagers want to discuss and receive information about health-related behavior, such as sex, drugs, protection against human immunodeficiency virus (HIV) and sexually transmitted disease and pregnancy prevention. Most teenagers or young adults, however, will not initiate such discussions. They depend on the care provider to begin a dialogue.

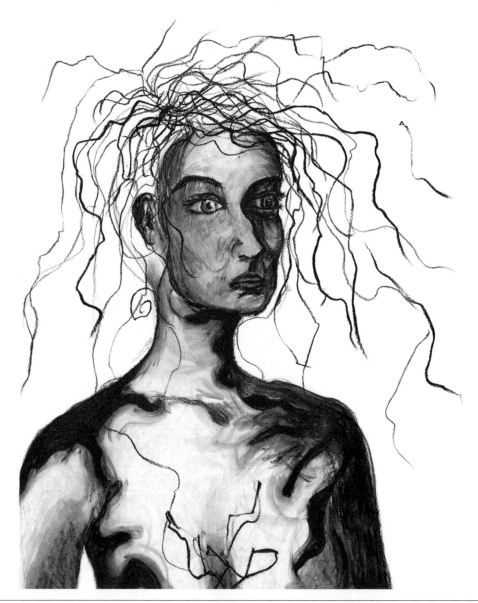

A 17-year-old's self-portrait conveys outward calm and sophistication, hiding the anxiety, tension and confusion that mark this important transition time. By Jessie Boilek (original 16 × 21 inches, charcoal).

HIV/AIDS

HIV risk assessment, counseling and testing have become routine among those providing health services to teenagers and young adults. Although teenagers constitute a relatively small proportion (approximately 1%) of acquired immunodeficiency syndrome (AIDS) cases nationally, the long incubation time (approximately 10 years) and the large proportion of AIDS cases affecting individuals in their third decade of life indicate that adolescents are at substantial risk for HIV infection. Adolescent rates of unprotected sexual intercourse, as measured by unwanted pregnancy and sexually transmitted diseases, substantiate this concern.

Clinicians should be knowledgeable about which groups are at highest risk and know the local HIV seroprevalence among teenagers. National data indicate that minority females, gay males and those practicing survival sex (having sex for money, food, drugs or shelter) are at greatest risk. Having sex with older partners, who themselves may have had multiple partners or used intravenous drugs, is the thread that connects teenagers at highest risk (Fig. 24–1). Many teenagers are concerned about their risk for HIV and are often encouraged to be tested without thought for the potential consequences. Reasons for requesting an HIV test frequently include health concern, guilt or anxiety about sexual experiences, media messages, school curriculum and peer group pressure. Everyone should be counseled that HIV does not preferentially infect stereotypical groups but is spread only by specific behavioral practices, all of which involve exchange of body fluid. Intravenous drug users should be advised to use sterile needles exclusively, and condom use should be advised for all who are sexually active. Special attention should be paid to the most vulnerable patients because they are usually the least able to handle the implications of HIV infection. It is always hoped that those who are HIV infected will alter their behavior to stay healthy and prevent others from becoming infected. This may not apply to those who are substance dependent, homeless or runaways. These teenagers are often disenfranchised and angry and have difficulty trusting adults. In this population, consideration about substance abuse treatment, housing, case management, social services and availability of medical services should be given before HIV testing.

DATA GATHERING

Life Transitions

COLLEGE. Ask about reasons for attending college, vocational goals and whether attendance is self-motivated. Discuss separation fears and potential benefits about moving away from home.

EMPLOYMENT/UNEMPLOYMENT. Ask about reasons for entering the workforce and about preparedness to accept financial independence and responsibility. Ask pregnant or parenting teenagers about plans to reenter school or the workplace.

MILITARY. Ask about reasons for enlisting and whether this is a career path or a means to developing a skill set. Discussion about exposure to alcohol, drugs and sex should be similar to that for those attending college.

INCARCERATION. Inquiry should be made about whether and where routine health care is obtained in the community.

HOMELESSNESS. Ask about the circumstance that led to homelessness.

	13–19 years old				20–24 years old			
	2001		Cumulative total		2001		Cumulative total	
Male exposure category	No.	(%)	No.	(%)	No.	(%)	No.	(%)
Men who have sex with men	231	(46)	1,442	(51)	988	(49)	7,606	(55)
Injecting drug use	13	(3)	126	(4)	70	(3)	736	(5)
Men who have sex with men and inject drugs	11	(2)	122	(4)	61	(3)	848	(6)
Hemophilia/coagulation disorder	2	(0)	102	(4)	3	(0)	85	(1)
Heterosexual contact	23	(5)	183	(6)	128	(6)	907	(7)
Sex with injecting drug user	*0*		*25*		*18*		*124*	
Sex with person with hemophilia	*0*		*2*		*0*		*0*	
Sex with transfusion recipient with HIV infection	*0*		*0*		*0*		*6*	
Sex with HIV-infected person, risk not specified	*23*		*156*		*110*		*777*	
Receipt of blood transfusion, blood components, or tissue	0	(0)	13	(0)	1	(0)	27	(0)
Risk not reported or identified	220	(44)	837	(30)	773	(38)	3,511	(26)
Male subtotal	500	(100)	2,825	(100)	2,024	(100)	13,720	(100)
Female exposure category								
Injecting drug use	36	(5)	269	(7)	74	(5)	865	(11)
Hemophilia/coagulation disorder	0	(0)	0	(0)	0	(0)	4	(0)
Heterosexual contact	241	(37)	1,838	(49)	440	(32)	3,419	(45)
Sex with injecting drug user	*18*		*279*		*69*		*704*	
Sex with bisexual male	*12*		*130*		*28*		*266*	
Sex with person with hemophilia	*1*		*24*		*3*		*44*	
Sex with transfusion recipient with HIV infection	*0*		*3*		*1*		*19*	
Sex with HIV-infected person, risk not specified	*210*		*1,402*		*339*		*2,386*	
Receipt of blood transfusion, blood components, or tissue	2	(0)	20	(1)	8	(1)	39	(1)
Risk not reported or identified	376	(57)	1,635	(43)	856	(62)	3,301	(43)
Female subtotal	655	(100)	3,762	(100)	1,378	(100)	7,628	(100)
Total[4]	**1,155**		**6,588**		**3,402**		**21,349**	

Figure 24–1 HIV infection cases in adolescents and young adults from areas with confidential HIV testing, by sex and exposure category through 2001. (From Centers for Disease Control and Prevention, National Center for HIV, STD, TB Prevention: *HIV/AIDS Surveillance Report, Year-End Edition*, 13, No. 2. Atlanta, Public Health Service, 2001.)

Organizing History

For organizational ease and consistency, to address current and potential health risk behavior and to provide health education, many recommend that the history be organized to follow the *HEADSS format—H(ome), E(ducation), A(ctivity), D(rugs), S(ex), (S)uicide.* Although most practitioners still depend on a verbal history for gathering data, recent investigation suggests that a history obtained via interactive computer software may be even more accurate.

Home

GOAL: Determine whether the patient lives independently, with family, with friends, in cohabitation with a significant partner, or at home with parents.

For college students, determine the living situation while at school and during vacations. If the patient is living with roommates, inquire about the household use of cigarettes, alcohol, and other drugs. It is generally difficult to live in a house with peers who use alcohol or other drugs heavily and have no personal use. In addition, determine the degree of financial independence, conflict resolution skills, and existence of household violence. If violence is present, determine whether the patient is a victim or perpetrator. Ask whether there are firearms in the residence. If there are, recommend that they be removed.

QUESTIONS: "Where are you living now?" and "Who else lives where you live?" Ask whether the living situation is satisfactory and whether the patient is exposed to potential health-compromising behavior. For instance, cigarette smoking by roommates may explain recurrent asthma exacerbations, or financial hardship may prevent proper diet and nutrition. Questions about household violence should include, "What happens when people in your household argue?" and "Does anyone ever get hurt during arguments?" This should be followed by, "Do arguments ever happen when someone has been drinking or is under the influence of drugs?" Ask about meals served at home (quality and availability of food). "Is health care available when you need it?"

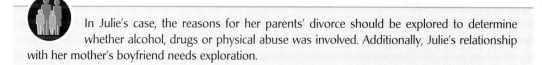

In Julie's case, the reasons for her parents' divorce should be explored to determine whether alcohol, drugs or physical abuse was involved. Additionally, Julie's relationship with her mother's boyfriend needs exploration.

Education and Vocation

GOAL: Evaluate current achievements, strengths and weaknesses and their realistic connection to future plans. Assess for unrecognized learning disabilities and stress or anxiety related to college admission or separation from family, school and community.

QUESTIONS: Discussion about educational or vocational status can initially be directed according to patient's age. For those still in school (high school or college), ask "What classes are you taking? How are your grades? How do your grades compare with last year?" Without specific questioning about classes or grades, most will typically respond that everything is "OK." Falling grades may indicate a mental health condition, a substance abuse problem or a conflict with the development of a personal identity (see Chapter 2). Generally speaking, teenagers who are performing well in school are less likely to participate in multiple health risk behaviors.

For those not in school, ask "Have you graduated from high school?" If not, ask "What is the last grade you completed? Why did you drop out of school? Do you have any plans to complete high school?" The spectrum of reasons why youngsters drop out of school includes some that relate to physical and mental health conditions. Answers to these questions may help uncover learning disabilities, severe family disruption or abuse by family or peers. For instance, an unrecognized learning disability may result in school termination because of recurrent poor performance, low self-esteem and ridicule. Teenagers may leave home before completing high school because they have been sexually victimized or because they reveal gay or lesbian sexual orientation and become ostracized by family, school and peers.

Activity

GOAL: Evaluate social interactions, interests and self-esteem.

QUESTIONS: "What do you do for fun?" or "Are you involved in any clubs, organizations, religious groups, sports or hobbies?" Because active participation is often linked to self-esteem, this may be a nonthreatening way to assess social skills and peer group and community connections. Adolescents who participate only in solitary activities may have difficulty with social skills, feel alienated or be depressed. For this reason, it is important to ask, "How much time do you spend on the Internet?" While the Internet can provide a wealth of information and be a source of entertainment, it can also be a cause of social isolation.

Evidence is strong that teenagers who feel closely connected to family, school and community are less likely to participate in health-compromising or delinquent behavior than peers who are not well connected. Depending on circumstances, also ask, "Do you belong to a fraternity, sorority, or religious youth group or to a gang?" These activities, to varying degrees, provide a sense of community and belonging. In some situations, they may also be sources of extreme peer pressure and result in inappropriate drug and alcohol use, sexual behavior or interpersonal violence. Gangs are a powerful source of identity for those who feel disempowered, disenfranchised and alienated.

Drugs

GOAL: Determine personal, environmental and genetic risks for substance use and abuse and current habits. Identify those whose substance use is likely to interfere with social, mental and physical performance. Injection drug use, uncommon in early and middle adolescence, usually begins in late adolescence or early adulthood, and identification is crucial. Reinforce the behavior of those who have chosen not to use drugs or alcohol.

QUESTIONS: By late adolescence, most American teenagers have had some personal experience with cigarettes, alcohol or other drugs. Among many teenagers, the use of substances is not considered abnormal or dangerous. Nonetheless, questions about substance use may seem threatening and intrusive. For that reason, initiating the discussion by asking first about use by peers is often preferable. Begin by acknowledging that it is common for teenagers to have some drug or alcohol experiences. Then ask, "Do any of your friends ever smoke cigarettes, drink alcohol or use other drugs?" This should be followed by "Have you ever tried any of these substances?" Those whose friends use are more likely to use themselves. Even if the answer is negative, permission has been given to ask questions in the future. Inquiry should address specific substances, such as cigarettes, alcohol, marijuana, stimulants (cocaine, crystal methamphetamine), hallucinogens (LSD, mescaline, ecstasy), prescription pills, anabolic steroids and opiates, as well as routes of ingestion such as intravenous, nasal or inhalation. If the patient reports use, ask for each substance, "How often do you use (daily, weekly, occasionally, rarely)? When was the last time you used? How much do you use at a time? Is your use increasing (to determine whether tolerance is developing)? What are the circumstances of your use (parties, friends, alone)?" Determining the level of use and whether a substantial problem exists can challenge the most experienced clinician. Recognition of a problem depends on the patient's willingness to share and the clinician's willingness to receive information about the use of drugs.

Prejudicial statements and negative body language or facial expression by a provider will hinder the diagnostic process. Evaluation should initially focus on adverse consequences associated with use. Ask "Have you ever had any physical consequences such as vomiting, blacking out or losing consciousness from use? Have you gotten into family, school or legal trouble because of use? Have you found it difficult to drive when using a drug?"

Most chemically dependent teenagers are polysubstance users. Untreated, polysubstance use will generally continue into adulthood with the development of a preference for a particular substance.

It is most important to differentiate teenagers at highest risk for developing adult problems from those whose use will moderate with time. Differentiation can often be achieved by searching for patterns of use common in adult users. Some classes of drugs, such as the stimulants (cocaine, crack, crystal methamphetamine) and the opiates (heroin), have had the basis of their addiction defined at the level of molecular receptors in the central nervous system. On this basis, physical addiction, defined by tolerance and withdrawal, develops in anyone who uses opiates or sympathomimetics at high enough doses for long enough periods. Anyone who becomes a regular user is likely to become dependent. Predicting who may try using these drugs can be difficult.

The same is not necessarily true of alcohol. For instance, many people consume wine daily and do not develop any signs or symptoms of alcohol abuse or dependency. Males who have a family history of alcoholism and those who begin use in early adolescence are at especially high risk for alcohol problems. These individuals should be identified by asking "How old were you when you first began using, and how old were you when you started using regularly?" Obtaining an accurate family history isn't always easy. Rather than asking whether a parent or grandparent has a drinking problem, it may be more efficient to ask, "Do your mother or father ever drink alcohol?" If so, "Have you ever seen either one intoxicated? Has either parent ever received treatment for a drug or alcohol problem or ever attended Alcoholics Anonymous?"

Convincing evidence exists that many alcoholics have high alcohol tolerance, are relatively insensitive to the effects of alcohol, and can consume extraordinary amounts without perception of adverse consequences. This should be evaluated by asking, "What is the most that you have drunk at one time? When you drink, can you stop after one or two drinks, or is your goal always to get drunk? Can you feel the effect of one or two drinks?" Although no data support counseling's efficacy or prevention benefit, those at high risk because of family history should receive it and be told of their risk. They should be advised that if they don't drink, they will not develop an alcohol problem. A variety of diagnostic tools are available to identify substance abusers. Although all have advantages and disadvantages, perhaps the tool most widely used in the office setting is the CAGE questions (Cut down, Annoyed, Guilty, Eye-opener [Box 24–1]).

Affirmative answers to two or more CAGE questions strongly suggest an alcohol or drug problem. Although their predictive value in teenagers is still uncertain, the sensitivity and

---

BOX 24–1   "CAGE" QUESTIONS FOR IDENTIFICATION OF ALCOHOL AND DRUG ABUSE

Pattern of Use

Have you ever felt the need to **CUT DOWN** on drinking (or drug use)?

Probe

What was it like? Were you successful? Why did you decide to cut down? Have you ever limited substance use in order to please someone?

Consequences

Have you ever felt **ANNOYED** by criticism about your drinking (drug use)?

Probe

Can you give me an example? What led to the criticism?

Consequences

Have you ever felt **GUILTY** about your drinking (drug use)? Have you ever felt **GUILTY** about something you said or did while you were drinking (using drugs)?

Probe

Tell me more about that. What happened? Can you give me an example of a specific event?

Pattern/Tolerance

Have you ever taken a morning **EYE-OPENER**?

Probe

Have you felt shaky or edgy after a night of heavy drinking (drug use)? What did you do to relieve the feeling? Have you ever had trouble getting back to sleep in the morning after a night of heavy drinking (drug use)?

From Cyr MG, Sherman SE: Screening, assessment, making the diagnosis. In Bigby J (ed): *Substance Abuse Education in General Internal Medicine*, SGIM, HRSA and ADAMHA Contract 240-91-0053, 1993.

Julie's change to an older peer group, withdrawal from family activities, moodiness, and the discovery of an empty alcohol bottle in her room—indicating nonsocial drinking—collectively strongly suggest a substance abuse problem. Whether concurrent depression is present is important to know so that it can be treated. However, treatment of depression will be hampered by continued substance use.

---

specificity of CAGE questions in adults are high enough to suggest that they might be integrated into every medical interview of young adults.

Sex

GOAL: Evaluate and counsel about sexual behavior, family planning, sexually transmitted diseases, HIV, and sexual abuse. Reinforce the decision of those who have decided to remain sexually abstinent.

QUESTIONS: Open-ended questions that do not assume sexual orientation, such as "Have you ever been involved sexually with anyone?" are a nonthreatening way to begin a discussion.

For those who report sexual involvement, to determine use of condoms and birth control, ask "How do you protect yourself from sexually transmitted diseases and pregnancy?" Ask females, "Have you ever been pregnant?" and ask males, "Have you ever fathered a child?" For those answering affirmatively, ask "What was the pregnancy outcome?" Ask about the age of the sexual partner. Those with older partners may be at greater risk for sexually transmitted diseases, including HIV. If condom use is reported, ask "Do you use condoms some of the time or all of the time?" Because it is surprising how often a history of pregnancy or sexually transmitted disease exists even in older teenagers who report always using a condom, it is worth reviewing safer sex, condom use and effective methods of pregnancy prevention with all teenagers. Also ask, "Do you ever have sex while under the influence of drugs or alcohol?" It is important to inform patients that condom use diminishes significantly, even in those with excellent HIV prevention knowledge, when they are intoxicated. In addition, patients should be informed that almost all date rape occurs while one or both dating partners are under the influence.

Although it is important to reinforce the decision of those who have chosen sexual abstinence, they should be allowed to ask questions and be reassured that if their sexual behavior changes, they have a source of information, advice and prevention resources.

PHYSICAL EXAMINATION

The *Guidelines for Adolescent Preventive Services* recommend that adolescents who have no disease or symptom-specific complaints receive a health maintenance visit to discuss disease-related and prevention behavior once during each period of adolescence—early, middle and late. In an adolescent with symptoms or signs of drug use or depression and other mental illnesses, more frequent office visits for an interval history, physical examination or counseling are usually necessary. The American Academy of Pediatrics' *Guidelines for Health Supervision III* recommends annual visits for health supervision and emphasizes that social, psychological, educational and vocational screening and counseling are a major part of the visit. In addition, these guidelines recommend that (1) all menstruating adolescents be screened once by laboratory evaluation of hematocrit or hemoglobin, (2) a urine dipstick for leukocyte esterase and nitrate be performed once as a screening test for sexually transmitted diseases and (3) a pelvic exam and Papanicolaou (Pap) smear be done as part of preventive health maintenance for patients between 18 and 21 years of age.

During examination of a late adolescent, attention should be directed to general condition, height, weight, blood pressure and pulse rate. General appearance and cleanliness often provide clues about self-esteem, and the type of clothing may indicate with which group or clique the teenager identifies. Look for tattoos and body piercing. Although tattoos are currently popular among many teenagers, pay attention to large tattoos of numbers or neighborhood names because they may indicate gang membership. Body piercing sites should be inspected for signs of infection, and inquiry should be made about whether the piercing was self-inflicted or performed professionally. If self-inflicted, assess risk for hepatitis B or HIV transmission. Tanner staging should be performed and any signs or symptoms of delayed puberty identified and evaluated. If not done in earlier adolescence, girls should be taught breast self-examination and boys taught testicular self-examination. Sexually active girls should receive a pelvic examination with a Pap smear yearly. Those with multiple partners should have a Pap smear every 6 months.

Laboratory Examination

Routine laboratory evaluation in an asymptomatic late adolescent is usually unnecessary. Sexually active teenagers should be routinely screened for sexually transmitted diseases. Urine screening by polymerase chain reaction (PCR) and ligase chain reaction (LCR) for chlamydia and gonorrhea means that this evaluation can be performed accurately (high specificity and sensitivity) without requiring a urethral swab or pelvic examination.

Cholesterol screening is controversial. Those with a family history of hypercholesterolemia or early adult heart disease should be screened at least once during adolescence. However, screening should always be accompanied by counseling about diet and exercise. Vision testing should be performed periodically, once every 3 years for youth without symptoms. Audiometry is recommended when hearing loss is suspected.

ANTICIPATORY GUIDANCE

Vocation Planning

For clinicians, discussion with a patient about future vocational plans may be useful as a catalyst to assess health risk behavior and to provide health education and anticipatory guidance. Almost all teenagers will be eager to have such a discussion if it occurs in a nonthreatening, nonjudgmental, and confidential manner.

 Julie undoubtedly would benefit from a discussion about many issues, including family, parents, future plans, goals and educational possibilities.

Transition Events

COLLEGE. Pressure to use alcohol and other substances, along with pressure for sexual relationships, should be discussed and integrated into conversation about disease prevention and health maintenance. All youth, especially those who excel scholastically, should be cautioned about school-related stress and anxiety.

PARENTHOOD OR TEEN PREGNANCY. Rapid return to school or work should be encouraged because this strongly decreases the likelihood of repeat pregnancy and increases the ability to achieve financial and social independence.

INCARCERATION. If a regular source of medical care does not exist, suggestions should be offered for where care can be obtained. This is especially important for minors requiring chronic medication, such as those with mental health problems. Compounding these problems, in most communities the medical and mental health systems are often difficult to navigate, thus making follow-up and prescription refills problematic.

HOMELESSNESS. Solving problems of homeless youth always requires help from social service and counseling organizations. Providers should be aware of local agencies with which they can work before providing care to homeless or runaway youth.

QUICK CHECK–17 TO 21 YEARS

✓ Separation from parents and decision about vocation/education

✓ Transitions to higher education, workforce or military and from incarceration or homelessness

✓ Developing intimate interpersonal relationships and sexual identity

✓ Evaluating and interviewing patients with substance use

✓ Taking a behavior-directed medical history

✓ Guidelines for physical examination and laboratory investigations

✓ Anticipatory guidance

HEADS UP–17 TO 21 YEARS

• Use the HEADSS format to interview.
• Understand the consent and confidentiality laws in your state—and explain them to your patient.
• Homeless adolescents need their issues prioritized. Usually, finding shelter and addressing substance-use issues come first.
• Ask open-ended questions that make patients feel they have permission to discuss sexuality, substance use, history of abuse or mental health concerns.
• Teenagers with chronic disease need to play an increasingly larger role in self-care throughout adolescence so that the transition is not abrupt in early adulthood.
• Alcohol is the "drug" most commonly abused by adolescents.
• Asking about the age of the oldest sexual partner is a quick way to assess HIV risk.
• Assess self-esteem and be aware of community resources that may help enhance self-esteem.
• Adolescents who feel connected to family, school and community are far less likely to participate in health-compromising behavior than those who feel disconnected.

Risk Factors for Substance Use and Abuse among Adolescents

Characteristics
• Family history
• Low self-esteem
• Learning disabilities
• Poor body image
• Gay/lesbian identity
• Chronic disease
• Physical, psychological or sexual abuse
• Depression or thought disorder
• Antisocial personality

Continued

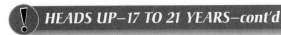

HEADS UP—17 TO 21 YEARS—cont'd

- Peer and cultural pressure
- Repeated thrill-seeking and risk-taking behavior
- Young age at initiation

Diagnostic Clues

- Change in peer group
- Increased school or work absences
- Decline in grades or work performance
- Increased interpersonal turmoil and arguments

Advice to Adolescents about Substance Abuse

Drug Use Status	Clinician's Action
Nonuser	Praise decision
Potential user	Praise decision and offer alternatives
Experimental user	Encourage quitting and set date
Committed user	Encourage quitting, set date and ask again at next encounter

RECOMMENDED READINGS

For Youth and Parents

nlm.nih.gov/medlineplus/childandteenhealth.html.
nlm.nih.gov/medlineplus/healthtopics.html.

For Youth

McCoy K, Wibbelsman C: *Life Happens: A Teenager's Guide to Friends, Failure, Sexuality, Love, Rejection, Addiction, Peer Pressure, Families, Loss, Depression, Change and Other Challenges of Living.* New York, Berkeley, 1996.

McCoy K, Wibbelsman C: *The Teenage Body Book.* New York, Perigee, 1999.

nlm.nih.gov/medlineplus/childandteenhealth.html—National Library of Medicine site for health-related facts.

Simons J, Finlay B, Yang B: *The Adolescent and Young Adult Fact Book.* Washington, DC, Children's Defense Fund, 1991.

For Parents

Adolescent health information and guidelines from the AMA. Available at http://www.ama-assn.org/adolhlth.

Kaufman M: *Mothering Teens: Understanding the Adolescent Years.* Chartottetown, Prince Edward Island, Canada, Gynergy Books, 1997.

Steinberg LD, Levin A: *You and Your Adolescent: A Parent's Guide for Ages 10 to 20.* New York, Harper & Row, 1990.

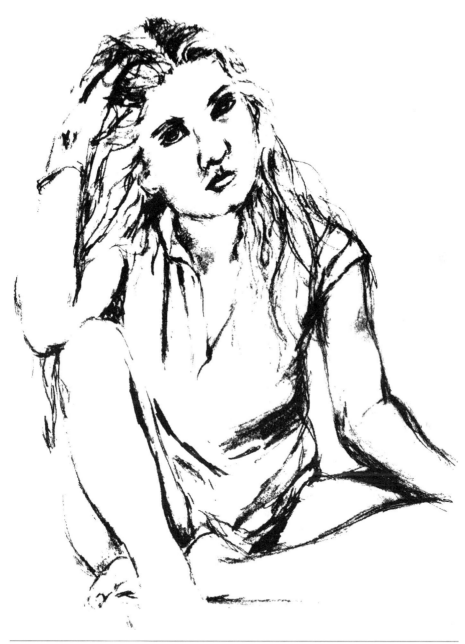

"Self-portrait." By Eileen Fitz, age 18.

CHAPTER 25

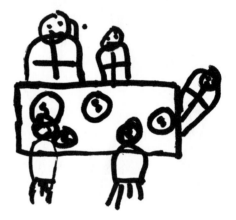

"mom at home by
heiself"

"me at the table with my
Dad, Donna (stepmom), and her
kids"

"I'm on the phone i my mon"

The stark division of lives is shown in this drawing by a child living with divorce.

Special Families

ROBERT D. WELLS and MARTIN T. STEIN

Social and economic patterns of change have a significant effect on family constellations. This chapter describes the impact of the family constellation on a child's behavior and development from infancy through adolescence.

Key Words

- **Divorce**
- **Stepfamilies**
- **Serious Illness of Parent**
- **Single Parents**
- **Adoption**
- **Foster Care**
- **Gay or Lesbian Parent**
- **Homeless Children**
- **Low-Income Families**

In addition to the traditional nuclear family composed of two biological parents and their children, many children today are raised in a variety of different family units, including step-families, single-parent families, gay and lesbian parent families and homeless families. Adopted children and foster children are other forms of child rearing. Pediatricians with a knowledge of the influence of a particular family structure on the development and behavior of children and their parents are in a position to provide more attention to both the medical and psychosocial aspects of health care. Recognition that family values and child-rearing principles that encourage the provision of concrete resources, discipline, expectations, modeling, and emotional support to children are important in all families, regardless of the specific constellation, is a critical feature of contemporary pediatric care.

WHAT IS A FAMILY?

The rapid changes in family constellations in the United States over the past 50 years have created considerable diversification in the makeup of families. The divorce rate has doubled since 1965, as has the number of mothers who are working full-time. Recognizing the changed meaning of the "family," the *American Heritage Dictionary* changed its 1992 definition of a "fundamental social group ... typically consisting of a man and woman and their offspring to "a fundamental social group ... typically consisting of one or two parents and their children" in the 2000 edition. If our definition of the typical family is restricted to homes with two biologically related parents, the majority of children come from special families. From 1990 to

Catherine, an 11-year-old girl, was seen by her pediatrician for recurrent abdominal pain. She lived with her mother, a 52-year-old nurse administrator, and her father, a 63-year-old retired physician. Catherine complained of abdominal pain almost daily for the past year. At first her parents dismissed it as "just nerves." When she was sent home from school, her parents became more concerned. Catherine was evaluated by her pediatrician, who did not find an apparent cause for her pain after an initial history, review of symptoms and complete physical examination. Results of screening laboratory tests, including a complete blood cell count, erythrocyte sedimentation rate, urinalysis, chemistry panel and stool examination for occult blood and ova and parasites, were normal. While performing the medical assessment, her pediatrician was impressed by Catherine's depressed and anxious demeanor. She was fidgety and often rolled her hair around a constantly moving finger. When a question was directed to Catherine, eye contact diminished, she looked down and a sad appearance came over her.

When Catherine's mother was interviewed alone, she quickly became tearful and disclosed that her husband was severely disabled by multiple sclerosis and was abusing opiates to control his pain and depression. Marital conflict was extremely high, and she admitted involvement in an extramarital affair, which Catherine had known about for 1 year. She also wondered how Catherine was coping with taking care of her dad after school.

Interviewed alone, Catherine indeed appeared quite depressed and worried. She described a recurrent fear that she would return home from school to find her father dead or severely injured. She hated having to take care of him and longed for her mother's return from work. She did not volunteer any information about her mother's affair but did admit to worrying about her mother's adjustment. She saw her as a "workaholic who was always stressed out" and quick to anger. It was clear that Catherine experienced a tremendous amount of stress and anxiety related to her special family circumstances.

The pediatrician referred Catherine and her mother to a pediatric psychologist. The mother was eventually referred to an adult psychiatrist for psychopharmacological treatment of significant depression. Through counseling, she made a decision to place her disabled husband in a chronic care facility. She recognized that she and Catherine were unable to sustain him at home.

Catherine was responsive to individual counseling. In the context of a warm, supportive relationship, she enjoyed the mutual detective work of understanding and modifying her stress and pain. After the third visit and without direct interpretation, Catherine verbalized the belief that her anxious state and frequent stress were associated with her abdominal pain. As she was helped to see the special nature of the stressors in her family, her feelings of anger, worry and sadness were now viewed as a natural outcome of stress overload. Her love for both parents was constantly reaffirmed in the counseling sessions, but she was also helped to get in touch with her anger and frustration at their excessive demands on her. Her abdominal pain declined steadily and resolved completely shortly after the nursing home placement of her father. She continued to visit him in the nursing home, where he was able to resolve his substance dependency.

2000, the proportion of children living in single-parent families increased from 24% to 30%. Only 42% of children currently live in a traditional nuclear family, and 22% live in a second marriage, two-parent family. By the time children reach their 18th birthday, 50% to 60% of them will be affected by divorce. It may well be that over the next decade, a child with both birth parents present will be seen as unusual.

No evidence proves that a particular family constellation is either "good" or "bad" for children. However, the way a family functions to support the growth and development of its children is important. Several family characteristics are important for children, regardless of the specific constellation:

- Regular provision of life necessities, including food, housing, clothing and medical care
- Demonstrated warmth, unconditional love and constructive limit setting for the child
- Continuity and stability in caregiving for the child
- Appropriate models of the development of healthy intimacy and sexuality
- Cooperation among involved caretaking adults
- Lack of violence toward and respect for all members in the family
- Lack of excessive stress, such as significant physical or mental illness of the caretaking adults, including depression, alcoholism and drug abuse
- Adequate support for caretaking adults from relatives, friends, neighbors and community
- Stimulation of cognitive development and opportunities to enhance moral reasoning
- Capacity for meaningful interpersonal relationships, good communication, problem-solving capacity and motivation to achieve
- Fostering of socialization by helping children function as cooperative members of society

These basic aspects of family functioning are necessary if children are to acquire a sense of security and self-esteem, learn to socialize, respond to rules, limit and control their anger and aggression and develop long-term achievable career goals.

All families provide varying levels of concrete resources, discipline, expectations, modeling and emotional support to their children. After significant acute or chronic loss, most families appear somewhat less able to meet the needs of their children (see Chapter 27). When the functional capacity of any special family is assessed, it is important to avoid value-laden expectations in favor of a more objective appraisal of relative strengths and weaknesses. Specifically, it is not important how different from the norm the family is, but how well it goes about meeting the needs of the various family members while remaining effective in the wider community.

WHAT MAKES A FAMILY SPECIAL?

The term *special families* is used in this chapter to delineate a variety of family constellations that may affect child health, behavior and development. Such a definition includes foster, adoptive, stepparent and single-parent families, in addition to families facing severe strain because of poor parental health or adjustment. Though differing from each other in important ways, the commonality of special families lies in **the effects of loss** on the children. In this manner, intact, nuclear families can be seen as "special" if they indeed subject the child to certain risks as a result of loss or threatened loss. Farm families who are facing bankruptcy, inner-city homeless families and immigrant families who have had to flee their homelands should be considered special because of the loss that their members experience. For clinicians, recognition of these special circumstances focuses our behavioral and developmental assessment on each family and promotes individually tailored anticipatory guidance to support all families in performing their essential functions.

Assessment of children in special families must take into account several dimensions of the loss situation:

- The extent of loss experienced
- The amount of time that has elapsed
- The child's age
- The degree to which stressors are acute, chronic or recurrent
- The adaptive capacity of the child, including his own temperament
- Parenting figures' ability to rally to the needs of the child

Although the clinician should be restrained from letting personal values and beliefs enter into the equation, the values of the family's community should also be considered. Unique family constellations are more or less acceptable in certain contexts. For example, teenage pregnancy in some middle-class neighborhoods is associated with greater ostracism than in a neighborhood where it is more common and acceptable. Similarly, having homosexual, adoptive or disabled parents will be less of a strain on children living in communities where it is not considered unusual.

Even when large numbers of families experience similar losses (e.g., after natural catastrophes), the actual experience in terms of severity of the loss is highly subjective. Some parents find that the **divorce process** is a considerable strain, whereas others find it eventually energizing and liberating. Death of a family member is typically stress producing, but a study of Amish families has documented that families with an Amish heritage show a relative ease of adjustment. Loss and stress clearly are subjectively determined experiences. The implication for clinicians is that the family and child must be asked about their own sense of the severity of loss or upheaval rather than the clinician relying on her own impression.

The amount of time that has elapsed since the change or loss is also important in determining the nature of an individual child and family's adjustment. Studies of bereavement and divorce indicate significant upheaval during the first year after the loss, with the majority of children returning to baseline functioning during the second year. Consequently, disruptions in a child's behavior or academic functioning during the first year after divorce are not unusual and may not signify serious maladaptation, whereas such behavior after the second year is of greater concern.

Age and developmental skills also play an important role in determining the child's state of adjustment to special family circumstances. Infants require responsive and predictable caregiving behavior, and the biological relationship of the caregiver is relatively unimportant. Separations or changes in caregivers are particularly stressful between about 8 and 18 months, when the developmental theme of attachment is prominent. Similarly, losses because of divorce or death during infancy and the preschool years are less obviously sensitizing than those that occur during the school-age and adolescent period, provided that there is consideration in meeting the child's physical and emotional needs. Divorce itself may not be so stressful for a preschool child, but the necessity to live in two homes may require significant adjustment and provoke heightened stress. The number of elements that changed for a child may be more salient than the divorce itself. In general, children will be more vulnerable to special family circumstances from elementary school age to middle adolescence.

The effects of multiple, chronic and severe stressors on children appear most dramatic and disabling. Ongoing domestic violence, parental substance abuse and dire poverty are particularly devastating and appear to have long-standing effects on child development and adjustment. Acute stressors such as natural catastrophes, divorce, sudden loss of income and death of a parent can also pose a profound challenge to the child and family. Longitudinal studies suggest that a period of adaptation follows the initial shock. For children and parents alike, this may lead to a decrease in academic and occupational functioning, moodiness, depression, anger, behavioral problems, psychosomatic complaints and sleep disturbances.

After the initial trauma, the quality of a child's adaptation is determined primarily by the parent's ability to model effective coping strategies while maintaining family rules and expectations. When the child's clinician focuses family energy toward the augmentation of parental recovery, she encourages the child's adaptation and recovery as well. Self-help groups, religious organizations, and more formal mental health services may be helpful, especially when the parent and the child have few friends or available family or community linkages.

IMPACT OF SPECIAL FAMILY MEMBERSHIP ON CHILDREN

Prediction of the developmental outcome of a particular child reared in one class of special families is not usually possible. However, some generalizations about the ways families influence children can be made from the available literature. Clear evidence exists that children can be successfully reared in special families despite some evidence that an intact family with both biological parents present and reasonably compatible provides children with the best opportunity for healthy growth and development. One study concluded that poor, single-parent families have the highest risk for social maladaptation and psychological problems in their children. The presence of second adults in these families did have important ameliorative functions. Families headed by mother and grandmother were nearly as effective in producing socially and emotionally healthy first graders as were mother-father families. The powerful ameliorative effects of social support have been clearly documented.

Developmental and behavioral problems in children may not be directly related to loss of the nuclear family. Rather, it is family discord and harsh parental discipline, associated with isolation, financial stress, and parental mental illness, that seem to lead to delinquent behavior in children. These all draw resources away from a child, including the psychological energy to keep the child's needs primary. Family discord may, of course, occur in either an intact family or a special family.

These general principles of understanding and determining the specific needs of an individual family and child should assist the child's clinician. The following sections provide more specific information about different types of special families.

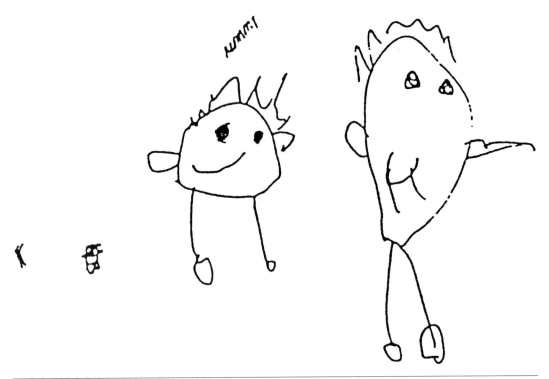

Figure 25–1   Joey, age 7, has drawn himself as a very small person next to his mother and her new boyfriend. When his mother saw the drawing, she became convinced that Joey should receive counseling to help him adjust to his parents' separation and probable divorce (see Case Study, p. 625). (From Stein MT: Challenging case: The use of family drawings by children in pediatric practice. *J Dev Behav Pediatr* 18:334, 1997.)

DIVORCING FAMILIES

The effect of the **divorce** process on the development of children has been studied extensively. Approximately 50% of children experience a divorce of their parents by the middle of adolescence. Most children respond to the initiation of separation and divorce with significant feelings of depression, anxiety and anger. Infants and preschool-age children appear less affected than their older counterparts, provided that their needs for physical and psychological nurturance are met. Notable declines in academic performance may occur in both boys and girls during the first year after the separation. Boys tend to respond to this loss with increased emotional outbursts, noncompliance and other external behavior problems (Fig. 25–1). Withdrawal, sadness and anxiety, characterized as internalizing behavior, are more commonly observed in girls, and their difficulties may be overlooked for longer periods. Some data also suggest that some young women suffer from a "sleeper" effect, whereby an initial adjustment is realized, but when these women enter young adulthood, a reawakening of anxieties regarding male-female relationships may occur.

When Joey's mother made an appointment for a health supervision visit just before his seventh birthday, she talked about his recent behavior change. During the past 6 months, his teacher phoned on several occasions with concerns about Joey's disruptive classroom behavior. He hit other children on two occasions, offered comments when not called on and frequently wandered aimlessly around the class, talking to other students and disrupting their work. He often did not complete his assigned work in school or at home. This behavior pattern was in contrast to his cooperative, interactive and productive style of learning and social interaction before this time.

The pediatrician discovered that Joey's parents had separated 6 months earlier. The marriage had been conflictual during the past 3 years. Verbal battles between the parents were common, and Joey witnessed physical spousal abuse on two occasions. Joey saw his father on weekends, but the parents' lingering distrust and anger surrounded the visits with ambivalence and stress. Joey would not talk to the pediatrician about the visits with his father. He was subdued and answered questions with a single word and limited eye contact. His physical examination was normal. When the pediatrician recommended a brief period of counseling to help Joey explore his feelings about the separation and his new living situation, his mother adamantly refused. She declared that "therapy would harm him more."

While Joey was waiting for the doctor, he was asked to draw a picture of his family. When the pediatrician showed the drawing to his mother, she cried immediately, followed by "Of course, you're right. Joey needs counseling to help him."

Joey drew himself as a very small person next to his mother and her new boyfriend (see Fig. 25–1). The visual image of a diminutive person with poor self-esteem helped his mother overcome her resistance to counseling by associating his behavior with a poor self-image. The drawing acted as a nonverbal trigger to seek help. After five sessions with a therapist, Joey's classroom behavior improved, and he was once again responsive to learning.

Recent evidence refutes the general belief that by the second year the majority of children adjust to their altered family circumstances. In a longitudinal study, 37% of children were doing poorly (i.e., academic underachievement and behavior problems at school, home or both) 5 years after divorce. At the 10-year follow-up, 41% were still maladjusted, which suggests that the years following a divorce continue to be stressful for many children.

Investigators studying the 10-year period after a divorce reported that only one in seven children saw their parents happily remarried, 50% experienced a new divorce, 60% felt rejected by at least one parent and 50% grew up in families in which the parents remained intensely angry at each other. The economic consequence of a divorce is also quite significant, with 25% of children who experienced a divorce living with a parent who had significantly reduced financial resources. How the divorcing parents as individuals and as partners in parenting make social, psychological and economic adjustments after the divorce determines the long-term effects on children.

The degree to which families are unable to develop their own parenting plan and custody decisions is an important predictor of child adjustment. When parents continue to litigate with emotional viciousness after divorce and children have frequent access to both parents, the children appear more depressed, withdrawn, aggressive, and prone to psychosomatic complaints.

Child transfers in a neutral setting (e.g., school or church), where parents need not be in direct contact with each other, may help reduce the extreme stress associated with this activity.

> Quinn was 3 years old when his parents arranged an appointment with the pediatrician to discuss different approaches to Quinn's child rearing. An abrupt separation had occurred 2 months before the visit. The parents expressed anger and hostility toward each other. Before the separation they worked with a marriage and family therapist for 3 months without resolution of differences. Quinn's mother did not want Quinn spending time with his dad, who was now living with another woman and her two children. Quinn's dad expressed a desire to continue his role as a father and wanted Quinn to stay with him at least 2 days each week.
>
> Note: The pediatrician's initial response can take the form of an active listener, giving Quinn's mother undivided attention (even when limited to a 15-minute visit). Allowing Quinn's mother to tell her story provides an opportunity for the clinician to understand the effect of the divorce on Quinn and his mother, as well as showing empathy. Quinn's recent development should be assessed for regressions and his behavior responses to his dad and mom. It may be a good opportunity to review the normal development and behavior expectations of a 3-year-old. The clinician can help Quinn's mother appreciate the value of both a mother and father in a young child's life, even when the original nuclear family has been lost. An opportunity to arrange an office visit with both mom and dad, where Quinn would be he focus of their mutual interest, should be offered.

A number of factors may predict the relative risk of maladaptation after divorce. Children exposed to continuing family discord either before or after a divorce are at much greater risk for conduct disturbances. If open family conflict decreases after divorce, better outcomes are predicted. In contrast, children who have been sheltered from parental conflicts and awaken to open conflict during and after the divorce are often the most grievously injured. Children whose parents demonstrate aggressive styles of resolving conflict with each other tend to have continued difficulty with behavioral problems and poor coping skills. Children who are able to experience a trend toward family stabilization after a divorce are more likely to return to their baseline functioning.

The emotional availability of one or both parents is often diminished during the separation and divorce process. If this continues, children face tremendous obstacles in meeting their own, their siblings' and their parents' needs. Although age (younger) and sex of the child (female) are predictors of a better outcome in general, appropriate ongoing relationships with both parents are the most important factor in supporting resilience. An easy child temperament, social support, physical health and intelligence also contribute to better outcomes.

The clinician's role in helping families who experience divorce should precede the actual separation if possible. During regular pediatric health supervision visits, families should be made aware of the clinician's interest and need to know about significant family events that might affect the child. Periodic focused questions that serve to update the clinician about family function will both inform and cement the relationship between the parents and the clinician. If marital separation occurs, specific guidelines can be offered regarding how and what to tell the child. Attention can be focused on ways to support the child's coping skills and to maintain appropriate contact with parents, friends and concerned others. Parents frequently need help in controlling their own emotional state, especially in the presence of their children.

Helping parents distinguish their own needs and feelings from those of their child is also important. Predicting the types of reactions they and their child may experience is usually helpful. Monitoring subsequent responses of the child and parent is then critical for effective clinical assessment, and at times referral to a mental health professional may be appropriate. Anticipatory guidance for a child whose parents have separated or divorced can be guided by recognition of predictable responses at each developmental stage (Table 25–1).

> Quinn's pediatrician recognized that both parents would benefit from individual counseling in order to learn strategies to manage their emotions at this difficult time. The pediatrician saw this as an opportunity not only to suggest an appropriate mental health referral but also to emphasize the parents' mutual desire to help Quinn through the family crisis and to be effective parents.

Relating to Two Separate Parents

When facing separated parents with a high degree of conflict, it is not unlikely that the clinician may find herself drawn into disagreements regarding concerns and treatments required by their child. A wise clinician will clarify who has physical and, perhaps more importantly, legal custody because this directly relates to issues of medical consent, information sharing, and withdrawal of consent for treatment. In most situations, both parents retain joint legal custody, and therefore the clinician should clearly state an interest in getting to know both parents and ensuring that all information is shared directly. At times, if the postdivorce conflict is under good control, it can be quite beneficial to the clinician and rewarding for the child to be accompanied by both parents to well-child exams. If the conflict is overly heated and neither parent nor the child can tolerate this arrangement, the clinician should arrange for visits so that the child is accompanied by each parent separately, in an alternating pattern. This strategy will allow the clinician to maintain an alliance with both parents and avoid the specter of seeming to favor one over the other. Specific policies about payment for visits should be directly discussed to avoid embroiling the office in the financial battles that are all too common.

The clinician should also be prepared to respond when one parent disagrees with the treatment plan. This can typically occur regarding psychotropic medications but may also arise around immunizations and other medical treatments. Whenever one parent with legal guardianship dissents while the other parent consents to treatment, the clinician should speak directly with each parent individually. After education and brief counseling, if the dissenting parent is not convinced of the treatment benefits, that parent should be asked to send a written letter formally withdrawing consent to use a specific treatment. This letter can then be shared with the assenting parent, and the clinician should suggest family therapy or legal consultation and advise that nonemergency treatments will be withheld until the conflict is legally remediated. Whenever possible, the clinician should avoid testifying on behalf of one parent over the other and should maintain a balanced posture in the child's best interest.

TABLE 25–1   Responses of Child to Parents' Divorce within the First Year

Developmental Status	Child's Response	Primary Care Clinician's Role
Preschool	Regressive behavior Sleep disturbance Tantrums Aggressive behavior Bowel and bladder difficulties Clinging Fears of abandonment	Encourage stable, predictable meal and bedtime routines Develop consistent patterns of joining and separating from child Continue contact with noncustodial parent Provide reassurance
Younger school age	Sadness Fearfulness Loyalty conflicts Attempts to determine responsibility Hopes for family reconciliation Declining school performance	Empathize with child's feelings Provide regular opportunities for child to talk Support child's continuing relationship with both parents Offer reassurance
Older school age/prepubertal	Grief, intense anger Declining school performance Disrupted peer relationships Attempts to clarify responsibility for divorce Caretaking of a parent	Express interest in and availability to the child Support child's school and peer involvement Provide clear acknowledgment and support for child's working through feelings about the divorce
Adolescence	Depression Anger Premature emancipation Increase in adolescent acting out Sleeper effects, particularly in females	Provide opportunities for discussion Offer appropriate supports within and outside the family, including peer involvement (such as in school-based family transition groups)

Modified from Wallerstein JS: Separation, divorce and remarriage. In Levine MD, Carey WB, Crocker AC (eds): *Developmental-Behavioral Pediatrics*, 2nd ed. Philadelphia, WB Saunders, 1992; and Kaplan-Janoff M. Divorce. In Parker S, Zuckerman B, Augustyn M. *Behavioral and Developmental Pediatrics: A Handbook for Primary Care*, 2nd ed. Philadelphia, Lippincott Williams and Wilkins, 2005, p 393.

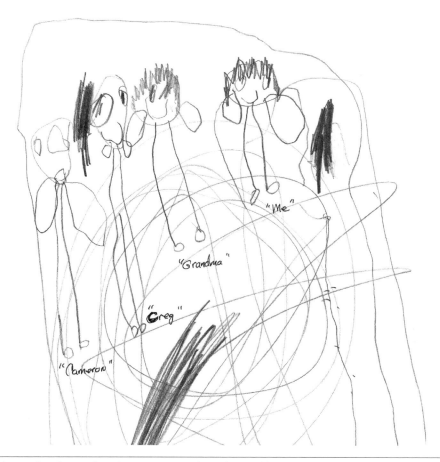

A home with grandmother as the primary care provider is depicted by this 5½-year-old. With three children with special needs, there is good reason why the family is surrounded by scribbled force lines by Jared Mell.

STEPFAMILIES

As the divorce rate remains high and that of remarriage continues to increase, **stepfamilies** have become an important part of our culture. Although these reconstituted families usually function as effectively as nuclear family units, a number of salient differences should be appreciated by responsive clinicians. Each member of the family has experienced significant losses. Children who are depressed and anxious after parental separation must now cope with sharing their biological parent with a new adult. The biological parent, who may also be functioning with diminished coping resources, must contend with playing a "middleman" role, thus leaving neither side satisfied. The stepparent will quickly appreciate that parent-child bonds precede his involvement; issues of loyalty and alliance in the biological parent may lead to a sense of isolation and rejection in the stepparent. Most stepchildren continue to visit the other biological parent. Differences in rules between the households and jealousies between the biological noncustodial parent and the stepparent may lead to further disruption.

Despite these challenges, studies suggest that children from stepfamilies do not differ significantly from children in other family structures. They can achieve effective family functioning with developmentally appropriate levels of adjustment and are equally prone to maladaptation in the face of family discord as occurs in wholly biologically related families. Family functioning is optimal with positive marital adjustment, strong parent-child attachment, generalized family cohesiveness and effective problem solving.

When stepfamilies are dysfunctional, they are characterized by strong parent-child coalitions (rather than parent-parent coalitions) and lack of mutual decision-making skills. Adolescents appear particularly vulnerable to developing problems when their stepfamilies are characterized by chaotic rules, punitiveness, excessive dependency and frequent major life changes.

A sensitive and alert clinician may at times become confused about the nature of the alliance between natural parents, stepparents and children. Attempts should be made to maintain contact with all adults who serve as psychological parents while complying with the legal rights and restrictions to information stipulated in custody agreements. Keeping in mind the nature of loss experienced by children in reconstituted families, expect some early adjustment difficulties, with eventual remission in the majority of cases. Specific attention should be paid to developing well-recognized rules of behavior in the home. Stepparents can be counseled to develop a role as an independent caregiver in addition to supporting the spouse's actions. It is important to counsel stepparents that they should not assume a larger disciplinary role than the biologically related parent. Children may be helped if the biologically related parent explains that she is the parent in charge but will be delegating authority to her new partner when she is unavailable.

Parents, children and the clinician should maintain hope that over time, rules and roles will become more comfortable and acceptable. The clinician should express clear support for the importance of the noncustodial parent's right to visit, obtain information about the children, and discuss concerns. Finally, the stepparent–biological parent couple should be encouraged to maintain nonparental, romantic and supportive roles with each other so that the alliance between the adults remains balanced and strong. When adjustment problems predominate or become chronic or when fixed maladaptive roles and alliances have developed, referral for family counseling is indicated and often helpful.

Jane, who was 13 years old when her mother remarried, always resisted talking to and sharing activities with her stepfather. At her 14th birthday, she proclaimed, "You're not my dad. I will only talk to mom and I don't want you to be my parent." At the same time, Jane's grades were declining and she missed curfew on two occasions. Note: Hearing Jane's story, her pediatrician discussed the challenges of stepfamily relationships with Jane and her mom, pointed out how difficult it can be for all kids to accept a new parent in their home and made a recommendation for referral to a family counselor.

Stepparents, as well as adoptive parents, may need considerable external validation of their roles as parents, and the child's clinician is often in a unique position to provide such support. In her role of advocate for the child's development, the clinician may assist these parents through timely support and guidance in understanding the changes the family is experiencing in terms of the best interest of the child or children, as well as the needs and emotional responses of the parents. Give some positive feedback when gains are made and some supportive comments when challenges remain.

SERIOUS ILLNESS OF PARENTS

The psychosocial effects of growing up with a parent who has a serious, life-threatening physical illness is perhaps one of the least studied stressful childhood events. In contrast, the effects of parental mental illness on children have been more extensively studied. Children who have a schizophrenic parent benefit significantly when they have a healthy relationship with a caring and predictable adult. This was also the conclusion for families with mothers in whom breast cancer, diabetes or fibrocystic breast disease was diagnosed. Children in these families showed the most adaptive behavior when fathers maintained frequent interactions with their children. Not surprisingly, marital harmony was also correlated with improved child functioning. A clinician will look for and encourage these parent figures when the biological parent is burdened with serious illness. It may be the other parent, another relative, a close family friend or a neighbor.

For the clinician treating children who have highly stressed, physically ill parents, special attention should be directed to guilt reactions in children. Psychosomatic conditions, school avoidance, separation anxiety and depression are common responses to a sudden threat to a parent's health. A temperamentally easy child may show a tendency to develop "pseudo-maturity," appearing to be the psychological parent for the family. Extra effort is needed to keep the child out of the family's decision-making process so that she experiences and benefits from a normal period of growth and development. Parents may have to be explicitly informed not to seek counsel from children acting in pseudomaturity, and they should be encouraged to develop more adaptive and supportive relationships with other adults and health care providers. Children should be encouraged to continue their normal scholastic and extracurricular activities. Family communication about the parent's illness and treatment should be encouraged, particularly when the focus is on the feelings and reactions that are naturally evoked.

The clinician may find it useful to maintain contact with the ill parent during the course of illness. The questions on the minds of the well parent and the ill parent are often different regarding what, how, and when to tell children about predictable and frightening events. In the majority of circumstances, open and honest communication with children is the best advice. Concerns about the death of a parent should be directly addressed to minimize the child's tendency to fantasize catastrophic outcomes or miraculous cures. Most importantly, the clinician should take the time to empathize with the child regarding her worries about her parent. She should be encouraged to ask questions about her parent's condition and to call for an appointment if she becomes confused, overwhelmingly anxious or depressed (see Chapter 27).

SINGLE-PARENT FAMILIES

Financial concerns are a serious problem faced by most **single parents**, a rapidly growing segment of our population. Earning a living and caring for the needs of children can easily consume the full-time energy of more than one adult. Remarkably, many single parents find ways to spend as much or more time with their children than they would if they were in a marriage, although certain sacrifices must be made. Frequently, single parents have to sacrifice some "adult time" that would ordinarily be spent meeting their own emotional needs to meet their financial and family obligations. When appointments are broken or arrival to the office is late, when anxiety levels are heightened or when payment for medical service is delayed, the child's clinician should be sensitive to these added stresses in single parents.

Clinicians can be helpful to single parents by accepting their families as healthy units that are capable of providing for the needs of their children, while being sensitive to the special pressures felt by single parents. Isolation from other adults is a particular problem for some single parents, and at times they need to share their experiences with another adult. The child's clinician may be the most respected and available adult. The physician can use this position therapeutically by providing feedback, empathy and validation of the parental role. More explicit directions, detailed action plans and direct feedback may be needed from the clinician in these circumstances.

Joy was 11 years old when she drew the picture in Figure 25–2 during a visit for a mild acute illness. She lived with her mother in a single-parent family since birth. She had no siblings. On the surface, her physical health, schoolwork and social development were satisfactory. However, Jessica made friends slowly. She was unusually cautious about leaving her mother to go to a friend's house. She preferred to have a friend come to her house and play in her mother's presence.

Jessica's pediatrician had been concerned that the close bond between Jessica and her mother had limited their emotional separation. At several previous office visits, the pediatrician unsuccessfully looked for an opportunity to discuss this observation with Jessica and her mother. The family drawing was an opening. When her mother was asked, "What do you think about this picture?" she initially responded with pride in her daughter's drawing skills. Then she said, "We are rather close, aren't we?" The pediatrician encouraged the mother to discuss that observation further. After 10 minutes alone with the pediatrician, Jessica's mother was motivated to help her daughter (and herself) discover ways to psychologically separate while maintaining their loving and close relationship.

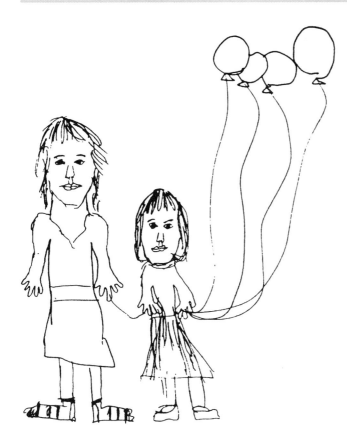

Figure 25–2 A drawing by Joy, age 11, reveals that her relationship with her mother may be too close. After talking about the drawing, the mother agreed with the pediatrician that she and her daughter should explore ways to separate more psychologically. (From Stein MT: Challenging case: The use of family drawings by children in pediatric practice. *J Dev Behav Pediatr* 18:334, 1997.)

Single parents can be encouraged to share some of their parenting obligations with other responsible adults. Depending on the situation, this might mean encouraging contact with grandparents or noncustodial parents or using the support of various social agencies, such as Big Brother/Big Sister organizations and single-parent clubs. The pediatric office can make available a directory of single-parent support groups in the community. Finally, a number of joys and strengths can result from single-parenting experiences (e.g., learning self-sufficiency as a parent), and the positive aspects of single parenting can be emphasized to members of single-parent households.

ADOPTIVE FAMILIES

Adoption provides a caring and responsive home and family for about 2% of U.S. children, who might not otherwise have a home, and provides children for couples who wish to parent. Like other special families, children and adults each bring their own unique strengths and liabilities together to create a warm environment for healing previous losses and developing new capacities. Although most adoptions occur when nonparental relatives become the adoptive parents, many unrelated families are adopting infants and older children with the help of adoption agencies and private attorneys. The clinician may be asked to help review the birth and health information of a soon-to-be-adopted child. The parents may have many questions regarding ways to guide their infant's or child's transition to a new family.

Adoptions outside the family involve at least three participants, referred to as "the adoption triangle." At one corner of the triangle is the biological parent or parents, often a single woman in her early 20s who has chosen adoption for her fetus or newborn. Frequently, she is under considerable emotional stress, supported by neither the biological father of the baby nor her own parents. Although many adoptions are arranged during pregnancy, a significant number of babies are placed after birth as a result of neglect or abuse. To avoid a tendency to blame or stigmatize the biological parent, the clinician should bear in mind the difficult circumstances in which many parents live. In general, the decision to relinquish a child demonstrates the parent's capacity to recognize the predominance of the child's needs. The biological parent's adjustment is aided by having the opportunity to know her neonate and "say good-bye." Reassurance of the child's well-being from the clinician also aids adjustment.

At another corner of the triangle are the adoptive parents, who may have dreamed of and contemplated the wonderful experience of raising a child. Although many families have been counseled by the time adoption becomes a reality, private adoptions may be completely free of counseling. Some couples may have unresolved feelings related to their decision to adopt, and most parents worry about their own reactions to the parenting role. Grief over infertility or unresolved anger at a spouse may also be operative. Over the years, adoption has become far less stigmatized, although some parents may still not experience support—from extended family members and friends. Adoptive parents may also live with unanswered questions about the child's biological and genetic background and the possibility of intrauterine substance exposure or other unknown pregnancy complications.

The adopted child forms the final part of the triangle. This child brings a particular genetic endowment that includes intellectual, temperamental and physical factors. The child may have experienced many prenatal stresses related to the biological mother's age, emotional state and physical health and habits during pregnancy. Placement for varying periods at critical ages in one or more foster homes may have occurred with its accompanying stress and disruptions of attachments. When adoption takes place within the first 6 months of life, the infant is likely to avoid the experience of significant loss that is often apparent in older children. The quality of care that children experienced before placement has significant effects on the level of trust they exhibit. Children with a background of abuse, neglect and unpredictability will come to the adoption setting with a very different set of expectations, and parents may find the attachment process to be lengthened and more complex. A striking example is children adopted from Romanian orphanages, who initially exhibited overinhibited behavior patterns that transitioned into disinhibited and externalizing (impulsive/oppositional) behavior about 3 years after adoption. Approximately 12% of these children developed autistic-like behavior.

The child's temperament is also an important aspect to consider when determining risk factors and level of adjustment, with easier temperaments leading to more rapid family integration. Ethnic differences, in appearance and cultural identification, may be additional challenges for a racially mixed adoptive family.

When caring for adopted children, clinicians should realize that all three parties in the adoption process have their own emotional needs and civil rights. Open adoptions are now becoming the norm, and all three members of the triangle are encouraged to maintain contact. In open adoption, the biological and adoptive parents agree beforehand on the level of involvement that each will have with the child. This can range from sending a school picture every spring to regular weekly visitations. In general, full awareness and select visitation with biological parents appear to be beneficial to all three parties involved; however, research on open adoptions is limited, and the long-term effects on children are not documented. In an open adoption, the biological parent may be helped to assuage concerns about the child's circumstances, and the adoptive parents may come to appreciate the character and heritage of their child. Just as with divorce, the child may be powerfully influenced by the ability of the biological and adoptive parents to form an effective alliance and to function without insecurity or jealousy.

Helping parents feel comfortable in talking with a child about his adoption is a matter in which clinicians can be quite helpful (Table 25–2). Families should be encouraged to include the child's adoption as an important part of the family's story. When parents tell a child about an adoption by age 3 or 4, the adopted child will grow up with true knowledge about his birth status. Children's books can be used to help talk about the adoption process. Even when children grow up with early knowledge of their adoption, it is in the school-age years that many first become aware that adoption meant loss and relinquishment by their biological parent. The child may demonstrate signs of mourning and will be helped by sensitive questions from the adoptive parent after either subtle or overt behavior or questions.

Clinicians will occasionally come in contact with school-age and adolescent patients who were adopted but have not yet been told, and parents will at this point seek consultation on when and how to break the news to their child. In most instances, families should be encouraged to share this information at the earliest opportunity to avoid a sense of rejection and mistrust. These exchanges should be done as a process over time and should be responsive

TABLE 25–2 **Issues of Adoption at Different Ages**

Age	Issue
Preschool	"Where did I come from?" Life and death issues Generally accepting of being adopted
School age (7–11 years)	"Why was I adopted when most people aren't?" Worried that their value as a person is less because they are adopted Concerns about being different Aware that they have lost someone who played an extremely important role in their life Imagines birth parents as rich, famous and more attractive than adoptive parents
Adolescence	Task of developing an identity and discovering how they are different and how they are connected to "their people" Concerns about family illness such as insanity, talents and physical appearance of birth family Interest in meeting birth parents

From Roizen N. In Parker S, Zuckerman B, Augustyn M (eds). *Behavioral and Developmental Pediatrics: Handbook for Primary Care*, 2nd ed. Philadelphia, Lippincott Williams and Wilkins, 2005, pp 376-   .

to the types of questions asked by the child. The clinician can be particularly useful in helping adoptive parents find ways to explain the reason for adoption and the difficulties experienced by the biological parent. Avoidance of the idea of having "been chosen" by the adoptive parents is important because this concept can introduce the thought that one can be "unchosen." Clinicians should avoid such pejorative terms as "natural" or "real" mother. The adoptive parents are real and natural; the term "birth mother" is preferred when referring to the biological mother.

FOSTER FAMILIES

In the United States, approximately half a million children receive **foster care** services. Foster care provides children with a home and family life when the child's parents are unable to do so, usually in the child's known community. At one time, foster care was used primarily to serve the needs of temporarily displaced children. Currently, children in foster care are likely to have been placed there because of severe psychological, social, or behavioral problems in the child, in the parents or in both. Unlike adoption, the goal of foster care placement, at least in theory, is to preserve and hopefully improve the child's relationship with the biological parents. Like adoption, this creates a triangle consisting of the child, the foster parents, and the biological parents. It will also contain a bevy of social workers, therapists, lawyers, court advocates, and others in social service agencies. Like a stepchild, a foster child may feel as though she is a member of two (or more) homes and families concurrently and that this circumstance is beyond her control.

Foster parents volunteer to take children into their homes and are infrequently given specific training in the complexities of foster parenthood. Foster parents must attempt to provide for the present needs of and perhaps even rehabilitate the children entrusted to their care. They must also make room in the family for the new child. The birth children of foster parents may experience feelings akin to sibling rivalry on the arrival of a foster child in their home. Conversely, they may benefit by exposure to children less fortunate or to infants who are the result of irresponsible behavior on the part of others. Foster parents must also maintain a collaborative relationship with the foster care agency and be open to investigation and periodic evaluation of their intimate family life. They must often advocate for services and deal with mounds of paperwork. The foster family may be required to establish a relationship with the birth parents of the child, and such relationships are often quite challenging. Finally, foster parents must work through issues of attachment and separation with their foster children and within themselves related to the continuous process of bonding with and separating from foster children.

When foster children present the foster family with challenging problems (and they almost always do), a variety of reactions can occur. Some foster parents distance themselves from these problems, citing the child's lack of biological relationship, as well as the previously poor conditions in which the child lived. Other foster families assume that the child's maladaptive behavior is a response to the foster family and feel frustrated or rejected. In working with these parents, the clinician should help them realize that children bring a significant history into foster family relationships. In fact, perhaps after a brief "honeymoon," the child may test to the limit the structure provided by the foster family. In some cases it may even appear that the child has set out to prove that he is unmanageable in any home and therefore should be returned to his biological parents. With a high rate of physical and mental illness and often unmet needs for care, these children meet these challenges with diminished resources.

In helping a foster child the health care provider must understand the effects of separation from natural parents on children at various developmental levels. Most children react to the loss of their relationship with the biological parent in the same ways that children react to the loss of a parent through divorce or death. Reactions include a period of grief, a sense of failure, angry feelings toward the present caretaker and perhaps behavioral acting out or depression and withdrawal. Many children will develop somatic complaints, and some may experience a loss of previously achieved developmental milestones. Children who are placed in foster care between the ages of 6 and 18 months may show the classic pattern of reaction to separation from parents that is described by Bowlby. This includes reactions of protest, despair and, finally, a period of "detachment" in which the child may appear to have adjusted to the new home but has become dangerously superficial in his relationships to important adults. These signs of infantile depression must be recognized and permanent placement sought with urgency. The clinician should advocate for no further changes, if possible, and certainly not during this critical period in emotional development.

A clinician may have a relationship with a child that continues despite the child's various living arrangements with natural or foster parents. Whenever possible, the clinician should develop a relationship with the child that allows the child to express feelings about foster placement and allows the clinician to help the child and foster parents deal with a variety of problems. The physician may act as the child's advocate in her relationship with the foster parents and the foster care placement agency in helping determine the individual child's needs and current state of development. The foster child's clinician should encourage continuity of medical records as the child moves from one foster home to the next or into an adopting family. Physicians should be supportive of the children in foster care by seeing them with priority, delineating their physical and mental health needs in detail and communicating these needs to the child welfare agency. The tendency to avoid these complex, often record-less cases should be resisted, and advocacy for the best interests of these at-risk children should be promoted.

GAY AND LESBIAN FAMILIES

Currently, 6 to 14 million children live with a **gay or lesbian parent**, with wide variation in the type of openness demonstrated to children and to the wider community. Some homosexual couples may become parents by using surrogates and insemination techniques, and these children grow up within the context of having two same-sex parents. Other families may develop through adoption and foster parenting. Additionally, a number of children may initially have been raised in a more conventional family, but after separation, divorce or death, one parent may acknowledge his or her homosexuality. Some of these families have full-time custody, whereas others may share custody with an ex-partner. As children grow up within these family units, they may face some of the same loss issues experienced by children in other special families, including concerns about being accepted by others in the wider community.

Health care professionals must be especially conscientious to avoid being insensitive to these new family constellations. Increased awareness and acceptance are needed in order to allow families and children to receive the same quality of care given to more mainstream families. Homophobia (fear and disapproval of homosexuality) and heterosexism (a belief that only heterosexual families are the appropriate setting for raising children) should be avoided to reduce the risk of insulting these individuals or isolating them from health care services. Parents are more likely to be open about their concerns if they perceive that the health care provider is nonjudgmental and open to nontraditional family structures. Gender-neutral terms such as "parent" or "family member" may be preferred on office forms and questionnaires to avoid the appearance of bias and prejudice.

In the past, common misconceptions were that children raised in gay- or lesbian-headed families would have an increased risk for emotional disorders or sexual dysfunction later in life. Recent research has demonstrated that children raised in such families are similar to children in traditional families and are equally likely to be well adjusted and to have positive self-esteem. Patterson, in her review of 12 studies involving more than 300 children of gay and lesbian parents, concluded that these children are not more likely to establish a homosexual preference than children raised in heterosexual-led families.

Children who are raised in communities that are tolerant of these differences probably experience less stress and concern about the reaction of others. The scientific literature suggests that they adjust to being raised by two same-sex parents by creating names to help distinguish them (e.g., Mommy Kate and Mommy Jane). When openness is encouraged at home, children may show very little concern about the different characteristics of their family. As adolescence approaches, issues of sexual identity and exploration can be discussed with the same sensitivity and openness that one hopes to find in more traditional families. It is likely that over time, health care professionals and our society at large will become more aware and sensitive to the needs of these children and their parents.

HOMELESS FAMILIES

Families are the fastest growing segment of the homeless population in America. More and more children are living in cars, vans, low-cost hotels or shelters or simply on the street. They are exposed to severe poverty, violence and profound deprivation. Approximately half of these children suffer from severe depression, anxiety and learning and behavior problems. Their parents are typically aware of these problems but do not have resources for dealing with them.

When treating **homeless children**, the clinician should pay particular attention to their school attendance and functioning. Collaboration with teachers, public health nurses, social workers, and mental health personnel is useful. Concrete recommendations for the parents about community resources often produce positive results when the pediatric office has an up-to-date list of available resources. Guidance about growth and development is important in this group of children because previous experience with pediatric continuity of care is often absent. With the high rates of violence and substance abuse among the homeless, these children should be screened carefully for developmental delays, depression, post-traumatic stress disorder, conduct problems, and substance exposure. Provide a copy of all medical encounters, the growth chart, and immunizations so that families can carry that with them.

As a result of the tremendous disorganization commonly found among homeless families, clinicians may become frustrated by the lack of follow-up during planned medical visits. It is useful to keep in mind Maslow's hierarchy, whereby motivation for higher goals of achievement, self-esteem and identity is based on achieving earlier goals of safety, comfort and love. As with all special families, issues of safety, predictability and organization can help overcome the effects of previous losses. It is likely that more children will be growing up in these disruptive environments, and clinicians will need to be particularly sensitive to the frustration experienced by parents who are unable to meet their child's needs because of extraordinary social circumstances.

LOW-INCOME FAMILIES

In the past 2 decades the number of children living below the poverty line has not changed significantly, and children now comprise the most impoverished group in the United States. Approximately 16% of all children and 19% of children younger than 6 years live in families with incomes less than the official federal poverty level ($14,351 for a family of three in 2002). While poverty affects all races, it is also clear that children of color are disproportionately represented, with 21% of African American and Latino children, 10% of Asian children and 7% of white children living in families who face daily struggles around basic resources. Clinicians who care for children living in poverty recognize the multiple sources of stress that face these families and their difficulties maintaining consistent and safe housing, available transportation, ample food and resources to pay for medical supplies.

Children who grow up in poverty are at risk for poor health (e.g., low birth weight, lead poisoning, growth failure and higher infant mortality), delayed development, learning challenges (e.g., learning disabilities, grade repetition, high school dropout) and psychiatric and behavioral disorders. In addition, parental depression is five times more common in families living in poverty. Depression in mothers of a young child, coupled with poverty, increased the risk for low birth weight, behavior problems, language delay and child depression.

With basic needs and security concerns in the forefront of their daily lives, it is not uncommon to find that low-income parents have difficulty securing time and the resources required for finding high-quality daycare, providing for involvement in extracurricular activities, and engaging in preventive health care services. The rate of failed appointments is often higher in clinics serving low-income families, and frequent moves and lack of telephone access often make it difficult to provide an effective reminder of upcoming health maintenance appointments. As a result, medical care of low-income children is often less continuous, and clinicians may need to provide well-child services in the context of episodic visits for acute illness and injuries. It is important to avoid "blaming the victim" when clinicians feel frustrated by the lack of follow-through and attention to the range of health, behavioral and developmental concerns. By focusing on concerns directly raised by the parent, clinicians can secure a more trusting therapeutic alliance and thus provide a high level of care and treatment. The principles of cultural competency can be applied when pediatricians care for children in low-income families (see Chapter 3).

CONCLUSION

The needs of children living in specific forms of special families (stepfamilies; single-parent, adoptive, foster care, and homeless families; and families with gay or lesbian parents) have been described. Other types of special families in which a child's development may be affected in unique ways are increasing in contemporary America. These include children living with a grandmother as a primary parent and low-income families. Openness, respect and a desire to talk about the effect of these special family environments on the development of children should be the goal of the child's clinician. Helping parents guide the development of children who live in special families is an appropriate goal—and challenge—in a developmentally focused clinical practice. The fundamental, shared functions of all family units must be kept clearly in mind when the circumstances in which a child lives, no matter how "special" they seem, are evaluated.

In the introduction to a recent report from the American Academy of Pediatrics on "Family Pediatrics," the case is made for making an effort to anticipate the role of the family in the provision of child health care: "The practice of pediatrics is unique among medical specialists in many ways... . Regardless of whether parents or other family members are physically present, their influence is pervasive. Families are the most central and enduring influence in children's lives. Parents are also central in pediatric care. The health and well-being of children are inextricably linked to their parents' physical, emotional and social health, social circumstances, and child-rearing practices." By including nonparental caretakers who care for children in special families, the significance of this statement for pediatric practice is expanded.

 HEADS UP–SPECIAL FAMILIES

- Sensitivity to the family constellation at each pediatric encounter enhances the quality of communication among clinicians, parents and children. Don't assume that each child comes with a biological set of parents living at home.
- An individual child or parent's response to loss is subjective; ask about their sense of the severity of loss or upheaval rather than rely on one's own impression.
- Don't underestimate the value of supportive care when working with special families, including asking empathic questions about the family constellation, discovering and commenting on family and child developmental strengths and informing families about community resources that will support the family and child's developmental needs.
- After a separation, divorce, adoption or entry into a new stepfamily, continue to ask about the effects of change on the child's development and behavior. Listing the change in family pattern as a separate problem in the medical record encourages continuous follow-up.
- Children who have lived through a divorce but still have significant behavioral concerns after 1 year need a mental health referral.
- All children in foster care need a comprehensive developmental assessment and behavioral evaluation.
- When separated parents remain in conflict with each other and about child rearing, clarify who has physical and legal custody, attempt to involve both parents in care decisions and avoid inappropriate support of one parent over the other.

Continued

HEADS UP–SPECIAL FAMILIES–cont'd

- Recognize the enormous stress placed on parents who raise children as a single parent or live in a homeless environment or in significant economic poverty. When appointments are broken or arrival to the office is late, when anxiety levels are heightened or when payment for medical service is delayed, the child's clinician should be sensitive to these added stresses.
- Children are resilient. Be attentive to the characteristics of children raised in special families that promote educational, psychological and social resiliency when developmental expectations are challenged. Support parents with positive feedback when these attributes are discovered.

QUICK CHECK–SPECIAL FAMILIES

✓ Only 42% of children currently live in a traditional nuclear family and 22% live in a second marriage, two-parent family. By the time children reach their 18th birthday, 50% to 60% of them will be affected by divorce.

✓ The emotional experience of loss is a central theme that guides children in many "special families." The sense of loss is especially important after a divorce, illness or death of a parent (or other close relative), entering a new stepfamily and frequent changes in foster families.

✓ Prediction of the developmental outcome of a particular child reared in one type of special family is not usually possible.

ACKNOWLEDGMENT

An early draft of this chapter was written with contributions from Nicholas Putnam, M.D.

RECOMMENDED READINGS

For Parents

Adoption: National Adoption Information Clearinghouse, (888) 251-0075, hhtp://naic.acf.hhs.gov.
Foster parents: National Foster Parent Association, (800) 557-5238, www.nfpainc.org.
Single parents: Parents Without Partners, (561) 391-8833, www.parentswithoutpartners.org.
Gay and lesbian families: Parents, Families and Friends of Lesbians and Gays, Inc., (202) 467-8180, www.pflag.org.
Stepparents: Stepfamily Association of America, (800) 735-0329, www.saafamilies.org.

For Clinicians

American Academy of Pediatrics: Coparent or second-parent adoption by same-sex parents. *Pediatrics* 109:339-340, 2002.
American Academy of Pediatrics: Family-centered care and the pediatrician's role. *Pediatrics* 112:691-696, 2003.
American Academy of Pediatrics: Families and adoption: The pediatrician's role in supporting communication. *Pediatrics* 112:1437-1441, 2003.
Cohen GJ: Helping children and families deal with divorce and separation. *Pediatrics* 110:1019-1023, 2002.

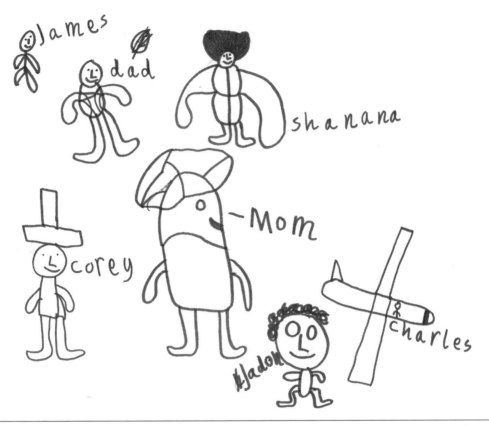

A complex adopting and extended family is shown, all with distinct hair styles. The artist, Corey, shows his older adopted brother in the upper left; his uncle is seen departing in the plane. It seems that Mom is at the center of things, holding it all together.

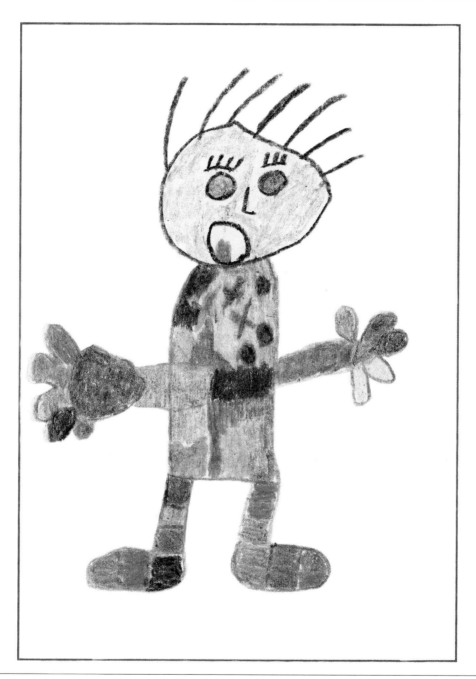

This self portrait is done by a 9-year-old adopted child, working on understanding his past. Although he shows himself with large hands and bright colors ("to be happy"), his yelling mouth and electric hair suggest that all is not calm inside. By CH, age 9.

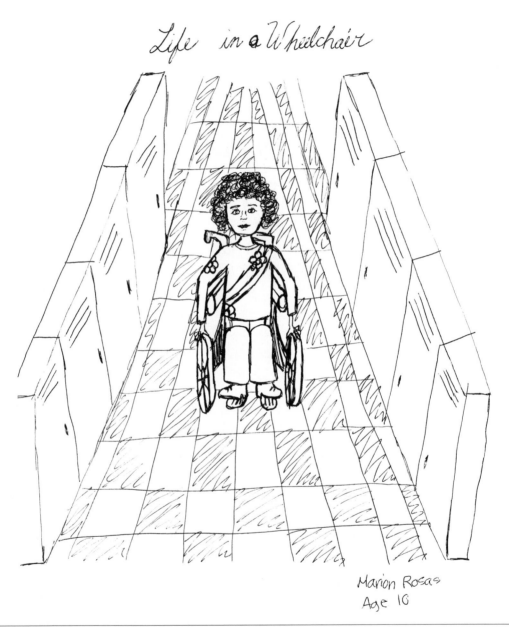

CHAPTER 26

Life in a Wheelchair

Marion Rosas
Age 10

A 10-year-old girl protrays her life as she moves around her school in a wheelchair. Some sense of loneliness in a seemingly cold environment is conveyed in this drawing. By Marion Rosas, age 10.

Encounters with Illness: Coping and Growing

MARTIN T. STEIN

Pediatricians can enhance the quality of care with an understanding about the developmental and psychosocial significance of illness episodes for both children and parents. An office visit for an acute illness offers an opportunity to enhance a child's social competency and independence, prevent a parental perspective of child vulnerability, and learn more about each child and family. The principles of chronic illness and developmentally specific responses to hospitalization and procedures are reviewed with recommendations for pediatric practice.

Key Words

- Acute/Chronic Disease
- Illness and Disease
- Social Competence
- Developmental Regression
- Patient and Parent Agenda
- Solution-Building Family Model
- Object Constancy
- Separation Experience
- Protest-Despair-Denial
- Explanatory Models of Illness

Accurate diagnosis of an acute physical illness is the hallmark of a pediatric clinician. It is an accomplishment that occurs repetitively as clinical experience generates greater precision. In addition to disease recognition and appropriate treatment, attention to the way a child and parent perceive a disease and the behavior and feelings that are a result of their illness and perceptions are important components of comprehensive care. By considering a child's development and behavior and the psychosocial profile of the family, the pediatric clinician not only broadens the data base on which to make treatment decisions but also brings a new dimension to the encounter.

An "illness" is the subjective experience of an altered physical state in contrast to the physical "disease" state. It can be viewed in the context of a particular child's development, as well as the family's experience with symptoms and disease and their expectations and resources. Parmelee has made the insightful observation that in some families "one may have a disease and not feel ill or feel ill and not have a disease." Although an illness may interfere with normal developmental processes, it may also be an opportunity for mastery and enhancement of self-esteem. With this understanding, the emphasis may no longer be limited to the disease process but can include perceptions and reactions to the diagnosis and treatments, stresses that accompany the illness and coping mechanisms available to the child and family.

649

In primary care pediatric practice, at least 50% of office visits are for an **acute illness**; about 10% to 15% of children have a **chronic disease**, and at least a few children are hospitalized each month. The impact of a disease on a child's behavior and developmental expectations is not limited to chronic disorders. Opportunities for the application of pediatric principles that inform our responses to and counseling about disease and illness are equally important during acute illness visits for common problems. Whether a child has a well-defined, limited illness (e.g., streptococcal pharyngitis) or a complicated, chronic disorder (e.g., poorly controlled asthma in a child with multiple hospitalizations and significant family stress), office management should make use of the fundamental principles of child development and the importance of family interactions. Doing this, as well as recognizing the distinction between disease and illness, is more likely to lead to success in meeting the needs of a child and family.

ACUTE MINOR ILLNESS

A Child's Understanding of Illness

Acute illness is a part of childhood. It occurs frequently and is usually self-limited or responsive to medical therapy. During the first 3 years of life, most children experience between six and nine illnesses each year; most illnesses are respiratory or gastrointestinal infections. Between 4 and 10 years old, children average four to six illnesses annually. The high transmission rate throughout a family means that a family with two adults and two children will average 21 illnesses per year. A child's early experiences with these inevitable parts of childhood potentially shape several aspects of her development.

Every pediatrician who enters an examination room has one major objective: to get the diagnosis right and prescribe the appropriate treatment. This goal, coupled with courtesy, empathy and the recognition that at least two patients are being treated (see Chapter 4), make up the core components of pediatric practice. The next level of understanding is to ask the question, "What is the child's understanding of her symptoms and the reason she has been brought to the doctor?" The child may think or say, "Why is mommy or daddy being asked all these questions? Why is the doctor putting a tube on my body and a Popsicle stick in my mouth? Am I going to get better? Will I get a shot? Do I have to take off my clothes?"

An understanding of a child's perspective on the acute illness visit is crucial for two reasons. First, it generates age-appropriate ways to communicate with children, a core pediatric value. Equally important is the clinician's recognition that *the experience of the office visit itself shapes the way a child learns about the body, physical symptoms and illness and the healing process*. Although limited research has been done in this area, it seems reasonable to assume that the cumulative experience of the way parents manage illnesses and the experience at the doctor's office contribute substantially to subsequent adult perceptions of physical and psychological symptoms, response to illness and perceptions of health care.

When Physical Symptoms Occur without an Explanation

Stacy, a 13-year-old, came to the office with concern about a sore throat of 3 days' duration without fever or other symptoms. This was Stacy's seventh office visit during the past year for the same symptoms. Physical examinations demonstrated mild erythema of the pharynx and tonsils without fever or adenopathy; at other times the oropharynx was normal. Throat cultures were consistently negative for group A beta-hemolytic streptococci, and Stacy was given a handout about viral respiratory illness. Note: this case illustrates an exaggerated response to a minor, frequently encountered illness. The understanding of the disease is easy; the question is why it is perceived as serious enough to warrant a physician visit. It's time to step back and look more widely.

This situation is familiar to all pediatric clinicians. An early adolescent comes to the doctor with frequent sore throats that are either mild and self-limited viral infections or exaggerated concerns of a mildly irritated throat. These office visits may reflect a parent's perspective of this child as fragile and vulnerable, or she may be growing up in a family where somatic complaints for minor problems among other family members are frequently brought to medical attention. She and her family may be worried about something serious, a concern that isn't stated. Any of these situations is an opportunity to go beyond taking yet another throat culture and labeling the problem viral pharyngitis. A focused medical history may reveal one or more encounters with illness that were perceived by Stacy's parents to be more serious than implied by the diagnosis. Alternatively, a family history may suggest a pattern of somatization in a parent and other members of the extended family. In this situation, chronic stress or acute situational stressors may trigger the onset of physical or emotional symptoms that are repeatedly brought to medical attention.

A pediatric intervention might start with the recognition that there is a problem in addition to a sore throat. The next step, depending on the intensity of the problem and the particular family, might be a few brief follow-up appointments with the pediatrician to explore the associations between minor physical symptoms and the family's responses. A referral to a mental health specialist would be useful when frequent visits for minor symptoms of a sore throat continue even after pediatric education, probing and counseling. A brief dismissal of each episode never really gets at the core issues and is unlikely to break an inappropriate pattern of care for such minor complaints.

Clinicians who care for children are generally empathic individuals. They have a genuine regard and understanding of the experience of their patient and his parents. To strengthen the capacity for empathy, it is useful to analyze the components of a child's experience as he encounters illness in his home and at the doctor's office (Table 26–1).

Periodic analysis of a patient's psychological and social responses to an illness will bring refreshing clinical insights into the process of providing primary care. These insights usually point to both strengths and vulnerabilities in a particular child and family. They often suggest language to use to strengthen a therapeutic alliance and help children adapt to illness. Most children adapt effectively to illness. Through a greater understanding of the emotional and social context that surrounds illness, clinicians will discover those children and families who experience greater stress or a sense of ongoing vulnerability during such an episode.

TABLE 26–1   **Components of the Experience of Acute Minor Illness**

Child's Experience	Parents' Experience
Physical discomfort of the illness and treatment	Emotional responses: guilt, fear, anger, depression, lethargy
Fantasies about illness	Loss of social contacts
Restrictions (bed rest, diet)	Decreased or altered sensory input
Change in relationship with parents (indulgent or hostile)	Increased child care responsibilities
Worry about body integrity	Expense of illness
Fear of serious illness	Interference with employment Sleep deprivation/fatigue
Decreased recreation	Effects on marital relationship
Fear, anger, guilt	Depression Distortions and misconceptions

Modified from Carey WB: Acute minor illness. In Levine MD, Carey WB, Crocker AC (eds): *Developmental-Behavioral Pediatrics*, 2nd ed. Philadelphia, WB Saunders, 1992, pp 295-296.

Perceptions about Illness Change with Cognitive Development

Children perceive the nature of their illness in a manner consistent with their cognitive level of development. The level of understanding of symptoms moves during childhood through a rapid developmental change from the magical responses ("You get sick because you eat too much candy.") of preschool children to early school-age children ("You get sick because you go out in the cold.") to older school-age children, who are able to generalize symptoms and show some understanding of the role of a germ in causing disease, as well as beginning awareness of their contribution to the nature of the experience (Table 26–2).

As clinicians develop a better understanding of a child's internal response to an illness, they are in a better position to offer individualized targeted suggestions. In addition, this knowledge strengthens the therapeutic alliance with children and their parents. Knowledge about frequently used coping strategies during an acute illness will bring some of these insights to the medical encounter. For example, it is important to understand that a child younger than 5 years often runs away from a clinician and hides behind or under an examination table. She may ask for a bandage or a kiss on a "boo-boo." These are direct coping mechanisms that reflect the child's magical thinking rather than the logical consequences of events. For a school-age child who may perceive a set of symptoms in concrete terms and may begin to show some understanding of causality, an astute clinician can make use of the new coping skills. Allowing the child to listen to his heart with a stethoscope and to ask questions about a medicine or an x-ray film and encouraging him to talk about his perceptions of the illness will give him an opportunity to use age-appropriate coping skills, as well as enhance the therapeutic relationship. The

TABLE 26–2 **Growth in a Child's Understanding of Illness**

Age	Understanding	Examples
4–6 yr	Circular, magical or global responses	"I got a boo-boo on my head because I didn't eat my soup!" (A child's reaction to a scalp laceration caused by falling and hitting his head on a table shortly after lunchtime, when his mother unsuccessfully encouraged him to eat tomato soup)
6–8 yr	Concrete, rigid responses with a "parrot-like" quality; little comprehension by the child; enumeration of symptoms, actions or situations associated with illness	"The cough is a bug that tickles my throat and makes me stay home and in bed. The bug can't play with my friends."
8–11 yr	Increased generalization, with some indication of the child's contribution to the response; the quality of invariant causation remains	"I get these headaches sometimes because I fight with my sister and won't let her play with my things." When asked about his symptoms during a mild gastroenteritis episode, Sammy responded, "I got it because I ate some poison, just like last year when we all got sick at the restaurant."
11–13 yr	Beginning use of an underlying principle; greater delineation of causal agents of illnesses	"Kids get sick when germs like a virus get into their body. It's the virus that makes us feel lousy, causes a fever and makes us want to sleep more."
Over 14 yr	Organized description of mechanism(s) underlying illness and recovery; abstract principles	"Last year I had mono along with three of my friends. I know it's caused by a virus that makes you sleepy and not want to eat and zaps energy. But my friends got better quickly. I stayed out of school for a month. It seems that the mono virus was harder on my body and tougher to get rid of. My mom thinks it's because we've had a lot of stress in the family. She may be right because I know I get better quicker from a cold when things at home are cool."

Modified from Perrin EC, Gerrity PS: There's a demon in your belly: Children's understanding of concepts regarding illness. *Pediatrics* 67:841, 1981. In Levine MD, Carey WB, Crocker AC (eds): *Developmental-Behavioral Pediatrics*, 2nd ed. Philadelphia, WB Saunders, 1992, p 306.

TABLE 26–3   **TEACHER–Method for Enhancing Communication with Pediatric Patients and Their Parents**

T	Trust	Build trust and rapport with the child by asking nonthreatening questions not related to the illness.
E	Elicit	Elicit information from the parent(s) and child regarding parental fears and concerns and the child's understanding of the reason for the visit.
A	Agenda	Set an agenda early in the visit to help ensure that the parents' concerns are addressed.
C	Control	Help the child feel control over the visit (e.g., knowing what will and will not happen) to help decrease fear and increase cooperation.
H	Health plan	Establish a health plan with the child and parent to meet the child's needs and limitations.
E	Explain	Explain the health plan to the child in a way he can understand.
R	Rehearse	Have the child rehearse the health plan as a way of assessing understanding; reinforce the child's jobs related to health care; explore any potential problems in the plan with the child and parent.

From Bernzweig J, Pantell R, Lewis CC: Talking with children. In Parker S, Zuckerman B (eds): *Behavioral and Developmental Pediatrics*. New York, Little, Brown, 1995, p 7.

TEACHER mnemonic is a useful technique to improve the quality of communication with children and their parents at the time of a pediatric illness visit (Table 26–3).

Further probing of the case of Stacy, the 13-year-old girl with recurrent sore throats, revealed several family members with irritable bowel syndrome, tension, headaches and chronic low back pain. Her maternal grandfather had acute rheumatic fever as a child, and her mother grew up in a family that feared the medical consequences of acute pharyngitis. A pattern of somatization, coupled with an exaggerated fear of a mild sore throat, suggested to the clinician that to break the generational transmission of vulnerability to minor illness, referral to a behavioral-developmental pediatrician or a family therapist was indicated.

Preventing a Parent's Misunderstanding about a Child's Condition

Pediatric clinicians can practice a form of preventive medicine in order to limit adverse psychosocial responses during the course of acute minor illnesses. Several strategies are available. Overdiagnosis of benign, often transient physical findings may lead to excessive parental concern or unnecessary restrictions. For example, a benign functional cardiac murmur may be managed in several ways: (1) do not mention it because it is so frequently found and inconsequential; (2) explain to the parents that it is a sound heard when listening to a normal heart in a healthy child, does not reflect any cardiac problems and will disappear as the child grows;

(3) tell the parents that "he has a murmur coming from the heart that is called a functional murmur … it's not really important and we won't worry about it." The latter explanation for some vulnerable families may predispose to "cardiac nondisease," a condition in which the parents leave the office uncertain of their child's cardiac status because of the vague explanation. Some parents may inappropriately restrict the child's activity or develop an inappropriate sense of vulnerability about the health of the child. Other physical findings that require clear explanation to prevent a "nondisease" problem include mild (physiological) adenopathy, tibial torsion, hydrocele, strawberry hemangioma and umbilical hernia. Such entities should be discussed cautiously and with careful thought. These "nondiseases" can easily create illness or a sense of vulnerability in a child, so "do no harm."

> Juan was born at 40 weeks' gestation after an uncomplicated labor and delivery. He was moderately jaundiced during his first office visit for a weight check after early discharge from the nursery. At 60 hours of age, his serum total bilirubin was 18 mg/dL, and he was 5% below his birthweight. Plans were initiated to begin home phototherapy, assist his mother with techniques for optimal breastfeeding and follow up his weight and bilirubin in 24 hours.

This case is an opportunity to educate parents about a problem that may appear serious or even life threatening to a parent but is characteristically benign and limited to the early neonatal period. Diagnostic and monitoring interventions (blood tests) and therapy (phototherapy accompanied by daily home nursing visits) are often overmedicalized by clinicians, nurses and other health personnel. In part this is because hyperbilirubinemia can be associated with serious consequences in some circumstances. However, a pediatrician should be able to manage the diagnosis and treatment of this condition with information for the parents that leaves little room for exaggerated worry. It is most likely a benign condition that will resolve spontaneously or with a few days of phototherapy, will not recur and will not have any lasting effect on the baby's growth and development. Without this kind of focused parent education, a common problem such as neonatal hyperbilirubinemia can induce in the new parents a lasting sense of vulnerability about the baby. A thoughtful clinician may want to review the neonatal course when the infant is 4 to 6 months old to be sure there is no distortion of events.

> Dr. Corsini saw a 9-month-old as a new patient. The parents reported that he was a "very small preemie," needed treatment for breathing problems and required phototherapy. They said they had to get his weight checked frequently. When the medical records arrived, they stated that the infant was born at $36^1/_2$ weeks, weight was appropriate for gestational age, and the baby was monitored in the neonatal intensive care unit for 12 hours after birth without problems. He underwent phototherapy for 24 hours with a peak bilirubin level of 13 mg/dL. Note: The parents experienced a serious neonatal illness in their child, whereas the clinician saw this as an excellent course. These opposing views need to be exposed and remodeled.

Direct, age-appropriate and honest explanations during acute illness visits help children and parents understand and adapt to each situation. Dishonesty ("the shot the nurse will give won't hurt you"), belittling a child's feelings ("your belly really doesn't hurt that much") and preoccupation with the disease (medical diagnosis) demonstrate limited attention to the patient's perceptions and style of coping with disease and are risk factors for adverse behavior in children. Separation of children from their parents during a procedure should be avoided. A parent's presence usually serves to anchor a frightened child.

Donnie came to the office for a health supervision visit at 3 years of age. His mother remarked that his behavior had changed dramatically in the past month. After a year of feeding himself and learning to use a cup and spoon, he now wanted his mother to help feed him. His language became "like a baby," and he used fewer words than before. He wanted to be held more often and cried when left with a sitter or about simple frustrations that he had managed with less emotional upset in the past.

His pediatrician, at first alarmed by the recent history of acute regression in social, motor and language milestones, asked a critical question, "Did anything out of the ordinary occur to Donnie just before the changes in his behavior?" In fact, he had been to the emergency room for treatment of a small scalp laceration from a fall onto a coffee table. Restraints were used during the procedure, and his parents (inappropriately) were asked to leave the treatment room.

After a normal physical examination, the pediatrician explained to Donnie's mother that Donnie most likely reacted to the stressful emergency room encounter with developmental regression ("He lost some of his skills as a way to cope with the stressful experience of the emergency department visit."), which is one of the few coping mechanisms available to a toddler. The pediatrician guided Donnie through a play experience with a doll (available in a drawer in the examining room) "who went to the doctor to get a hurt fixed up." His mother was encouraged to use the play technique at home a few times. She phoned the pediatrician 2 weeks later and reported resolution of the regression and reestablishment of his previous developmental skills.

POSITIVE ASPECTS OF ACUTE ILLNESS

Parmelee has suggested that the multiple experiences with acute illness, a characteristic of everyone's childhood, guides the process of **social competence**. The manner and style of each family's response to an illness shape the child's sense of self and his coping strategies. From an experience with overindulgence in response to a simple cold to denial of the symptoms when a child is uncomfortable or in pain ("let's move on, get well and return to school"), children are exposed to a variety of adult responses to symptoms as they experience an illness associated with fatigue and vulnerability (Box 26–1). Discovering the nurturing value of chicken soup must be balanced against the risk of overindulgence. Children learn what it means to be sick, what rituals are involved in that state and that they will get well with time. A sense of the body and what it means to be cared for by a parent are the positive aspects of an illness.

Children often regress in their development in response to even minor illness. Those milestones that have been achieved most recently are vulnerable to temporary loss. Expressive language and self-regulation skills such as feeding, sleeping and toilet training are most

---

BOX 26-1 WHAT CHILDREN CAN LEARN DURING ACUTE ILLNESS

An important social lesson learned is that there is an appropriate time to let others take care of us so that we may recover as rapidly as possible and resume our usual activities. Making the decision to let others care for us in timely fashion is essential to restoring wellness. Learning when and how to do this is one of the aspects of general social competence that is learned in childhood.

From Parmelee AJ Jr: Illness and development of a social conscience. *J Dev Behav Pediatr* 18:120, 1997.

---

vulnerable. Parents can be guided to anticipate some degree of **developmental regression** in all children during an illness. Parents may get a chance to "baby" a child again, an indulgence that they may miss from an earlier time.

Tiffany, a healthy 8-year-old girl, developed acute vomiting, diarrhea and a low-grade fever. She visited her pediatrician, who diagnosed acute viral gastroenteritis and prescribed fluids, a bland diet and bed rest. Her mother stayed home from work for 2 days and provided the prescribed nutrition and emotional comfort. She read stories and watched video movies as Tiffany improved. Tiffany enjoyed her mom's attention. She regressed to baby talk on occasion.

By the third day, Tiffany's symptoms had improved, with only mild loose stools. When her mother said it was time to return to school, Tiffany responded, "I want to stay home with you." Her mother then praised her for getting well quickly, noted that her healthy body healed without medication and let her daughter know how much she enjoyed helping her get well. Tiffany returned to school and the baby talk resolved.

Clinicians can help parents achieve a balance between reasonable indulgence and maintaining a goal of recovery. It is a delicate balance that should encourage the healing process while the child learns about the value of being cared for by another individual. For many families, various healing rituals that are transferred through generations provide positive expectations that teach coping mechanisms (see Chapter 3). The "sick role" and the "caretaker role" are defined by personal and cultural norms. Children learn these roles through such experiences.

CHRONIC ILLNESS

Primary care pediatric clinicians have considerably less experience with chronic illness than with acute illness in children. With the exception of asthma and attention deficit/hyperactivity disorder, conditions that have a prevalence of 5% and 6% to 9% in school-aged children, respectively, primary care clinicians who care for children typically do not see specific chronic disorders frequently. However, most pediatric practices are filled with one or more children with various chronic disorders managed by the pediatrician along with specialists. Caring for the psychosocial needs of children with chronic illness and their families can be guided effectively by a set of principles that simultaneously account for developmental considerations and the biology of the disease. A biopsychosocial approach to chronic illness does not require specific knowledge of a particular disorder's impact on a child. Substantial clinical benefits are derived from a generic approach to children and families with chronic disorders rather than an approach that views each disorder as distinct. Principles of managing a child with a chronic illness include

- Availability to answer family questions
- Helping families set specific goals in areas related to the child's condition and its effects on daily activities
- Ensuring coordination of health and other services
- Monitoring care over time, including specific plans for follow-up
- Updating and monitoring family knowledge on a periodic basis
- Counseling regarding family response to the condition
- Linking families with other families who have children with similar chronic conditions

Certain characteristics are common to all chronic health conditions; they transcend the specific nature of the illness. For example, respect psychological concerns. Behavioral problems and psychological disorders occur twice as often in children with most chronic illnesses as in children without a chronic illness. Effects on parents' work schedules, job stability, marriage and family finances are seen to variable degrees regardless of the specific illness. A family's adjustment to a child with a chronic illness does not correlate with the severity of the illness. Individual, family and community factors have a tremendous impact on adaptation and adjustment.

To establish a therapeutic alliance in which mutual trust guides the clinical dialogue and decision-making process, following guidelines for working with children and their families facing chronic illness can be useful (Table 26–4). After the initial assessment it is critical that the child's clinician begin to convey the impact of a chronic disorder on a child's patterns of living (at school, at home, with friends and with the family). When a cure is not the goal, realistic expectations for the amelioration of symptoms and adaptations to living should be made clear, even if only a short time frame is known. For treatment strategies to be effective, they must fit the daily activities of a child and family. The primary care clinician can negotiate and adapt schedules and regimens that are stressful or impossible without unduly compromising the quality of care. To be effective, this kind of planning requires knowledge about family life, family members and those who provide child care at different times.

Although identification of parental concerns (the parent's agenda for the visit) is critical to all pediatric clinical encounters, it is especially important when working with a child who has a chronic disorder. Ask the parent and child to identify those things that they most want to see changed. Ask them to establish the care priorities. Encouraging them to identify three concerns often leads to the discovery of one that can be relatively easy to address.

Eric, a boy with autism, was becoming increasingly disruptive in school and couldn't participate in his speech program. His family was fearful of working on a medication change with the psychiatrist because Eric's sleep had been disrupted by medication in the past. They felt they couldn't cope at all if Eric didn't sleep at night. The primary care physician helped them start a sleep diary and wrote a note to the psychiatrist about the family's priority and the school's concern.

TABLE 26–4   **Biopsychosocial Approach to Chronic Disease**

Approach	Action
Recognition of a chronic disorder	Help the child and family understand fluctuating symptoms, good days and bad days, amelioration of symptoms (vs. cure)
Treatment that should fit the pattern of the child's and family's daily activities	Use knowledge about family life, family members, schedules, roles, decision making, who provides care at various times
Assisting the child and family in identifying major concerns, priorities in care and outcome	Child, family and clinician have shared agenda Ask "What would you like to see changed?" Initially address only three concerns
Valuing and building on small successes	Set small goals, specific measures of progress

Effective use of a clinician's
  Skill
 	
  Patience
 	
  Persistence
	
	Help child and family articulate problems, strengths and goals
	Set realistic goals
	View the illness as chronic disorder for biological and psychosocial aspects of illness
	Plan follow-up visits, phone calls, periodic assessment

Adapted from Stein MT, Meltzer EO, Stein REK: Challenging case: Recurrent episodes of asthma in a 10 year old. *J Dev Behav Pediatr* 19:44, 1998.

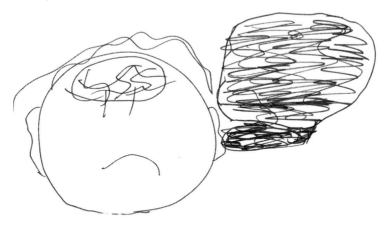

A migraine headache

A 12-year-old boy was asked to draw a picture of his (migraine) headache. The picture tells a great deal about the illness experience. By BL.

Success in working on a problem that the family perceives as important improves the opportunity to then work on more difficult problems and those that are important to the clinician as well. A clinician's sensitivity to treatable symptoms, whether they are physical, psychological or social, brings further opportunities to achieve these goals. Building a therapeutic relationship with a family through successful negotiation of realistic goals leads to small and large gains. Encouragement and reinforcement of each small success improve adherence to therapies and problem-solving skills.

POOR COMPLIANCE

When working with some parents of children with chronic disorders, it is not uncommon to find either poor adherence to a treatment or suboptimal adaptation to an illness after appropriate medications, advice, and education have been tried. This means it's time to pull back and approach the situation differently. These situations are opportunities to reframe the nature of the problem and try some new approaches. Returning to the **patient and parent agenda** model, it is useful to discuss with the child and family their perceptions of the illness and their experiences with trying to solve specific problems. The goal is to reframe the individual problems of the child with a disease as family problems that require a joint effort. Epstein has observed that "just as rapport and empathy facilitate self-disclosure and trust with individual patients, developing rapport by 'joining' the family and demonstrating understanding of each family member's perspective on a problem can facilitate collaborative problem solving. By adopting an attitude of active curiosity in learning each member's point of view, the clinician can convey a genuine interest in the family." This is the foundation for better compliance with any care plan or therapeutic effort. Participation of the family in the problem-solving process is illustrated when the traditional biomedical model is contrasted with a solution-building

Text continued on page 662

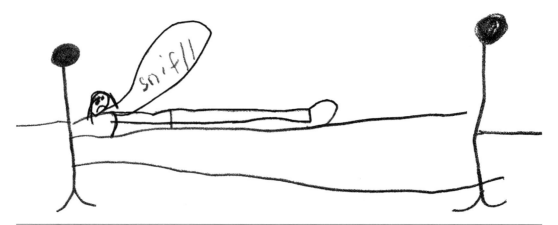

A girl draws a picture of what it is like to be sick with a cold. The bed seems stark and confining and the expression very sad. These "cinema noir" pictures are typical of children with acute illness. A brighter picture and a more sophisticated figure would be expected when she recovers. By Louise Dixon, age 7.

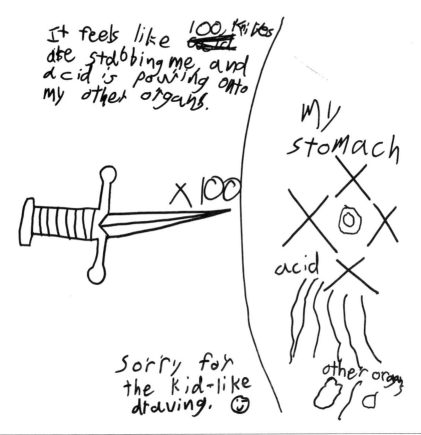

It feels like 100, ~~acid~~ knives ~~are~~ stabbing me, and acid is pouring onto my other organs.

× 100

My stomach

acid

Sorry for the kid-like drawing. 😊

other organs

A 12-year-old boy with severe abdominal pain illustrates it in this drawing. He lives with conflict between two families. His mom is severely ill.

TABLE 26–5   **Comparison of Approaches to Patients**

Issue	Biomedical	Solution Building with Family
Patient role	"Sick" patient; passive partner	Equal and active participants
Patient focus	Problems, dilemmas	Solutions
Expert	Clinician	Clinician, patient and family as problem solvers and solution builders
Encounter focus	Deficits, pathology of the individual; extended history of the problem	Strengths, competence of the family system; brief history of the problem; detailed history of goals and solutions
Therapeutic focus	Clinician's decisions	Clinician, patient and family develop solutions

Modified from Stein MT, Coleman WL, Epstein RM: We've tried everything, and nothing works: Family centered pediatrics and clinical problem solving. *J Dev Behav Pediatr* 18:118, 1997.

model that relies on the strength and competencies of the family (Table 26–5). Finally, when clinicians are sensitive to their own emotional reactions to families of children with a chronic illness, self-reflection helps them use their own particular strengths as they work within the **solution-building family model** of communication (see Chapter 4).

HOSPITALIZATION AND PROCEDURES

Hospitalization of a child involves removal of that child from a characteristically safe and nurturing environment within the home to a place populated by strangers, to a crib or bed that is unfamiliar, to a place with walls and floors that are different from home colors and to sounds that are new and, at times, cacophonous. The child may see people in uniforms for the first time. Procedures, examinations and treatments may be perceived as frighteningly invasive or affrontive. Any hospitalization, no matter how well managed, is stressful for the child. That stress can be a source of growth in experience and competence or can create additional illness complications and delay healing in its broadest sense.

The behavioral patterns of hospitalized children have received increasing attention in the past 50 years from research, clinical and child advocacy vantage points. In association with the emergence of hospitals and wards designed specifically for the needs of children, more attention has been given to the emotional needs and developmental capacities of children in hospitals. The American Association for the Care of Children in Hospitals has provided leadership in making these changes. Hospitals in general are better able to respond to the unique needs of children now than ever before. Family visiting and involvement, child life programs, school involvement and attention to psychosocial needs are now nearly routine. However, the clinician cannot rely on the institution alone to be supportive of the patient during the stress of hospitalization.

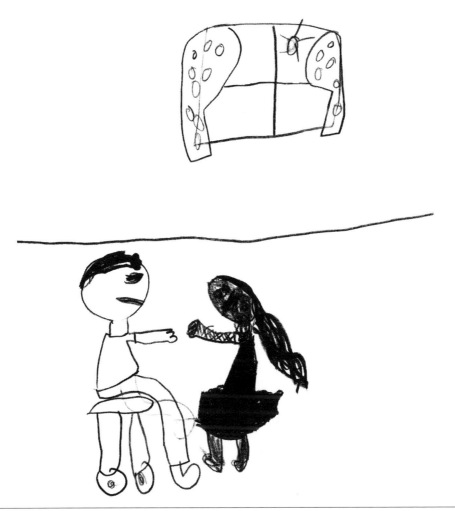

A girl shows a doctor applying an arm cast. The doctor is drawn only in outline, whereas the patient has long brown hair, a purple dress, red lips, blue eyes and a summer tan. Detail and color often signal importance, and the patient is clearly the center here. By Louise Dixon, age 7.

Impact of Hospitalization

The impact of hospitalization is significant when viewed from the perspective of a sudden environmental change. A hospital environment brings predictable alterations to a child's relationships with family members, peers and school activities. Perhaps most significantly, going to the hospital means a loss of the independence that is appropriate to the child's developmental level. Because the quest for independent activity and psychological autonomy begins at birth and is the energizing force that fuels development, most children are affected by the loss of independence when hospitalized. In addition, they may be stripped of their usual patterns of coping with stress (e.g., withdrawing to the bedroom, a temper tantrum at dinnertime, asking for and receiving more nurturing time from parents). This leaves them in a vulnerable, psychologically naked position. We expect their behavior to be altered.

Children develop attachments to important people throughout childhood. A child relies on these attachments to carry him through developmental hurdles and times of stress. The hospitalization experience varies among children, depending in some measure on the quality of those attachments and the developmental level of each child. In this context, the experience of separation (from mother, father or another significant caretaker) is the major psychological event that occurs when a child is hospitalized. She is deprived of the trust and security of having the loving person or persons present and responsive at all times of need. The psychological and physiological effects of separation are mediated to some extent by the child's ability to maintain the image of the primary caretaker or caretakers in her mind. This milestone in development is known as **object constancy** (see Chapter 13). It is a necessary cognitive skill, but it is not sufficient help for the child to weather the separation without stress. With this skill the child may be able to call forth the image of the primary caretaker without experiencing an overwhelming feeling of abandonment. The attachment figure's presence is maintained throughout the separation if the separation is relatively short and if the bond has been a strong one.

INFANT. When younger than 6 months, most infants seem to tolerate hospital experiences with minimal long-term behavioral or physiological reactions to **separation experiences**. Very young infants do distinguish parents and strangers in social interactions, so some transient change in behavior and responsiveness should be expected. The clinician will appreciate behavioral differences in the child when cared for by the parent rather than a nurse. These differences are data to support or refute the attachment between the parent and child. Although the close bond with the mother is described as "symbiotic," an infant younger than 6 months has not reached the stage of perceiving herself as an independent being to the point that separation appears threatening. A young infant may show behavioral reactions (fussiness, inconsolability, sleep disturbances) or physiological reactions (vomiting, constipation, poor weight gain, poor feeding) in response to a hospital experience. Young infants will begin to establish new relationships with sensitive, consistent caretakers and will build on these very quickly. Similarly, they will reestablish patterns of interactions with parents quickly after the separation, if it is brief. Alterations in sleep patterns and feeding may show the impact of hospitalization on the child's schedule and state regulation. The more that stays the same for the infant—schedules, objects and people—the less the stress.

TODDLER. Behavioral changes in a toddler are more dramatic and require a longer recovery phase. As she develops independence, the child has an accompanying awareness of the stress of separation. This response is particularly acute between the age of 8 months and 18 months. The toddler's concern is, "Will mommy come back?" She appreciates cognitively and emotionally that a strange environment without the parent's presence is threatening and overwhelming. She also lacks a sense of time, so she cannot appreciate a promise of a prompt return by the parent. Her anxiety remains chronically high. Temper tantrums, listlessness, refusal to eat, and sleep disturbances are characteristic responses of a normal toddler to a hospital setting without the presence of the parent. It is testimony to appropriate psychological growth. Regressive behavior in this situation should be seen as adaptive and appropriate because it allows for conservation of energy and a bid for help during this "crisis" situation. It usually subsides after hospitalization as long as the separation experience has not been too intense or prolonged and the attachment process has evolved normally before the hospitalization.

Normal toddlers who experience abrupt or prolonged separation from parents undergo a progression of behavioral patterns. Originally described by Bowlby, these phases allow the clinician to monitor the child's response to stress:

- **Protest** reaction—tantrums, refusal to eat, aggressive behavior.
- **Despair**—a quiet, withdrawn, sad appearance.
- **Denial**—the previously depressed, despairing toddler now appears outgoing and responsive to everyone indiscriminately and shows no differential response to familiar care providers.

This third stage attests to severe stress for the child, who is now resistant to engaging in deep relationships or unwilling to risk wide excursions into either negative or positive emotions. It is a conservative psychological mechanism and is evidence of the severity or chronicity of the insult to consistent caretaking. Red flags should appear when a child becomes the favorite of every nurse on the floor, offers no objection to examinations or makes extraordinary efforts to elicit interactions with every passerby. A sad, withdrawn toddler or one who is "too good" is a warning that there has been a serious psychological assault.

Language may play an important role in the toddler's reaction to hospitalization. Before the age of 18 months, the child's expressive language is limited; he may not understand hospital personnel, or they may not understand him. After 1 year of age, the toddler becomes acutely aware of this dissonance. After age 18 months to 2 years, the acceleration of expressive and receptive language provides the toddler the equipment to interact with others in a more advanced form and therefore to understand, at least in part, some of the strange people and events around him.

PRESCHOOLER. In contrast to the toddler's experience, a preschool child's response to hospitalization may call forth newly developed skills of imagination, verbal questioning and magical thinking to understand and deal with the acute stresses of a strange environment. A 4- to 5-year-old can tolerate the absence of parents for a longer period because she now understands that "out of sight is not out of mind." Her memory is better developed, and she can use words to call up images, talk about planned events and elicit conversations with hospital personnel. At the same time, cognitive thinking may produce distortions about causality, with associated fears, fantasies and body distortions. Children at this age may feel personally responsible for their illness or that they did something wrong that caused their parents to bring them to the hospital. Causal relationships may depend on the child's perception of the temporal or spatial placement of events. Linkage occurs automatically as the child generates her own hypotheses regarding events around her. These **"explanatory models"** may be resistant to change, no matter how many "facts" the parent or clinician provides.

SCHOOL-AGE CHILD. A hospitalized school-age child is often able to develop peer group friendships and attachments to nurses, physicians and other personnel that may buffer the feelings arising from a separation. Increasing verbal skills and the capacity to understand causality allow a school-age child to gain more mental control over the situation. He understands the basic causes of illness and the logic of treatment. Multidimensional causal models will be beyond his understanding. One thing causes a specific problem in his mind. However, the child may be able to exercise more options in his treatment and participate in his own care if these options are concrete and specific and make some sense to him, given his own understanding of the disease.

The hospital experience may become stressful for a school-age child because he may experience a lack of control and feelings of guilt and anger. A loss of internal control, with subsequent behavioral manifestations of depression, anxiety or behavioral regression, can be expected. The concept of *locus of control* (a feeling of either internal or external control of events or an illness) may at times be useful in understanding and navigating a child through a stressful hospital experience. This approach encourages greater clarity of what's happening and what control and choices he has. The loss of school relationships and fear of getting behind scholastically and socially may add to the distress for a child of this age.

ADOLESCENT. As the child reaches adolescence, the toddler theme of independence versus dependence takes on a more advanced stage of negotiation in the form of a quest for personal identity separate from the family. A hospital experience, as well as the disease process, confronts the adolescent's identity directly. The loss of an idealized self as a result of the disease, coupled with an abrupt separation from peer group and activities, may bring about psychological distress in a hospitalized teenager. The disease process, coupled with invasive hospital procedures, may distort the adolescent's concept of body image and disrupt future plans, real or imagined. Although an adolescent possesses the cognitive ability to understand multiple and somewhat abstract causality with regard to illness and the need for hospitalization and treatment, the psychological turmoil may be dominant. Fantasies of the future may be encroached on by visions of deformities and disabilities. Age-appropriate independence may be distorted by the need for care, increased dependence and disruptions of social support.

Developmental Regression

Children of all age groups can be expected to demonstrate a loss of some developmental milestones during and after a hospital experience (see Table 24–3). The intensity and duration of developmental regression are controlled by several determinants that have both preventive and therapeutic implications for the clinician:

- The child's developmental level with regard to social and language skills.
- Personality and temperament—what kind of child was she before hospitalization? The quality of the reaction to a separation experience will vary not only with the developmental level but also with the unique temperament of each child (see Chapter 2).
- Previous styles of coping with new situations.

- Characteristics of the illness—duration, acuteness, severity, invasive procedures, immobilization, isolation.

- Family's response to the illness—the behavioral reactions of close relatives may influence the child's behavior. Is denial, rejection or overpermissiveness apparent?

- Fears and fantasies—Ask the child, "What do you think is wrong with you?" or "Why are you in the hospital?" Observation of play or review of the child's drawings (see Chapter 5) or fantasies that are based on her own explanatory model of the illness.

In an attempt to lessen the adverse reactions of children to the hospital experience, pediatric professionals should not lose sight of the fact that *developmental regression symbolizes both a stress and a protective maneuver* to defend against the loss of parent or parents and settle into the hospital experience. In this sense, behavioral alterations in the hospital may be adaptive and represent a healthy response to the experience. For example, a toddler's mild to moderate protest is an appropriate adaptation to a strange new world that is inhabited by a new crib, an intravenous line and numerous nurses and physicians. Preparing parents for these responses to hospitalization may help them understand their adaptive significance.

MEASURES TO HELP CHILDREN WITH HOSPITALIZATION AND PROCEDURES

Pediatricians and other providers of health care for children may be advocates for their patients when hospitalization or a painful procedure is being considered by attending to the following issues:

- *Avoid hospitalization when possible.* When diagnostic or therapeutic procedures can be accomplished without hospital admission, do not hospitalize the child. Outpatient procedures usually allow more parent participation, which may lessen the stress on the child. Outpatient surgical units for children provide the child a hospital experience without an overnight stay. Short stays with home nursing follow-up will also lessen the impact.

- *Provide parents and the child with an age-appropriate explanation for the hospitalization.* Ask a verbal child, "Why do you think you must come to the hospital?"

- *For elective procedures (e.g., hernia repair, cardiac catheterization, myringotomy), provide the child with a description of the hospital setting and the procedures that will be encountered before anesthesia.* Children's books, coloring books and doctor-nurse toys may assist the child in preparing for the new experience. Some hospitals arrange tours through the children's facility to acquaint parents and children with the setting, uniforms and routines before hospitalization. Tours have been shown to lessen fears, fantasies and behavioral symptoms during the following year for children in the preschool years and beyond.

- *Encourage a rooming-in policy for parents and encourage family members to be present as much as possible.* The parent's presence in the hospital may assist the child in his adaptation to the new setting by helping him master separation anxiety and self-control. Rooming-in may give parents the opportunity to assist in the care of the child and may lessen parental feelings of losing control over their child. Parent participation in hospital care is so beneficial to the well-being of children that it outweighs the occasional problems that parents may bring to the nursing or medical staff. When one nurse from each shift cares for the child during the entire hospitalization, the child and the parents may benefit by developing feelings of attachment and trust. It is the practice in some hospitals that serve children to involve parents during the induction of anesthesia. This is carried out in a special room adjacent to the operating room. Although it is difficult to document a beneficial behavioral effect from these child-oriented interventions, they deserve consideration in planning hospital policies along with further careful study.

- *Hospitalize children in a pediatric setting that is appropriately designed for children.* Colors and pictures on the walls should be child oriented. Toys in a play room that provide flexibility of movement should be available; play is the "work" of childhood, and in this role it provides children with an opportunity for symbolic expression of concerns and fantasies. The mere act of playing can be therapeutic.

- Encourage the parents to bring a few familiar toys and books or a "lovey" as a way to lessen the effects of the separation. Keep as many things as possible the same.

- Pediatricians must have knowledge about the need to improve recognition and management of pain in children. Recently, the American Academy of Pediatrics endorsed the policy that "Acute pain is one of the most common adverse stimuli experienced by children, occurring as a result of injury, illness and necessary medical procedures. It is associated with increased anxiety, avoidance, somatic symptoms and increased parent distress. Despite the magnitude of effects that acute pain can have on a child, it is often inadequately assessed and treated. . . . Pediatricians are responsible for eliminating or assuaging pain and suffering in children when possible."

- Be truthful about procedures. Children are not helped by statements such as, "It won't hurt," if it will. Mistrust builds anxiety. When painful procedures are planned, an explanation just before the procedure that "it will hurt for a moment" prepares a child older than 2 in an honest manner.

- Provide realistic options for the child and age-appropriate opportunities for her to participate in her own care by making as many choices as possible. Set clear, simple limits and expectations on behavior as much as possible. For anxious parents, clear directions for their participation can ease anxiety.

- When possible, allow the child to participate in medical care. Child-centered health care allows children to feel that they have some control over their bodies, even at a time of illness. For example, ask an older child, "Which arm would you like the blood test from?" "What color gown do you want today?"

- Identify sensory information, cognitive interventions and coping strategies. A description of each part of a planned procedure and the purpose behind it may focus on particular sensations that the child will experience. Relaxation techniques, self-talk and distracting imagery can be combined to block out unpleasant sensations. Distraction reduces pain by redirecting the child's attention away from the painful stimulus and toward a pleasant experience. During a painful procedure, children can be distracted by blowing bubbles, hand holding, whistling, singing, storytelling, puppets and visual or auditory engagement with toys. Unpleasant procedures experienced by infants can be modified by rocking, singing, sucking and even playing peek-a-boo.

- *Pain management.* In some pediatric centers, pain management has reached sophisticated levels in the form of hypnosis and other distraction-relaxation techniques. Many of these techniques can be adapted to pediatric office practice. Children can be engaged in these techniques. Though particularly beneficial in children who experience recurrent painful or aversive procedures (e.g., cancer treatment, renal dialysis), distraction-relaxation techniques can be used successfully during common outpatient procedures such as injections, heel sticks, intravenous placement, venipuncture, bladder catheterization and lumbar puncture. After the induction of a relaxed physical state through slow, deep breathing and progressive relaxation, a child's fantasy and imagination can be used in the form of guided imagery to modify unpleasant or painful experiences.

- *Use safe medications to eliminate or modify pain during procedures.* Examples of this practice include topical analgesia for venipuncture and intravenous line insertion (e.g., a eutectic mixture of lidocaine and prilocaine, EMLA) and a dorsal penile block for circumcision. Oral sucrose is an effective analgesic in newborn infants. When the pain-relieving effect of oral sucrose is enhanced with non-nutritive sucking and holding by a parent during immunizations, crying and parental stress are significantly reduced.

The desired outcomes for a hospitalized child are that the child heal as quickly and completely as possible, that he be supported in an appropriate manner through recognition of his developmental needs and that he be given the opportunity to grow from the experience. The clinician's role is to understand and support the child's developmental work while caring for the child's physical illness. The clinician must monitor the environment to ensure that it is providing the appropriate support. The parents must be provided with expectations for their child's physical and psychological recovery. They should emerge from the experience of their child's hospitalization as better parents, as better observers of their child's physical and mental health, as better participants in the healing process and with an enhanced sense of competency as guardians of their child's health. The child's physician must support these processes through knowledge and sensitivity.

HEADS UP–ILLNESS

- Be mindful of the difference between an illness and disease at each medical encounter. It's the difference between a child's/parent's perception of the experience of being ill and the medical formulation of the problem.
- Regressions in development and/or behavior during an illness are common and often necessary to support self-esteem and the integrity of the family.
- When adherence to a therapeutic recommendation is poor, reevaluate the parent's agenda and priorities, consider a culturally dependant explanatory model for the disease that is different from your own and make use of the solution-building family model of negotiation and dialogue.

Continued

HEADS UP–ILLNESS–cont'd

- Frequently ask, "Have I considered that the experience of this office visit is shaping the way this child learns about her body, physical symptoms, illness and the process of healing?" Asking the question is the initial step in changing communication techniques and procedures to enhance social competency and self-esteem.
- Recognize the child who is brought to your office frequently for minor somatic or behavioral concerns. When a medical assessment consistently rules out physical illness, is it an opportunity to explore acute or chronic stress in the family (social, economic and psychological) or the presence of a vulnerable child syndrome.
- Medical problems that are benign or self-limited are often perceived as more serious by parents who then inappropriately restrict activities and perceive their child as fragile. Examples include a benign cardiac murmur, uncomplicated neonatal jaundice or an umbilical hernia. Anticipatory guidance that focuses on clarification of the benign or self-limited nature of the problem goes a long way in preventing unnecessary long-term anxiety or restrictions.
- Behavioral problems and psychological disorders occur twice as often in children with most chronic diseases. Monitor behavior carefully in these children.
- A hospital experience is a major psychosocial shift in the experience of all children and adolescents. Clinicians who are aware of the developmental significance of this experience at different stages in development are prepared to provide education and anticipatory guidance while helping the parents and hospital staff understand and ameliorate difficult behavior and regressions.
- Cognitive and behavioral strategies, as well as the use of safe pain-relieving medications, should be considered during routine office procedures, hospitalizations or outpatient procedures.

RECOMMENDED READINGS

For Children

Berenstain S, Berenstain J: *The Berenstain Bears: Go to the Doctor.* New York, Random House, 1981 (4–8 years).
Cole J, Degan B: *The Magic School Bus: Inside the Human Body.* New York, Scholastic, 1990 (6–9 years).
Jennings S, Clark B, Bourgeois P, Southern S: *Franklin Goes to the Hospital.* New York, Scholastic, 2000.
Walker R: *Encyclopedia of the Human Body.* London, Dorling Kindersley, 2002 (school age and adolescence).

For Parents

Prentice R, Keene N: *Your Child in the Hospital: A Practical Guide for Parents,* 2nd ed. O'Reilly & Associates, Sebastopol, CA, 1999. Available at http://www.oreilly.com.

For Clinicians

Bergman AB, Stamm SJ: The morbidity of cardiac nondisease in school children. *N Engl J Med* 276:1008, 1967.
Kharasch S, Saxe G, Zuckerman B: Pain treatment: Opportunities and challenges. *Arch Pediatr Adolesc Med* 157:1054, 2003.
Parmelee AJ Jr: Illness and the development of social competence. *J Dev Behav Pediatr* 18:120, 1997.
Perrin EC, Gerrity PS: There's a demon in your belly: Children's understanding of concepts regarding illness. *Pediatrics* 67:841, 1981.
Sugarman LI: Hypnosis: Teaching children self-regulation. *Pediatr Rev* 17:5, 1996.

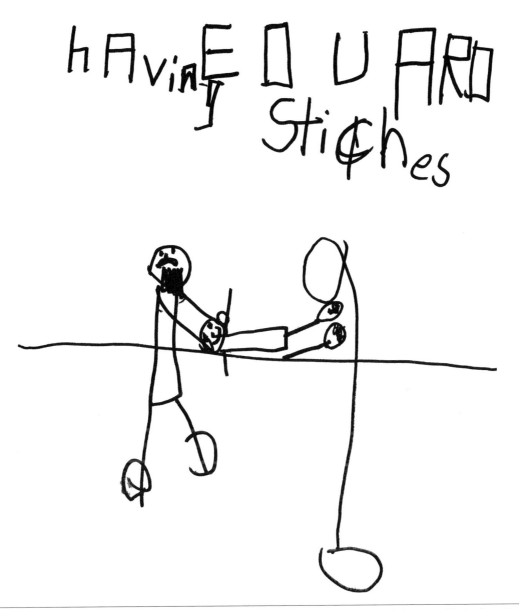

"Having stitches." A boy, age 6, shows his doctor fixing him up. The nurse is less well drawn and is faceless. The lack of hands and disconnected leg might suggest a sense of losing control, of powerlessness in the situation.

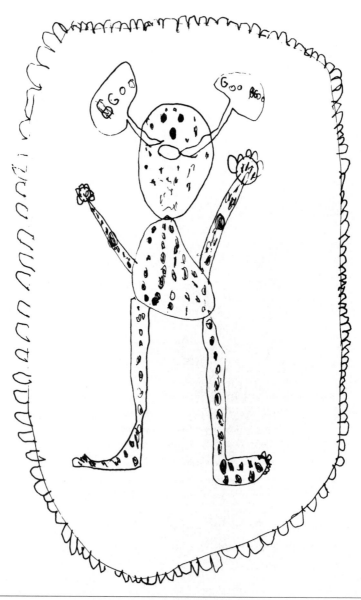

A boy, age 7, draws his baby brother with chickenpox. The blanket serves as an enclosure, perhaps reflecting the boy's distancing himself from the baby's predicament.

CHAPTER 27

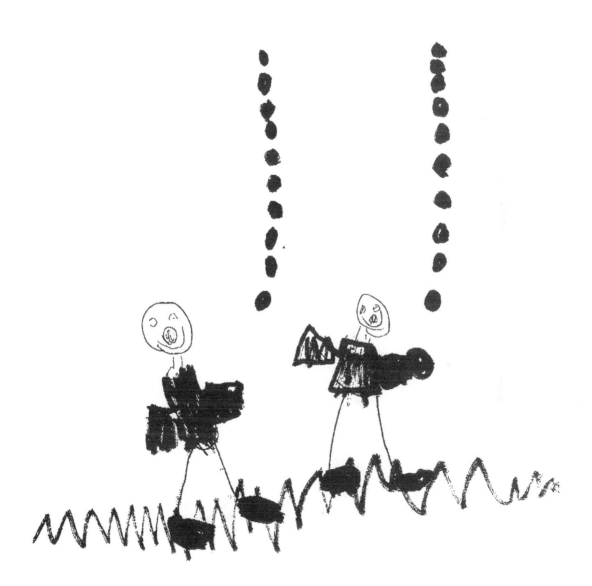

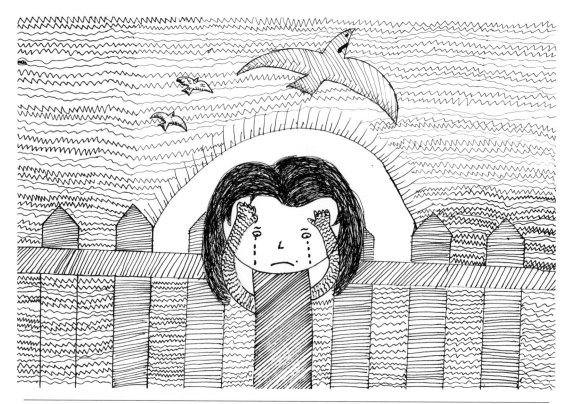

A teen uses simple geometrical shapes to convey a sense of hope (as well as sorrow). By Sherey Harris, age 18.

Stressful Events: Separation, Loss, Violence and Death

MARIA TROZZI and SUZANNE DIXON

This chapter describes children's emotional responses to the significant loss events that touch their lives, including their responses to death, family disruption and exposure to violence.

Key Words

- Children's Understanding of Death
- Grief Reactions
- Suicide
- Sibling Loss
- Divorce and Separation
- Parental Loss
- Violence and Trauma
- Terrorism

Losses are an inevitable part of the landscape of childhood. Examples are the first time an infant is aware of her mother's momentary absence, a toddler's struggle with separation at bedtime and a preschooler's brave leap from a safe, known environment to the bigger world of a school. However, with each loss comes an opportunity for growth, and in each successful resolution and adaptation to loss come increased coping skills and a greater sense of self.

In contrast to the normal losses we expect as part of the progress of normal development, a death—even though an inevitable part of the life cycle—presents a true crisis to a child. Exposure to extraordinary events such as violence close to home and terrorism near or far brings special challenge. The Chinese express the concept of crisis when they write the word as a combination of two pictographs—one representing danger and the other, opportunity. A child usually needs help to realize the opportunity in any loss situation. The clinician can help by seeing any of these crises through a child's eyes and then mobilizing support for the child as needed. A risk will then become an opportunity for growth.

This chapter focuses on the conceptual assumptions, interventions and insights that will help clinicians provide monitoring and assistance to bereaved children and their families. Age-specific stressors of childhood are discussed in the context of loss and grieving in order to guide support by a clinician. We discuss developmental responses associated with the death of a close family member to provide a framework of how a child experiences losses in general. These fundamental concepts should inform the clinician of how a child might experience other losses.

675

CHILDREN'S UNDERSTANDING OF DEATH: DEVELOPMENTAL PERSPECTIVE

A simple child
That lightly draws its breath
And feels its life in every limb
What should it know of death?
       —WORDSWORTH

For adults, death is a disruption in their usual "steady state" and results in a sense of disequilibrium. **Children's understanding of death** is different, however. For children, death usually also represents a developmental interference that results in a suspension of their ongoing cognitive and emotional growth. It is this "stall factor" that must be taken into account for children at different developmental stages. The goal of clinical intervention with children is to get them "unstuck," to help them get through, over, under or around a temporary barrier to their normal and healthy forward movement. The health provider should view the child's ability to cope with a significant loss or death in relation to specific factors (Box 27–1).

BOX 27–1   INDIVIDUAL FACTORS THAT INFLUENCE ABILITY TO COPE WITH LOSS

- The child's ability to make sense of the death from the perspective of his own developmental level
- The child's history of loss and death
- Repeated and/or multiple losses that diminish capacity to cope
- The child's normal ability to cope with change, temperament and situational stress

---

DEVELOPMENTAL FRAMEWORK

Much of our understanding about how children perceive death is derived from Piaget's theories about children's cognitive development (see Chapter 2). This framework is a helpful starting point in assessing a child's reaction to the death of a loved one. Remember, however, that children regress under stress such as a major loss, and changes in the age and stage boundaries to more "primitive" responses may be seen in such circumstances. These changes in response to death are meant as broad guidelines only and are presented in Table 27–1.

Infants (0 to 2 Years)

Before age 3, infants and toddlers have no cognitive conceptualization of death. Its effect on them is linked to what is lost, to the relationship to a significant other and to the consistency that is or is not part of their life. Bowlby made a significant contribution to our thinking about attachment and loss by pointing out that even infants and toddlers who experience maternal separation grieve:

TABLE 27–1   **Children's Understanding of Death at Different Ages**

Age	Understanding
Infants	Have no cognitive understanding of death. Death is the same as a significant separation
0–2 yr	Respond to changes in routine, caregivers, emotional chaos of family situation Experience separation anxiety, irritability and regression
Preschoolers (3–5 yr)	Death is temporary, reversible, living under different circumstances Literal thinking about causes Link seemingly unrelated factors to the death (transductive reasoning) Use magical thinking to explain death
School age (6–8 yr)	Death is final, irreversible, but not universal See death as a person or spirit that catches you Death "catches" the elderly, disabled, klutzes May be contagious Concerned with safety, predictability Need for details
Preadolescents (9–12 yr)	Adult understanding: death is final, irreversible, universal Disconnect between thinking and emotions Understand the biological aspects of death Interested in rituals, roles, ceremonies Understand causality: may feel guilty about contributing to it Intellectualize death: thoughts more available than feelings
Adolescents (13–18 yr)	Adult understanding: death is final, irreversible, universal Engage in high-risk activities (challenge own mortality) Understand existential implications of death Reject adult rituals and support May see some aspects of stigma

If a child is taken from his mother's care at this age (18 to 24 months), when he is so possessively and passionately attached to her, it is indeed as if his world has been shattered. His intense need of her is unsatisfied, and the frustration and longing may send him frantic with grief. It takes an exercise of imagination to sense the intensity of this distress. He is as overwhelmed as any adult who has lost a beloved person by death. To the child of 2 with his lack of understanding and complete inability to tolerate frustration, it is really as if his mother had died. He does not know death, but only absence; and if the only person who can satisfy his imperative need is absent, she might as well be dead (Bowlby, 1969).

It seems indisputable that infants and toddlers react strongly to the loss of a meaningful person and show their **grief reactions** in alterations in behavior. However, what is controversial is whether the very youngest child is capable of mourning without a mature understanding of the meaning of the loss. Behavioral change indicative of internal stress is expected when an infant loses a significant care provider. Consistency in care, attentiveness, and emotional responsiveness are needed if the infant is to continue to thrive. These are the essential elements that are lost to an infant who loses a primary care provider.

A significant loss in an infant may be expressed as irritability, whining, loss of self-care abilities such as self-feeding, withdrawal, increases in aggression, poor feeding, and sleep disturbances.

The following suggestions may be useful in the case of loss of a parental figure:

- If the deceased was the infant's primary caregiver, identify a permanent surrogate caregiver as soon as possible. Don't divide the job or delay in this designation if at all possible. Consistency is key to coping.

- Learn the deceased caregiver's routines; keep the same as much as possible.

- Provide a consistent, nurturing, dependable environment. Overindulgence may actually impede the infant's adjustment.

- Be prepared for regression in behavior and developmental competency. This regression may even have a delayed onset.

Preschooler (3 to 5 Years)

Preschoolers have a concept of death, but they view it as temporary or reversible, as going someplace else or as changing in a reversible way.

 Four-year-old Alexandra, whose grandfather died the previous Christmas, proudly showed her aunt a picture she had drawn on Christmas Eve and said, "Last year Papa was very sick and he died. But this year he's coming back on Christmas." With that said, she placed her little drawing under the Christmas tree, awaiting his return.

Children this age want and expect to continue a relationship with their deceased loved one through prayers, writing or engaging in one-sided conversations. They think the person is coming back. Children who place the deceased loved one in heaven want to visit, call or write to him. Their thinking tends to be egocentric, that the death was caused by or was linked to their own actions or that the cause is magical. They often attribute faulty thinking to the death or define associations based on their own rule structure and make spurious associations.

When a 3-year-old child died in daycare after choking on a grape, her little classmates concluded that "Sally died because she ate her dessert before her sandwich."

Preschoolers need simple, straightforward explanations of death, what it means in concrete forms. "Grandpa died. His body totally stopped working." Many preschoolers will need help to operationally define death by answering specific questions: "Can he eat? Can he sleep? Does he still dream? Does he go to the bathroom? Will he breathe under the ground? Can he hear me in heaven? Does he need his wheelchair still?" Be particularly careful to respond with concrete, simple explanations to these kinds of queries. Avoid euphemisms like "lost," "sleeping," "passed," "with the angels." At best they confuse young children. At worst, they terrify them.

In explaining death to their young children, adults often jump immediately to their own spiritual beliefs. Although this can be comforting and in general should be part of the process, it may also be confusing. For instance, preschool children are perplexed by how the body and spirit can simultaneously be in the grave and in heaven. One preschooler found for himself an adequate explanation: "The insides go up, and the outsides go down!" Adults should be careful of elaborate stories about heaven that suggest a composite of Disney World and Nintendo or stories about Uncle Henry dancing with angels. Children in the preschool age take these stories completely literally. Although religious beliefs need to be shared with young children, they usually require some explanation and many opportunities to bring up the child's specific questions, no matter how concrete or even disturbing they may be to the adults.

A bereaved parent told her 5-year-old child that "the angels came down and took your baby sister," after the baby had died of sudden infant death syndrome during the Christmas season. Six weeks later, 5-year-old Jeffrey was taken to a counselor because of an inability to sleep at night. When asked to tell the counselor about his baby sister, he said, "I don't want to talk about her. I want to talk about angels. There's two things to know about angels. There are lots of them, and they're on the loose at Christmas. And, they don't have headlights. So you can't see them coming and you have to stay awake at night so they won't get you."

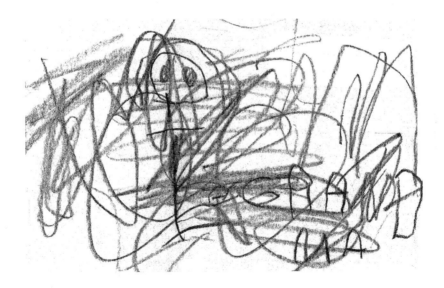

A 4-year-old girl draws her grandmother in the year after her death. The figure is primitive compared with the writing beside it. It is orange, but scribbled all over with gray. The drawing level often goes down when stressful emotions are being expressed. Scribbled over scenes often mean depression or sadness. By Louise Dixon, age 4.

School Age (6 to 8 Years)

Children of school age understand death to be final and irreversible, but *not universal.* They know that people who die stay dead, but they don't think that they themselves will die. Death is often personalized, perceived as a male Darth Vader–like character who can grab you at any unsuspected time, a dangerous and wily presence. Those who are vulnerable can't run (e.g., elderly, physically disabled). All the others who get caught must be klutzes. This explanation works at this age to allow the child to distance and defend himself from death. However, unlike younger children, a death presents him with the challenge of questioning his and others' safety. "Is life still safe?" becomes an overriding question. An ongoing sense of impending disaster or unpredictable happenings exists unless the safety issue is addressed. Disruption of one's own life is also seen as a threat to safety. So again, reassurance of continuity and consistency adds to a sense of safety.

Six-year-old Beth was vacationing with her parents when her mother was struck by a car while crossing a Vermont country road at dusk and died. Beth reasoned thereafter that crossing the street led to disaster. Understandably, she refused to cross any streets after her mother's death. At the September start of school, her teachers were worried about how to handle this issue, especially because the temporary playground was across a busy street. Their solution was to allow her to stay in at recess with the school nurse. After consultation with a mental health professional, they understood that being motherless is isolating enough; any further separation would not only exacerbate the isolation but also ultimately lead to the challenge of weaning her from this temporary solution. They decided instead to "normalize" her fear of crossing the street and allow her and her classmates to strategize ways to stay safe while crossing. This plan was not only successful the first day of school, but within the first week, Beth had taken on the role of "crossing guard" for her class! What an opportunity for healing!

Predictability, that is, what will be the same versus what will be different because of this death, is an inescapable concern confronting a school-age child. The child needs direct, simple answers to what changes will happen that will affect her life. She may ask after a sibling's death, "Will I have my own room now? Can I have Jimmy's Nintendo?" Although adults may initially view these questions as egotistical and completely unfeeling, the child is really asking how his world will change fundamentally because of this death. Both the specifics and the general concern should be answered directly with support and assurance.

Other typical concerns prompted by a parent's death are illustrated by comments such as the following: "If Beth's mom died, are you (i.e., the parent) going to die also? Who will take care of me? Am I safe? Will I be safe?" Parents, particularly those in single-parent households, should face these important questions directly and seriously. It would *not* be useful to respond, "Don't worry about that" or "I'm too healthy to die." Remind the child that *everyone* dies some-day, but that unlike Beth's mom, most people live to be very, very, very old. "If I were to die, your Aunt Susie is prepared to care for you until you are grown up." Children are generally satisfied with that response, and it teaches them that you can talk about death, thus opening the door for more questions and voiced concerns.

Although discussing the details of a death, particularly the gross and grubby ones (e.g., What happens to the body? Was there blood? What did she look like?), is difficult for adults, most school-age children have a need for some details about these events to help them feel more in control of the overwhelming event by learning the specifics. What seems to be morbid curiosity to an adult is really the way for a child to get a handle on an incomprehensible situation. The emotional response will come later.

Adults in the child's life have an opportunity to face these questions with her, and by doing this, they are telling their child that they can face stressful life events together. In contrast, to refuse to discuss issues or to give flip answers sends the wrong message. "If it's unmentionable, it's unmanageable." Children are left with uncertainty, fear and no place to go to get their questions answered and their needs met. Emotional coping comes out of the knowledge base at this age, so first the facts, then the hugs.

Preadolescents (9 to 11 Years)

Preadolescents have an adult understanding of death: it is final, irreversible and universal. Most youngsters this age understand that everyone dies someday, even them, and that it is forever. This new awareness may actually heighten anxiety for youngsters this age as the result of an increased sense of vulnerability at this stage. They may view death as a punishment for bad behavior as they begin to explore moral development at this age. They are able to understand the biological aspects of death, such as what happens if the heart has a blockage or what effect a brain tumor has on life function. So physical causability is usually understood at this age, at least as final cause of death. In addition, they can understand the concept of specific and possible multiple causes and effects. That leads them to wonder about what part, if any, they may have played that contributed to a death. They may feel guilty in ways that they may not even understand; adults need to help them process such complicated ideas and emotions.

Preadolescents are fascinated with the religious and cultural rituals that surround death and display a curiosity about topics such as cremation, burial, embalming and the afterlife. Adults in their lives may find these questions disarming, particularly if they are without any coherent emotional display or if posed at inappropriate times. However, if approached in a straightforward way, youngsters are reminded that they can trust adults to give them useful information about "difficult to talk about" topics.

The Smiths were vacationing in Florida when they learned from their adult baby-sitter that their 4-year-old child had died after running into the street and being hit by a car. Bewildered and overcome with grief, they returned home on the next plane. When 12-year-old Christine faced her parents at the door, she smiled and asked," What did you bring me from Florida?"

This response, though infuriating to her parents, protected her from a display of overwhelming grief. Christine knew how to handle her parents' anger because she had probably seen it before; she was less prepared to respond to their presumable expression of overwhelming grief. "After all, if they fall apart, then who will take care of me?" was her unconscious motivation for turning around the emotional climate of the family. The 12-year-old's comments brought more predictable attention and energy from her parents.

Many preadolescents respond without a display of emotion or may even be sarcastic when faced with a loved one's death. They intellectualize death because *their thoughts are often more available to them than their feelings*. This bewilders and concerns most adults, who think that their typically sensitive and caring 11-year-old has been replaced with an insensitive creep. Feelings are typically buried under a very unattractive demeanor at this age. It takes a long time for youngsters at this age to identify and let out feelings.

Even adolescents continue to use magical thinking in their formulations of death, ideas that may be hidden but have profound effects on young people.

> Bob, 15, and his older brother Ted, 17, were playing basketball against the side of their grandmother's brick apartment building. Several times she opened the window of her third floor apartment and asked them to stop. Finally, she angrily yelled to them, "For the last time, stop. You boys will be the death of me!" Sadly, the next day, grandma suffered an aneurysm and died. In therapy, one of the boys revealed that he thought that they had killed their grandmother.

At any age, magical thinking should be uncovered and challenged. Simply ask the question, "What made your (mother, father, friend, pet) die? Why do you think he died?" Offer a simple statement of your own belief around the issue. And then wait. The child or adolescent has been given fuel to reconstruct his thinking and a supportive place to discuss it. The clinician may respond with, "Many young people have ideas like that—it's a way of saying we cared. But wishes do not make things happen. Bad thoughts can't harm people."

A preadolescent is dependent on the adults in her life to make life feel safe for her, especially in times of crisis such as a death. This may be very hard at this age because much behavior is as confusing as the thoughts and emotions of the child. Parents and other support people should remember to do the following:

- Be authentic. Kids pick up platitudes, gloss-overs and ambivalence like radar.
- Verbalize that in spite of your grief, you are still able to care for them. Help them feel that they are safe and that their lives will go on.
- Give them repeated opportunities to discuss the death, but don't push too hard. It will take weeks to months to get at feelings. Provide openings and then wait.
- Talk about your own grief and how your feelings influence your own behavior. Provide a prototype of how to behave with a loss.

> One winter morning, shortly after her father had died, Terry was removing a gallon of milk from the refrigerator door when it slipped out of her grasp and crashed to the floor. The children, seated at the kitchen table, were shocked to hear their mother scream and then sob. They quickly started to help with the cleanup. When Terry stopped crying, she faced her children and explained, "I'm having a bad morning. I am missing your Grampa terribly." She proceeded to help the children with the cleanup, and together they sat down to breakfast.

Children can face intensely difficult emotional times if the adults in their life continue to make them feel safe throughout. If this mom had run out of the room, leaving them without breakfast and without an explanation, the children may have felt abandoned by her. Explaining her display of emotion and continuing to care for them in spite of her feelings teaches them that grief and its intense emotions can be faced with the adults in their lives.

Adolescents (12 to 18 Years)

This period brings in several new cognitive abilities, emotional processes and developmental gains that have an impact on the experience of death.

- Adolescents are actively engaged in the normal developmental task of separation from the significant adults in their lives. A close death, such as the death of a parent or sibling, can derail this intense separation-individuation process and make the maturational process scary and overwhelming.

- Adolescents often engage in high-risk behavior, almost as though they need to "flirt with death." They are fascinated with death, but may be overwhelmed when it intrudes closely on their lives. This is hard for them to admit.

- Paradoxically, adolescents intellectually have an adult's understanding of death, but they behave as though they themselves were immortal. Many adolescents during this period will face the death of a peer, and it shatters all their fantasies of immortality. The intellectualization cover that is typical at this age may make it harder to get at such a devastating developmental and emotional experience. Peer loss is a huge event.

- Adolescents are capable of understanding the existential implications of death as they gain the ability to think abstractly. However, they may not have fully formed their understanding at this level before confronting a death. So these abstractions for the reasons, consequences and meaning of death may not be available to them on a personal level.

- Adolescents are interested in exploring society's attitudes about life and death. They will monitor how their immediate circle of family and friends, as well as the broader society, responds to, explains and grieves a death. They look to others to help make sense of these overwhelming events while seeming to ignore the usual conventions or to challenge beliefs.

Although teens often reject traditional adult rituals surrounding death and create their own with the help of their peers, they do need adults in their life to help them sort out the often colliding feelings of sadness, anger, disbelief and isolation. Adults may feel rejected when attempting to provide emotional support at this age. However, just their continued presence and availability during the crisis are therapeutic. Adults must interpret this distancing as developmentally appropriate and respect it while remaining available for reassurance and support.

Brendan, 16, became furious when his parents said they would attend the funeral of his beloved teacher who had died suddenly. The parents would have liked to attend the ceremony because they too knew the teacher. Brendan insisted that he was going with his friends and preferred that his parents not go. That evening he asked to play cards with his mom and just "hang out" at home. He said the service was "fine," making no further comments. Note: His parents would be wise to just leave the topic alone and deal the cards. Feelings and reactions will come later.

Parental Death; Long-Term Consequences

Parental loss has long-term consequences no matter when it occurs. For infants younger than 2 who lose parents, there is a risk of attachment disorders and serious emotional, cognitive and developmental problems unless someone steps in quickly. For preschoolers, a variety of somatic complaints, anxiety symptoms, clinginess and aggressive behavior would be typical. They may be overly responsible to take care of the surviving parent or blame themselves for the parent's death. This may take time to resolve or may linger as anxiety, depression or separation phobias.

Middle childhood parental loss may deal a blow to self-esteem and set up a child for short- and long-term emotional problems. Academic achievement and friendships are at risk, and they may even have a fear of being stigmatized by peers. The key here is the mental health of the surviving parent. An overly adult demeanor may mean the child feels too much responsibility. Difficulties with relationships may be present into adulthood.

Children older than 12 may become very anxious, have long-term difficulty with trust and may feel alienated from peers. They may harbor guilt about past behavior and are prone to a variety of complex emotional problems into adulthood. Help from outside as well as inside the family is usually needed.

SPECIAL CASE OF SUICIDE

Adolescent **suicide** is becoming an increasingly frequent tragedy. Statistics reveal that every day in this country, many youth between the ages of 13 and 25 will attempt suicide, and many will succeed. Why do so many adolescents attempt to kill themselves? Why, if they have an adult understanding of death, can they see "ending their lives" as an option? Unfortunately, adolescents deny the *physical* consequences of suicide. They are often unable to look beyond the act itself and fail to fully comprehend that the consequences of death are final and irreversible.

> Seventeen-year-old Amy was a senior at a prestigious prep school. She was bright and popular and had recently been accepted at her first-choice Ivy League college. One afternoon, three of her girlfriends betrayed her in a powerful secret. She was humiliated. That evening, she slashed her wrists in an attempted suicide. When the therapist asked her what she was thinking when she was hurting herself, she replied, "All I could think was, won't my friends be upset when they walk by the casket and see me lying there."

Adults who care for, teach and live with adolescents must help them face the stark reality of the act of suicide through clear discussion with them whenever a suicide is in the news or happens in their school or neighborhood. Conversation should emphasize facts such as the following:

- Suicide is killing yourself.
- People who commit suicide don't know how to get help to solve problems.
- You don't come back.

- It will not glorify your memory.
- It is a permanent solution to a temporary problem.
- Adolescents need to look for help with problem solving.
- No problem is solved by suicide.

CHILDREN'S GRIEF REACTIONS—SPECIAL CHARACTERISTICS

Children of all ages have *grief responses* that are different from those of adults. Their behavior must be understood as indicating grief so that appropriate support can be provided.

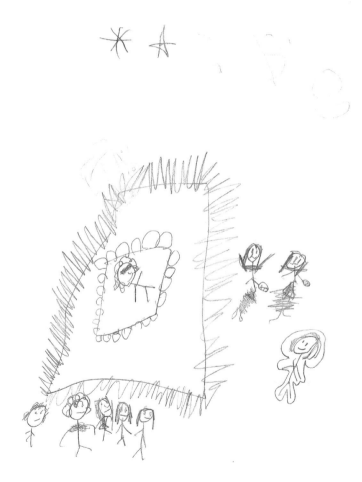

A 5-year-old shows her grandmother's burial. The coffin, on wheels, is placed in the grassy grave. Her grandmother is visible in the drawing, but her eyes are masked. The family is gathered at the bottom of the page. To the side we see Jesus and two angels, dancing, soon to be joined by grandma. By Dori Dedmon, age 6.

- *Children grieve in spurts.* Children fluctuate between expressions of anger, sadness, anxiety and confusion and then, in a moment, resumption of their normal behavior. They do not continuously show overt signs of grieving. This leads some to believe that children do not recognize the loss or understand its implications and therefore do not grieve appropriately. The behavior is adaptive, however, because children have a limited capacity to tolerate emotional pain and will pull away from it cognitively and emotionally when it all becomes too much for them. Adults might mistrust the child's intermittent display of intense feelings and see them as disingenuous. Children, even very young children, experience intensely painful responses that adults must understand within a developmental framework.

- *Children grieve longer than adults, contrary to popular thinking.* They *regrieve* the loss over and over again at each new stage in development as they change their perspective on themselves and the world around them and make more mature meaning of the significance of the past loss. The grief process recurs over and over.

> Kate was barely 5 when her mother died of lung cancer. Her only memories of her mother were of the illness. Now, 6 years later, she and her brother have adjusted to life with dad as the primary caregiver. However, when 11-year-old Kate brought home the school notice for the mother-daughter "Learning About Our Bodies" evening, she angrily threw it on the kitchen counter and said, "I'm not going!" When her father offered to go with her, Kate began to cry inconsolably. She ran upstairs to her room, slammed her door and refused to talk to her father for the rest of the evening. Note: As Kate grows through each developmental stage, being a "motherless daughter" takes on new meaning. Each event that marks her growing up, such as the first signs of puberty, the prom, graduation from high school, marriage, pregnancy and giving birth, also restimulates her grief of mother loss. Clinicians should keep past losses in mind when considering behavioral problems.

- **Childhood grief is manifested in *qualitatively different ways*.** Adults often think the child is not grieving after a loss because the emotions and behavior don't match the sad demeanor we expect. However, there may be marked changes in the child's behavior. Difficulty concentrating, heightened sibling squabbles, inappropriate and aggressive behavior, moodiness, withdrawal, disorganization, and temper tantrums are symptoms of grieving in childhood. Because of differences in cognitive ability and temperament, children are apt to use more primitive defense mechanisms than adults do, particularly denial and regression. Common psychosomatic symptoms include headaches, stomachaches, bowel and bladder difficulties and sleep disturbances. The clinician can interpret such behavior as manifestations of grief for baffled families and school personnel.

MONITORING THE GRIEF PROCESS

A prolonged duration or intensity of these normal behavioral responses and symptoms may indicate the need for clinical intervention, whereas brief periods of turmoil are usually

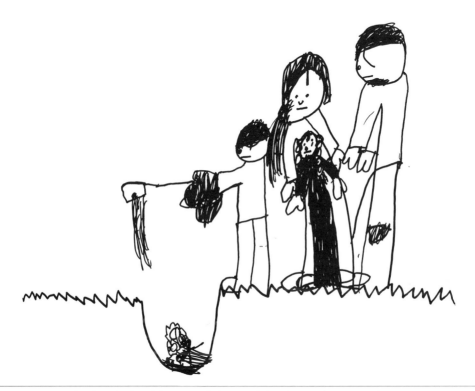

This picture depicts the burial of a child's grandfather. Each family member places dirt in the grave. The artist draws her brother doing this. By E. O., a girl aged 7.

evidence of expected grief work. Chronic depression or hostility, longing to join the deceased, persistent fear or panic and chronic loss of appetite or ability to sleep indicate the need for professional referral. For a school-age child, regular communication with the teacher regarding the child's classroom behavior is recommended because this should show gradual normalization after a brief period of disruption. Especially during the first several months after a loss, caring adults can help the grieving child significantly by providing a stable environment and well-defined behavioral boundaries, but doing so with empathy. Well-intentioned teachers who become more permissive do not serve the grieving child, particularly because the school environment is often the only place that feels the same for the child. Similarly at home, the same level of expectation, routine and pattern is more supportive than a more permissive or lenient approach. A significant adult who is physically and emotionally available to the child over time is essential to recovery. Six months to a year is a reasonable time frame for resolution of acute grief reactions. A longer duration or lack of progress in resolution will require a mental health referral.

CHALLENGES TO SUCCESSFUL GRIEVING

For a child to grieve a loss, he must perceive his world to be safe and "back to normal." Often, one loss leads to secondary losses that may, in effect, have a more profound influence on a child's sense of loss. For example, when a parent dies and the surviving parent goes to work full-time or when the family must move or there is a financial downturn, it may be these events that complicate and prolong the grief process. A deceased parent may be fantasized as away on a trip, but the immediacy of moving, leaving friends, changing schools and so forth goes beyond the child's ability to use denial as a coping strategy. Especially during the first few months following a loss within the family unit, family dynamics are apt to change because of explosive emotions, significant depression, financial stress and new schedules. This is all part of the predictable "grief" landscape that a clinician must consider in seeing the stresses from the child's point of view. The more blown apart the landscape, the more serious the threat to the child.

Certain other factors can significantly derail the child's mourning process and require clinical intervention:

- The inability of the significant adult in the child's life to mourn. Stony silence is devastating to a child's sense of safety. There has to be emotional space in which to mourn.

When Brian's father committed suicide, Brian's world and that of his three brothers changed forever. The day after the funeral, all family photos that included dad were put away; mom never talked about dad again. Shortly after dad died, mom went to work for the first time, took a computer course at night and moved the family from the only home that Brian had ever known.

- The significant adult's inability to tolerate the child's expression of grief. A "stiff upper lip" is not to be encouraged.

Julie's eighth birthday would be especially bleak this year because her twin sister had died 6 months earlier. When she cried while discussing party plans with her parents, dad immediately started in with his routine response, "Let's not be sad; we must be grateful to be alive!"

- Forced hypermaturity of the child; requirement to exemplify adult behavior, such as to take care of siblings and prepare meals.

 Fourteen-year-old Charlie refused free tickets to the Red Sox game that evening; he knew his mom would be alone if he went.

- Overwhelming secondary losses or a history of unresolved losses.

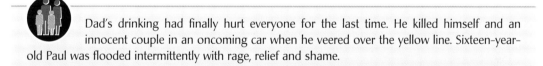 Jaime had to move to Texas to live with his grandmother after his mother died. His sister quit high school and went to work. His two brothers went to live with aunts.

- Ambivalence toward the deceased person or confusion about details of the death.

 Dad's drinking had finally hurt everyone for the last time. He killed himself and an innocent couple in an oncoming car when he veered over the yellow line. Sixteen-year-old Paul was flooded intermittently with rage, relief and shame.

- Inability to make meaning of the loss, lack of ability to accept the finality of the loss, fantasy ideas beyond a few weeks.

Each time 9-year-old Rebecca looked at the video of her family's vacation, it assured her that her baby brother would be at the cottage when the family returned next summer.

RITUALS AROUND DEATH

Clinicians must view a child's conception of death and grief reaction in religious and cultural contexts that are determined by the child's family and tradition.

Most bereavement specialists agree that it is of assistance to children to attend funerals and other rituals associated with the death of a loved one. However, an adult, not necessarily an immediate family member but a familiar and supportive person, should prepare the child for the experience directly and without euphemisms, accompany the child and be available to answer questions. A child should be told what her role will be and that she can leave if she needs to do so (this rarely happens). For a child to benefit from this experience, she must be old enough to make sense of the event and be assured of an adult for direct support. Keeping a child separate from the family and community during this time is usually more harmful to a child older than 4 than inclusion is. Abandonment at a time of family upheaval can be stressful for a young child. Her fantasies about the death and the funeral are more scary than anything that will happen in reality. Participation in all or part of the grieving ritual is to be supported in the vast majority of cases. If given support, children will leave if it gets overwhelming.

Enrique went to the backyard to his swing while the funeral lunch continued in the house. He swung for a while and then came in "for dessert" he said to his aunt.

SPECIAL ISSUES IN LOSS

Pet Loss

Few if any children will grow up without facing the painful experience of "losing" their pet. Some parents, in an effort to shield their children from the pain, mistakenly disallow the child the opportunity to face the grief that is a necessary byproduct of affection and connection to their beloved pet. How many adults can remember being told as children that Rover was sent to a "farm in Iowa where he can run and breathe fresh air." Why did parents think that that information would not be equally devastating? No better are the all-too-familiar stories of children returning home from school to learn that while they were gone, Rover was taken to the veterinarian and "put to sleep." The unexpected and hidden aspect of the event makes it difficult for a child to profit from this learning opportunity (or to sleep securely himself!).

In fact, the death of a pet provides a rich opportunity for a youngster to strengthen coping skills and learn how to face losses. The family can grieve together, naming the feelings and recognizing and respecting each family member's individual way of dealing with feelings. Finally, the family can engage in the rituals involved in saying good-bye. Parents and other caring adults serve their children by not trivializing or denying their feelings of grief but, at the same time, by not being overwhelmed by them or exaggerating them. Simple, clear and short rituals and discussions are best.

Sibling Loss

The death of a sibling presents an enormous challenge to the surviving child. She has weathered the death of her brother or sister, a contemporary whose loss will continue to be felt throughout her life. She also has lost her parents as she knew them because the complicated mourning process that parents face in this circumstance is more intense and prolonged than any other. Marital conflict, depression, guilt, social isolation and possible resentment of the surviving children may exacerbate parents' grief and further inhibit their ability to be emotionally available to their surviving children. To gain affection and ease their parents' pain, the surviving child may attempt to "replace" a deceased sibling, thereby compromising the youngster's own identity development. Some children will hold in their grief until they see parental grief resolve and feel safer in revealing their own feelings. An explosion of emotion may occur weeks to months down the line. This often confuses and angers parents. Too often, the tendency to idealize the dead child also makes it difficult for the surviving siblings to deal with their own ambivalent feelings (e.g., unresolved sibling rivalry) or with anger at the deceased or at their parents (e.g., for not preventing the death or for seeming to care more about the deceased child). Finally, a survivor's guilt is commonly felt by the surviving sibling and must be challenged. Many times brief counseling is needed to explore these issues, separate from any group family therapy. Sibling survivor groups may be an additional help. This issue will need to be revisited over time.

Parental Loss

It is not clear exactly how many children experience the death of a parent, but estimates are about 5% to 8%, and about three fourths of these deaths are anticipated. The death of a parent affects the child's development profoundly in the short and long term. All such children are depressed or dysphoric at 3 months after a parent's death, and 20% have continuing serious problems at 1 year. Anticipate that about a third of such children will have behavioral problems that require mental health referral. In addition to the child's developmental age at the time of death (see earlier), the next most important consideration is the emotional availability of the surviving parent or other supportive adult. Children can do their necessary grief work only if and when life feels safe again, and sometimes that is delayed if a lot of family disruption takes place. The acute grieving period, usually 2 to 3 years, is a time of adjustment because each family member feels a real need to be understood and has the least capacity to give understanding.

> A month after 9-year-old Molly's mother died of amyotrophic lateral sclerosis, Molly and her dad were at a drive-through at McDonald's. When he grabbed for his wallet, he realized that he had left it at home and had no money to pay for dinner that night. Molly became hysterical, thinking that they were poor now that mommy had died.

Children may idealize and overidentify with the deceased parent while distorting their view of the remaining parent. They are particularly concerned about any perceived vulnerability of the remaining parent. Depending on the cause of death, safety or health issues may become exaggerated. A common concern for the surviving parent is whether a young child will remember the deceased parent. Looking at family photos and videos and storytelling are not universally welcomed by the children, who may fear the surviving parent's strong display of emotion. Letting children take it in at their own pace is the best way to handle this. The health and adjustment of the surviving parent are key to the child's ability to cope. When a child faces a life-threatening illness or injury, a new crisis must be faced by the child, family and clinician. Although family members are all grieving the same person, that person had a unique relationship with each of them.

The Dying Child

Before the 1970s, most professionals used a protective approach regarding disclosure of information to a dying child. Today, most researchers and clinicians agree that an open approach with disclosure about diagnosis, treatment and prognosis promotes coping skills and adaptive behavior for most children and families. In a recent study, none of the parents who talked to their dying child about death expressed any regrets; in contrast, 27% of parents who did not talk with their child expressed regret. Children should be given information that allows them to understand the illness and treatment. The child may vacillate between denial and acceptance of the situation. With some people, the child may practice mutual pretense, with both parties ignoring the illness, whereas with others, he may be open about the seriousness of his illness and his fears and fantasies of impending death. Listening to the child and taking cues from him mitigate his sense of isolation. Spinetta suggests five factors that should be considered by caregivers before discussing the illness or death with a dying child (Box 27–2).

BOX 27–2   FACTORS TO CONSIDER BEFORE DISCUSSING DEATH WITH A DYING CHILD

- Parents' **philosophical stance** on death. What are their religious and cultural views about life, death and the afterlife? These should be supported but within a developmental framework.
- Parents' **emotional stance** on death. Is either parent in denial about death as an eventuality? Is either parent likely to be stoic or hyperemotional?
- Child's **age, experience and level of development**.
- Family's **coping strategies**. What history of crisis or illness can predict its ability to cope with this illness? What are the other stressors a family is facing?
- Child's **perception of participation or control**. Does the child require detailed information about procedures or treatment? Can she look at "the big picture"?

A child's understanding of death will depend on his developmental stage (see earlier). Most children with a prolonged illness will actually advance in their understanding of death as they face it. Some children in middle childhood will acquire a very adult notion of death and dying. A few may regress. The clinician should regularly pose open-ended questions to allow the child to reveal her understanding of her circumstances and have a place to pose concerns and worries.

Today, a dying child is often actively involved with the treatment team. Because many children will die at home, the parents play a much more active role in treatment as well. When curative therapy has been replaced by palliative care, the treatment team should take special care to not abandon the child or family, because this will compound the loss. The primary care clinician's role is central to this support by identifying the needs of the child and the treatment choices and assisting with decision making. In this way, the primary care clinician's work is complementary to a specialist caring for the child. The natural tendency is to withdraw from the child and family because most clinicians feel defeated by death and helpless to do anything. That's the wrong thing to do—it makes the loss for the child and family even worse.

GETTING HELP

When a child is facing the death of himself or someone close, the primary clinician should be a source of personal support but also a source of community resource information. Developmentally appropriate grief groups are outstanding supports for children and the parent or parents who bring them. Children can be helped to express their grief through individual and group play, artwork (see the artwork in this chapter), journaling and sharing time. Selected books and videos can be particularly helpful to a bereaved child. The Good Grief Program at Boston Medical Center offers an annotated bibliography that catalogs books by the type of loss and the reading level (see "Recommended Readings" at the end of this chapter).

CHILDREN AND TRAUMA

Children in the United States are exposed to **violence** in epidemic proportions. Each day in the United States, 9 children are murdered, 30 children are wounded by guns and 307 children are arrested for violent crimes. Children are also often witnesses to domestic and community violence.

The media have brought school violence home to every household in America. Domestic violence occurs in rural and urban areas without regard to class or ethnicity. A study of 6-year-old children by Schuler and Nair indicated that 43% of these young children had seen a beating, 13% saw a knife threat, and 7% saw an actual stabbing or shooting. Young children are deeply affected by witnessing violence, particularly when the perpetrator or victim is a family member.

What is the effect on children who live with violence in their world? Lenore Terr defined childhood psychological **trauma** as "the mental result of one blow or a series of blows, rendering the young person temporarily helpless and breaking past ordinary coping and defensive operations." The child's reaction to violence, the trauma experienced, will depend on a number of factors, including her age, previous exposure to violence, whether the perpetrator and/or the victim is known and whether the violence is a single incident or is chronic. Children exposed to violence have an increased level of aggression, are more anxious and have higher rates of delinquency and social problems. Children are usually more affected than adults suspect. Most children communicate their fear and uncertainty about their lives through behavior rather than language.

The following are clinical clues that a child or adolescent may have witnessed overwhelming violence:

- Hypervigilance, jumpiness
- Hyperactivity, frantic activity
- Nightmares
- Separation anxiety, clinginess
- Risk-taking behavior
- Withdrawal, isolation
- Emotional numbing

Post-traumatic stress disorder (PTSD) develops in a significant percentage of children who experience violence (Box 27–3). Studies of the etiology of PTSD in children have shown that

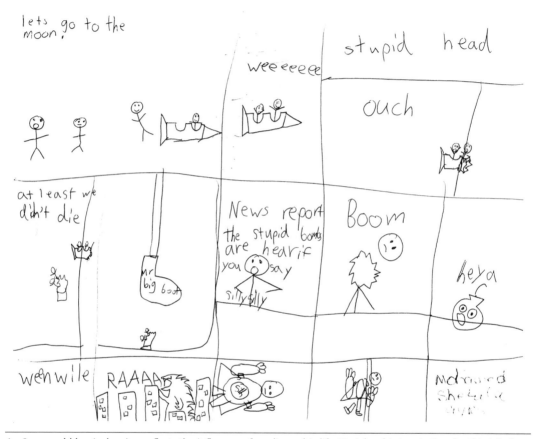

An 8-year-old boy's drawing reflects the influence of media on his life. He takes his inspiration for this tale from a website for kids. A space journey starts and is interrupted by a crash, but one that has no lasting consequence. A news report is embedded in his story; a bomb knocks the head off the reporter. The story continues with more bombs, threatening menaces directed at tall city buildings and a disembodied person who has crashed into a pole. By Mohammed Shetula.

BOX 27–3   DIAGNOSTIC CRITERIA FOR POST-TRAUMATIC STRESS DISORDER

A. The person has been exposed to a traumatic event in which both of the following were present:
   1. The person experienced, witnessed or was confronted with an event or events that involved actual or threatened death or serious injury or a threat to the physical integrity of self or others.
   2. The person's response involved intense fear, helplessness or horror. Note: In children, this may be expressed instead by disorganized or agitated behavior.

B. The traumatic event is persistently re-experienced in one (or more) of the following ways:
   1. Recurrent and intrusive distressing recollections of the event, including images, thoughts or perceptions. Note: In young children, repetitive play may occur in which themes or aspects of the trauma are expressed.
   2. Recurrent distressing dreams of the event. Note: Children may have frightening dreams without recognizable content.
   3. Acting or feeling as though the traumatic event were recurring (includes a sense of reliving the experience, illusions, hallucinations and dissociative flashback episodes, including those that occur on awakening or when intoxicated). Note: In young children, trauma-specific reenactment may occur.
   4. Intense psychological distress at exposure to internal or external cues that symbolize or resemble an aspect of the traumatic event.
   5. Physiological reactivity on exposure to internal or external cues that symbolize or resemble an aspect of the traumatic event.

C. Persistent avoidance of stimuli associated with the trauma and numbing of general responsiveness (not present before the trauma), as indicated by three (or more) of the following:
   1. Efforts to avoid thoughts, feelings or conversations associated with the trauma
   2. Efforts to avoid activities, places or people that arouse recollections of the trauma
   3. Inability to recall an important aspect of the trauma
   4. Markedly diminished interest or participation in certain activities
   5. Feeling of detachment or estrangement from others
   6. Restricted range of affect (e.g., unable to have loving feelings)
   7. Sense of a foreshortened future (e.g., does not expect to have a career, marriage, children or a normal life span)

D. Persistent symptoms of increased arousal (not present before trauma), as indicated by two (or more) of the following:
   1. Difficulty falling or staying asleep
   2. Irritability or outbursts of anger
   3. Difficulty concentrating
   4. Hypervigilance
   5. Exaggerated startle response

E. Duration of the disturbance (symptoms in criteria B, C and D) is longer than 1 month.

F. The disturbance causes clinically significant distress or impairment in social, occupational or other important areas of functioning
   Specify if
   • Acute: duration of symptoms is less than 3 months
   • Chronic: duration of symptoms is 3 months or more
     Specify if delayed onset: onset of symptoms is at least 6 months after the stressor

From American Psychiatric Association: *Diagnostic and Statistical Manual of Mental Disorders*, 4th ed–text revision (DSM-IV TR). New York, American Psychiatric Association, 2000.

witnessing domestic violence is as traumatic as being the victim of sexual abuse. Clinical experience suggests that PTSD can be a chronic problem and a source of ongoing problems in school, relationships and emotional development. One of the unmistakable symptoms of chronic exposure to violence is the child's foreshortened view of the future. They cannot imagine next year's vacation or what they will be when they grow up.

> Although Jeremy was legally old enough to take driver's education classes, he couldn't see the point. His best friend, Joshua, had not lived long enough to get his license; his older brother, Rene, was also killed before he was able to buy a car that he was saving to buy. What were the chances he would live long enough to have a car the way things were going in his neighborhood?

Because the scars carried by children who are chronically exposed to violence are invisible and because their immediate caregivers may also be victims or perpetrators, it is incumbent on the clinician to recognize symptoms and ask questions that can lead to intervention. Think about PTSD when evaluating a child with behavior or learning problems who has witnessed a violent event any time in the past.

Asking about violence takes little time, doesn't require special expertise and demonstrates concern. The following are indications that a referral to a community resource such as a mental health specialist, the department of social services or the police should be made:

- The child's safety is at immediate risk. The child must be protected now.
- Symptoms have persisted for more than 6 months. Behavioral change with distress lasting less than 3 months is labeled adjustment disorder, but it should be gradually improving across that time.
- The trauma was particularly violent or involved the death or departure from the home of a parent or primary caretaker.
- Continuing revisualization of the violent event.
- The child's caretakers are unable to empathize with or support the child.

PTSD requires a mental health referral, with other agencies involved as indicated. About 20% to 30% of child survivors of serious trauma will need extended mental health care. It is unclear why PTSD does not develop in some children who are exposed to chronic violence. However, resiliency factors such as the presence of a strong role model and activities that promote competence and self-esteem (see Box 27–4) remind us that an understanding, nurturing parent, a dedicated coach or a member of the clergy who works with youth can positively change the child's view of himself. Some children who have weathered severe violence with apparent good resolve may suffer from symptoms years later. The clinician may have to probe the past to identify the source of current emotional, social or behavioral complaints.

WHEN VIOLENCE OCCURS AT HOME

Children who experience violence within the home are at even greater risk than those who see it in the community. Estimates indicate that as many as 10% of youngsters witness such

---

BOX 27–4 FACTORS THAT INFLUENCE A CHILD'S ABILITY TO COPE WITH SERIOUS TRAUMA OR VIOLENCE

Enhanced Risk

- Predisposition to anxiety and/or depression in self or family
- Preexisting family and school problems
- Preexisting developmental and/or physical disabilities
- No stable family member as a support
- Poor economic security
- Moving, immigration, cultural or family isolation

Protective Factors

- Higher intellectual abilities
- Enhanced language skills
- Special talents, abilities
- School success. Other experience with success and mastery
- Participation in outside activities, e.g., scouting, sports, church groups, special camps
- Physical and emotional availability of an adult support person

---

violence. Although much is associated with substance abuse, it occurs in all communities worldwide. The children in such homes are at serious risk of being physically abused themselves, but they are also likely to have anxiety, depression and enhanced aggressive behavior. Over the long term they are at increased risk for anxiety and depression, poor school performance and substance abuse. Behavior problems of both the internalizing and externalizing type are seen in a large proportion of children 6 to 18 years old who have witnessed domestic violence. Unfortunately, many will become perpetrators.

Most child health care clinicians have limited knowledge about or rarely screen for domestic violence among families in their practices. This can be remedied by asking at health encounters whether a parent feels or has felt at risk. A referral to a community resource should be available. A high level of suspicion for domestic violence as a possible cause of childhood behavioral concerns needs to be part of the clinician's thinking. It can be accomplished during a clinical interview or through a psychosocial parent questionnaire that includes an assessment of domestic violence (see Kemper and Kelleher, 1996, in "References").

WHEN CATASTROPHE STRIKES

Many children may face the threat of natural disasters such as hurricanes or earthquakes, and all children today face the fears and insecurities that accompany world terrorism (Box 27–5). The feelings experienced by children, even very young children, include anxiety, confusion, fear, irritability and depression. Very young children may suffer symptoms of stress such as crying and whining, repressive behavior, separation anxiety and fear of being alone, sleep disorders, illness, changes in normal patterns of behavior, aggression and fear.

Why some children in a family appear to be resilient and others suffer permanent psychological scars in the wake of an overwhelming event is a subject of much inquiry. However, experts all

BOX 27–5   **POST 9/11: WHAT DID IT MEAN FOR CHILDREN?**

The terrorist attacks of 9/11/01 profoundly changed America and the world. These catastrophic events permanently changed our sense of safety; the recurring media depiction of these events imprinted indelible images on our minds and hearts. Children all over the world witnessed these events over and over themselves and soaked up the profound emotional responses of the adults around them.

Clinicians seeing children in the immediate area around the World Trade Center have identified that the majority of children expressed significant distress in word and behavior, with over a fourth having severe post-traumatic stress disorder (PTSD). Children most affected were those who lost a parent or another loved one or those who had antecedent mental health concerns. Chronic worry, anxiety and a variety of school and behavioral problems continue long after the events.

Most local clinicians admitted they were woefully ill prepared to deal with the issues presented: death and dying, disruption of lives and loss and continuing mental health concerns in over 10% of patients. PTSD was unfamiliar to many and largely absent from the pediatric literature before these events.

September 11 unmasked the huge unmet needs for child mental health care. For example, nearly 90% of physicians dealing with children in this aftermath identified serious barriers to mental health care, and only a small minority of children with frank PTSD had any professional counseling or therapy.

These events were, in the words of David Schonfeld,* a wake-up call to the unmet mental health care needs of children. They revealed the long-standing inadequacies of care and training and a stark lack of preparedness for severe psychological threats. The magnitude of these events was without precedent. The everyday lack of resources for children with horrific events to face in their lives preceded and, unfortunately, followed these September events.

---

*Schonfeld DJ: Supporting children after terrorist events: Potential role for pediatricians. *Pediatr Ann* 32:182-187, 2003.

agree what resilience is *not*. It is not rare; most children have the capacity to be resilient. Second, people are not born resilient. Resilience is developed.

What, then, are the strategies that parents can use when children are facing threats that may be imminent or threats that are more nebulous, such as a "yellow alert" terrorism watch? The following strategies are important for helping toddlers and young children manage the stress of exposure to man-made and natural disasters: Clinicians should be aware of these strategies to assist if the occasion warrants it.

- **Infants and children** younger than 6 years rely exclusively on the emotional competence of their primary caregiver. How a parent communicates about escaping to safety from a disaster, the emotional tone that is set and the age-appropriate explanations about what will happen in the next few minutes or hours will determine the child's reaction. Communicate in a clear, calm voice, hold the child close physically when possible and reassure the child that you, the adult, are in charge and will make everything all right.

- Exposure to the media should be avoided at all costs since very young children have no capacity to distinguish real-time action from the replay displays of destruction. There is no sense of distance or time in the presentations of these images at a young age.

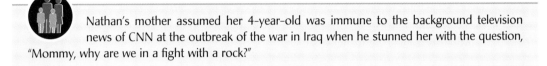 Nathan's mother assumed her 4-year-old was immune to the background television news of CNN at the outbreak of the war in Iraq when he stunned her with the question, "Mommy, why are we in a fight with a rock?"

- **Elementary-aged children** will understand the life event or threat not just from their primary caregiver's perspective but also from that of their peers and other adults. They worry about the safety of their limited world of home, neighborhood and school. It is critical to assure these children that you are in charge, that you will do your best to keep them safe and that other helping professionals, such as police officers and mayors, will do their best to keep everyone safe as well.

Seven-year-old Ben was terrified when the family's SUV was stopped and a police officer's large flashlight peered into the windows as they were about to cross the Golden Gate Bridge to return home from their weekend at Nana's. The nation was at yellow alert, which Ben didn't understand. Why did he need to look in the back space and open the suitcases? Had his dad done something wrong? Would they be able to return home? Were the terrorists on the bridge? Would they be in his hometown when he got home?

- **Preadolescents** view themselves as members of a more complex world; they are part of a family, a community of school and sports, a religious and an ethnic group and a citizen of a town, a state and a nation. They have the capacity to worry in times of threat about their immediate safety, as well as how the event or the threat will change their future.

Eleven-year-old Martha couldn't sleep again and went into her mom's bedroom looking for comfort. Everyone at the airbase was talking about who would be deployed next month, and she was scared that her dad's company was on the list. She had been born on a military base but had never really worried until now about her dad going to war. For the first time, she hated being a military kid.

- **Adolescents** are caught in the middle between the understandable feelings of terror and their own imposed pressure to be mature in the face of a threat. They rely on the adults in their lives to make them feel safe and yet may want to participate in creating safety nets for others. They may be philosophical and/or political in their attempts to make sense of the event.

Sixteen-year-old Ali's stomach kept doing somersaults as she and her sister made emergency preparations for the mandatory 3 PM evacuation from her home to a neighboring community shelter. Her father had said she had to pack everything in her overnight roller suitcase, and it was just not possible to choose what to leave behind. How could she leave Scout, her dog, behind? It wasn't fair. It was too scary, but there wasn't time to do anything but pack. Hurricane Ivan was coming, no matter what.

In summary, for any age child, adults whom they know and trust will provide the most safety and security in times of crisis and stress. Adults should never promise anything that they can't control, but they should reassure children that they are doing everything to make them safe and secure. They should explain action plans, a crisis response and immediate future events, all with confidence and competence. For older children who may want to watch and listen to the media, parents should join them so that they can respond to any concerns. They should preserve whatever routines can be maintained in their children's lives such as bedtime rituals. They should anticipate the symptoms of stress in their children and be available to comfort them.

RECOMMENDED READING

American Academy of Pediatrics, George Cohen (lead author): Helping children and families deal with divorce and separation. *Pediatrics* 110:1019-1023, 2002.

Books and Videos on Loss for Children and Adolescents: An Annotated Bibliography. Boston, The Good Grief Program, One Boston Medical Center Place, Boston, MA 02118, 1996.

Galeo S, Ahera J, Resnick H, et al: Psychological sequelae of the September 11 terrorist attacks in NYC. *N Engl J Med* 346:982-987, 2002.

Lamberg L: In the wake of tragedy: Studies track psychological response to mass violence. *JAMA* 291:587-589, 2003.

Sourkes B: *Armfuls of Time: The Psychological Experience of the Child with a Life-Threatening Illness.* Pittsburgh, University of Pittsburgh Press, 1995.

Stein MT, Heyneman EK, Stern EJ: Recurrent nightmares, aggressive doll play, separation anxiety and witnessing domestic violence in a nine year old girl. *J Dev Behav Pediatr* 25:419-422, 2004.

Swick S, Dechant E, Jellinek M: Children of victims of September 11th: A perspective on the emotional and developmental challenges they face and how to help meet them. *J Dev Behav Pediatr* 23:378-384, 2002.

Tanner JL: Parental separation and divorce: Can we provide an ounce of prevention? *Pediatrics* 110:1007-1009, 2002.

Terr L: *Too Scared to Cry.* New York, Basic Books, 1990.

Walman-vander, Molen JW: Violence and suffering in television news: Toward a broader conception of harmful television content in children. *Pediatrics* 113:1771-1775, 2004. (See this whole issue to read about this topic in more detail.)

Winston F, Kassam-Adams N, Garcia-Espana F, et al: Screening for risk of persistent posttraumatic stress in injured children and their parents. *JAMA* 290:643-649, 2003.

Resources for Children and Families

Grollman EA: *Talking about Death: A Dialogue between Parents and the Child.* Boston, Beacon Press, 1990.

Mundy M: *Sad Isn't Bad: A Good Grief Guidebook for Kids Dealing with Loss.* St Meinrad, IN, Abby Press, 1998.

The Dougy Center for Grieving Children: *35 Ways to Help a Grieving Child.* Portland, OR, The Dougy Center for Grieving Children, 1999. www.dougy.org.

See Good Grief Program (above), Boston Medical Center, for a complete bibliography.

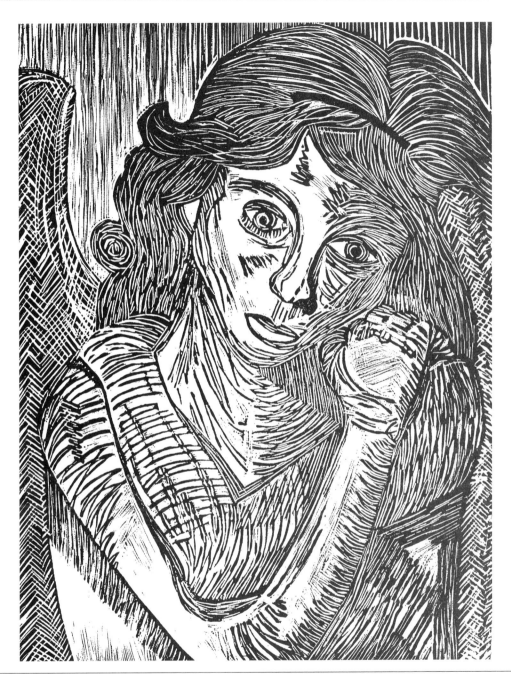

An 18-year-old girl depicts herself, with her evident sense of loss after the death of her father. She used her substantial artistic talent to explore and express this monumental loss in her life. A woodcut by Loni Blankenship, age 18.

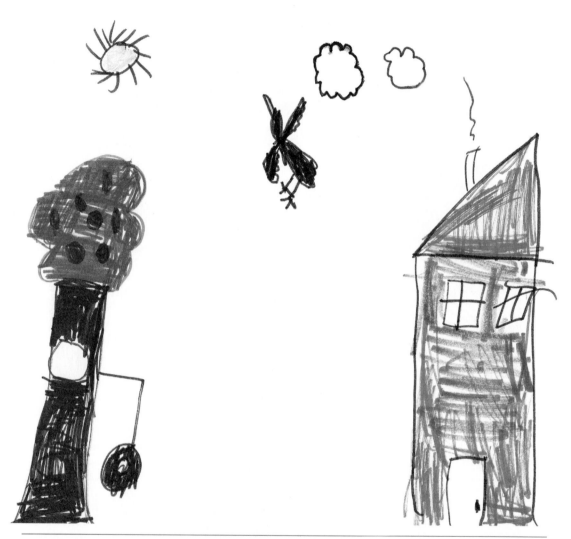

This boy draws an empty house when asked to draw his family. Mom was away seeking work and he and his siblings were staying with grandma. Empty houses are common in the drawings from children under stress. By Cameron M.

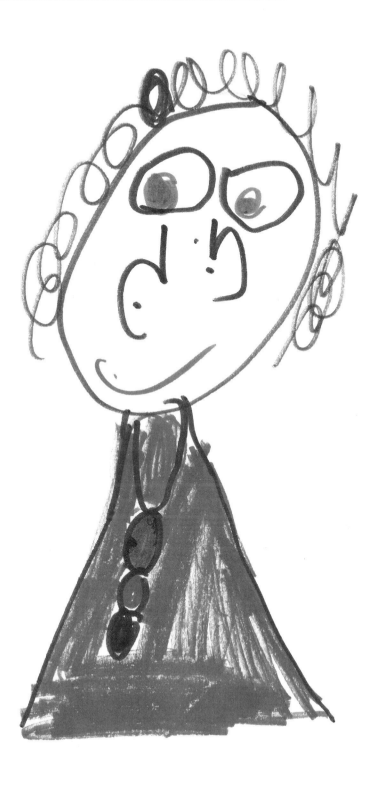

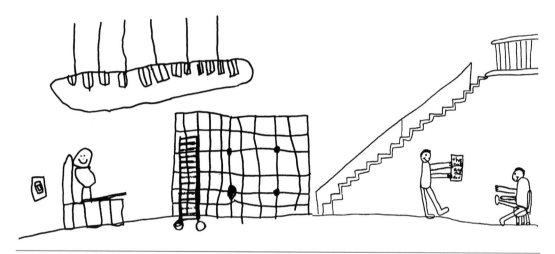

"Reading together." Left illustration by Ben Stein, age 5. Right illustration by Josh Stein, age 8.

Resources for Families: An Annotated Bibliography

MARTIN T. STEIN and SUZANNE D. DIXON

> *A professional's role is to help parents locate tools within themselves so they can understand their own need and the needs of their children and become aware that they are the real experts with their children.*
> LEON HOFFMAN, M.D., NEW YORK TIMES, 4/9/03

Pediatric professionals recommend books for parents to read for various reasons. Books often serve as an adjunct to the teaching done in the office. Some parents need or request additional information on topics discussed briefly in the office visit. Books can provide a reinforcing or differing view, as needed. Parents of children with special needs may be especially appreciative of such resources. **Books do not substitute for direct, personal guidance, but are an important adjunct to care.**

Several factors should be considered before recommending a book, such as the following:

- Parents' particular need
- Child's developmental level
- Parents' ability to use written material
- What is affordable and available
- Parental motivation

Clinicians should be clear about the goals to be achieved in recommending books. A pernicious belief exists that parenting can be done only by professionals and that more information automatically ensures better parenting. The clinician can unconsciously support that belief and add to anxiety by wholesale or routine reading suggestions. Giving people confidence is the goal here—not overwhelming them with "professionalism."

Maximal availability of the books will offer the opportunity for ready use. Strategies include keeping copies of selected books in the waiting room or examining room, having books available to purchase at cost in the office, compiling a lending library and requesting a nearby bookstore to stock selected favorites. A printed reading list can be developed, but it should be given out with *specific* notation from the clinician to point parents in a good direction.

A few cautions are in order. First, it is essential for the clinician to read the books. One must be familiar with an author's philosophy and recommendations to determine whether the book would be compatible with the clinician's own philosophy and information as imparted to parents in the office.

Second, the list in this chapter has been selected from the vast and ever-growing literature available for parents. Many books that are no doubt excellent escaped our review. The clinician should periodically peruse the child development section at the local bookstore to be familiar with the most current books. A few we have found helpful are listed below by category and alphabetically by first author.

BIBLIOGRAPHY FOR PARENTS

Child Development

Ames LB, Ilg F: *Your One Year Old: The Fun Loving Fussy* (1982); *Your Two Year Old: Terrible or Tender* (1976); *Your Three Year Old: Friend or Enemy* (1976); *Your Four Year Old: Wild and Wonderful* (1976); *Your Five Year Old: Sunny and Serene* (1979); *Your Six Year Old: Loving and Defiant* (1980). New York, Dell Books. Codirectors of the Gesell Institute of Child Development, these authors display their knowledge, experience and sense of humor in their uncanny skill of depicting accurate portraits of children's behavior. Very practical advice combined with a reassuring style makes these books invaluable reading for a frustrated parent. Although they are now more than 2 decades old, their insights have passed the test of time and are still applicable.

Brazelton TB: *Infants and Mothers*. New York, Dell, 1969. In describing the behavior of three normal babies, Dr. Brazelton makes extremely clear how different infants can be. His descriptions of the interactions between average, quiet and active babies and their families during the first year of life make worthwhile reading for new parents and also for parents who make frequent comparisons between their infant and other babies. This has been updated somewhat. Highlights individuality and temperament. Now a "classic" in infant development.

Brazelton TB: *Touchpoints: Your Child's Emotional and Behavioral Development: Birth-3: The Essential Reference for the Early Years*. New York, Harper Collins, 1992. An easy-to-read reference book in which parents' questions and concerns about their child's behavior, development and feelings are anticipated and answered in chronological (part I) as well as problem (part II) form.

Brazelton TB, Sparrow JD: *Touchpoints 3-6*. Cambridge, MA, Perseus Publishing, 2002. An extension of Dr. Brazelton's original book, *Touchpoints*, that now extends the age from 3 to 6 years. There are few books on normal development and behavior in preschool children for parents and clinicians. This one fills the gap.

Caplan F (ed): *The First Twelve Months of Life*, 2nd ed. New York, Grosset & Dunlap, 1993. In this new edition Caplan has continued to use much of the most recent research on infants in an effort to help parents understand why babies behave as they do. Descriptions of a baby's month-by-month development, numerous photographs and growth charts make the book reader friendly. Like the first edition, this excellent book has a wealth of information that is both fun to discover and helpful to know.

Comer JP, Poussaint AF: *Raising Black Children*. New York, Penguin Books, 1992. A revision of *Black Child Care*, this general guide to parenting focuses on special concerns of black families. More ethnic specific than the first edition with the main focus still on child development.

Fraiberg S: *The Magic Years*. New York, Charles Scribner's Sons, 1959. Now a child development classic—a "must read" for students of early childhood! Child psychoanalyst Fraiberg discusses early psychological development (birth to 6 years) as though the reader were experiencing the child's inner world. More theoretical than most books in this list, it discusses typical developmental problems and their management. Very sensible observations. A big favorite for pediatricians, both in the making and established.

Gopnik A, Meltzoff AN, Kuhl PK: *The Scientist in the Crib: What Early Learning Tell Us About the Mind*. Perennial, 2001. Written by three pioneer researchers in infant cognitive science, a journey through the discoveries about how much babies and young children know, how available they are to learn and how much parents teach them during everyday activities. Among the best reviews of contemporary early development research for parents and clinicians—and easy to read.

Greenspan S, Greenspan NT: *First Feelings*. New York, Viking, 1985. This book chronicles the stages of emotional and cognitive development from birth through age 4. Six stages in the emotional life of a young child are seen as critical to healthy development: awakening of the infant, discovery of communication, deepening of relationships, developing of a sense of self, ability to create new ideas and development of complex feelings. Descriptions of children and families are strategically used to clarify each stage. Practical advice assists parents as they encounter the range of children's emotions, fears and struggles. College-educated audience.

Klaus M, Kennell J, Klaus P: *Bonding*. Reading, MA, Addison-Wesley, 1995. A readable text for parents and professionals that discusses the formation of emotional bonds between parent and child from pregnancy through early infancy. Sensitive and insightful coverage of premature births and birth defects. Includes a discussion of the benefits of a doula, a social support person for the laboring mother.

Klaus M, Klaus P: *Your Amazing Newborn*. Reading, MA, Perseus Books, 1998. A photographic journey into the readiness of newborns to engage and be engaged by their environment. The authors make research in early child development available to parents with clear narrative and photographs on nearly every page.

Klaus, MH, Klaus JH, Kennell PH: *The Doula Book: How a Trained Labor Companion Can Help You Have a Shorter, Easier, and Healthier Birth*, 2nd ed. Cambridge, MA Perseus Publishing, 2002. Published earlier as *Mothering the Mother*, this small book explains the role of the doula as a support during childbirth and summarizes some of the research on the advantages of such an assistant.

Kutner L: *Toddlers and Preschoolers*. New York, William Morrow, 1994. Easy, practical, small book. Short chapters, issues of temperament, choosing a preschool.

Levine M: *A Mind at a Time*, New York, Simon & Schuster, 2002. Written by a developmental pediatrician with an emphasis on the recognition of individual differences in learning. Through case studies, Dr. Levine focuses on each child's intellectual, emotional and physical strengths as the foundation for successful learning. The book provides parents with clues to the identification of individual learning patterns and ways to use a child's strengths to enhance learning.

Parenting

Barkeley RA, Benton CM: *Your Defiant Child: 8 Steps to Better Behavior*. New York, Guilford Press, 1998. A discussion about the causes and behavioral treatments of disruptive behavior in children with a focus on impulsiveness, hyperactivity and defiance. Specific approaches to behavior management that are supported by research are outlined in clear formats for use by parents.

Brazelton TB, Sparrow JD: *Calming Your Fussy Baby* (2003); *Discipline* (2003); *Sleep* (2003); *Toilet Training* (2004). Cambridge, MA, Da Capo Press. Short monographs written in a comforting style for parents as they experience normal fluctuations in development.

Brown J, Davis J: *No More Monsters in the Closet*. New York, Crown Publishers, 1995. A guide for teaching a child to use imagination to overcome every fear from doctors to nightmares, social situations, school plays and relatives visiting. The perspective and writing are reader friendly. Helpful for motivated parents and professionals who are interested in imagery.

Coles R: *The Moral Intelligence of Children*. New York, Plume Books, 1997. This book focuses on the connection between the behavior of parents and teachers and raising children with a spirit of generosity and empathy. A major contribution to parent guides.

Elkind D: *The Hurried Child: Growing Up Too Fast Too Soon*, 3rd ed. Cambridge, MA, Perseus Publishing, 2001. A revised edition of a classic book on how and why many parents encourage children to grow up too fast, both emotionally and intellectually. An articulate statement about the downside of exposing children to adult pressures and excessively high expectations for achievement.

Faber A, Mazlish E: *Siblings Without Rivalry*. New York, Avon Books, 1987. This book offers practical guidelines supplemented with the views and experiences of parents in a parenting workshop. Thought-provoking ideas for role-playing. Helpful comic strips and reminder strips on how to handle different situations make this book a good source for parents and professionals.

Ferber R: *Solve Your Child's Sleep Problems*. New York, Simon & Schuster, 1985. Excellent explanations of the developmental basis of sleep disturbances in a family context. Specific, sensible suggestions for solving problems from sleep rhythm disturbances to enuresis. Highly recommended; for educated parents only.

Frankel F, Wetmore B: *Good Friends Are Hard to Find: Help Your Child Find, Make and Keep Friends*. Glendale, CA, Perspective Publishing, 1996. Teaches parents empirically tested social skills techniques for helping school-age children make friends and solve problems with other kids. Addresses teasing and bullying for the child who is picked on and for the one who bullies. This book can be extraordinarily helpful for parents.

Ginott HG, Gonott A (ed), Goddard W (ed): *Between Parent and Child: The Bestselling Classic That Revolutionized Parent-Child Communication*. New York, Three Rivers Press, 2003. An update of a widely read book originally published over 30 years ago. One of the first parent guides with an emphasis on transmitting values, responsibility and the power of words. Lots of examples of parent-child dialogue leading to effective communication.

Gordon T: *P.E.T.: Parent Effectiveness Training*. New York, Plume Books, 1975. One of the best books in presenting the basic, essential communication skills needed in families: how to listen, how to communicate your feelings, how to solve conflicts. Recipe format. Gives parents a concrete place to manage issues and sets up an approach to solving problems. May be too prescriptive for some families, just right for others.

Green RW: *The Explosive Child: A New Approach for Understanding and Parenting Easily Frustrated, Chronically Inflexible Children*, 2nd ed. New York, HarperCollins, 2001. From an experienced child psychologist who offers specific guidelines for parents who face a child with frequent "meltdowns." Offers practical ways to reduce hostility and antagonism between child and parent with an emphasis on communication and collaborative problem solving.

Greenspan S: *The Challenging Child*. New York, Addison-Wesley, 1995. A valuable book for motivated parents of "difficult" children that gives insight to the child while offering child-rearing guidelines. Dr. Greenspan describes five personality patterns and devotes a chapter to each (sensitive child, self-absorbed child, defiant child, inattentive child, active-aggressive child). A nice neutral chapter of environmental and dietary influences on children's behavior is also included.

Greenspan S, Greenspan NT: *The Essential Partnership*. New York, Penguin, 1989. This book builds on the information presented in *First Feelings*, offering guidelines on everyday child-rearing issues from infancy through age 4. The authors discuss relationship building, self-esteem, independence, anger, aggression, tantrums and peer relationships. Case histories, including ones from single- and dual-career families, clarify concepts and offer practical advice. Offers an excellent discussion on the use of play time or "floor time" as an opportunity to observe and learn about children.

Hopson DP, Hopson D: *Different and Wonderful: Raising Black Children in a Race Conscious Society*. New York, Prentice Hall, 1990. Black children in America are born into a society with strong racist undercurrents that can damage self-esteem and reduce control over their environment. Black parents are faced with the challenge of raising children with a positive sense of self-worth in a society that judges them as less intelligent, attractive and trustworthy. This book guides black parents through each phase of child development in the context of race issues and self-esteem. Explores tough issues affecting black middle-class families. Provides parents with practical tools for recognizing their own racial attitudes, instilling ethnic pride and discussing race-related issues. Offers a resource guide to direct parents toward children's books and toys that celebrate African American culture.

Hulbert A: *Raising America: Experts, Parents, and a Century of Advice About Children*. New York, Knopf, 2003. The author takes the reader on a historical journey of child-rearing advice by experts over the past century. Fascinating reading about the influence of personal experience of individual experts and cultural values of their time on the advice they offered.

Kurcinka MS: *Raising Your Spirited Child: A Guide for Parents Whose Child Is More Intense, Sensitive, Perceptive, Persistent and Energetic*. New York, HarperCollins, 1991. An encouraging book for parents that addresses understanding, working, living with and enjoying "difficult" children. Emphasis is on the positive aspects of these children. Good for frustrated parents who are willing to follow good, solid advice.

Phelan T: *1-2-3 Magic: Effective Discipline for Children 2-12 Years*, 3rd ed. Parent Magic, 2003. A simple, proven method of discipline that uses counting to help parents stop unwanted behavior and start wanted behavior without arguing, yelling or spanking. Easy-to-follow steps for a very motivated parent.

Pipher M: *Raising Ophelia: Saving the Selves of Adolescent Girls*. New York, Ballantine Books, 1994. The theme of this book is that many girls experience a loss of spirit and self-esteem as they enter adolescence. The author points to cultural values and expectations as the source of change. She illustrates her ideas with cases from her practice as a child psychologist. The emphasis is on prevention.

Schneider-McClure V: *Infant Massage: Handbook for Loving Parents*. New York, Bantam Books, 1989. This small book places infant massage into the context of the infant's sensory world and then gives practical, how-to advice.

Turecki S: *The Difficult Child*. New York, Bantam Books, 1989. Parents have found this book to be useful to help them understand their child with difficult-to-manage behavior. Practical strategies are described for behavior change in the child and family.

Turecki S, Wernick S: *The Emotional Problems of Normal Children*. New York, Bantam Books, 1994. The authors describes emotional difficulties that can happen to typical children and offers management strategies for parents to help children overcome these challenges. Best for educated, highly motivated parents.

Parenting Teenagers

Greydanus D (ed): *Caring for Your Adolescent*. New York, Bantam Books (for American Academy of Pediatrics), 1995. The third of a three-book series developed by the American Academy of Pediatrics. Well-written and easy-to-use comprehensive guide for parents of 12- to 21-year-olds. Practical advice on everything from typical development to nutrition to school failure to family conflicts. Straightforward coverage of sexuality, signals of substance abuse, sexually transmitted diseases, birth control and eating disorders. Reader-friendly format and illustrations make it informative for all parents.

Kutner L: *Making Sense of Your Teenager*. New York, William Morrow, 1997. Straightforward and easy-to-read book that offers insights and tools to help parents understand their teenagers and find solutions to common problems.

Pruitt DB: *Your Adolescent: Emotional, Behavioral and Cognitive Development from Early Adolescence through the Teen Years*. New York, HarperCollins, 2000. A publication from the American Academy of Child and Adolescent Psychiatry, this is a valuable resource for parents that covers a wide range of frequently encountered adolescent developmental issues. In addition, it covers information on more serious obstacles in adolescent development, such as depression, eating disorders, substance abuse and disruptive behavioral disorders.

Wolf AE: *Get Out of My Life, but First Could You Drive Me and Cheryl to the Mall? A Parent's Guide to the New Teenager*. New York, Farrar, Straus & Giroux, 2002. An accurate description of the behavior of teenagers and the psychological aspects behind such behavior. The humorous approach makes it easy and enjoyable to read.

Child and Health Care

Blocker A: *Baby Basics: A Guide for New Parents*. Minneapolis, MN, Chronimed Publishing, 1997. Straightforward, practical advice for new parents that covers a wide range of topics, such as planning for the arrival of the baby, investing in the future, making wills, nutrition, baby proofing and clothing. Good checklist and resource list in each chapter. Very easy to use.

Cohen G (ed): *Guide to Your Child's Sleep*. New York, Villard and Elk Grove Village, IL, American Academy of Pediatrics, 1999. Very nice summary of the science of sleep, as well as practical suggestions for parents' concerns with a heavy emphasis on infancy. Problems presented as parents would state them and solid suggestions offered.

Eisenberg A, Murkoff HE, Hathaway SE: *What to Expect the First Year*, 2nd ed. New York, Workman Publishing, 2003. Comprehensive guide to newborn and infant care. Offers up-to-date practical information. Format is easy to read with chapters that identify issues at monthly stages. Useful sections on nutrition, language development and safety.

Leach P: *Your Baby and Child: From Birth to Age 5*, revised ed. New York, Alfred A Knopf, 1997. Developmental psychologist Penelope Leach has written an outstanding encyclopedia for parents of children from birth to 5 years. Leach uses an approach to everyday care and common behavioral issues that is based on development of the child and the family. Subtitles within the chapter, many excellent drawings and pictures and a superb index with definitions facilitate reading this comprehensive book and make it accessible to most parents.

Leach P: *Your Growing Child*. New York, Alfred A Knopf, 1989. An encyclopedia of child care issues, from health to nutrition to development. Solid and clear, although brief sections. Alphabetical format a bit difficult to use. However, it does cover issues through adolescence, with a strong section on teenage issues.

Nathanson LW: *The Portable Pediatrician: A Practicing Pediatrician's Guide to Your Child's Growth, Development, Health and Behavior, from Birth to Age Five*, 2nd ed. New York, HarperResource, 2002. A practical guide for parents of young children, written in an engaging style by an experienced pediatrician. Drawings and highlighted advice make this an easy and informative read (including morsels of humor). New edition updated with contemporary medical concerns.

Pantell R, Fries JF, Vickery DM: *Taking Care of Your Child: A Parent's Guide to Medical Care*, 6th ed. New York, Perseus Publishing, 2002. Pediatrician Pantell and his colleagues outline many aspects of health promotion, approaches to common symptoms and home management for parents. Through a series of algorithms designed for parents faced with specific symptoms, the format is especially lucid and practical. Updated edition includes many new health concerns and recommendations for parents.

Schiff D, Shelov S (eds): *Guide to Your Child's Symptoms*. New York, Bantam Books (for American Academy of Pediatrics), 1997. A home reference developed by the American Academy of Pediatrics to aid parents in assessing a problem and deciding what action should be taken. Easy to use, with an alphabetical listing of symptoms accompanied by age-specific charts with questions to consider, possible cause and actions to take. Illustrated first-aid manual section is practical and comprehensive.

Schmitt BD: *Your Child's Health: The Parents' Guide to Symptoms, Emergencies, Common Illnesses, Behavior, and School Problems*, revised ed. New York, Bantam Books, 1991. A revision of the first guidebook on children's common illnesses, behavior problems, and health promotion from infancy through adolescence. Offers parents appropriate and safe home remedies and guidelines for seeking emergency and nonemergency medical care. The behavior modification protocols for common developmental problems are readily accessible and practical for most parents. It is especially valuable for parents who will benefit from specific, detailed recommendations.

Schor E (ed): *Caring for Your School Age Child*. New York, Bantam Books (for American Academy of Pediatrics), 1995. The second in a three-book series developed by the American Academy of Pediatrics. Well-written and easy-to-use comprehensive guide for parents of 5- to 12-year-olds. Useful information on typical health and physical, social and personal development. Extensive coverage of emotional, behavioral and discipline problems and family and school matters, as well as health problems. Reader-friendly format and illustrations make it informative for all parents.

Shelov S (ed): *Caring for Your Baby and Young Child: Birth to Age 5*. New York, Bantam Books (for American Academy of Pediatrics), 1991. Written especially for new parents, this well-written guide was developed by the American Academy of Pediatrics. Details about physical and psychological growth, development and common problems of early childhood are described in appropriate detail to be of help to all parents. The index and organization of the book provide quick access to questions and concerns.

Spock B, Needlman R: *Dr. Spock's Baby and Child Care*, 8th ed. New York, Pocket Books (softcover), EP Dutton (hardcover), 2004. This 8th edition of Dr. Spock's classic guide to parenting and child rearing is a compilation of information on child development, parenting skills and common medical conditions. Dr. Spock's advice on parenting (captured in the book's opening statement, "Trust yourself. You know more than you think.") has engaged parents for three generations. New sections include contemporary issues in child care. The index is particularly useful for rapid retrieval of information by concerned parents.

Tristram C, Tristram L: *Have Kid Will Travel: 101 Survival Strategies for Vacation with Babies and Young Children*. Kansas City, KS, Andrews McMeel, 1997. Practical advice on planning trips and traveling with children. Excellent points on where not to go, how to baby proof a hotel room and how to fly with small children. Good list of references.

Weisbluth M: *Healthy Sleep Habits, Happy Child*, 3rd ed. New York, Ballantine Books, 2003. A popular parent guide to understanding natural sleep cycles, ways to promote restful sleep and problems related to sleep. Emphasis on individual temperaments.

Wilkoff W: *Coping With a Picky Eater. Fireside, 1998*. Small book that looks at eating as an interaction and sets advice in that context. Commonsense material for the general reader. Some small points don't always fit with the official guidelines (e.g., flavoring milk), but overall, this book gives some useful advice.

Daycare

Katzev AR, Bragdon NH: *Child Care Solutions*. New York, Avon Books, 1990. Comprehensive guide for the selection of daycare from infancy to after-school care. Identifies strategies for parents to use as they search for, evaluate and choose among various child care environments. Includes practical advice for parents as they manage day-to-day child care issues and strive to work effectively with providers.

US Department of Health and Human Services, Office of Human Development Services, Daycare Division: *A Parent's Guide to Daycare*, DHHS Publication No (OHDS) 80-30254. Washington, DC, Superintendent of Documents, US Government Printing Office. A practical, readable and inexpensive booklet for parents. Part I discusses the components of quality daycare and pragmatic considerations to be made before seeking it. Part II details the step-by-step process of finding daycare. The checklists are particularly valuable. In addition to noting the age-related needs of children and individual parent preferences, special situations such as nighttime care, single parenting and children with special needs are considered. Part III covers a multitude of common daycare problems and suggestions for management. Part IV offers resources of organizations and agencies that may be useful when selecting daycare for children with disabling conditions. In addition to the manual's reasonable length (75 pages), sections are designed to ease finding the particular information needed by having headlines in the left column and boldface headings in the text. Highly recommended.

Woolever E (ed): ***Your Child: Selecting Day Care***. Des Moines, IA, Better Homes and Gardens Books, 1990. Brief, but thorough review of issues that parents face as they evaluate and select child care. Includes checklists for evaluating child care providers, identifying quality of programs and safety. Provides excellent information on parent–child care provider relationships.

Families with Special Needs

Prematurity

Harrison H, Kositsky A: ***The Premature Baby Book***. New York, St Martin's Press, 1983. Parents will appreciate this book as the most complete compilation of information about preemies. Written by the mother of a preemie with extensive consultation from neonatology experts, this is a superb resource. Numerous vignettes of families' responses and adaptation make this a must for neonatal staff as well. Some medical issues may be dated, but the essence here is still sound.

Ludington-Hoe S, Golant S: ***Kangaroo Care***. New York, Bantam Books, 1993. A guide to the kangaroo care holding program. The book reviews the program's history, the research supporting its benefits, who can follow the program, and how. This book also has excellent coverage of life in the neonatal intensive care unit for parents and the baby. Recommended for parents who would like to participate more in the care of their premature infant.

Tracy, AE, Maroney DI, Bernbaum JC (ed), Groothuis J (ed): ***Your Premature Baby and Child: Helpful Answers and Advice for Parents***. New York, Berkeley Press (Penguin Putnam), 1999. Very informative. Written as parent to parent but quite authoritative in content.

Wechsler Linden D, Trenti Paroli E, Wechsler Doron M: ***Preemies: The Essential Guide for Parents of Premature Babies***. New York, Pocket Books (Simon & Schuster), 2000. Easy to read, too complex for some families. On target but digest in small doses.

Twins

Friedrich E, Rowland C: ***The Parent's Guide to Raising Twins: From Pre-Birth to First School Days—The Essential Book for All Those Expecting Two or More***. New York, St Martins Press. 1984. Still good, reliable and takes you from the multiple-birth pregnancy and beyond into childhood.

Gromada K, Hulburt M: ***Keys to Parenting Twins***. New York, Barrons, 1992. Written by parent educators and mothers of twins who publish a newsletter for parents of twins, this guide touches on baby basics (feeding, sleeping, family adjustment) with emphasis on individuality. Most topics are briefly covered; however, a good resource list for more in-depth coverage is provided.

Disabled

Charkins H: *Children with Facial Difference: A Parents' Guide*. Bethesda, MD, Woodbine House, 1996. Informative book that covers all aspects of having a child with a facial difference, from basic genetics to emotional challenges. Written by the mother of a child born with Treacher Collins syndrome, in collaboration with professionals. It offers the support and resources that only a parent who has been there can offer. A must for parents of a child born with a facial difference.

Freeman RD, Carvin CF, Boese RJ: *Can't Your Child Hear? A Guide for Those Who Care for the Deaf*. Baltimore, University Park Press, 1981. Complete, clear guide for a child with any degree of hearing impairment from birth onward. Good resource for professionals, too.

Miller N: *Nobody's Perfect: Living and Growing with Children Who Have Special Needs*. Baltimore, Paul F Brooks, 1994. Excellent practical, insightful and supportive book for parents of children with special needs; it addresses the theoretical (model for adapting) to the practical (how to handle parents, friends, going out in public etc.). Many anecdotes from mothers of children with special needs. A helpful list of readings and resources is included.

Schleichkorn J: *Coping with Cerebral Palsy*, 2nd ed. Austin, TX, ProEd, 1993. This paperback book provides concise guidelines toward an understanding of the issues, facing children with cerebral palsy, definitions of medical terms, psychosocial issues and educational concerns. It has a particularly valuable section describing issues that affect the older child and adult and a further list of readings. Appropriate for beginning a discussion with a family after an initial postdiagnosis adjustment period.

Thompson CE: *Raising a Handicapped Child*. New York, Ballantine Books, 1987. Written by a pediatrician and mother, this book addresses issues facing a family with a child who has a major handicapping condition. A significant portion is dedicated to the feelings of parents and helpful approaches to coping. Strategies for working with medical and educational systems are discussed. This book is for parents of a child with an established disability, particularly for those in a "dawn time" of grief, frustration or hopelessness.

The **Woodbine House Special Needs Collection** has books covering many topics, such as visual impairments, Down syndrome, autism, Tourette syndrome and teaching communication skills to children with special needs, all of which are well written and practical (for information, phone 800-843-7323).

Attention Deficit/Hyperactivity Disorder

Barkley R: *Taking Charge of ADHD*, revised ed. New York, Guilford Press, 2000. A well-organized guide of suggestions for helping children with ADHD. Practical lists of suggestions and charts. The text can get a bit technical, but the advice given is excellent. Good for motivated, well-educated parents.

Hallowell E, Ratey J: *Driven to Distraction*. New York, Touchstone, 1994. A best-selling book that any parents who think they or their children have ADHD probably will have read. The authors use stories from their patients to demonstrate the different forms of ADHD. It offers sound advice on how to identify ADHD and what to do about it.

Jensen PS: *Making the System Work for Your Child with ADHD*. New York, Guilford Publications, 2004. A guide for parents through the typically difficult process of obtaining professional services for their child with ADHD, including health care, educational and community services. Medication decisions and knowing about educational rights in the public schools are among the many practical topics in this book.

Levine M: *The Myth of Laziness*. New York, Simon & Schuster, 2003. Case studies of children with ADHD (and often other behavior problems) labeled "lazy" who have a neurodevelopmental source that affects their productiveness (e.g., difficulty with writing, memory, oral expression, organization). These children experience "output failure" because of different neuro-developmental weaknesses that are remediable with appropriate educational interventions.

Nadeau KG, Littman EB, Quinn PO: *Understanding Girls with ADHD*. Silver Spring, MD, Advantage Press, 2000. An important contribution to our understanding of girls with ADHD from preschool through high school. A developmental perspective guides the interpretation of ADHD behavior and educational issues unique to girls.

Quinn P, Stern J: *Putting on the Brakes: Young People's Guide to Understanding Attention Deficit Hyperactivity Disorder*, revised ed. New York, Magination Press, 2001. A book written for 8- to 13-year-olds that uses wonderful analogies to explain what ADHD is and how to address the problems that it presents. Practical and straightforward.

Reiff MI: *ADHD: A Complete and Authoritative Guide*. Elk Grove Village, IL, American Academy of Pediatrics, 2004. An excellent guide written for parents of school-age children and adolescent youth with ADHD. Clear descriptions of behavior associated with ADHD, coexisting psychological and learning problems, and medications. Considerable attention to behavioral management, classroom accommodations and ways for parents to advocate for the child in the school.

Bilingual Families

Harding-Esch E, Riley P: *The Bilingual Family: A Handbook for Parents*, 2nd ed. New York, Columbia University Press, 2003. Organized as a guide to help parents identify factors that will influence their decision to bring up their children in a bilingual home. Practical examples of families who have raised bilingual children followed by responses to commonly asked questions.

Gifted Children

Yahnke S, Walker SY, Pernu C: *The Survival Guide for Parents of Gifted Kids: How to Understand, Live with, and Stick up for Your Gifted Child*, revised ed. Minneapolis, MN, Free Spirit Publishing, 2002. Although this book does not offer too many recommendations for overcoming problems, it does have a good list of other references at the end of each chapter and a good "when to worry" list. A chapter on educational programs and advocacy is included.

Divorce and Stepfamilies

Bernstein AC: *Yours, Mine and Ours*. New York, WW Norton, 1990. This book explores how families change when remarried parents have a child together. Based on the author's experiences as a stepmother and family therapist and on interviews with "mixed" families, this book explores the psychology and social influences of stepfamilies. Bernstein details the interdependent roles of each member in a stepfamily and analyzes the issues of resentment, competition and anger.

Boyd H: *The Stepparent's Survival Guide*. London, Ward Lock, 1998. Small paperback with all the issues clearly identified. British words a little distracting to the American reader, but no problem with the content.

Brown LK, Brown M: *Dinosaurs Divorce*. New York, Little, Brown, 1986. Cartoon dinosaurs explain in a straightforward, easy-to-understand fashion what divorce is, why it happens and what the child can expect in the future. The familiar illustrations by Marc Brown make it reader friendly for the elementary school–age child.

Evans MD: *This is Me and My Single Parent* (1989), *This is Me and My Two Families* (1988). New York, Magination Press. Fill-in-the-blanks workbooks for parent(s) and children to do together to open up discussion on the stress points in these special families.

Ives S, Fassle D, Rash M: *The Divorce Workbook: Guide for Kids and Families*. Burlington, VT, Waterfront Books, 1985. A workbook for parents, relatives or counselors to use with elementary school–age children. Explains marriage, separation, divorce, legal "stuff" and feelings. Encourages creative expression of thoughts and feelings through picture drawing. Good for use in conjunction with therapy.

Kalter N: *Growing up with Divorce*. New York, Free Press, 1990. Informative discussion of the impact of divorce on children at specific ages with practical suggestions for parents. Focus is on observing the individual child, respecting the stage of development and communicating clearly. Case histories provide insight into children's perceptions of the immediate and long-term issues in divorce and the ways families have learned to cope with their children's anger, fears and maladaptive behavior.

Neuman GM: *Helping Your Kids Cope with Divorce*. New York, Random House, 1999. Provides parents with ideas and tools for protecting children caught in parental struggles during and following a divorce. Emphasis on practical suggestions with many children's drawings that describe conflicts and resolutions.

Wallerstein J, Blakeslee S: *Second Chances: Men, Women, and Children a Decade after Divorce*, revised ed. New York, Mariner Books, 1996. The authors interviewed 60 families with 131 children at the time of their divorce and again at 5- and 10-year intervals. The long-term psychological effects and economic impact of divorce are analyzed. Descriptions of the effects of divorce on children's thoughts and feelings, social relationships, work, family life and economic stability are candid and comprehensive. The psychological stages of divorce are defined for children and adults. Case vignettes add a valuable personal dimension to the research findings. This is really a scholarly work for families who wish to explore the issue at this depth.

Adoption

Adesman A, Adamec C: *Parenting Your Adopted Child: A Positive Approach to Building a Strong Family*. New York, McGraw-Hill, 2004. Written by a pediatrician who suggests ways to explain adoption to children at different stages of development. Provides helpful tools for families to understand and counter common myths about adoption that may be harmful to their children.

Cole J: *How I Was Adopted*. New York, HarperTrophy, 1999. A straightforward story that explains to early school-age children what adoption is and how it happens.

Hicks R: *Adopting in America*, 4th ed. Sun City, CA, Wordsing Press, 2004. A comprehensive book that covers the technicalities of adoption. It explains different types of adoption, lists resources in every state, reviews laws and procedures and includes sample letters.

Register C: *Are those Kids Yours? American Families with Children Adopted from Other Countries*. New York, Free Press, 1991. Comprehensive look at the issues for families who are contemplating interracial adoption or for those with multiethnic families. Explores real issues facing such families as they mature together.

Schaffer J, Lindstrom C: *How to Raise an Adopted Child*. New York, Plume Press, 1991. An age-correlated guide that covers physical and psychological development from birth to adolescence and the special needs of adoptive children. Answers many common questions. Somewhat dense.

Gay and Lesbian Families

Garner A: *Families Like Mine: Children of Gay Parents Tell It Like It Is*. New York, Harper Collins, 2004. An informative, well-written discussion by a daughter who grew up with her gay father. Also includes interviews of 50 children of gay/lesbian parents who discuss coping with prejudice, homophobia, and stresses of growing up with a gay parent.

Serious Illness and Death

Good Grief Program: *Books and Videos on Loss for Children and Adolescents: An Annotated Bibliography*. Boston, Boston Medical Center, 1996.

Grollman EA: *Talking about Death: A Dialogue Between Parent and Child*, 3rd ed. Boston, Beacon Press, 1991. A frank guide for parents. The book begins with a straightforward read-along "story" explaining what death is. The rest of the book explains to parents how children view and react to death and how they can help. Excellent list of resources parents can use locally, as well as nationally.

Grollman E (ed): *Bereaved Children and Teens*. Boston, Beacon Press, 1995. A comprehensive guide for parents who are helping their children cope with the death of someone they know. Each chapter is written by an authority and covers, in a developmentally appropriate fashion, everything from how to talk about death and dying to how bereavement affects a child to different religious customs about death and how to explain them to children. The last section addresses useful treatments and therapies that can help children cope with death and alerts parents to signs that a child needs professional care. The in-depth style makes it valuable for highly educated parents and professionals.

Kübler-Ross E: *On Children and Death*, reprint ed. New York, Scribner, 1997. From the person who gave the classic descriptions of the grieving process, this book explains children's understanding of death and how to assist in the process.

Trozzi M: *Talking with Children about Loss: Words, Strategies and Wisdom to Help Children Cope with Death, Divorce, and Other Difficult Times*. New York, Putnam, 1999. Intended for parents and professionals, this book gently leads the reader through the most difficult terrain: how to help your child deal with the painful feelings of significant loss in a way that actually enhances healthy psychological development. This easy-to-read book uses lots of examples: facing the death of a family member or a pet, divorce, chronic illness, and welcoming a new sibling born with special needs, as well as the inevitable losses and changes that all children face. Practical suggestions for management and intervention are included. Good for parents who need this perspective and for teachers and other professionals who deal with children facing the death of themselves or family members.

Child Safety Resources

The following organizations and agencies provide pamphlets and leaflets dealing with child safety resources:

Action for Child Product Safety, 358 Woburn St, Lexington, MA 02173.

Action for Children's Television (ACT), 20 University Road, Cambridge, MA 02138. An advocacy group that continues to be legislatively active, to provide ongoing monitoring of television and to provide educational materials. A good mailing list to be on.

Committee on Accident and Poison Prevention, American Academy of Pediatrics (AAP), 141 Northwest Point Blvd, Elk Grove Village, IL 60009.

Parents' Choice, Box 185, Newton, MA 02168. Awards for books, magazines, computer games, television shows and toys.

US Consumer Product Safety Commission (Washington, DC 20207): *Because You Care for Kids* (numerous hazards); *Safety Sampler* (baby equipment and toys); *Super Sitter* (advice to baby-sitters).

Nutrition

Baker S, Henry R: *Boston Children's Hospital Parents' Guide to Nutrition.* Reading, MA, Addison-Wesley, 1989. Comprehensive, sensible and usable information on nutritional issues from infancy to adolescence. The authors review the latest research, demystify fad diets and provide nutritional recommendations. The format is easy to read, and recipes are included.

Brazelton TB, Sparrow JD: *Feeding.* Cambridge, MA, Da Capo Press, 2004. Feeding patterns from the newborn to the 5-year-old are described in the context of developmental abilities and family expectations. Also reviews common feeding problems and solutions.

Dietz WH, Stern L (eds): *Guide to Your Child's Nutrition.* New York, Villard (for the American Academy of Pediatrics), 1999. Collaborative effort sponsored by the American Academy of Pediatrics to provide the best nutritional information. Detailed, for newborns to adolescents. Common and uncommon problems. Lots of charts, practical ideas. For the physician or the very interested family.

Ikeda J, Naworski P: *Am I Fat? Helping Young Children Accept Differences in Body Size.* Santa Cruz, CA, ETR Associates, 1993. This perceptive and colorful storybook helps parents and children talk about differences in body sizes and shape. It is easy and fun to read and provides an entry for talking about other kinds of physical differences.

Lansky V: *Feed Me: I'm Yours.* Oldhaven, NJ, Simon & Schuster, 1996. This is a practical book with an emphasis on feeding toddlers.

Piscatella J: *Fat-Proof Your Child.* New York, Workman Publishing, 1997. An in-depth guide for parents that emphasizes parents being the most influential factor on how active and healthy their children will be. Sound advice on diet and exercise. Some parts a bit technical (e.g., figuring out basal metabolic rate).

Satter E: *How to Get Your Kid to Eat—But Not Too Much.* Palo Alto, CA, Bull, 1987. This practical resource shows parents how to help children develop good eating behavior. It also discusses childhood distortions about eating and feeding that may be precursors to eating disorders in later life.

Satter E: *Child of Mine: Feeding with Love and Good Sense*, 3rd ed. Palo Alto, CA, Bull, 2000. This nutritional guidebook offers information on the developmental and social aspects of feeding from infancy through adolescence. Types of behavior that encourage the formation of healthy eating patterns are reviewed, and technical nutrition information is translated into practical and basic concepts.

Tamborlane W (ed): *The Yale Guide to Children's Nutrition*. New Haven, CT, Yale University Press, 1997. A comprehensive reference that addresses all aspects of nutrition (e.g., eating disorders, childhood obesity, diabetes, cholesterol, food allergies), using the most current research findings. Reader friendly with charts and tables that provide information on everything from healthy snacks to nutrition for the breastfeeding mother. Good for professionals and parents who like to be well informed.

Sports and Child Development

Schreiber LR: *The Parent's Guide to Kids' Sports*. Boston, Little, Brown, 1990. This book provides essential information on the physical, psychological and social issues in children's sports. Parental involvement, coaching, competition, and girls' participation in sports are emphasized. Exercise, nutrition and injury prevention are also reviewed. It is a useful guide to the equipment needs, costs and injuries in common sports. A bibliography and resource list is included.

BOOKS FOR CHILDREN

Developmental and Situational Conflicts

Berenstain S, Berenstain J: First Time Books: *The Berenstain Bears: Go to the Doctor; Go to Visit the Dentist; Moving Day; and the Sitter; Get in a Fight; Trouble with Friends; Trouble with Money; and the Messy Room; Learn About Strangers; and Too Much TV; and Too Much Junk Food; Go Out for the Team; and Mama's New Job; Forget their Manners; and the Truth; Get Stage Fright; Trouble at School; in the Dark; and the Bad Habit*. New York, Random House, 1981 to 1997. Inexpensive picture books that highlight some stressful experiences. Written for older toddlers and preschoolers in a pleasant and reassuring manner. Available in bookstores and children's stores.

Berger T: *I Have Feelings*. New York, Human Sciences Press, 1977. Nice, reflective book for kindergarten through sixth grade. An example of several books that help children to reflect on themselves through another child's eyes.

Cole J, Degan B: *The Magic School Bus: Inside the Human Body.* New York, NY: Scholastic, 1990. For ages 6 to 9 years.

Lansky V: *It's Not Your Fault Koko Bear*. Minnetonka, MN: Book Peddlers, 1998. For ages 3 to 6 years. A sensitive story about why Koko Papa must get his own den after parents' separation.

Perrin EC, Starr S: Addressing common pediatric concerns through children's books. *Pediatr Rev* 21:130-138, 2000. A pediatrician and educator annotate over 100 books for children.

Frequently encountered developmental and behavioral concerns are outlined by specific topics. Very useful for pediatric clinicians—for the waiting room and to recommend to parents.

Rockell L: *Good Enough to Eat: A Kid's Guide to Food and Nutrition.* New York, Harper Collins, 1999. Written in a question-answer format for kids 4 to 8 years old with an emphasis on eating right.

Stern Z, Stern E: *Divorce is Not the End of the World: Zoe and Evan's Coping Guide for Kids.* Triangle Press, 1997. For ages 6 to 10 years. Written from a child's perspective with lots of humor and practical advice.

Viorst J Lobel A: *I'll Fix Anthony*, 2nd ed. Aladdin, 1988. A classic tale of an older brother who is mean and the younger brother who dreams of revenge.

Walker R: *Encyclopedia of the Human Body.* London, Dorling Kindersley Publishing, 2002. For school-age children and adolescents. Beautifully illustrated guides to teach children and youth about the anatomy and function of he human body.

BOOKS FOR TEENAGERS

Lindsay JW: *Pregnant Too Soon: Adoption Is an Option.* Buena Park, CA, Morning Glory Press, 1980. This soft-cover book uses case histories of pregnant teenagers to illustrate the problems of young women who become mothers in their teen years. The author emphasizes the option of adoption, and this book serves as a good resource for pregnant teenagers who want to learn or read more about the process of adoption.

Mayle P: *What's Happening to Me?* Secaucus, NJ, Lyle Stuart, 1975. This delightful, slim, inexpensive soft-cover book is described as a guide to puberty and is produced by the same authors who wrote *Where Did I Come From?* With amusing drawings and a brief, compassionate narrative, the authors present various aspects of pubertal development from breasts to erections. This book is probably best suited for those in early adolescence.

McCoy K, Wibbelsman C: *The Teenage Body Book*, revised ed. New York, Perigee Books, 1999. This book is based on questions commonly asked by teenagers concerning their bodies and bodily changes. The authors are a former editor of *Teen Magazine* and a physician who specializes in adolescent medicine. The authors cover a wide range of topics, including normal physical development and birth control. Case vignettes and examples of letters from teens are used to illustrate various problems. Detailed line drawings are plentiful and excellent. This book is more appropriate for those in mid to late adolescence; it may be too sophisticated for younger adolescents.

• Riera M: *Surviving High School.* Berkeley, CA, Celestial Arts Publishing, 1997. This book, written for 13- to 20-year-olds, covers all aspects of adolescence—sex, parents, safety, money and college. The format of teenagers' commentaries intermixed with explanations and questions from a counselor sets a friendly tone. Riera encourages reflections through "think about it" questions at the end of each chapter.

SEX EDUCATION

Basso MJ: *The Underground Guide to Teenage Sexuality*, 2nd ed. Minneapolis, MN, Fairview Press, 2003. The classic guide to teen sexuality—updated and expanded with information on sexually transmitted diseases, contraception, sexual abuse, healthy relationships and resources.

Cole J, Tiegreen A: *Asking about Sex and Growing Up: A Question-and-Answer Book for Boys and Girls*. New York, HarperTrophy, 1988. An illustrated book for kids 7 to 11 years old, it has accurate information and is intended for both boys and girls.

Fenwick E, Smith T: *Adolescence: The Survival Guide for Parents and Teenagers*. New York, DK Publishing, 1996. A comprehensive discussion of concerns of most adolescents and parents with an appealing writing style.

Haffner DW, Tartaglione AH: *Beyond the Big Talk: Every Parent's Guide to Raising Sexually Healthy Teens from Middle School to High School and Beyond*. New York, New Market Press, 2002. Sections on early, middle and later adolescent development are organized by the age appropriateness of sexual information. Encourages looking for "teachable moments" to engage teens in talks with parents about sexuality.

Harris RH, Emberley M: *It's Perfectly Normal: Changing Bodies, Growing Up, Sex and Sexual Health*, Cambridge, MA, Candlewick Press, 1994. A wonderful book for preteens and their parents. Informative, easy to read, accurate and unbiased. Nice cartoons and illustrations.

Harris RH, Emberley M: *It's So Amazing! A Book about Eggs, Sperm, Birth, Babies, and Families*. Cambridge, MA, Candlewick Press, 1999. Similar format written for younger children (kindergarten through fourth grade).

Maderas L: *What's Happening to My Body? A Book for Girls: A Growing-Up Guide for Parents and Daughters*, 3rd ed New Market Press, New York, 2000 and *What's Happening to My Body? A Book for Boys: A Growing-Up Guide for Parents and Sons*, 3rd ed. New York, New Market Press, 2000. Excellent comprehensive books to be read with preadolescents. The new edition has information on AIDS and sexually transmitted diseases.

Philothea T Sweet, RN, Obstetrics Clinic, Outpatient Department, University of Minnesota Hospitals; Minneapolis, MN. Eight-page annotated **bibliography of books on sex education** (and sibling preparation and rivalry), with age-level recommendations developed by and available from this nurse-mother. A free, annotated resource list of sex education books is available from the local Planned Parenthood Association. The list has separate sections for parents, teens and children. Free reprints of some articles are also available.

Stoppard M: *Sex Ed*. New York, DK Publishing, 1997. In a comic book fashion, Dr. Stoppard debunks myths and encourages safe sex and contraception. Strong emphasis on seeking additional help.

INTERNET RESOURCES

The Internet offers the opportunity to find information readily and easily. This is a growing avenue to provide parent education, referral and a lot of valuable information. Caution must be exercised, however, because no overall process for review or oversight exists. Some information may reflect personal or ideological viewpoints that are not mainstream or in line with the goals and values of a family. This must be evaluated for each site. Some services purport to identify legitimate sources of medical information on the Web, but they may not have kept up with the rapid influx of information.

The clinician cannot stop families from getting information from the Web. Honest interaction about this issue and joint review of material will help clinicians and parents use the information together. The following are some things to consider that will help the health care provider and a family evaluate Internet advice on a parenting or child care site:

- **Who is writing the material?** In addition to the name of the author(s), the site should provide the background and credentials of the contributors. These should be highly qualified professionals with specific education and training in the issues on which they write.

- **The organizational affiliates should all be identified.** These should be mainstream, professional and official linkages, not just "the author is a member of. . . ." Clear distinctions between organizational backing versus individual perspective alone is important.

- **The site sponsorship should be identified.** Who is paying for site development and oversight? The *.org* address suffix, indicating supposedly nonprofit organizational sponsorship, is not a guarantee of legitimacy. Conversely, a *.com* suffix doesn't mean that the material is invalid because of commercial sponsorship. Sometimes these sites have the best material because resources are available to develop and maintain the site at a high level of excellence. For commercially sponsored sites, the commercial components should be explicit ad units, clearly demarcated from the content as one would see in a magazine. The *.edu* designation indicates an educational entity as the base site. These, too, call for scrutiny of content, although commercialization is less likely.

- **The processes for the development, oversight and updating of content should be available for review** so that the reader knows how the material is scrutinized before being posted. This gives some assurance that it is not just the views of one individual.

- **The dating of the material should be stated.** This ensures the timeliness of the information. Archival material can be of great worth, but one should be able to find out how old the material is and how often it is reviewed and updated.

These criteria are similar to those developed for the appraisal of medical information in general as stated in a multidisciplinary conference on the uses of the Web in medical practice. Physicians should develop ways to address the use of the Internet in their practices because it will probably have an increasing impact on their work.

Families should be encouraged to bring in the material that they get on the Internet for review with the child health care provider. They can look it over together, and sharing of the materials with other families can be facilitated if the material looks good to the clinician. Dismissal of this growing medium as a resource will result only in hiding of the material from this shared review.

Sites Offering General Parenting and Child Care Advice to Parents

http://www.pampers.com—This site contains an encyclopedia of information about pregnancy to age 3 on development, health, safety and current news issues; it also has a question and answer section, monthly age-adjusted e-mail newsletters and a lot of special features. Sponsored by Proctor and Gamble, Pampers division, it brings high-level and seasoned professionals and organizations together to provide to provide a wealth of information.

http://www.babycenter.com—This site focuses largely on pregnancy and the first year. Many features on this site change daily, including polls, news, games and the largest baby name reference available. Monitored chat, questions and answers and lots of special features. Well written and reviewed. Webby award winner: "Best on the Web" several years in a row.

http://www.parentime.com—A Time/Warner production, this site contains a lot of material from several sources, much of it archived. Under renovation at the time of this review.

http://www.parentsoup.com—Lots of good things here from a lot of different perspectives. Needs some wading through. Parent and professional contributions. Quality varies widely.

http://www.aap.org/parents.html—The American Academy of Pediatrics site, contains abstracts from *Pediatrics*, AAP policy statements and important news that affects children, families and clinicians who provide care for children and adolescents.

http://www.aacap.org/publications/factsfam/index.htm—The American Academy of Child and Adolescent Psychiatry developed Facts for Families to provide concise and up-to-date information on psychological issues that affect children, teenagers and their families. Each statement is available in English, Spanish, German, French, Polish and Icelandic.

http://www.naspcenter.org/teachers/teachers.html—National Mental Health and Education Center's website for parents, teachers and clinician on behavioral and educational issues of school-age children. Well organized and well written.

http://med.umich.edu/1libr/yourchild—Resources for parents from developmental and behavioral pediatricians at the University of Michigan. Well-researched, accessible and in-depth information on a range of topics with links to other information, organizations and support groups.

http://www.talkingwithkids.org—Talk with Kids about Tough Issues, a project of Children Now and the Kaiser Family Foundation.

http://www.4girls.gov—Resources on caring for adolescent girls.

http://www.advocatesforyouth.org/parents/—An excellent site providing anticipatory guidance for parents on adolescents.

http://www.aacap.org/publications/factsfam/index.htm—Excellent site that provides fact sheets on adolescent and mental health issues from the American Academy of Child and Adolescent Psychiatry. English and Spanish.

http://www.pflag.org—Parents, Families and Friends of Lesbians and Gays.

Teen Websites

http://www.advocatesforyouth.org/teens—Information on teen health, sexual health and other topics.

http://www.iwannaknow.org—Information from the American Social Health Association for teens on sexuality, sexual transmitted infections and related topics with a parent's guide and great links.

http://www.kidshealth.org/teen—A great site for teens on health with separate sections geared toward boys and girls. From the Nemours Foundation.

http://teengrowth.com—Interactive website for teens on health and development. Board-certified physicians give advice on topics such as obesity, diet, emotions, alcohol, drugs, family, friends, school, sex and sports.

http://www.advocatesforyouth.org/glbtq.htm—Great site that includes fact sheets and links on issues for gay, lesbian, bisexual and questioning youth. English and Spanish.

http://www.4girls.gov—Information geared toward younger female teens.

http://www.iemily.com—Site for teenage girls about health-related matters.

http://www.youngwomenshealth.org—Site from the Center for Young Women's Health, Children's Hospital Boston. English and Spanish.

http://mysistahs.org—A site for and by young women of color.

http://www.freevibe.com—Excellent site to get information on drugs, alcohol, and tobacco that is teen friendly.

http://www.teenpregnancy.org/teen/default.asp—Website from the National Campaign to Prevent Teen Pregnancy. A good site for anyone (teen, parent, professional) wanting information on teen pregnancy.

Other sites may be identified through search engines by using *parenting, healthcare, newborn, child health, child development* and *baby care* in a search. Sites that deal with specialty information can be searched through identification by the term or professional organization.

ADDITIONAL READING ABOUT THE USE OF INTERNET RESOURCES IN MEDICAL PRACTICE

Hancock L: *Physicians' Guide to the Internet.* Philadelphia, Lippincott-Raven, 1996.

Kiley R: *Medical Information on the Internet.* New York, Churchill Livingstone, 1998.

Smith RP, Edwards MJA: *The Internet for Physicians.* New York, Springer, 1997.

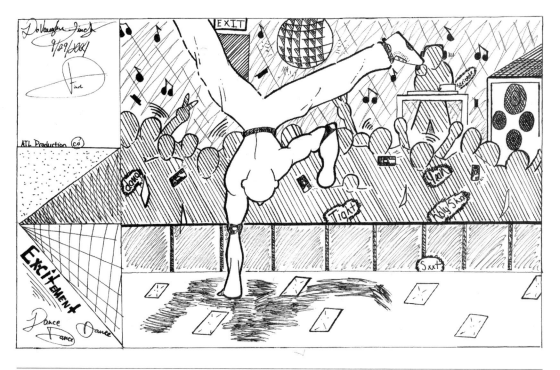

"Parenting can make one seem like you can dance on your hands." By DeVaughn Finch, age 18.

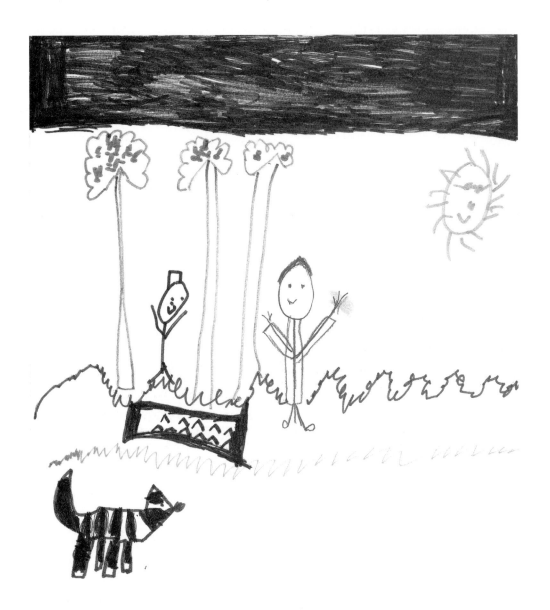

Dogs are very important to children and frequently appear in drawings, often not the least or last but central to the action. A 6-year-old boy shows himself with his dad and his dog. The dog crossed the stream and is off on his own. By T.M.M.

Section I: Screening Checklists as Aids to Interview

A fundamental principle that guides the recommendations found in this book is that the acquisition of information about development, behavior and family function is acquired optimally from interviewing children, youth and parents. We focus on a major developmental or behavioral theme at each health supervision visit as an organizing method in order to guide our observations, questions, assessment and anticipatory guidance. With practice, it becomes the most effective and efficient way to screen for developmental and behavioral problems. The clinical interview, at its best, forms the foundation for a therapeutic relationship with child and parents.

Many clinicians have discovered the benefits of selected screening checklists as a way to supplement or focus the clinical interview. These tests, when administered before seeing a child, can trigger questions, raise issues and prevent omissions in data collection. Most of the tests have been evaluated for validity, reliability and predictive value. However, a screening test is not diagnostic. Rather, it suggests a problem that must then be evaluated further through a comprehensive and focused interview by a primary care clinician. Referral for a developmental assessment or a mental health consultation may follow, depending on the clinician's interpretation of the screening test and clinical interview. Perrin and Stancin observed that "screening instruments are clinical tools that are useful to help identify and quantify parent's concerns, (developmental delays), and worrisome child behavior or feelings efficiently ... as long as their limitations are recognized." Rating scales for behavioral conditions (e.g., depression) cannot take the place of a careful clinical interview. They are often helpful in the assessment of severity of symptoms and monitoring progress over time.

As we make use of screening checklists, it is useful to keep in mind both the advantages and limitations of these instruments. They provide a standardized database that serves to organize a health supervision visit. Screening tests prevent omissions that may occur during an interview alone. They provide potential educational value as a parent or older child answers questions that raise a concern that may not have been considered previously. They may help parents become better observers of their child's developmental changes and behavior. Maintaining copies of the screening checklist in the medical record leads to quality assurance. A potential disadvantage of using a checklist alone is missing a parent's agenda for the visit by not permitting an individualized focus for the visit. A checklist without a therapeutic interview encourages an emphasis on content at the expense of process and a false sense of completeness (see Chapter 4).

When a screening test is used, it is the clinician's responsibility to interpret the results accurately and convey the information to the parents and/or child clearly. Screening for developmental and behavioral conditions should always be done with current knowledge about available referral sources in the community.

Every assessment is an interaction between the examiner and the child. The state, temperament and availability of the child, as well as the training, ease, skill and style of the examiner, influence it. The results of screening tests must always be interpreted with these factors in mind. They should never be a substitute for face-to-face clinical encounters in primary care practice. Screening tests serve as an adjunct, a time saver and a structure on which to focus behavioral and developmental concerns.

REFERENCES

Blackman JA: Developmental screening: Infant, toddler and preschooler. In Levine MD, Carey WB, Crocker AC (eds):
    Developmental-Behavioral Pediatrics, 3rd ed. Philadelphia, WB Saunders, 1999, pp 689-695.

Glascoe FP: Early detection of developmental and behavioral problems. *Pediatr Rev* 21:272-280, 2000.

Jellinek M. Patel B, Froehle M: *Bright Futures in Practice: Mental Health.* Arlington, VA, National Center for Education
    in Maternal and Child Health, 2002.

Perrin EC: Ethical questions about screening. *J Dev Behav Pediatrics* 9:350-352, 1998.

Perrin EC, Stancin T: A continuing dilemma: Whether and how to screen for concerns about children's behavior.
    Pediatr Rev 23:264-275, 2002.

TABLE A–1 Standardized Developmental-Behavioral Screening Instruments

Tool, Source And Price	Age Range	Description	Scoring	Accuracy	Time Frame
Child Development Inventories (formerly Minnesota Child Development Inventories), 1992. Behavior Science Systems, Bx 580274, Minneapolis, MN 55458 (ph: 612-929-6220) ($41.00 + s/h)	3–72 mo	Three separate instruments, each with 60 yes/no descriptions. Can be mailed to families, completed in waiting rooms, administered by interview or by direct elicitation.	A single cutoff tied to 1.5 standard deviations below the mean	Sensitivity in detecting children with difficulties is greater than 75% (across studies), and specificity in correctly detecting normal development is 70% (across studies).	About 10 minutes
Parents' Evaluations of Developmental Status (PEDS), 1997. Ellsworth & Vandermeer Press, Ltd. 4405 Scenic Dr., Nashville, TN, 37204 (ph: 615-386-0061/ fax: 615-386-0346) http://edge. net/~evpress ($30.00 + s/h)	Birth to 8 years	Ten questions eliciting parents' concerns. Can be administered in waiting rooms or by interview in Spanish and English. Determines when to refer, provide a second screen, counsel, reassure or carefully monitor development, behavior and academic progress	Identifies levels of risk for various kinds of emotional and developmental problems and delays	Sensitivity ranges from 74% to 79%, and specificity ranges from 70% to 80% across age levels.	About 2 minutes
Ages and Stages Questionnaire (formerly Infant Monitoring System), 1994. Paul H. Brookes Publishers, P.O. Box 10624, Baltimore, MD 21285 (ph: 800-638-3775) ($130.00 + s/h)	0–60 mo	Clear drawings and simple directions help parents report on children's skills. Separate copyable forms of 30 items for each age range (tied to well-child visit schedule). Can be used in mass mailings for child-find programs.	Single pass/fail score	Sensitivity ranges from 70% to 90% at all ages except the 4-month level, and specificity ranges from 75% to 91%.	About 7 minutes

Continued

TABLE A–1 **Standardized Developmental-Behavioral Screening Instruments**–cont'd

Tool, Source And Price	Age Range	Description	Scoring	Accuracy	Time Frame
Pediatric Symptom Checklist, Jellinek MS, Murphy JM, Robinson J, et al: Pediatric Symptom Checklist: Screening school age children for psychosocial dysfunction. *J Pediatr* 112:201, 1988. (Test is included in the article.)	4–16 yrs	Thirty-five short statements of problem behavior, including both externalizing (conduct) and internalizing (depression, anxiety, adjustment, etc.). Ratings of never, sometimes or often are assigned a value of 0, 1 and 2, and scores above cutoffs indicate when referrals are needed.	Single refer/nonrefer score	All but one study showed high sensitivity (80%–95%) but somewhat scattered specificity (68%–100%).	About 7 minutes
Denver II (1990), Denver Developmental Materials (DDM), PO Box 6169, Denver, CO 80206 (ph: 303-355-4729)	0–6 yr	Administered by trained person, who asks parents questions and assesses child's skills in motor, language and social domains. A helpful visual aid of a child's development for parents. Helps clarify concerns. Gives a structure for observation.	Scoring chart with bar graphs that display 25th to 90th percentile for each milestone; produces a single score—normal, suspect and untestable.	It is not meant to predict specific developmental conditions. Rather, the validity is based on its accuracy to detect the normal range of each developmental milestone.	20 minutes

Modified with permission from Glascoe FP: *Collaborating with Parents*. Nashville, TN, Ellsworth & Vandermeer, 1998.

Developmental and Behavioral Screening Tests In Pediatric Practice

The screening tools listed below are those that we find adaptable to primary care pediatrics. Some were designed specifically for office and clinic-based practices. Others have been used in different settings in addition to primary care. With few exceptions, these instruments have sensitivities and specificities above 75% with good validity and reliability. From the perspective of a primary care clinician, the *language* used in the behavioral screening questions can become a part of a clinical interview. With experience, pediatric clinicians can tailor an interview to make use of questions suitable to a particular age and situation. The examples of screening tests are shown as a way to introduce the reader to different formats. For many tests, formal scoring systems are available from the publisher of the instrument.

Developmental Screening

- Ages and Stages Questionnaire*
- Child Development Inventories
- Denver II*
- Parents' Evaluation of Developmental Status (PEDS)*
- Early Language Milestone Scale-2*

Behavioral Screening

- Ages and Stages Questionnaire: Social-Emotional
- Beck Depression Inventory-II
- Carey Temperament Scales*
- Children's Depression Inventory (CDI)
- Edinburgh Postnatal Depression Scale (maternal depression)*
- Pediatric Symptom Checklist*
- Family Psychosocial Screening*

Attention Deficit/Hyperactivity Disorder and Learning Disorders (see Chapter 20)

- NICHQ Vanderbilt Assessment Scale. American Academy of Pediatrics/National Initiative for Children's Healthcare Quality (NICHQ). ADHD: *Caring for Children with ADHD: A Resource Toolkit for Clinicians.* http://www.nichq.org/resources/toolkit/
- Einstein Assessment of School-Related Skills

Autism

- Modified Checklist for Autism in Toddlers (M-CHAT)*
- Pervasive Development Disorder Screening Test-II
- Guides to Pediatric Visits (American Academy of Pediatric's Guidelines for Health Supervision Visits III)*

---

*Examples of screening instruments in the Appendix

AGES & STAGES QUESTIONNAIRE (8 mo sample)

	YES	SOMETIMES	NOT YET	

COMMUNICATION   *Be sure to try each activity with your child.*

1. If you call to your baby when you are out of sight, does he look in the direction of your voice?   ❑ ❑ ❑ ____

2. When a loud noise occurs, does your baby turn to see where the sound came from?   ❑ ❑ ❑ ____

3. If you copy the sounds your baby makes, does your baby repeat the same sounds back to you?   ❑ ❑ ❑ ____

4. Does your baby make sounds like "da," "ga," "ka," and "ba"?   ❑ ❑ ❑ ____

5. Does your baby respond to the tone of your voice and stop her activity at least briefly when you say "no-no" to her?   ❑ ❑ ❑ ____

6. Does your baby make two similar sounds like "ba-ba," "da-da," or "ga-ga"? (He may say these sounds without referring to any particular object or person.)   ❑ ❑ ❑ ____

COMMUNICATION TOTAL ____

GROSS MOTOR   *Be sure to try each activity with your child.*

1. When you put her on the floor, does your baby lean on her hands while sitting? (If she already sits up straight without leaning on her hands, check "yes" for this item.)   ❑ ❑ ❑ ____

2. Does your baby roll from his back to his tummy, getting both arms out from under him?   ❑ ❑ ❑ ____

3. Does your baby get into a crawling position by getting up on her hands and knees?   ❑ ❑ ❑ ____

4. If you hold both hands just to balance him, does your baby support his own weight while standing?   ❑ ❑ ❑ ____

5. When sitting on the floor, does your baby sit up straight for several minutes *without* using her hands for support?   ❑ ❑ ❑ ____ *

6. When you stand him next to furniture or the crib rail, does your baby hold on without leaning his chest against the furniture for support?   ❑ ❑ ❑ ____

GROSS MOTOR TOTAL ____

If gross motor item 5 is marked "yes" or "sometimes," mark gross motor item 1 as "yes."

Ages & Stages Questionnaires, Bricker et al.
© 1995 Paul H. Brookes Publishing Co.

ASQ   **8 months**

	YES	SOMETIMES	NOT YET

FINE MOTOR *Be sure to try each activity with your child.*

1. Does your baby reach for a crumb or Cheerio and touch it with her finger or hand? (If she already picks up a small object, check "yes" for this item.) ❑ ❑ ❑ ___

2. Does your baby pick up a small toy, holding it in the center of his hand with his fingers around it? ❑ ❑ ❑ ___

3. Does your baby *try* to pick up a crumb or Cheerio by using her thumb and all her fingers in a raking motion, even if she isn't able to pick it up? (If she already picks up a crumb or Cheerio, check "yes" for this item.) ❑ ❑ ❑ ___

4. Does your baby pick up small toys with only one hand? ❑ ❑ ❑ ___

5. Does your baby *successfully* pick up a crumb or Cheerio by using his thumb and all his fingers in a raking motion? (If he already picks up a crumb or Cheerio, check "yes" for this item.) ❑ ❑ ❑ ___

6. Does your baby pick up a small toy with the *tips* of her thumb and fingers? (You should see a space between the toy and her palm.) ❑ ❑ ❑ ___ *

FINE MOTOR TOTAL ___

*If fine motor item 6 is marked "yes" or "sometimes," mark fine motor item 2 as "yes."

PROBLEM SOLVING *Be sure to try each activity with your child.*

1. Does your baby pick up a toy and put it in his mouth? ❑ ❑ ❑ ___

2. When she is on her back, does your baby try to get a toy she has dropped if she can see it? ❑ ❑ ❑ ___

3. Does your baby play by banging a toy up and down against the floor or table? ❑ ❑ ❑ ___

4. Does your baby pass a toy back and forth from one hand to the other? ❑ ❑ ❑ ___

✿ASQ **8 months**

	YES	SOMETIMES	NOT YET	

PROBLEM SOLVING   *(continued)*

5. Does your baby pick up two small toys, one in each hand, and hold onto them for about 1 minute? ❑ ❑ ❑ ____

6. When holding a toy in his hand, does your baby bang it against another toy on the table? ❑ ❑ ❑ ____

PROBLEM SOLVING TOTAL ____

PERSONAL-SOCIAL   *Be sure to try each activity with your child.*

1. While lying on her back, does your baby play by grabbing her foot? ❑ ❑ ❑ ____

2. When in front of a large mirror, does your baby reach out to pat the mirror? ❑ ❑ ❑ ____

3. Does your baby try to get a toy that is out of reach? (He may roll, pivot on his tummy, or crawl to get it.) ❑ ❑ ❑ ____

4. While on her back, does your baby put her foot in her mouth? ❑ ❑ ❑ ____

5. Does your baby drink water, juice, or formula from a cup while you hold it? ❑ ❑ ❑ ____

6. Does your baby feed himself a cracker or a cookie? ❑ ❑ ❑ ____

PERSONAL-SOCIAL TOTAL ____

OVERALL   *Parents and providers may use the bottom of the next sheet for additional comments.*

1. Do you think your child hears well? YES ❑ NO ❑

If no, explain: _____

2. Does your baby use both hands equally well? YES ❑ NO ❑

If no, explain: _____

3. When you help your baby stand, are her feet flat on the surface most of the time? YES ❑ NO ❑

If no, explain: _____

Ages & Stages Questionnaires, Bricker et al.
© 1995 Paul H. Brookes Publishing Co.

●ASQ   **8 months**

OVERALL   (continued)

4. Does either parent have any family history of childhood deafness or hearing impairment?   YES ☐   NO ☐

    If yes, explain: _____

5. Has your child had any medical problems in the last several months?   YES ☐   NO ☐

    If yes, explain: _____

6. Does anything about your child worry you?   YES ☐   NO ☐

    If yes, explain: _____

♥ASQ   **8 months**

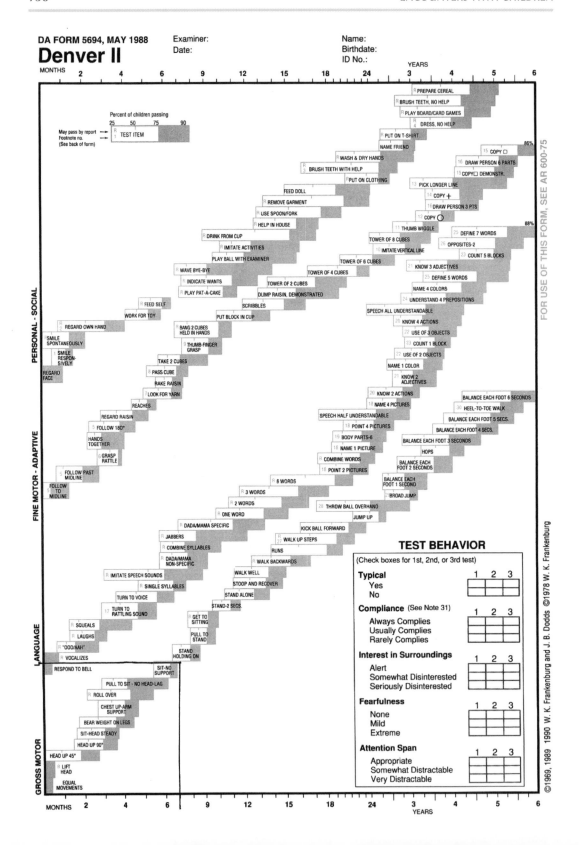

DA FORM 5694, MAY 1988

Denver II

Examiner:
Date:

Name:
Birthdate:
ID No.:

TEST BEHAVIOR

(Check boxes for 1st, 2nd, or 3rd test)

Typical
Yes
No

Compliance (See Note 31)
Always Complies
Usually Complies
Rarely Complies

Interest in Surroundings
Alert
Somewhat Disinterested
Seriously Disinterested

Fearfulness
None
Mild
Extreme

Attention Span
Appropriate
Somewhat Distractable
Very Distractable

DIRECTIONS FOR ADMINISTRATION

1. Try to get child to smile by smiling, talking or waving. Do not touch him/her.
2. Child must stare at hand several seconds.
3. Parent may help guide toothbrush and put toothpaste on brush.
4. Child does not have to be able to tie shoes or button/zip in the back.
5. Move yarn slowly in an arc from one side to the other, about 8" above child's face.
6. Pass if child grasps rattle when it is touched to the backs or tips of fingers.
7. Pass if child tries to see where yarn went. Yarn should be dropped quickly from sight from tester's hand without arm movement.
8. Child must transfer cube from hand to hand without help of body, mouth, or table.
9. Pass if child picks up raisin with any part of thumb and finger.
10. Line can vary only 30 degrees or less from tester's line. $\lor$
11. Make a fist with thumb pointing upward and wiggle only the thumb. Pass if child imitates and does not move any fingers other than the thumb.

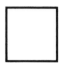

| 12. Pass any enclosed form. Fail continuous round motions. | 13. Which line is longer? (Not bigger.) Turn paper upside down and repeat. (pass 3 of 3 or 5 of 6) | 14. Pass any lines crossing near midpoint. | 15. Have child copy first. If failed, demonstrate. |

When giving items 12, 14, and 15, do not name the forms. Do not demonstrate 12 and 14.

16. When scoring, each pair (2 arms, 2 legs, etc.) counts as one part.
17. Place one cube in cup and shake gently near child's ear, but out of sight. Repeat for other ear.
18. Point to picture and have child name it. (No credit is given for sounds only.)
    If less than 4 pictures are named correctly, have child point to picture as each is named by tester.

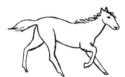

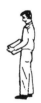

19. Using doll, tell child: Show me the nose, eyes, ears, mouth, hands, feet, tummy, hair. Pass 6 of 8.
20. Using pictures, ask child: Which one flies?... says meow?... talks?... barks?... gallops? Pass 2 of 5, 4 of 5.
21. Ask child: What do you do when you are cold?... tired?... hungry? Pass 2 of 3, 3 of 3.
22. Ask child: What do you do with a cup? What is a chair used for? What is a pencil used for?
    Action words must be included in answers.
23. Pass if child correctly places <u>and</u> says how many blocks are on paper. (1, 5).
24. Tell child: Put block **on** table; **under** table; **in front of** me, **behind** me. Pass 4 of 4.
    (Do not help child by pointing, moving head or eyes.)
25. Ask child: What is a ball?... lake?... desk?... house?... banana?... curtain?... fence?... ceiling? Pass if defined in terms of use, shape, what it is made of, or general category (such as banana is fruit, not just yellow). Pass 5 of 8, 7 of 8.
26. Ask child: If a horse is big, a mouse is __? If fire is hot, ice is __? If the sun shines during the day, the moon shines during the __? Pass 2 of 3.
27. Child may use wall or rail only, not person. May not crawl.
28. Child must throw ball overhand 3 feet to within arm's reach of tester.
29. Child must perform standing broad jump over width of test sheet (8 1/2 inches).
30. Tell child to walk forward, ∞∞∞∞➤ heel within 1 inch of toe. Tester may demonstrate.
    Child must walk 4 consecutive steps.
31. In the second year, half of normal children are non-compliant.

OBSERVATIONS:

DENVER PRESCREENING DEVELOPMENTAL QUESTIONNAIRE II

9-24 MONTHS
(PDQ-II)

Child's Name _____

Person Completing PDQ-II _____

Relation to Child _____

For Office Use			
Today's Date	___ yr	___ mo	___ day
Child's Birthdate	___ yr	___ mo	___ day
Subtract to get Child's Exact Age	___ yr	___ mo	___ day
PDQII Age:		___ mo	___ completed wks

CONTINUE ANSWERING UNTIL 3 "NOs" ARE CIRCLED

	For Office Use 90% 75%

28. Mama/Dada, Non-Specific
Does your baby make either "mama" or "dada" sounds?
YES NO — 9 7-3 L

29. Pulls To Stand
When in a crib or beside furniture, can your baby pull herself up to a standing position without help?
YES NO — 9-3 9 GM

30. Gets to Sitting
When crawling or lying down, can your baby get into a sitting position without help?
YES NO — 9-3 9 GM

31. Combines Syllables
Does your baby repeat the same sounds several times in a row like "dadadada," or "gagagaga"?
YES NO — 10 7-1 L

32. Thumb-Finger Grasp
When your baby picks up a tiny object, such as a raisin, does he do so by squeezing it between his thumb and at least one finger like either of these pictures?
YES NO — 10 9 FMA

33. Plays Pat-A-Cake
Can your baby play "pat-a-cake" with someone without any help, such as helping him clap his hands?
YES NO — 11-1 10-1 PS

34. Stands - 5 Seconds
Can your baby stand alone (without having to hold on to something) for about 5 seconds?
YES NO — 11-2 10-3 GM

	For Office Use 90% 75%

35. Jabbers
When your baby is playing alone, does he jabber as though really talking? This jabbering does not have to be understandable.
YES NO — 12 8-1 L

36. Indicates Wants
Can your child let you know what she wants without crying or whining? Examples of this are pointing, or pulling on you.
YES NO — 12-3 11 PS

37. Mama/Dada Specific
Does your child say "Dada" when he wants or sees his father? Does your child say "Mama" when he wants or sees his mother? Circle YES if your child says either one.
YES NO — 13-1 11 L

38. Stands Alone
Can your child stand alone (without having to hold on to something) for 15 seconds or more?
YES NO — 13-3 12-2 GM

39. Puts Toy in Cup
Can your child put a small object (such as finger food or a toy) into a cup, letting go of it and leaving it there for at least a few seconds?
YES NO — 13-3 12-1 FMA

40. Waves Bye-Bye
When you or someone else waves and says "bye-bye" to your child, can your child wave back without help?
YES NO — 14 9 PS

41. Stoops and Recovers
Without holding on to something or touching the floor, can your child bend over or stoop to pick up a toy or other object on the floor and stand up again?
YES NO — 14-2 13-1 GM

(Please turn page)   ©Wm. K. Frankenburg, M.D., 1975, 1986, 1998

CONTINUE ANSWERING UNTIL 3 "NOs" ARE CIRCLED

	For Office Use
	90% 75%

42. Walks well
Can your child walk all the way across a large room without falling or wobbling from side to side? **YES NO**
14-3 13-2 GM

43. One Word
Does your child say at least one *other* word besides "Mama," "Dada" and names of family members or pets? **YES NO**
15 13-1 L

44. Plays Ball
If you roll a small ball to your child, can she roll or throw it back to you? If your child only hands the ball to you, or if you have never tried this, circle **NO**. **YES NO**
15-3 11-3 PS

45. Scribbles
Without moving his hand or showing him how to do it, give your child a pencil and see if he will scribble on a piece of paper. If he bangs or mouths the pencil, Circle **NO**. Circle **YES** only if he scribbles without help. **YES NO**
16-1 14-3 FMA

46. Two Words
Does your child say 2 or more words *other than* "Mama," "Dada" and names of family members or pets? **YES NO**
16-2 14-2 L

47. Drinks from a Cup
Can your child hold a cup or glass by herself and drink from it without spilling much? The cup should not have a spout or lid. **YES NO**
17 15 PS

48. Helps in House
Does your child do things to help you, such as picking up his toys or bringing something to you when asked? **YES NO**
17-1 15-3 PS

49. Three Words
Does your child say three or more words *other than* "Mama," "Dada" and names of family members or pets? **YES NO**
18 15-3 L

	For Office Use
	90% 75%

50. Dumps Raisin
Can your child dump something small such as a raisin or piece of cereal from a small bottle, glass or cup? If she has not had the opportunity to try this, Circle **NO**. **YES NO**
19-1 15-3 FMA

51. Uses Spoon/Fork
Does your child feed himself with a spoon or fork without spilling much? **YES NO**
19-3 17-2 PS

52. Runs
Can your child run across a room without falling or tripping? **YES NO**
19-3 17-3 GM

53. Tower of 3 Cubes
Can your child stack three or more small blocks on top of each other? If she has never tried this, Circle **NO**. **YES NO**
20-2 17 FMA

54. Six Words
Does your child say six or more words *other than* "Mama," "Dada" and names of family members or pets? **YES NO**
21-1 18-3 L

55. Kicks Ball Forward
Without holding on to anything, can your child kick a small ball (like a tennis ball)? Circle **YES** only if you have seen your child do this with a *small* ball. **YES NO**
23 20-3 GM

56. Removes Garment
Can your child take off any of his clothes, such as pajamas (tops or bottoms) or pants? Do not count diapers, hats, socks or shoes. **YES NO**
23-3 20-1 PS

Catalog #1210

©Wm. K. Frankenburg, M.D., 1975, 1986, 1998

PEDS RESPONSE FORM

Child's Name __Billy Morris__   Parent's Name __Linda Morris__

Child's Birthday __4/17/94__   Child's Age ___3___   Today's Date __4/27/97__

Please list any concerns about your child's learning, development, and behavior.

He's kind of quiet and doesn't say very much. Seems to prefer

watching to interacting.

Do you have any concerns about how your child talks and makes speech sounds?

Circle one: No   Yes   (A little)   COMMENTS:

As I said, I don't think he talks as well as he should for his age. Otherwise, he's just a great

little boy, very loving, watches everything carefully. Figures things out quickly. Very bright!

Do you have any concerns about how your child understands what you say?

Circle one: (No)   Yes   A little   COMMENTS:

Do you have any concerns about how your child uses his or her hands and fingers to do things?

Circle one: (No)   Yes   A little   COMMENTS:

Do you have any concerns about how your child uses his or her arms and legs?

Circle one: (No)   Yes   A little   COMMENTS:

Do you have any concerns about how your child behaves?

Circle one: (No)   Yes   A little   COMMENTS:

Do you have any concerns about how your child gets along with others?

Circle one: (No)   Yes   A little   COMMENTS:

Do you have any concerns about how your child is learning to do things for himself/herself?

Circle one: (No)   Yes   A little   COMMENTS:

Do you have any concerns about how your child is learning preschool or school skills?

Circle one: (No)   Yes   A little   COMMENTS:

Please list any other concerns.

None.

Child's Name ___Billy Morris___   Birthday ___4/17/94___

PEDS INTERPRETATION FORM

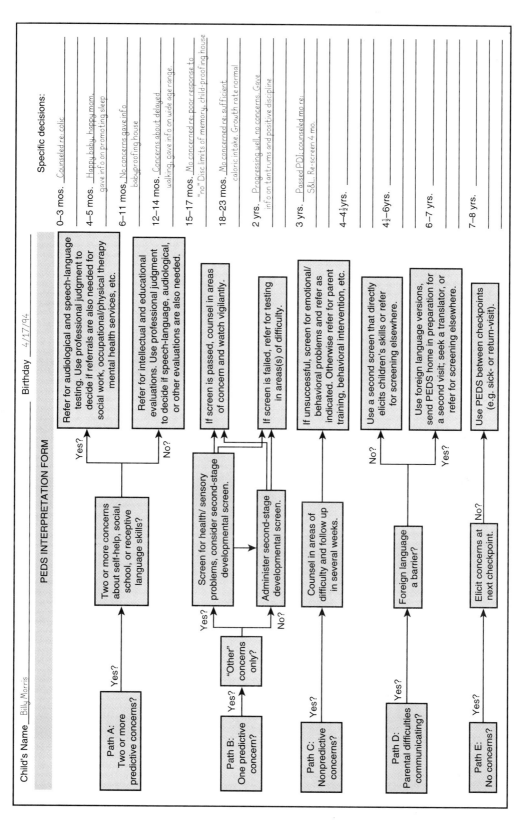

Path A:
Two or more predictive concerns? — Yes? → Two or more concerns about self-help, social, school, or receptive language skills?

Yes? → Refer for audiological and speech-language testing. Use professional judgment to decide if referrals are also needed for social work, occupational/physical therapy mental health services, etc.

No? → Refer for intellectual and educational evaluations. Use professional judgment to decide if speech-language, audiological, or other evaluations are also needed.

Path B:
One predictive concern? — Yes? → "Other" concerns only?

Yes? → Screen for health/ sensory problems, consider second-stage developmental screen. → Administer second-stage developmental screen.

No? →

If screen is passed, counsel in areas of concern and watch vigilantly.

If screen is failed, refer for testing in areas(s) of difficulty.

Path C:
Nonpredictive concerns? — Yes? → Counsel in areas of difficulty and follow up in several weeks.

If unsuccessful, screen for emotional/ behavioral problems and refer as indicated. Otherwise refer for parent training, behavioral intervention, etc.

Path D:
Parental difficulties communicating? — Yes? → Foreign language a barrier?

No? → Use a second screen that directly elicits children's skills or refer for screening elsewhere.

Yes? → Use foreign language versions, send PEDS home in preparation for a second visit; seek a translator, or refer for screening elsewhere.

Path E:
No concerns? — Yes? → Elicit concerns at next checkpoint.

No? → Use PEDS between checkpoints (e.g. sick- or return-visit).

Specific decisions:

0–3 mos. ___Counseled re: colic___

4–5 mos. ___Happy baby, happy mom, gave info on promoting sleep___

6–11 mos. ___No concerns, gave info babyproofing house___

12–14 mos. ___Concerns about delayed walking, gave info on wide age range.___

15–17 mos. ___No concerned re: poor response to "no" Disc limits of memory, child-proofing house___

18–23 mos. ___No concerned re: sufficient caloric intake. Growth rate normal___

2 yrs. ___Progressing well, no concerns. Gave info on tantrums and positive discipline___

3 yrs. ___Passed PDI; counseled mo re: S&L. Re-screen 4 mo.___

4–4½yrs. _____

4½–6yrs. _____

6–7 yrs. _____

7–8 yrs. _____

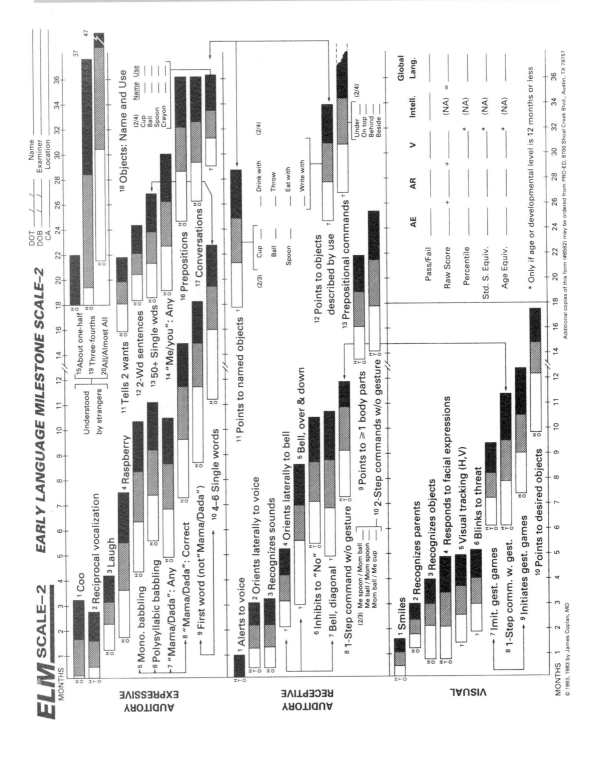

EARLY LANGUAGE MILESTONE SCALE-2

ELM SCALE-2

I. General Instructions

25% 50% 75% 90%   Percentage of Children Passing Item

Item may be elicited by

H = History
T = Direct Testing
O = Incidental Observation

• Always start with H, where allowed.
• Child passes item if passed by any of the allowable means of elicitation for that item.
• Basal = 3 consecutive items passed (work down from age line).
• Ceiling = 3 consecutive items failed (work up from age line).

II. Auditory Expressive (AE)
A. Content

AE 1. H: Makes prolonged musical vowel sounds in a sing-song fashion (ooo, aaa, etc.), not just grunts or squeaks.

AE 2. H: Does baby watch speaker's face and appear to listen intently, then vocalize when the speaker is quiet? Can you "have a conversation" with your baby?

AE 3. H: Blows bubbles or gives "Bronx cheer"?

AE 4. H: Makes isolated sounds such as "ba," "da," "ga," "goo," etc.

AE 5. H: Makes repetitive string of sounds: "bababababa," or "lalalalala," etc.

AE 6. H: Says "mama" or "dada" but uses them at other times besides just labelling parents.

AE 7. H: Child spontaneously, consistently, and correctly uses "mama" or "dada," just to label the appropriate parent.

AE 9, AE 10, AE 13. H: Child spontaneously, consistently, and correctly uses words. Do not count "mama," "dada," or the names of other family members or pets.

AE 11. H: Uses single words to tell you what he/she wants. "Milk!" "Cookie!" "More!" etc. Pass = 2 or more wants. List specific words.

AE 12. H: Spontaneous, novel 2-word combinations ("Want cookie" "No bed" "See daddy" etc.) Not rotely learned phrases that have been specifically taught to the child or combinations that are really single thoughts (e.g., "hot dog").

AE 14. H: Child uses "me" or "you" but may reverse them ("you want cookie" instead of "me want cookie," etc.)

AE 17. H: "Can child put 2 or 3 sentences together to hold brief conversations?"

AE 18. T: Put out cup, ball, crayon, & spoon. Pick up cup & say "What is this? What do we do with it? (What is it for?)" Child must name the object and give its use. Pass = "drink with," etc., not "milk" or "juice." Ball: Pass = "throw," "play with," etc. Spoon: Pass = "Eat" or "Eat with," etc., not "Food," "Lunch." Crayon: Pass = "Write (with)," "Color (with)," etc. Pass item if child gives name and use of 2 objects.

B. Intelligibility

AE 15, AE 19, AE 20. "How clear is your child's speech? That is, how much of your child's speech can a stranger understand?"

—Less than one-half
—About one-half (AE 15)
—Three-fourths (AE 19)
—All or Almost All (AE 20)

[Pick one (H, O)]

To score:
If less than one-half: Fail all 3 items in cluster.
If about one-half: Pass AE 15 only.
If three-fourths: Pass AE 19 and AE 15.
If all or almost all: Pass all 3 items in cluster.

III. Auditory Receptive (AR)

AR 1. H, T: Any behavioral change in response to noise (eye blink, startle, change in movements or respiration, etc.).

AR 2. H, T: What does baby do when parent starts talking while out of baby's line of sight? Pass if any shift of head or eyes to voice.

AR 3. H: Does baby seem to respond in a specific way to certain sounds (becomes excited at hearing parents' voices, etc.)?

AR 4. T: Sit facing baby, with baby in parent's lap. Extend both arms so that your hands are behind baby's field of vision and at the level of baby's waist. Ring a 2"-diameter bell, first with 1 hand, then the other. Repeat 2 or 3 times if necessary. Pass if baby turns head to the side at least once.

AR 5. T: See note for AR 4. Pass if baby turns head first to the side, then down, to localize bell, at least once. (Automatically passes AR 4.)

AR 6. H: Does baby understand the command "no" (even though he may not always obey)? T: Test by commanding "(Baby's name), no!" while baby is playing with any test object. Pass if baby temporarily inhibits his actions.

AR 7. T: See note for AR 4. Pass if baby turns directly down on diagonal to localize bell, at least once. (Automatically passes AR 5 and AR 4.)

AR 8. H: Will your baby follow any verbal commands without you indicating by gestures what it is you want him to do ("Stop" "Come here" "Give me" etc.)? T: Will child do what you ask him to do if you say "(Baby's name), give it to me." Pass if baby is playing with any test object, then say "(Baby's name), give it to me." May repeat command 1 or 2 times. If failed, repeat the command but this time hold out your hand for the object. If baby responds, then pass item V 8 (1-step command with gesture).

AR 9. H: Does your child point to at least 1 body part on command? T: Have mother command baby "Show me your..." or "Where's your..." without pointing to the desired part herself.

AR 10. H: "Can child do 2 things in a row if asked? For example 'First go get your shoes, then sit down'?" T: Set out ball, cup, and spoon, and say "(Child's name), give me the spoon, then give the ball to mommy." Use slow, steady voice but do not break command into 2 separate sentences. If no response, then give each half of command separately to see if child understands the following: "(Child's name), give me the ball and give mommy the spoon." May repeat once but do not break into 2 commands. Then "Give mommy the ball, then give me the cup." Pass if at least two 2-step commands executed correctly. (Note: Child is credited even if the order of execution of a command is reversed.)

AR 11. T: Place a cup, ball, and spoon on the table. Command child "Show me/where is/give me... the cup/ball/spoon." (If command is "Give me," be sure to replace each object before asking about the next object.) Pass = 2 items correctly identified.

AR 12. T: Put cup, ball, spoon, and crayon on table and give command "Show me/where is/give me... the one we drink with/eat with/draw (color, write) with/throw (play with)." If the command "Give me" is used, be sure to replace each object before asking about the next object. Pass = 2 or more objects correctly identified.

AR 13. T: Put out cup (upside down) and a 1" cube. Command the child "Put the block under the cup." Repeat 1 or 2 times if necessary. If no attempt, or if incorrect response, then demonstrate to the child. Then give command "See, now the block is under the cup." Remove the block and hand it to the child. Then give command "Put the block on top of the cup." If child makes no response, then repeat command 1 time but do not demonstrate. Then command "Put the block behind the cup," then "Put the block beside the cup." Pass = 2 or more commands correctly executed (prior to demonstration by examiner, if "under" is scored).

AR4

AR5

AR7

IV. Visual

V 1. H: "Does your baby smile—not just a gas bubble or a burp but a real smile?" T: Have parent attempt to elicit smile by any means.

V 2. H: "Does your baby seem to recognize you, reacting differently to you than to the sight of other people? For example, does your baby smile more quickly for you than for other people?"

V 3. H: "Does your baby seem to recognize any common objects by sight? For example, if bottle or spoon fed, what happens when bottle or spoon is brought into view before it touches baby's lips?" Pass if baby gets visibly excited, or opens mouth in anticipation of feeding.

V 4. H: "Does your baby respond to your facial expressions?" T: Engage baby's gaze and attempt to elicit a smile by smiling and talking to baby. Then scowl at baby. Pass if any change in baby's facial expression.

V 5. T: Horizontal (H): Engage child's gaze with yours at a distance of 18". Move slowly back and forth. Pass if child turns head 60° to left and right from midline. Vertical (V): Move slowly up and down. Pass if child elevates eyes 30° from horizontal. Must pass both H & V to pass item.

V 6. T: Flick your fingers rapidly towards child's face, ending with fingertips 1-2" from face. Do not touch face or eyelashes. Pass if child blinks.

V 7. H: Does child play pat-a-cake, peek-a-boo, etc., in response to parents?

V 8. T: See note for AR 8 (always try AR 8 first; if AR 8 is passed, then automatically give credit for V 8).

V 9. H: Does child spontaneously initiate gesture games?

V 10. H: "Does your child ever point with index finger to something he/she wants? For example, if child is sitting at the dinner table and wants something that is out of reach, how does child let you know what he/she wants?" Pass only index finger pointing not reaching with whole hand.

Temperament (See Chapter 2)

The Carey Temperament Scales were designed for use in pediatric primary care offices. They are questionnaires to be completed by a parent and are available for infants, toddlers, children 3 to 7 years old and those in middle-childhood. A selected group of questions from the Revised Infant Temperament Questionnaire (4 to 11 months) illustrates the information that taps temperament.

Using the scale below, please mark the space that tells how often the infant's recent and current behavior has been like the behavior described by each item.

1. Almost never   4. Variable, usually doe

2. Rarely   5. Frequently

3. Variable, usually not   6. Almost always

Children's Depression Inventory (CDI). Written at the first grade level, the CDI Short Version is a screening tool for depression in children and youth 7 to 17 years old. It is also available in a longer 27-item self-report format, as well as teacher and parent versions. The published formats include scoring by age and gender to generate a T score, a guide to clinically significant problems. These forms are available at the address listed at the end of the questionnaire.

The infant is fussy on waking up and going to sleep (frowns, cries).	1 2 3 4 5 6
The infant plays with a toy for under a minute and then looks for another toy or activity.	1 2 3 4 5 6
The infant plays continuously for more than 10 minutes at a time with a favorite toy.	1 2 3 4 5 6
The infant indicates discomfort (fusses or squirms) when diaper is soiled with a bowel movement.	1 2 3 4 5 6
The infant lies quietly in the bath.	1 2 3 4 5 6
The infant objects to being bathed in a different place or by a different person, even after 2 or 3 tries.	1 2 3 4 5 6
The infant is pleasant (coos, smiles, etc.) during procedures like hair brushing or face washing.	1 2 3 4 5 6
The infant continues to cry despite several minutes of soothing.	1 2 3 4 5 6
The infant adjusts easily and sleeps well within 1 or 2 days with changes of time or place.	1 2 3 4 5 6
The infant cries for less than 1 minute when given an injection.	1 2 3 4 5 6
The infant shows much body movement (kicks, waves arms) when crying.	1 2 3 4 5 6

Used by permission from Behavioral-Developmental Initiatives, 14636 N. 55th Street, Scottsdale, AZ 85254; phone: 800-405-2313 fax: 602-494-2688; website: *http://www.b-di.com/catalogueCTSqs.html.* Temperament scales available for early infancy (EITQ), infancy (RITQ), toddler (TIS), 3 to 7 years (BSQ), and middle childhood (MCTQ).

Edinburgh Postnatal Depression Scale

Please read each group of statements carefully and then circle the one in each group that describes the way you have been feeling during the past week.

1	I have been able to laugh and see the funny side of things
	0 as much as I always could
	1 not quite so much now
	2 definitely not so much now
	3 not at all
2	I have looked forward with enjoyment to things
	0 as much as I ever did
	1 rather less than I used to
	2 definitely less than I used to
	3 hardly at all
3	I have blamed myself unnecessarily when things went wrong
	3 yes, most of the time
	2 yes, some of the time
	1 not very often
	0 no, never
4	I have been anxious or worried for no good reason
	0 no, not at all
	1 hardly ever
	2 yes, sometimes
	3 yes, very often
5	I have felt scared or panicky for no very good reason
	3 yes, quite a lot
	2 yes, sometimes
	1 no, not much
	0 no, not at all
6	Things have been getting on top of me
	3 yes, most of the time I haven't been able to cope at all
	2 yes, sometimes I haven't been coping as well as usual
	1 no, most of the time I have coped quite well
	0 no, I have been coping as well as ever
7	I have been so unhappy that I have had difficulty sleeping
	3 yes, most of the time
	2 yes, sometimes
	1 not very often
	0 no, not at all

Continued

8	I have felt sad or miserable
3	yes, most of the time
2	yes, quite often
1	not very often
0	no, not at all

9	I have been so unhappy that I have been crying
3	yes, most of the time
2	yes, quite often
1	only occasionally
0	no, never

10	The thought of harming myself has occurred to me
3	yes, quite often
2	sometimes
1	hardly ever
0	never

Used by permission from Cox JL, Holden JM, Sagovsky R: Detection of postnatal depression: Development of the 10-item Edinburgh Postnatal Depression Scale. *Br J Psychiatry* 150:782-786, 1987. © 1987 The Royal College of Psychiatrists. The Edinburgh Postnatal Depression Scale may be photocopied by individual researchers or clinicians for their own use without seeking permission from the publishers. The scale must be copied in full and all copies must acknowledge the following source: Cox, J.L., Holden, J.M., & Sagovsky, R. (1987) Detection of postnatal depression. Development of the 10-item Edinburgh Postnatal Depression Scale. British Journal of Psychiatry, 150, 782-786. Written permission must be obtained from the Royal college of Psychiatrists for copying and distribution to others or for republication (in print, online or by any other medium).

Translations of the scale, and guidance as to its use, may be found in Cox, J.L. & Holden, J. (2003) Perinatal Mental Health: A Guide to the Edinburgh Postnatal Depression Scale, London: Gaskell.

PEDIATRIC SYMPTOM CHECKLIST
Please mark under the heading that best fits your child:

	Never	Sometimes	Often
1. Complains of aches or pains	☐	☐	☐
2. Spends more time alone	☐	☐	☐
3. Tires easily, little energy	☐	☐	☐
4. Fidgety, unable to sit still	☐	☐	☐
5. Has trouble with a teacher	☐	☐	☐
6. Less interested in school	☐	☐	☐
7. Acts as if driven by a motor	☐	☐	☐
8. Daydreams too much	☐	☐	☐
9. Distracted easily	☐	☐	☐
10. Is afraid of new situations	☐	☐	☐
11. Feels sad, unhappy	☐	☐	☐

Continued

	Never	Sometimes	Often
12. Is irritable, angry	☐	☐	☐
13. Feels hopeless	☐	☐	☐
14. Has trouble concentrating	☐	☐	☐
15. Less interest in friends	☐	☐	☐
16. Fights with other children	☐	☐	☐
17. Absent from school	☐	☐	☐
18. School grades dropping	☐	☐	☐
19. Is down on him or herself	☐	☐	☐
20. Visits doctor with doctor finding nothing wrong	☐	☐	☐
21. Has trouble sleeping	☐	☐	☐
22. Worries a lot	☐	☐	☐
23. Wants to be with you more than before	☐	☐	☐
24. Feels he or she is bad	☐	☐	☐
25. Takes unnecessary risks	☐	☐	☐
26. Gets hurt frequently	☐	☐	☐
27. Seems to be having less fun	☐	☐	☐
28. Acts younger than children his or her age	☐	☐	☐
29. does not listen to rules	☐	☐	☐
30. Does not show feelings	☐	☐	☐
31. Does not understand other people's feelings	☐	☐	☐
32. Teases others	☐	☐	☐
33. Blames others for his or her troubles	☐	☐	☐
34. Takes things that do not belong to him or her	☐	☐	☐
35. Refuses to share	☐	☐	☐

Procedures and Scoring criteria for the Pediatric Symptoms Checklist (PSC)

For children 4 and 5 years of age, responses to items 5, 6, 17, and 18 are not counted due to their emphasis on school issues which may not be relevant.

The value of 0 is assigned to "never," 1 to "sometimes," and 2 to "often." Add these values to obtain a score for the entire test.

The presence of significant behavioral or emotional difficulties is suggested when children ages 4–5 years receive 24 or more points, and when children 6–16 years receive 28 or more points.

To determine what kinds of mental health problems are present, determine the three factor scores on the PSC:

PSC Attention Subscale consists of these five items.

4. Fidgety, unable to sit still

7. Acts as if driven by motor

8. Daydream too much

9. Distracted easily

14. Has trouble concentrating

Children who receive 7 or more points on these five items need a work up for attention deficit hyperactivity disorder. The American Academy of Pediatrics recently revised its recommendations on how to diagnose ADHD, and the article is in the May 2000 issue of *Pediatrics*–a must read.

PSC Internalizing Subscale consists of these five items:

11. Feels sad

13. Feels hopeless

19. Is down on self

22. Worries a lot

27. Seems to have less fun

It is a screen for depression and anxiety. Children who receive 5 or more points on these five items need to be referred for counseling and may eventually need to be considered for anti-depressives, anxiolytics etc.

PSC Externalizing Factor consists of these seven items:

16. Fights with other children

29. Does not listen to rules

31. Does not understand other's feelings

32. Teases others

33. Blames others for his troubles

34. Takes things that do not belong to him or her

35. Refuses to share

It is a screen for conduct disorder, oppositional defiant disorder, rage disorder, etc. Children who receive 7 or more points on these seven items need behavioral intervention.

PSC Developmental/Academic Screening (33)

If a child fails the whole test, also refer for academic/developmental assessment. Children with mental health problems almost invariably have academic problems, and children with developmental or academic problems are at high risk of mental health problems.

Parents whose children pass the PSC but endorse numerous items should benefit from in-office counseling. If this has been tried and not found to be successful, such families should be referred for such services as parent training classes and behavior intervention programs.

Those with academic failure and difficulties (whose parents endorse items about poor school performance, absence from school, etc.), whether or not the PSC is passed, should be referred for intellectual and educational testing.

A short form of the Pediatric Symptom Checklist is available: Gardner W. *et al.* The PSC-17: A brief pediatric symptom checklist for psychosocial problem subscales: A report from PROS and ASPN. *Ambulatory Child Health.* 1999; 5:225-236.

FAMILY PSYCHOSOCIAL SCREENING

This office is dedicated to providing the best possible care for your child. In order for us to serve you better, please take a few minutes to answer the following questions. Your answers will be kept strictly confidential as part of your child's medical record. Ongoing evaluations of our care may involve chart reviews by qualified persons, but neither your name, nor your child's name will ever appear in any reports.

Child's Name _____ Today's Date _____

Circle either the word or the letter for your answer where appropriate. Fill in answers where space is provided.

Are you the child's:

A. Mother   B. Father.   C. Grandparent   D. Foster Parent

E. Other relative   F. Other   G. Self (Are you the patient?)

What is the highest grade you have completed?

1   2   3   4   5   6   7   8   9   10   11   12   (High School GED)

Some college or vocational school   College Graduate   Postgraduate

---

How many times have you moved in the last year?

_____ times

Where is the child living now?

A. House or apartment with family   B. House or apartment with relative or friends

C. Shelter   D. Other

What is your current monthly income, including public assistance? $ _____

Besides you, does anyone else take care of the child?   YES NO

If yes, who?

_____

Has child received health care elsewhere?   YES NO

If yes, what?

_____

Does the child have any allergies to any medications?   YES NO

If yes, what?

_____

Has the child received any immunizations?   YES NO

Which ones? _____

Where? _____

Has the child ever been hospitalized?   YES NO

When? _____

Where? _____

Why? _____

How would you rate this child's health in general?

A. Excellent   B. Good   C. Fair   D. Poor

Do you have any concerns about your child's behavior or development?   YES NO

If yes, what:

_____

What are your main concerns about your child?

_____

How old are you? _____ years old

Are you:

A. Single   C. Separated   B. Married   D. Divorced   E. Other

---

FAMILY MEDICAL HISTORY

Does the child's mother, father, or grandparents have any of the following? If yes, who?

High blood pressure	YES No	_____
Diabetes	YES No	_____
Lung problems (asthma)	YES No	_____
Heart problems	YES No	_____
Miscarriages	YES No	_____
Learning problems	YES No	_____
Nerve problems	YES No	_____
Mental Illness (depression)	YES No	_____
Drinking problems	YES No	_____
Drug problems	YES No	_____
Other	YES No	_____

(please specify) _____

FAMILY HEALTH HABITS

How often does your child use a seatbelt (carseat)?

A. Never   B. Rarely   C. Sometimes   D. Often   E. Always

Does your child ride a bicycle?   YES No

If yes, how often does he/she use a helmet?

A. Never   B. Rarely   C. Sometimes   D. Often   E. Always

Do you feel that you live in a safe place?   YES No

In the past year, have you ever felt threatened in your home?   YES No

In the past year, has your partner or other family member pushed you, punched you, kicked you, hit you or threatened to hurt you   YES No

What kind of gun(s) are in your home?

A. Handgun   B. Shotgun   C. Rifle   D. Other   E. None

Does anyone in your household smoke?   YES No

Do you currently smoke cigarettes?   YES No

If yes, how many cigarettes do you smoke per day?

_____ cigarettes/day

When you were a child

Did either parent have a drug or alcohol problem?   YES NO

Were you raised part or all of the time by foster parents or relatives (other than your parents)?   YES NO

How often did your parents ground you or put you in time out?
   A. Frequently   B. Often   C. Occasionally   D. Rarely   E. Never

How often were you hit with an object such as a belt, board, hairbrush, stick, or cord?
   A. Frequently   B. Often   C. Occasionally   D. Rarely   E. Never

Do you feel you were physically abused?   YES NO

Do you feel you were neglected?   YES NO

Do you feel you were hurt in a sexual way?   YES NO

Did your parents ever hurt you when they were out of control?   YES NO

Are you ever afraid you might lose control and hurt your child?   YES NO

Would you like more information about free parenting programs, parent hot lines, or respite care?   YES NO

Would you like information about birth control or family planning?   YES NO

Family Activities

How strong are your family's religious beliefs or practices?
   A. Very strong   B. Moderately strong   C. Not strong   D. N/A

What religion/ church/ temple?

_____

How often do you read bedtime stories to your child?
   A. Frequently   B. Often   C. Occasionally   D. Rarely   E Never

How often does you family eat meals together?
   A. Frequently   B. Often   C. Occasionally   D. Rarely   E. Never

What does your family do together for fun?

_____

How often in the last week have you felt depressed?
   0   1–2   3–4   5–7 days

In the past year, have you had two weeks or more during which you felt sad, blue, or depressed, or lost pleasure in things that you usually cared about or enjoyed?   YES NO

Have you had two or more years in your life when you felt depressed or sad most days, even if you felt okay sometimes?   YES NO

Drinking and Drugs

In the past year have you ever had a drinking problem?   YES NO

Have you tried to cut down on alcohol in the past year?   YES NO

How many drinks does it take for you to get high or get a buzz?
   1   2   3   4   5   6   7 or more

Have you ever had a drug problem?   YES NO

Have you used any drugs in the last 24 hours?   YES NO

If yes, which ones?
Cocaine   Heroin   Methadone
Speed   Marijuana   Other

Are you in a drug or alcohol recovery program now?   YES NO

If yes, which one(s)?

_____

Would you like to talk with other parents who are dealing with alcohol or drug problems?   YES NO

Help and Support

Whom can you count on to be dependable when you need help: (just write their initials and their relationship to you)

A.   No one   B. _____   C. _____

D. _____   E. _____   F. _____

G. _____   H. _____   I. _____

How satisfied are you with their support?
   A. Very satisfied   B. Fairly satisfied   C. A little satisfied
   D. A little dissatisfied   E. Fairly dissatisfied   F. Very dissatisfied

Who accepts you totally, including both your best and worst points?

A.   No one   B. _____   C. _____

D. _____   E. _____   F. _____

G. _____   H. _____   I. _____

How satisfied are you with their support?
   A. Very satisfied   B. Fairly satisfied   C. A little satisfied
   D. A little dissatisfied   E. Fairly dissatisfied   F. Very dissatisfied

Whom do you feel loves you deeply?

A.   No one   B. _____   C. _____

D. _____   E. _____   F. _____

G. _____   H. _____   I. _____

How satisfied are you with their support?
   A. Very satisfied   B. Fairly satisfied   C. A little satisfied
   D. A little dissatisfied   E. Fairly dissatisfied   F. Very dissatisfied

The questionairre and scoring criteria can be found at:
http://pedstest.com/links/files/fampsych.pdf

M–CHAT (THE MODIFIED CHECKLIST FOR AUTISM IN TODDLERS) (18–24 MONTHS OF AGE)

Please fill out the following about how your child **usually** is. Please try to answer every question. If the behavior is rare (e.g., you've seen it once or twice), please answer as if the child does not do it.

1. Does your child enjoy being swung, bounced on your knee, etc.?	Yes No
2. Does your child take an interest in other children?	Yes No
3. Does your child like climbing on things, such as up stairs?	Yes No
4. Does your child enjoy playing peek-a-boo/hide-and-seek?	Yes No
5. Does your child ever pretend, for example, to talk on the phone or take care of dolls, or pretend other things?	Yes No
6. Does your child ever use his/her index finger to point, to ask for something?	Yes No
7. Does your child ever use his/her index finger to point, to indicate interest in something?	Yes No
8. Can your child play properly with small toys (e.g. cars or bricks) without just mouthing, fiddling, or dropping them?	Yes No
9. Does your child ever bring objects over to you (parent) to show you something?	Yes No
10. Does your child look you in the eye for more than a second or two?	Yes No
11. Does your child ever seem oversensitive to noise? (e.g., plugging ears)	Yes No
12. Does your child smile in response to your face or your smile?	Yes No
13. Does your child imitate you? (e.g., you make a face-will your child imitate it?)	Yes No
14. Does your child respond to his/her name when you call?	Yes No
15. If you point at a toy across the room, does your child look at it?	Yes No
16. Does your child walk?	Yes No
17. Does your child look at things you are looking at?	Yes No
18. Does your child make unusual finger movements near his/her face?	Yes No
19. Does your child try to attract your attention to his/her own activity?	Yes No
20. Have you ever wondered if your child is deaf?	Yes No
21. Does your child understand what people say?	Yes No
22. Does your child sometimes stare at nothing or wander with no purpose?	Yes No
23. Does your child look at your face to check your reation when faced with something unfamiliar?	Yes No

© 1999 Diana Robins, Deborah Fein, & Marianne Barton

Please refer to: Robins, D., Fein, D., Barton, M., & Green, J. (2001). The Modified Checklist for Autism in Toddlers: An initial study investigating the early detection of autism and pervasive developmental disorders. *Journal of Autism and Developmental Disorders, 31* (2), 131-144.

Modified Checklist for Autism in Toddlers (M-CHAT)

M-CHAT SCORING INSTRUCTIONS

A child fails the checklist when 2 or more critical items are failed OR when any three items are failed. Yes/no answers convert to pass/fail responses. Below are listed the failed responses for each item on the M-CHAT. Bold capitalized items are CRITICAL items.

Not all children who fail the checklist will meet criteria for a diagnosis on the autism spectrum.

However, children who fail the checklist should be evaluated in more depth by the physician or referred for a developmental evaluation with a specialist.

1. No	6. No	11. Yes	16. No	21. No
2. NO	**7. NO**	12. No	17. No	22. Yes
3. No	8. No	**13. NO**	18. Yes	23. No
4. No	**9. NO**	**14. NO**	19. No	
5. No	10. No	**15. NO**	20. Yes	

Section II: Second Stage Screening and Common Tests

Some pediatricians will want to have available developmental screening and assessment tools that are more expansive, detailed, or specific. Many others will see the results of such tests in reports on patients whom they send for referral and would like to know about these tools. Research in this area may use some of these as outcome measures or predictor variables.

Some of these tools are described below along with the amount of training generally needed.

- **MacArthur Communicative Developmental Inventories (CDI):** Detailed parent questionnaire of language competencies, including gestures, comprehension, production, complexity and semantics. 8–30 months. English, Spanish and Italian forms. Gives percentiles on dimensions based on large norming sample. Age equivalent reported for delayed language. (Development Psychology Lab, Department of Psychology, San Diego State University, San Diego, CA 92182, http://www.pbrookes.com/store/books/fenson-cdi/)

- **Achenbach Child Behavior Check List (CBCL):** Parent questionnaire of behavioral concerns. Ages 2–3 and 4–18. Scores for internalizing and externalizing behavior. Broad-based measure; not diagnostic. Teacher forms also available. Computer scoring recommended. (Center for Children, Youth and Families, University of Vermont, 1 South Prospect Street, Burlington, VT 05401, http:/www.agsnet.com)

- **ANSER:** Detailed parent and teacher questionnaires to characterize development, behavior, attentional and learning concerns. Formal scoring in research settings. Can be used clinically as an inventory of concerns. (http://www.epsbooks.com/dynamic/catalog/mellevine.asp?subject=15S)

- **Bayley Scales of Infant Development (BSID)** editions 1 and 2: Developmental test of children from the ages of birth to 36 months on mental and motor scales. Yields quotient scores for age, the MDI (Mental Development Index), and PDI (Performance Development Index). Behavioral record component yields good observations collected during the assessment. Training required. An abbreviated form using a subset of items is now available. (The Psychological Corporation, Harcourt Brace Jovanovich, http://www.psychcorp.com.au/bayley.html

- **Beery Developmental Test of Visual-Motor Integration (VMI):** Hand-eye coordination in figure drawing. An expansion of the simple figure copying presented in Chapter 5. Gives an age equivalent. Minimal training and familiarization. Ages 3–18 (adult). (Modern Curriculum Press, 13900 Prospect Road, Cleveland, OH 44136)

- **Peabody Picture Vocabulary Test—Revised (PPVT-R)**: A series of pictures of increasing difficulty shown to a child to establish language age level. Ages 22 months to adult (33+ years). Yields a language score. Familiarization and cultural issues may alter the results somewhat. Some training required. (American Guidance Service, Circle Pines, MN 55041-1796, http://www.agsnet.com/Group.asp?nGroupInfoID=a12010)

- **Revised Developmental Screening Inventory (Knobloch):** An adaptation of the Gesell schedules designed for use in risk populations aged 4 weeks to 36 months. Yields a performance level in each of five areas. A Developmental Quotient is reported by area, and an overall classification of normal, questionable or abnormal is presented, weighted to motor performance. Some training required. (Developmental Evaluation Materials, Inc., Department of Pediatrics, Albany Medical College, Albany, NY 12208)

- **Hawaii Early Learning Profile (HELP):** Developmental screening for early childhood, curriculum based. Divided by area, showing progression. Good to use as a base for individual intervention. Ages birth to 3 years. Less useful in population studies. Form itself is seen as an intervention. Familiarization and some training required. (VORT Corporation, PO Box 60132, Palo Alto, CA 94306, http://www.vort.com/profb3.htm)

- **Battelle Developmental Inventory Screening Test:** Measures developmental competency for ages 6 months to 8 years in five areas. Yields age competency in each area assessed. Moderate training required. Takes 30–45 minutes; really a lot more than a screening. (http://www.riverpub.com/products/clinical/bdi/home.html)

- **Einstein Assessment of School-Related Skills (EASRS):** Grade-level brief achievement screenings. Examiner forms script the directions, so little training is needed. (Modern Curriculum Press, 4350 Equity Drive, Columbus, OH 43216)

For Psychologists or Those with Special Training to Administer

- **Wechsler Intelligence Scale for Children (WISC):** Standard intelligence test. Yields verbal, performance and full-scale or overall IQ measurement with 100 as the norm for age. Subscale scores are also reported to identify any existing discrepancies. Fully trained psychologist required. Ages 6–16.

- **Wechsler Preschool Primary Scale of Intelligence-Revised (WPPSI-R):** Ages 3–7. Yields IQ measures, full, performance and verbal.

- **Leiter Test of Nonverbal Intelligence:** Individual test to evaluate nonverbally mediated skills. Useful when there is a known language impairment. Fully trained psychologist required.
- **Wide Range Achievement Test (WRAT):** A measure of what a child knows in several academic areas. A reflection of learning, not necessarily ability. Discrepancy between ability and achievement defines learning difficulties in many school jurisdictions.
- **Woodcock Johnson Psychoeducational Battery—Revised:** Gives performance levels in basic academic areas. Ages 2 to adult.
- **Neonatal Behavioral Assessment Scale (NBAS):** A measure of neonatal behavior on 27 dimensions with a 9-point scale for each. Scores are reported by item and are clustered into three to four dimensions from worrisome to optimal. Valid from birth to 30 days old. Adaptations available for preterm infants. Strict training required for research use. Clinical adaptations of parts of the assessment are useful.
- **School-Based Achievement Tests.** Group-administered measure of what a child has learned and can put down in the timed test situation. Multiple tests:
  — California Achievement Tests
  — Iowa Test of Basic Skills
  — Stanford Achievement Test
  — ACT Proficiency Examination
  — Comprehensive Test of Basic Skills

Section III: A Pediatrician's Book Shelf

Recommended readings for pediatricians and other primary care clinicians who care for children and adolescents are presented.

The authors have found the following books to be insightful and clinically useful in their own development as pediatricians; they are part of the "classics" in this field. These books are recommended for those who choose to explore the wide range of behavior and developmental issues in children that are beyond the scope of this book.

Brazelton TB: *Infants and Mothers: Individual Differences in Development.* New York, Delacourt, 1969.

Bronfenbrenner U: *The Ecology of Human Development: Experiments by Nature and Design.* Cambridge, MA, Harvard University Press, 1979.

Erikson EH: *Childhood and Society,* 2nd ed. New York, WW Norton, 1963.

Fraiberg S: *The Magic Years: Understanding and Handling the Problems of Early Childhood.* New York, Scribner, 1959.

Freud A: *Normality and Pathology in Childhood: Assessments of Development.* New York, International Universities Press, 1965.

Illingsworth RS: *The Development of the Infant and Young Child: Normal and Abnormal.* London, Livingstone, 1960.

Kagan J: *The Nature of the Child.* New York, Basic Books, 1994.,

Spock B, Needlman R: *Dr. Spock's Baby and Child Care*, 8th ed. New York, Pocket Books (softcover), EP Dutton (hardcover), 2004.

Thomas A: *Temperament and Development.* New York, Brunner-Routledge, 1977.

Werner EE: *Cross-Cultural Child Development: A View from Planet Earth.* Monterey, CA, Brooks-Cole, 1979.

Whiting B, Whiting JWM: *Children of Six Cultures: A Psychocultural Analysis.* Cambridge, MA, Harvard University Press, 1975.

Winnicott DW: *The Child, the Family and the Outside World*, 2nd ed. Reading, MA, Addison-Wesley, 1992.

Though too recent for "classic" status, two publications are approaching a must-read status in developmental and behavioral pediatrics:

Gopnik A, Meltzoff AN, Kuhl PK: *The Scientist in the Crib.* New York, William Morrow, 1999.

Shonkoff JP, Phillips D (eds): *From Neurons to Neighborhoods.* Washington, DC, National Academy Press, 2000.

Section IV: Parent and Child Guides for Pediatric Visits

The Parent and Child Guides to Pediatric Visits can be filled out by parents and older children and adolescents before a health supervision visit. They are intended to inform parents and kids about normal aspects of development, as well as provide a checklist for concerns about behavior, development and other areas of health care. The guides were developed by the American Academy of Pediatrics and are published in the appendix of *Guidelines for Health Supervision III*. They are available from the American Academy of Pediatrics, Publications Department, 141 Northwest Point Blvd., PO Box 927, Elk Grove Village, IL 60009-0927 (phone: 888-227-1770; fax: 847-228-1281).

Guide to Pediatric Visits

Children 6 TO 11 YEARS OLD

In the past year or two you have learned a lot of new information and skills, both at home and at school. You can now do more on your own and you probably are involved in a lot of activities. You may have discovered new people and new experiences that are important to you.

You are also becoming able to make good decisions about your health and safety. For example, you can remember to *wear your helmet* when you are riding your bike, *buckle up your seat* belts anytime you ride in a car, *brush your teeth, eat nutritious foods, and avoid alcohol and tobacco use.* You can also let your doctor know how you are feeling, and ask any questions you have about your health, your friends, school, your family, or experiences you have had.

It would be helpful if you could take a few minutes now to think about what things you would like to discuss during your visit with your doctor today. The following list is intended to give you a few suggestions.

What is one thing you are proud of about yourself?

Please put a check (✔) by all areas you would like to discuss:

_____ 1. Your general health, or particular symptoms or concerns

_____ 2. Your physical growth

_____ 3. Questions about any aspect of your medical care or what will happen at today's visit

_____ 4. Your school work

_____ 5. Sports and other activities

_____ 6. Urinating or having bowel movements

_____ 7. Your appetite or diet

_____ 8. Your sleeping

_____ 9. Your energy or activity level

_____ 10. How you get along with other children

_____ 11. How you get along with your brothers and sisters

_____ 12. How you get along with your mother and father

_____ 13. Any aches and pains you have frequently

_____ 14. Any things you have been worrying about

_____ 15. Any injuries you have had

_____ 16. The effects of tobacco, alcohol, and other drugs of abuse

Are there any *other* concerns you would like to be able to talk about with the doctor or nurse?

Your name:	Today's date:
Date of birth:	
Parent(s)' name(s):	
Other people in the household:	

Reprinted with permission from the American Academy of Pediatrics. *Guidelines for Health Supervision Visits III.* May not be reproduced without permission from the American Academy of Pediatrics.

Guide to Pediatric Visits

Younger Adolescents II TO 15 YEARS OLD

As an adolescent, during your visits to the pediatrician, you will have the opportunity to meet with the doctor or nurse to talk confidentially about issues that concern you.

It is common for young adolescents to have concerns about their rapid physical growth and sexual development (puberty). It is important to feel accepted among your peers over standards for dress, recreation, behavior, and values. Adolescents experiment with many risk-taking behaviors. Conflicts with parents over issues of independence are common.

During these visits, you may bring up for discussion anything that concerns you. Some issues that commonly worry children and teenagers are listed below. Be assured that confidentiality will be maintained unless the doctor or nurse is concerned that you are going to hurt yourself or someone else.

What are some of the things that make you feel proud of yourself?

Please put a check (✔) by all areas you would like to discuss:

_____ 1. Any health issue, specific symptom or concern

_____ 2. Your eating or weight

_____ 3. Sleeping pattern and routines

_____ 4. Bowel and urine elimination

_____ 5. For girls — menstrual history (regularity/length of period/pain) For boys — "nocturnal emissions" (wet dreams)

_____ 6. School grades

_____ 7. Any problems with school

_____ 8. Sports, hobbies, or other activities

_____ 9. Your friends

_____ 10. Interactions with your brothers and sisters

_____ 11. Interactions with your parent(s)

_____ 12. Responsibilities at home, chores, household rules

_____ 13. Feelings of sadness, mood changes

_____ 14. Worrying a lot

_____ 15. Trouble concentrating

_____ 16. Frequent aches and pains

_____ 17. Feeling angry or hopeless

_____ 18. Taking unnecessary risks

_____ 19. Use of tobacco or alcohol

_____ 20. Other drugs

_____ 21. Sexual activity, contraceptives, sexually transmitted diseases

_____ 22. Your sexual orientation

_____ 23. Fears

_____ 24. Family problems, such as money problems, violence, alcohol or other drug abuse, conflicts between parents or separation

_____ 25. Death or illness of a family member

_____ 26. Any trauma or abuse you have experienced

Are there any *other* concerns you would like to be able to talk about with the doctor or nurse?

Your name: _____ Today's date: _____

Date of birth: _____

Parent(s)' name(s): _____

Other people in the household: _____

Reprinted with permission from the American Academy of Pediatrics. *Guidelines for Health Supervision Visits III.* May not be reproduced without permission from the American Academy of Pediatrics.

Guide to Pediatric Visits

Older Adolescents 16 TO 21 YEARS OLD

As an older adolescent, we would like to acknowledge your individuality by examining you without your parents present. We promise you confidentiality. We will inform your parents about our discussions only if you are doing or thinking things that pose a serious risk to yourself or to others. We may encourage you to discuss some issues openly with your family. We can brainstorm with you about how to do this.

During these years, teens typically show increasing intellectual, moral, social, and emotional independence. You may have substituted your own or your friends' standards for your family's value system. You may be experimenting with behaviors that put you at physical, psychological, or social risk. Many teens develop intimate relationships during this age and begin thinking about sexual activity. The possibility of conflict within the family increases in this period.

It would be helpful if you could take a few minutes to think about what things you would like to discuss during your visit today; the following list is intended to offer a few suggestions.

What are you happy about or proud of in yourself?

Please put a check (✔) by all areas you would like to discuss:

____ 1. Your overall health, or specific symptoms or concerns

____ 2. Your physical development or stage of puberty

____ 3. Menstrual patterns or problems

____ 4. Your social and emotional needs

____ 5. Appetite, eating patterns, or nutrition

____ 6. Your sleeping patterns

____ 7. Emotional problems, such as depression or anxiety

____ 8. Family problems, such as money problems, violence, alcohol or other drug use, separation or divorce

____ 9. Communication patterns in your family

____ 10. Problems with your parents

____ 11. Any problems at school

____ 12. Your school performance

____ 13. Preparation for future education or job

____ 14. Sports participation

____ 15. Your friends and peer group

____ 16. Angry or irritable moods

____ 17. Smoking

____ 18. Fears or anxiety you may have

____ 19. Alcohol use

____ 20. Use of other drugs

____ 21. Your sexual orientation

____ 22. Your sexual activity

____ 23. Unsafe, high-risk activities or practices

____ 24. Immunizations required at this age

____ 25. Special screening tests

____ 26. Any abuse or trauma you have experienced

____ 27. Planning for job or further education

Are there any *other* concerns you would like to be able to talk about with the doctor or nurse?

Your name: _____   Today's date: _____

Date of birth: _____

Parent(s)' name(s): _____

Other people in the household: _____

The information contained in this publication should not be used as a substitute for the medical care and advice of your pediatrician. There may be variations in treatment that your pediatrician may recommend based on individual facts and circumstances.   HE0230

©1997 American Academy of Pediatrics

Reprinted with permission from the American Academy of Pediatrics. *Guidelines for Health Supervision Visits III.* May not be reproduced without permission from the American Academy of Pediatrics.

Infants BIRTH TO 12 MONTHS

Children do best when their parent(s) and their doctors and nurses *work together* to observe them, listen to them, and understand them.

Your first year with your baby is one of the most exciting and important times you will have. It can also be one of the hardest. All babies are different. Perfectly healthy babies have different styles and schedules for eating, sleeping, reacting to noise and touch, and calming themselves when they get upset. Some babies will be very active, and some will seem more calm. Most will enjoy being cuddled, but some will feel more comfortable when they are not held so much. As you watch your baby, you will become the expert on what he or she does more easily, and what your baby needs more help with. Your doctor and nurse can help you with ways to make feeding, sleeping, and discovering the world go well. However, they will need to rely on your report of how your baby does things and what will work best in your household.

As babies grow, they become more regular about when and how long they sleep, when and how they eat, and how they react to you and other important people in their world. You should see signs that your baby hears even soft sounds and sees light and faces. Your baby may turn toward them, watch them, smile at them, and even imitate them. As your baby grows, you will see him or her lifting his/her head, pushing his/her upper body up, and even holding himself/herself up to sit — all so she/he can do even more to see you and the sights and sounds around him/her. If you have a "gut feeling" that there is something wrong or unusual about the way your baby does these things, be sure to talk to your pediatrician about it. Any observation or concern you have is important, and discussing it may help you do even more to help your baby.

It would be helpful if you could take a few minutes to think about what things you would like to discuss during your visit today; the following list is intended to offer a few suggestions.

What are you enjoying most about your baby?

Please put a check (✔) by all areas you would like to discuss:

_____ 1. The baby's health, specific symptoms or concerns

_____ 2. Questions about shots (immunizations) the baby needs

_____ 3. Vision, and how the baby reacts to things she/he sees

_____ 4. Hearing, and how the baby reacts to things she/he hears

_____ 5. How it feels to hold the baby — does she/he feel "tense" or "floppy" or in any way uncomfortable?

_____ 6. When the baby sleeps and for how long

_____ 7. What the baby eats and how often

_____ 8. How active and alert the baby seems to be

_____ 9. Concerns about spoiling the baby

_____ 10. Questions about when the baby might do new things, like sitting or talking

_____ 11. The baby's moods

_____ 12. Questions about bathing or diapering the baby

_____ 13. Questions about child care

_____ 14. Questions about how brothers or sisters interact with the baby

_____ 15. Recovery from pregnancy; questions about family planning or avoiding another pregnancy

_____ 16. Death or illness of a family member

_____ 17. Depression or other psychological problems in a family member

_____ 18. Any accidental injury, trauma, or abuse the child or a parent may have experienced

_____ 19. Other family problems, such as money problems, violence, alcohol, or other drug abuse, conflict between parents, or separation

Are there any *other* concerns you would like to be able to talk about with the doctor or nurse?

Child's name:	Today's date:
Date of birth:	
Your name:	
Your relationship to child:	
Other people in the household:	

Toddlers 12 TO 36 MONTHS

Children do best when their parent(s) and their doctors and nurses *work together* to observe them, listen to them, and understand them.

The toddler years are fascinating, exciting, and challenging for parents and children alike. Children are learning to do so many new things so quickly — to walk, to talk, to use the toilet, and to play with other children! They are learning to be more independent and to "have a mind of their own." Children are more and more interested in looking at books and having stories read to them as they advance through the toddler period.

Most parents of toddlers have seen a tantrum, and have had experience with a child who refused to cooperate. Some parents are surprised at how angry they feel under these circumstances. Discussing these issues with family members, friends, or physicians may help parents to think about their preferred approach to discipline.

It would be helpful if you could take a few minutes to think about what things you would like to discuss during your visit today; the following list is intended to offer a few suggestions.

What are you enjoying most about your child at this age?

Please put a check (✔) by all areas you would like to discuss:

_____ 1. The child's health, specific symptoms or concerns

_____ 2. Questions about necessary screening tests or immunizations

_____ 3. Vision or hearing

_____ 4. Appetite or eating patterns

_____ 5. Sleeping patterns and routines, naps

_____ 6. The child's energy or activity level

_____ 7. The child's overall development

_____ 8. The child's ability to speak and be understood

_____ 9. The child's ability to walk, run, climb

_____ 10. Toilet training

_____ 11. Good ways to discipline

_____ 12. Temper tantrums

_____ 13. Fears

_____ 14. How the child behaves with adults

_____ 15. How the child behaves with other children

_____ 16. How the child plays; good ideas for toys and activities

_____ 17. Child care or preschool

_____ 18. The child's relationship with brothers or sisters

_____ 19. Death or illness of a family member

_____ 20. Depression or other psychological problems in a family member

_____ 21. Other family problems, such as money problems, violence, alcohol or other drug abuse, conflicts between parents, or separation

_____ 22. Any trauma or abuse the child may have experienced

_____ 23. Any issues about your own childhood that you think may affect your parenting

Are there any *other* concerns you would like to be able to talk about with the doctor or nurse?

Child's name:	Today's date:
Date of birth:	
Your name:	
Your relationship to child:	
Other people in the household:	

Parents' Guide to Pediatric Visits

Preschool Children 3 TO 5 YEARS OLD

Children do best when their parent(s) and their doctors and nurses *work together* to observe them, listen to them, and understand them.

The preschool years are busy and exciting times for both parents and children. Children now want to do more and more things for themselves and need help to learn the best ways to dress and feed themselves, take care of bathing and toileting needs, and to explore and play safely. Often they feel "big" enough to try things on their own, but they still need a lot of teaching, supervision, and limits. They are beginning to understand some important learning concepts — numbers, letters, sounds, colors, and shapes. They also are beginning to consider concepts of how to get along — waiting, politeness, sharing, helping, resting. They may be having important experiences of "leaving home" for preschool or recreation activities. There are many differences in how quickly children learn at this age, and their attitudes and interests may be different from those of their brothers, sisters, and friends. They and their parents are learning together about their special skills, interests, and personalities.

It would be helpful if you could take a few minutes to think about what things you would like to discuss during your visit today; the following list is intended to offer a few suggestions.

What are you enjoying most about your child at this age?

Please put a check (✔) by all areas you would like to discuss:

____ 1. The child's health, specific symptoms or concerns

____ 2. Questions about necessary screening tests or immunizations

____ 3. Vision or hearing

____ 4. Appetite or eating patterns

____ 5. Sleeping patterns and routines, naps

____ 6. The child's overall development

____ 7. The child's ability to speak and be understood

____ 8. The child's ability to walk, run, and climb

____ 9. The child's ability to draw, play with blocks and puzzles

____ 10. The child's energy or activity level

____ 11. Fears

____ 12. The child's ability to pay attention to directions or tasks

____ 13. Toilet training

____ 14. Sexual behavior or masturbation

____ 15. Temper tantrums

____ 16. Good ways to discipline

____ 17. Child care or preschool arrangements, plans for kindergarten

____ 18. How the child plays; good ideas for toys and activities

____ 19. How the child behaves with adults

____ 20. How the child behaves with other children

____ 21. The child's relationship with brothers or sisters

____ 22. Death or illness of a family member

____ 23. Depression or other psychological problems in a family member

____ 24. Other family problems, such as money problems, violence, alcohol or other drug abuse, conflicts between parents, or separation

____ 25. Any trauma or abuse the child may have experienced

____ 26. Any issues from your childhood that you think may affect your parenting

Are there any *other* concerns you would like to be able to talk about with the doctor or nurse?

Child's name:	Today's date:
Date of birth:	
Your name:	
Your relationship to child:	
Other people in the household:	

Reprinted with permission from the American Academy of Pediatrics. *Guidelines for Health Supervision Visits III.* May not be reproduced without permission from the American Academy of Pediatrics.

Parents' Guide to Pediatric Visits

School-age Children 6 TO 11 YEARS OLD

Throughout the school years, children are becoming increasingly independent individuals. They are rapidly obtaining new skills, knowledge, and interests. Experiences outside of the home contribute increasingly to their psychological and social growth. During this period, children become increasingly able to make important decisions that influence their health.

The health supervision of school-age children includes attention to their physical, psychological, and social well-being. Health supervision visits provide opportunities to help children gain knowledge about their health and bodies and feel growing responsibility for making healthy decisions. For this reason, it is often helpful for children to be involved directly in discussions during these visits.

It would be helpful if you could take a few minutes to think about what things you would like to discuss during your visit today; the following list is intended to offer a few suggestions.

What are you enjoying most about your child at this age?

Please put a check (✔) by all areas you would like to discuss:

_____ 1. The child's general health, including specific symptoms or concerns

_____ 2. Physical growth and development

_____ 3. Questions about necessary screening tests, immunizations, or the physical examination

_____ 4. Gross- or fine-motor skills

_____ 5. The child's ability to communicate

_____ 6. Bowel and bladder function

_____ 7. Appetite or diet

_____ 8. Sleeping patterns and difficulties

_____ 9. Energy or activity level

_____ 10. Mood (sad, angry, hopeless)

_____ 11. Discipline strategies

_____ 12. School performance or adjustment

_____ 13. School absences

_____ 14. Fears

_____ 15. How the child gets along with other children

_____ 16. How the child interacts with adults

_____ 17. The child's interests and activities

_____ 18. Frequent aches and pains

_____ 19. Questions about sexuality

_____ 20. Annoying habits (like biting nails, sucking thumb)

_____ 21. The child's ability to deal with frustrations

_____ 22. The child's ability to be independent

_____ 23. Attention span

_____ 24. Child care or after-school arrangements

_____ 25. Relationship among family members

_____ 26. Death or illness of a family member

_____ 27. Depression or other psychological difficulties in a family member

_____ 28. Other family stresses (like employment issues, money problems, violence, alcohol or other drug use, conflicts between parents, separation)

_____ 29. Any trauma or abuse the child may have experienced

_____ 30. Any issues from your own childhood that you think might affect your parenting

Are there any *other* concerns you would like to be able to talk about with the doctor or nurse?

Child's name: _____ Today's date: _____

Date of birth: _____

Your name: _____

Your relationship to child: _____

Other people in the household: _____

Parents' Guide to Pediatric Visits

Younger Adolescents 11 TO 15 YEARS OLD

As children mature, they become much more interested in and capable of assuming responsibility for their own health needs. They show increased concern with their developing body and compare themselves with peers to reassure themselves that they are "normal." Psychological and social independence is increasing, and often teenagers begin to show unwillingness to participate in some family activities. They concentrate instead on peer relationships and social activities. Their social and emotional life can greatly influence their physical health. Risk-taking behaviors are more commonly observed during these years. Early adolescence may be a particularly trying time for both parents and adolescents.

During these years, it becomes appropriate to emphasize the opportunity for adolescent-initiated visits and confidential discussion/ examination without a parent present. It is also important for the parent(s) to speak with the pediatrician alone to communicate your observations and concerns.

What are some of the things that make you especially proud of your adolescent?

Please put a check (✔) by all areas you would like to discuss:

_____ 1. Health, specific symptoms or concerns

_____ 2. Appetite, eating habits, nutrition

_____ 3. Physical growth and development

_____ 4. Sexual development, sexual behavior, or sexual orientation

_____ 5. Sleeping patterns and routines

_____ 6. School performance this year (grades, frequency of absences)

_____ 7. Participation in sports

_____ 8. Friendships/response to peer pressures

_____ 9. Relationships with brothers and sisters

_____ 10. Interactions with parent(s)

_____ 11. Disciplinary methods, privileges, chores

_____ 12. Communicating feelings and concerns

_____ 13. Sadness, depression

_____ 14. Use of tobacco, alcohol, or illicit drugs

_____ 15. Family problems, such as money problems, violence, alcohol or other drug abuse, conflicts between parents or separation

_____ 16. Death or illness of a family member

_____ 17. Any trauma or abuse the adolescent may have experienced

_____ 18. Any particular fears

_____ 19. Your experience as a teenager and the impact it has on your parenting

Are there any *other* concerns you would like to be able to talk about with the doctor or nurse?

Adolescent's name:	Today's date:
Date of birth:	
Your name:	
Your relationship to adolescent:	
Other people in the household:	

Reprinted with permission from the American Academy of Pediatrics. *Guidelines for Health Supervision Visits III.* May not be reproduced without permission from the American Academy of Pediatrics.

Parents' Guide to Pediatric Visits

Older Adolescents 16 TO 21 YEARS OLD

Adolescents 16 to 21 years of age typically show increasing intellectual, moral, social, and emotional independence. Many teenagers substitute their own or their friends' standards for their family's value system. They may experiment with behaviors that put them at physical, psychological, or social risk. They enter into intimate relationships. Parents are excited and challenged by these developments. Conflicts within the family may occur during this period.

Adolescents do best when their parents and their doctors and nurses respect their autonomy and offer nonjudgmental support and advice. We demonstrate our respect for teenagers by examining them without their parents present and by promising them confidentiality. We want to assure you we will inform you if your adolescent poses a serious risk to himself or herself or to others. We will answer your questions as completely as possible without violating confidentiality. We usually encourage adolescents to discuss issues openly with their families.

It would be helpful if you could take a few minutes to think about what things you would like to discuss during your visit today; the following list is intended to offer a few suggestions.

What are you enjoying most about your adolescent at this age?

Please put a check (✔) by all areas you would like to discuss:

_____ 1. Your adolescent's overall health, or specific symptoms or concerns

_____ 2. Physical growth, development, or stage of puberty

_____ 3. Menstrual patterns or problems

_____ 4. Psychological and social development

_____ 5. Appetite, eating patterns, or nutrition

_____ 6. Sleeping patterns

_____ 7. Emotional outbursts or withdrawal

_____ 8. Evidence of depression or anxiety

_____ 9. Conflicts in the family

_____ 10. Family problems, such as money problems, violence, alcohol or other drug use, separation or divorce

_____ 11. School attendance or performance

_____ 12. Stealing or taking things that do not belong to him/her

_____ 13. Sports participation

_____ 14. Fears

_____ 15. Friends and peer group

_____ 16. Angry or irritable moods

_____ 17. Smoking

_____ 18. Alcohol use

_____ 19. Use of other drugs

_____ 20. Sexual orientation

_____ 21. Sexual activity

_____ 22. Unsafe activities or practices

_____ 23. Immunizations required at this age

_____ 24. Special screening tests

_____ 25. Any trauma or abuse

_____ 26. Planning for job or further education

Are there any *other* concerns you would like to be able to talk about with the doctor or nurse?

Adolescent's name:	Today's date:
Date of birth:	
Your name:	
Your relationship to adolescent:	
Other people in the household:	

The information contained in this publication should not be used as a substitute for the medical care and advice of your pediatrician. There may be variations in treatment that your pediatrician may recommend based on individual facts and circumstances.

©1997 American Academy of Pediatrics

HE0226

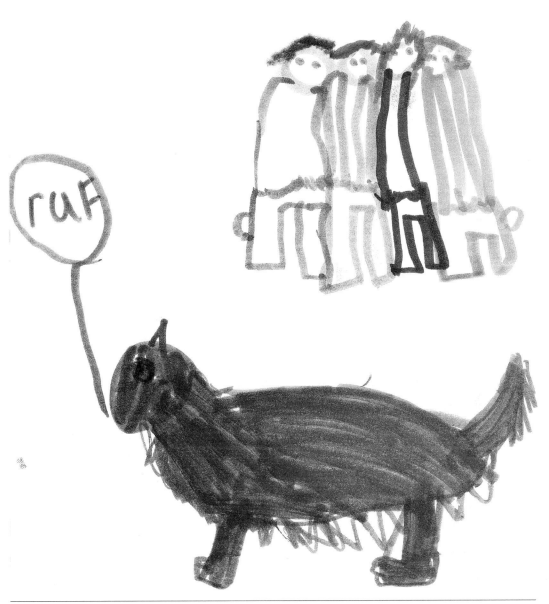

And finally, the tail wags. By a boy, age 5.

References

Chapter 1

American Academy of Pediatrics: Developmental surveillance and screening of infants and young children. *Pediatrics* 108:192, 2001.

American Academy of Pediatrics: *Guidelines for Health Supervision, III.* Elk Grove Village, IL, American Academy of Pediatrics, 2002.

Cole M, Cole SR: *The Development of Children,* 3rd ed. New York, WB Freeman, 1996.

Coury D, Berger SP, Stancin T, Tanner JL: Curricular guidelines for residency training in developmental-behavioral pediatrics. *J Dev Behav Pediatr* 20(2 Suppl):S1-S38, 1999.

Dworkin PH: Enhancing developmental services in child health supervision: An idea whose time has truly arrived. *Pediatrics* 114:827-831, 2004.

Glascoe FP, Macias M: How you can implement the AAP's new policy on developmental and behavioral screening. *Contemp Pediatr* 20:85-88, 93-102, 2004.

Halfon N, McLearn KT, Schuster MA (eds): *Child Rearing in America.* New York, Cambridge University Press, 2002.

Hall DMB, Elliman D: *Health for All Children,* 4th ed. Oxford, Oxford University Press, 2003.

Herschkowitz N, Kagan J, Zilles K: Neurobiological bases of behavioral development in the first year. *Neuropediatrics* 28:296, 1997.

Levine MD, Carey WB, Crocker AC (eds): *Developmental-Behavioral Pediatrics,* 2nd ed. Philadelphia, WB Saunders, 1992.

Lewis M (ed): *Child and Adolescent Psychiatry.* Philadelphia, Williams & Wilkins, 1997.

Parker S, Zuckerman B: *Handbook of Developmental and Behavioral Pediatrics,* 2nd ed. Boston, Little, Brown, 2004.

Regalado M, Halfon N: Primary care services: Promoting optimal child development from birth to three years. *Arch Pediatr Adolesc Med* 155:1316-1322, 2001.

Schor EL: Rethinking well-child care. *Pediatrics* 114:210-216, 2004.

Shonkoff JP, Phillips D (eds): *From Neurons to Neighborhoods: The Science of Early Child Development.* Washington, DC, National Academy Press, 2000.

Shore R: *Rethinking the Brain: New Insights into Early Development.* New York, Families and Work Institute, 1997.

Chapter 2

Bandura A: Influence of model's reinforcement contingencies on the acquisition of imitative responses. *J Pers Soc Psychol* 1:589, 1965.

Bandura A: *Psychological Modeling.* Chicago, Atherton, Aldine, 1971.

Bandura A: *Self-Efficacy and the Exercise of Control.* New York, Freeman Press, 1997.

Berk L: *Child Development,* 6th ed. Boston, Allyn & Bacon, 2003.

Bronfenbrenner U, Ceci S: *The Ecology of Human Development: Experiments by Nature and Design.* Cambridge, MA, Harvard University Press, 1979.

Bronfenbrenner U, Ceci S: Nature-nurture reconceptualized in developmental perspective: A bioecological approach. *Psychol Rev* 101:568, 1998.

Carey WB, McDevitt SC.: *Coping with Children's Temperament: A Guide for Professionals.* New York, Basic Books, 1995.

Chess S, Thomas A: *Origins and Evolution of Behavior Disorders.* New York, Brunner/Mazel, 1984.

Cole M, Cole SR: *The Development of Children*, 4th ed. New York, WH Freeman, 2001.

Dasan PR (ed): *Piagetian Psychology: Cross-Cultural Contributions*. New York, Gardner Press, 1977.

Elkind D: *A Sympathetic Understanding of the Child: Birth to Sixteen*, 3rd ed. Boston, Allyn & Bacon, 1994.

Elman JL, Bates EA, Johnson MH, et al: *Rethinking Innateness: A Connectionist Perspective on Development*. Cambridge, MA, MIT Press, 1996.

Emde R: Individual meaning and increasing complexity: Contributions of Sigmund Freud and Rene Spitz to developmental psychology. *Dev Psychol* 28:347, 1992.

Erikson EH: Identity and the life cycle. In Klein GS (ed): *Psychological Issues*, vol 1, New York, International Universities Press, 1959.

Erikson EH: *Childhood and Society*, 2nd ed. New York, WW Norton, 1963.

Freud S: Three contributions to the theory of sex. In Brill AA (translator): *The Basic Writings of Sigmund Freud*. New York, Modern Library, 1905.

Freud S: *Collected papers*, vols 2–5. New York, Basic Books, 1959.

Gardner H: *Frames of Mind: The Theory of Multiple Intelligence*. New York, Basic Books, 1993.

Gesell A: *The Embryology of Behavior*. New York, Harper & Row, 1945.

Gesell A: The ontogenesis of infant behavior. In Carmichael L (ed): *Manual of Child Psychology*. New York, John Wiley & Sons, 1946.

Gesell A, Amatruda C: *Developmental Diagnosis*, 2nd ed. New York, Harper & Row, 1965.

Gesell A, Ilg F: Infant and child in the culture of today (1943). In Gesell A, Iig F (eds): *Child Development*. New York, Harper & Row, 1949.

Ginsburg H, Opper S: *Piaget's Theory Of Intellectual Development*. Englewood Cliffs, NJ, Prentice-Hall, 1969.

Illingworth RS: *The Development of the Infant and Young Child: Normal and Abnormal*. London, Williams & Wilkins, 1966.

Kagan J: *The Nature of the Child*. New York, Basic Books, 1984.

Kagan J, Snidman N, Zentner M, Peterson E: Temperament and anxious symptoms in school age children. *Dev Psychopathol* 11:209-224, 1999.

Knobloch H, Stevens F, Malone A: *A Manual of Developmental Diagnosis: The Administration and Interpretation of the Revised Gesell and Amatruda Developmental and Neurologic Examination*. Hagerstown, MD, Harper & Row, 1980.

Kohlberg L: Development of moral character and moral ideology. In Hoffman ML, Hoffman LW (eds): *Review of Child Development Research*, vol 1. New York, Russell Sage Foundation, 1974.

Levine RA, Dixon SD, Levine S, et al: *Child Care and Culture: Lessons from Africa*. Cambridge, England, Cambridge University Press, 1994.

Lewis MD: The promise of dynamic systems approaches for an integrated account of human development. *Child Dev* 71:36-43, 2000.

Mahler MS, Pine F, Bergman A: *The Psychological Birth of the Human Infant: Symbiosis and Individuation*. New York, Basic Books, 1975.

McDevitt SC, Carey WB: *The Carey Temperament Scale*. Scottsdale, AZ, Behavioral Developmental Initiatives, 1995.

McGraw M: *The Neuromuscular Maturation of the Human Infant*. New York, Columbia University Press, 1943.

Morton JB, Munakata Y: What's the difference? Contrasting modular and neural network approaches to understanding developmental variability. *J Dev Behav Pediatr* 2005 (in press).

Pavlov IP: *Conditioned Reflexes*. London, Oxford University Press (translated and edited by GV Anrep), 1927.

Piaget J: *Play, Dreams and Imitation in Childhood*. New York, WW Norton, 1951.

Piaget J: *The Origins of Intelligence in Children*. New York, WW Norton (translated by M Cook), 1952.

Piaget J, Inhelder B: *The Psychology of the Child*. New York, Basic Books (translated by H Weaver), 1969.

Quinlan PT: *Connectionist Models of Development*. East Sussex, NY, Psychology Press, 2003.

Rothbart MK, Bates JE: Temperament. In Damon W, Eisenberg N (eds): *Handbook of Child Psychology*, 5th ed. New York, John Wiley & Sons, 1998, pp 105-176.

Rutter M: *Fifteen Thousand Hours: Secondary Schools and Their Effects on Children.* Cambridge, MA, Harvard University Press, 1979.

Saudino KJ: Behavioral genetics and child temperament. *J Dev Behav Pediatr* 2005 (in press).

Skinner BF: *About Behaviorism* (1927). New York, Alfred A Knopf, 1974.

Thelan E, Smith LB: Dynamic systems theories. In Lemer RE (ed): *Handbook of Child Psychology,* vol 1, 5th ed. New York, John Wiley & Sons, 1998, pp 563-634.

Thomas A, Chess S: *Temperament and Development.* New York, Brunner/Mazel, 1977.

Watson JB: *Behaviorism* (1924). New York, WW Norton, 1970.

Werner EE: *Cross-cultural Child Development: A View from the Planet Earth.* Monterey, CA, Brooks-Cole, 1979.

Werner EE: A cross-cultural perspective on infancy. *J Cross Cult Psychol* 19:96, 1988.

Chapter 3

Adib S: From the biomedical model to the Islamic alternative: A brief overview of medical practices in the contemporary Arab world. *Soc Sci Med* 58:697-702, 2004.

Aguirre-Molina M, Molina C: Latino populations: Who are they? In Molina C, Aguirre-Molina M (eds): *Latino Health in the US: A Growing Challenge.* Washington, DC, American Public Health Association, 1994.

American Academy of Pediatrics, Committee on Pediatric Workforce: Culturally effective pediatric care: Education and training issues (RE9753). *Pediatrics* 103:167, 1999.

Barrios L: DCFS Services to Latino Families: Latino Families and Parenting, December 2000.

Bartz KW, Levine ES: Child rearing by black parents: A description and comparison to Anglo and Chicano parents. *J Marriage Family* 40:708-720, 1978.

Beckwith L, Cohen SE: Home environment and cognitive competence in preterm children during the first five years. In Gottfried A (ed): *Home Environment and Early Cognitive Development.* New York, Academic Press, 1984.

Children's Defense Fund: *A Vision for America's Future: An Agenda for the 1990s* (policy statement). Washington, DC, Children's Defense Fund, 1990.

Condon EC, Peters JY, Sueiro-Ross C: *Special Education and the Hispanic Child: Cultural Perspective.* New Brunswick, NJ, Teacher's Corp Mid Atlantic Network, 1979.

Crummer GC: Indian Health Council, Inc., Valley Center, CA, personal communication, 2004.

Culture Clues: Communicating with Your African American Patient. UWMC Patient and Family Education Services, 2001.

Curran WJ: The Tuskegee syphilis study. *N Engl J Med* 289(14):730-731, 1973.

Delgado, Gaitan C: Socializing young children in Mexican-American families: A intergenerational perspective. In Greenfield PM Cocking RR (eds): *Cross-Cultural Roots of Minority Child Development.* Hillsdale, NJ, Lawrence Erlbaum Associates, 1994.

deVries MW, deVries MR: Cultural relativity of toilet training readiness: A perspective from East Africa. *Pediatrics* 60:170-177, 1977.

Eapen V, Ghubash R: Help-seeking for mental health problems of children: Preferences and attitudes in the United Arab Emirates. *Psychol Rep* 94:663-667, 2004.

Ernst E, Pittler MH: Efficacy of ginger for nausea and vomiting: A systematic review of randomized clinical trials. *Br J Anaesth* 84:367, 2000.

Fajardo BF, Friedman DG: Maternal rhythmicity in three American cultures. In Field TM, Sostek AM, Vietze P, Liederman PH (eds): *Culture and Early Interactions.* Hillsdale, NJ, Lawrence Erlbaum Associates, 1981.

Flores G: Culture and the patient-physician relationship: Achieving cultural competency in healthcare. *J Pediatr* 136:14, 2000.

Fortin AH 6th: Communication skills to improve patient satisfaction and quality of care. *Ethn Dis* 12(4):S3-58-S3-61, 2002.

Frye BA: Use of cultural themes in promoting health among Southeast Asian refugees. *Am J Health Promotion* 9:269, 1995.

Garcia Coll CT: Developmental outcome of minority infants: A process-oriented look into our beginnings. *Child Dev* 61:270-289, 1990.

Gonzalez V: The role of socioeconomic and sociocultural factors in language minority children's development: An ecological research view. *Bilingual Res J* 25(1 and 2), 2001 (on-line at http://brj.asu.edu/v2512/articles/art2.html).

Gorski PA: Toilet training guidelines: Clinicians—the role of the clinician in toilet training. *Pediatrics* 103(6 Suppl), 1999.

Greenfield PM, Suzuki L: Culture and human development: Implications for parenting education, pediatrics and mental health. In Siegel I, Renninger K (eds): *Handbook of Child Psychology*, vol 4, 5th ed. New York, John Wiley & Sons, 1998.

Guarnashelli J, Lee J, Pitts FW: "Fallen fontanel" (caida de mollera): A variant of the battered child syndrome. *JAMA* 222:1545, 1972.

Harriman AE, Lukosius PA: On why Wayne Dennis found Hopi infants retarded in age at onset of walking. *Percept Mot Skills* 55:1, 1982.

Harry B: *Developing Cultural Self-Awareness.* CASAnet Library on Cultural Competency, 1992.

Heyadat KM, Pirzadeh R: Issues in Islamic biomedical ethics: A primer for the pediatrician. *Pediatrics* 108:4, 2001.

Hoang GN, Erickson RV: Guidelines for providing medical care to Southeast Asian refugees. *JAMA* 248:710, 1982.

Jambunalhan S, Burts DC, Pierce S: Comparison of parenting attitudes among five ethnic groups in the United States. *J Comp Family Studies* 31:395-406, 2000.

Johnson CE, DeHertogh MB: *Understanding Cultural Diversity and Its Implication for Programming.* PEN pages College of Agricultural Sciences, 1999.

Johnson-Powell G, Yamamoto J (eds): *Transcultural Child Development.* New York, John Wiley & Sons, 1997.

Kleinman A: *Patients and Healers in the Context of Culture.* Berkeley, CA, University of California Press, 1980, p 106.

Laffrey S, Meleis AI, Lipson JG, et al: Assessing Arab-American health care needs. *Soc Sci Med* 29:877-883, 1989.

LeVine R, Dixon S, LeVine S, et al: *Child Care and Culture: Lessons from Africa.* New York, Cambridge University Press, 1994.

Lindsay J, Narayan MC, Rea K: Nursing across cultures: The Vietnamese client. *Home Healthcare Nurse* 16:693, 1998.

Lynch EW: Developing cross-cultural competence. In Lynch EW, Hanson MJ (eds): *Cross-cultural Competence: A Guide for Working with Young Children and Their Families*, 2nd ed. Baltimore, Paul H Brooks, 1998.

Mattson S: Culturally sensitive perinatal care for Southeast Asians. *J Obstet Gynecol Neonatal Nurs* 24:335, 1995.

Mattson S, Lew L: Culturally sensitive prenatal care for Southeast Asians. *J Obstet Gynecol Neonatal Nurs* 21:48, 1992.

McDavis RJ, Woodrow MP, Parker WJ: Counseling African Americans. In Vace NA, Devaney SB, Wittmer J (eds): *Experiencing and Counseling Multicultural and Diverse Populations*, 3rd ed. 1995, pp 217-248.

Mikhail BI: Hispanic mothers' beliefs and practices regarding selected children's health problems. *West J Nurs Res* 16:623, 1994.

Mosier CE, Rogoff B: Privileged treatment of toddlers: Cultural aspects of individual choice and responsibility. *Dev Psychol* 39:1047, 2003.

Native American medicine, wholehealthmd.com 2004.

Nuttall P, Flores F: Hmong healing practices used for common childhood illnesses. *Pediatr Nurs* 23:247, 1997.

Omran AR: Children's rights in Islam from the Qur'an and Sunnah. *Popul Sci* 9:77-88, 1990.

Pachter LM: Culture and clinical care: Folk illnesses beliefs and behaviors and their implications for health care delivery. *JAMA* 271:690-694, 1994.

Pachter LM, Dworkin PH: Maternal expectations about normal child development in 4 cultural groups. *Arch Pediatr Adolesc Med* 151:1144-1150, 1997.

Rairdan B, Higgs ZR: When your patient is a Hmong refugee. *Am J Nurs* 3:52, 1992.

Reid R, Rhoades ER: Cultural considerations in providing care to American Indians. In Rhoades ER (ed): *American Indian Health: Innovations in Health Care, Promotion and Policy.* Baltimore, Johns Hopkins University Press, 2000.

Risser AL, Mazur LJ: Use of folk remedies in a Hispanic population. *Arch Pediatr Adolesc Med* 149:978-981, 1995.

Rothbaum F, Weisz J, Pott M, et al: Attachment and culture: Security in the United States and Japan. *Am Psychol* 55:1093-1104, 2000.

Schmitt BD: Toilet training and getting it right the first time. *Contemp Pediatr* 21(3):105, 2004.

Slonim MB: *Children, Culture, and Ethnicity: Evaluating and Understanding the Impact.* New York, Garland Publishing, 1991.

Small MF: *Kids: How Biology and Culture Shape the Way We Raise Our Children.* New York, Doubleday, 2001.

Steward MS, Steward DS: The observation of Anglo-Mexican and Chinese-American mothers teaching their young sons. *Child Dev* 44:327-337, 1973.

Stopes-Roe M, Cochrane R: The child-rearing values of Asian and British parents and young people: An inter-ethnic and inter-generational comparison in the evaluation of Kohn's 13 qualities. *Br J Social Psychol* 29:149, 1990.

U.S. Census Bureau: Current Population Reports, March 2000.

Voices of the Arab Community. Cross Cultural Health Care Program. Seattle, Pacific Medical Center, 1996.

Voices of the Cambodian Community. Cross Cultural Health Care Program. Seattle, Pacific Medical Center, 1996.

Voices of the Lao Community. Cross Cultural Health Care Program. Seattle, Pacific Medical Center, 1996.

Watson WH: *Black Folk Medicine: The Therapeutic Significance of Faith and Trust.* New Brunswick, NJ, Transaction Books, 1984.

Weiss AL, Van Haren MS: What pediatricians should know about normal language development: Ensuring cultural differences are not diagnosed as disorders. *Pediatr Ann* 32:7, 2003.

Werner EE: *Cross-Cultural Child Development: A View from the Planet Earth.* Monterey, CA, Brooks-Cole, 1979.

West C: *Race Matters.* New York, Vintage Books, 1994.

Zahr LK, Hattar-Pollara M: Nursing care of Arab children: Consideration of cultural factors. *J Pediatr Nurs* 13:6, 1998.

Chapter 4

Allmond BW Jr, Tanner JL, Gofman HF: *The Family Is the Patient,* 2nd ed. Baltimore, Williams & Wilkins, 1999.

American Academy of Pediatrics: *Guidelines for Health Supervision III.* Elk Grove Village, IL, American Academy of Pediatrics, 2002.

American Academy of Pediatrics: Family pediatrics. *Pediatrics* 111(Suppl):1539, 2003.

American Academy of Pediatrics: AAP Task Force on the Family. *Pediatrics* 111(Suppl):1541-1569, 2003.

Bass LW, Cohen RL: Ostensible versus actual reasons for seeking pediatric attention: Another look at the parental ticket of admission. *Pediatrics* 70:870, 1982.

Boggs SR, Eyberg S, Reynolds LA: Concurrent validity of the Eyberg Child Behavior Inventory. *J Clin Child Psychol* 19:75, 1990.

Borowsky IW, Mozayeny S, Ireland M: Brief psychosocial screening at health supervision and acute care visits. *Pediatrics* 112:129-133, 2003.

Casey PH, Bradley RH: The impact of home environment on children's development: Clinical relevance for the pediatrician. *J Dev Behav Pediatr* 3:146, 1982.

Cohen SE, Parmelee AH: Prediction of five-year Stanford Binet scores in preterm infants. *Child Dev* 54:1242, 1983.

Costello EJ: Primary care pediatrics and child psychopathology: A review of diagnostic treatment and referral practice. *Pediatrics* 78:1044, 1986.

DiMatteo MR, Prince LM, Hays RD: Nonverbal communication in the medical context: The physician-patient relationship. In Blanck PD, Buck R, Rosenthal R (eds): *Nonverbal Communication in the Clinical Context.* University Park, PA, Pennsylvania State University Press, 1986, pp 74-98.

Dodds M, Nicholson L, Muse B 3d, Osborn LM: Group health supervision visits more effective than individual visits in delivering health care information. *Pediatrics* 91:668, 1993.

Epstein RM: Mindful practice. *JAMA* 282:833-839, 1999.

Gates LG Jr: Forward. In West C: *Restoring Hope.* Boston, Beacon Press, 1997.

Gordon T: *Parent Effectiveness Training.* New York, PH Wyden, 1970.

Green M (ed): *Bright Futures: Guidelines for Health Supervision of Infants, Children, and Adolescents,* 2nd ed. Arlington, VA, National Center for Education in Maternal and Child Health, 2002.

Green M, Solnit AJ: Reaction to the threatened loss of a child: A vulnerable child syndrome. *Pediatrics* 34:58, 1964.

Healthy Steps Interactive Multimedia Training & Resource Kit Brochure, an Approach to the Primary Care of Children Birth to Three. http://www.healthysteps.org/healthysteps/homepage.nsf

High P, Hopman M, La Grasse L, Linn H: Evaluation of a clinic-based program to promote book sharing and bedtime routines among low-income urban families with young children. *Arch Pediatr Adolesc Med* 152:459, 1998.

Jellinek MS, Murphy JM: Screening for psychosocial disorders in pediatric practice. *Am J Dis Child* 142:1153, 1988.

Johnson TM, Hardt EJ, Kleinman A: Cultural factors in the medical interview. In Lipkin ML Jr, Putman SM, Lazare A (eds): *The Medical Interview: Clinical Care, Education, and Research.* New York, Springer-Verlag, 1995, pp 153-162.

Kemper KJ, Kelleher KJ: Family psychosocial screening: Instruments and techniques. *Ambulatory Child Health* 4:325, 1996.

Kleinman A: *Patients and Healers in the Context of Culture.* Berkeley, CA, University of California Press, 1980, p 106.

Klineman A, Eisenberg L, Good B: Culture, illness and care. *Ann Intern Med* 88:251, 1978.

Korsch BM, Freemon B, Negrete VF: Practical implications of doctor-patient interactions and analysis for pediatric practice. *Am J Dis Child* 12:110, 1971.

Lipkin ML Jr, Putnam SM, Lazare A (eds): *The Medical Interview—Clinical Care, Education, and Research.* New York, Springer-Verlag, 1995.

Liu YH, Stein MT: Talking with children. In Parker S, Zuckerman B (eds): *Developmental and Behavioral Pediatrics: A Handbook for Primary Care,* 2nd ed. Boston, Little, Brown, 2004.

Minkovitz C, Strobino D, Hughart N, et al: Early effects of the Healthy Steps for Young Children program. *Arch Pediatr Adolesc Med* 155:470-479, 2001.

National Center for Education in Maternal and Child Health: *Bright Futures in Practice: Mental Health,* vols 1 and 2. Arlington, VA, National Center for Education in Maternal and Child Health, 2002.

Patcher LM: Practicing culturally sensitive pediatrics. *Contemp Pediatr* 14:139, 1997.

Roberts JM: Belief in the evil eye in world perspective. In Maloney C (ed): *The Evil Eye*. New York, Columbia University Press, 1976, p 223.

Rutter M, Tizard J, Whitmore K: *Education, Health and Behaviour*. New York, John Wiley & and Sons, 1970.

Schor EL: Families, family roles and psychological diagnoses in primary care. *J Dev Behav Pediatr* 9:327, 1988.

Spock B, Needleman R: *Dr. Spock's Baby and Child Care*, 8th ed. New York, Pocket Books, 2004.

Stancin T (ed): Pediatric mental health services in primary care settings. *J Pediatr Psychol* 24(5), 1999.

Stein MT: Preparing families for the toddler and preschool years. *Contemp Pediatr* 15:88, 1998.

Stein MT, Jellinek M, Wells RD: The difficult parent: A reflective pediatrician's response. *J Dev Behav Pediatr* 24:434-437, 2003.

Stein M: The providing of well baby care within parent-infant groups. *Clin Pediatr (Phila)* 16:825, 1977.

Weinstein CM, David TG: *Spaces for Children: The Built Environment and Child Development*. New York, Plenum Press, 1987.

Werner E, Honzik MP, Smith RS: Prediction of intelligence and achievement at ten years from twenty-month pediatric and psychological examinations. *Child Dev* 39:1063, 1968.

Willoughby JA, Haggerty RJ: A simple behavioral questionnaire for preschool children. *Pediatrics* 34:798, 1964.

Zuckerman B, Parker S: Teachable moments: Assessment as intervention. *Contemp Pediatr* 14:41, 1997.

Chapter 5

Burns RC, Kaufman SH: *Actions, Styles and Symbols in Kinetic Family Drawings: An Interpretive Manual*. New York, Brunner/Mazel, 1972.

Clatworthy S, Simon K, Tiedeman ME: Child drawing: Hospital—an instrument designed to measure emotional status of hospitalized school-aged children. *J Pediatr Nurs* 14:2, 1999.

DiLeo JH: *Young Children and Their Drawings*. New York, Brunner/Mazel, 1970.

DiLeo JH: *Interpreting Children's Drawings*. New York, Brunner/Mazel, 1983.

Gardner H: Artful scribbles: *The Significance of Children's Drawings*. New York, Basic Books, 1980.

Gillespie J: *The Projective Use of Mother-and-Child Drawings: A Manual for Clinicians*. New York, Brunner/Mazel, 1994.

Goodenough FL: *Measurement of Intelligence by Drawings*. New York, World Books, 1926.

Harris DB: *Children's Drawings As Measures of Intellectual Maturity*. New York, Harcourt, 1963.

Instone SL: Perceptions of children with HIV infection when not told for so long: Implications for diagnosis disclosure. *J Pediatr Health Care* 14:235, 2000.

Kellog R: *Analyzing Children's Art*. Palo Alto, CA, National Press, 1969.

Koppitz EM: *Psychological Evaluation of Children's Human Figure Drawings*. New York, Grune & Stratton, 1968.

Luquet GF: *Les Dessins d'un Enfants: Etude Psychologique*. Paris, Alcain, 1917.

O'Brien RP, Patton WW: Development of an objective scoring method for kinetic family drawings. *J Pers Assess* 58:156, 1974.

Spinetta J, et al: The kinetic family drawing in childhood cancer: A revised application of an age-independent measure. In Spinetta J, Deasy-Spinetta P (eds): *Living with Childhood Cancer*. St Louis, CV Mosby, 1981, pp 86-120.

Stafstrom CE, Rostasy K, Minster A: The usefulness of children's drawings in the diagnosis of headache. *Pediatrics* 109:46, 2002.

Stein MT: Challenging case: The use of family drawings by children in pediatric practice. *J Dev Behav Pediatr* 18:334, 1997.

Vohr B, Garcia-Coll CT: Neurodevelopmental and school performance of very low birth weight infants: A seven year longitudinal study. *Pediatrics* 76:345, 1985.

Chapter 6

American Academy of Pediatrics: What pediatricians really think about working mothers. In Rubenstein C Elk Grove Village, IL (ed): *Working Mothers*. April 1990 (reprinted in *AAP News*, May 1990).

American Academy of Pediatrics, Committee on Psychosocial Aspects of Child and Family Health: The Elk Grove Village, IL prenatal visit. *Pediatrics* 97:141, 1996.

American Academy of Pediatrics: Family pediatrics. *Pediatrics* 111(6 Suppl), June 2003.

American Academy of Pediatrics: The prenatal visit. In Morris Green (ed): *Bright Futures*. Arlington, VA, National Center for Education in Maternal and Child Health, 1994, 2004, pp 13-17.

Bibring GL, Valenstein AF: Psychological aspects of pregnancy. *Clin Obstet Gynecol* 19:357, 1976.

Bittman SJ, Zalk SR: *Expectant Fathers*. New York, Hawthorn Books, 1978.

Bowlby J: *Attachment and Loss*, vol 1, *Attachment*. New York, Basic Books, 1969.

Brazelton TB: *On Becoming a Family: The Growth of Attachment*. New York, Delacorte Press–Seymour Lawrence, 1992.

Caplan G: *Emotional Implications of Pregnancy and Influences on Family Relationships in the Healthy Child*. Cambridge, MA, Harvard University Press, 1976.

Deutsch H: *Psychology of Women*. New York, Grune & Stratton, 1944.

Dixon S: Helping siblings adjust to the new baby. In Jellinek M, Patel BP, Froehle MC (eds): *Bright Futures in Practice: Mental Health*, vol 2, *Tool Kit*. Arlington, VA, National Center for Education in Maternal and Child Health, 2002.

Dixon SD: *Economic, Social and Medical Risk Profiles of Pregnant, Addicted Women with and without Case Management Services*. Sacramento, CA, State of California, Department of Drug and Alcohol Services, 1998.

Earls F: The fathers (not the mothers): Their importance and influence with infants and young children. *Psychiatry* 39:209, 1976.

Egeland B, Sroufe LA: Attachment and early maltreatment. *Child Dev* 52:44, 1981.

Freed GL, Fraley JK, Schanter RJ: Attitudes of expectant fathers regarding breastfeeding. *Pediatrics* 90:224, 1992.

Gorski P: Perinatal outcome and the social contract: Interrelationships between health and humanity. *J Perinatol* 18:297, 1998.

Handfield B, Bell R: Do childbirth classes influence decision making about labor and postpartum issues? *Birth* 22(3):153, 1995.

Hepper PG: Fetal psychology: An embryonic science. In Nijhuis JG (ed): *Fetal Behavior: Development and Perinatal Aspects*. New York, Oxford University Press, 1992.

Hepper PG: Fetal habituation: Another Pandora's Box? *Dev Med Child Neurol* 39:274, 343, 1997.

Heymans H, Winter ST: Fears during pregnancy. *Isr J Med Sci* 11:1102, 1975.

Holtzman LC: Sexual practices during pregnancy. *J Nurs Midwifery* 21:29, 1976.

Hott JR: The crisis of expectant fatherhood. *Am J Nurs* 76:1436, 1976.

Kennell JH: The physiologic effects of a supportive companion (doula) during labor. In Klaus MH, Robertson MO (eds): *Birth, Interaction and Attachment*. Pediatric Round Table Series. Skillman, NJ, Johnson and Johnson Baby Products Co, 1982.

Legg C, Sherick I, Wadland W: Reaction of preschool children to the birth of a sibling. *Child Psychiatry Hum Dev* 5:3, 1974.

Leifer M: Psychological changes accompanying pregnancy and motherhood. *Genet Psychol Monogr* 95:55, 1977.

LeVine RA, Dixon SD, LeVine S, et al: *Child Care and Culture: Lessons from Africa*. Cambridge, England, Cambridge University Press, 1994.

Liebenberg B: Prenatal counseling. In Shereshefsky PM, Yarrow LJ (eds): *Psychological Aspects of a First Pregnancy and Early Postnatal Adaptation*. New York, Raven Press, 1973.

Monk C, Myers MM, Sloan, RP, et al: Effects of women's stress-elicited physiological activity and chronic anxiety on fetal heart rate. *J Dev Behav Pediatr* 24:32-38, 2003.

Nijhuis JG (ed): *Fetal Behavior: Developmental and Perinatal Aspects.* Oxford, England, Oxford University Press, 1992.

Obrzut LE: Expectant fathers' perception of fathering. *Am J Nurs* 76:1440, 1976.

Parke RD: Fathers. In Bruner J, Cole M, Lloyd B (eds): *The Developing Child Series.* Cambridge, MA, Harvard University Press, 1981.

Parke RD, Power TG, Tinsley BR, Hymel S: The father's role in the family system. *Semin Perinatol* 3:25-34, 1979.

Petre-Quadens O, De Barsy AM, Devos J, Sfaello Z: Sleep in pregnancy: Evidence of fetal sleep characteristics. *J Neurol Sci* 4:600-605, 1967.

Rubin R: Maternal tasks in pregnancy. *J Adv Nurs* 1:367, 1976.

Sanders L, Condon WM, Berk J: Primary prevention and some aspects of temporal organization in early infant-caretaker interactions. In Rexford EN, Sanders LW, Shapiro T (eds): *Infant Psychiatry.* New Haven, CT, Yale University Press, 1975, pp 187-204.

Sciacca JP, Dube DA, Phipps BL, Ratliff MI: A breastfeeding education promotion program: Effects on knowledge, attitudes and support. *J Community Health* 20:473-490, 1995.

Stadtler A: Fostering family adjustment prenatally. In Jellinek M, Patel BP, Froehle MC (eds): *Bright Futures in Practice: Mental Health,* vol 2, *Tool Kit.* Arlington, VA, National Center for Education in Maternal and Child Health, 2002.

Stainton MC: Parents' awareness of their unborn infant in the third trimester. *Birth* 17(2):92, 1990.

Uddenberg N, Fagerstroom CF, Hakanson-Zaunders M: Reproductive conflicts: Mental symptoms during pregnancy and time in labor. *J Psychosom Res* 20:575, 1976.

Van DenBergh BRH: Maternal emotions during pregnancy and fetal and neonatal behavior. In Nijhuis JG (ed): *Fetal Behavior: Development and Perinatal Aspects.* New York, Oxford University Press, 1992.

Wallerstein E: *Circumcision: An American Health Fallacy.* New York, Springer, 1980.

www.marchofdimes.org: Fetal development, prematurity prevention, healthy pregnancy tips.

www.pampers.com: Weekly pregnancy calendar with fetal pictures and ultrasounds, expert-authored articles on pregnancy and monthly electronic newsletters.

Yamamoto KJ, Kinsey DK: Pregnant women's ratings of different factors influencing psychological stress during pregnancy. *Psychol Rep* 39:203, 1976.

Zwelling E: Psychological responses to pregnancy. In Nichols F, Zwelling E (eds): *Maternal-Newborn Nursing: Theory and Practice.* Philadelphia, WB Saunders, 1997.

Chapter 7

Adams RJ, Maurer D, Davis M: Newborn discrimination of chromatic from achromatic stimuli. *J Exp Child Psychol* 41:267, 1986.

American Academy of Pediatrics: Breastfeeding guidelines. *Pediatrics* 100:1035, 1997.

American Academy of Pediatrics Joint Committee on Infant Hearing: Position statement, 1995. *Pediatrics* 95:152, 1994.

American Academy of Pediatrics, American College of Gynecologists: *Guidelines for Perinatal Care,* 4th ed. Elk Grove Village, IL, American Academy of Pediatrics, 1997.

Anand KJS, Hickey PR: Pain and its effects in the human neonate and fetus. *N Engl J Med* 317:1321, 1347, 1987 (commentary by A. Fletcher).

Borenstein MH, Sigman MD: Continuity in mental development in infancy. *Child Dev* 57:251, 1986.

Bower TGR: *The Perceptual World of the Child.* Cambridge, MA, Harvard University Press, 1977.

Brazelton TB: *Infants and Mothers: Individual Differences in Development.* New York, Delacorte, 1969.

Brazelton TB: *Neonatal Behavioral Assessment Scale,* 2nd ed. London, Spastics International Medical Publications, 1984.

Brazelton TB: A window on the newborn's world: More than two decades of experience with the Neonatal Behavioral Assessment Scale (NBAS). In Meisels S, Fenichel E (eds): *New Visions for the Developmental Assessment of Infants and Young Children.* Washington, DC, Zero to Three, 1996.

Brazelton TB, Nugent JK: *Neonatal Behavioral Assessment Scale.* London, MacKeith Press, 1995.

Bronson G: The postnatal growth in visual capacity. *Child Dev* 45:887, 1974.

Broussard E, Sergay M, Hartner S: Further considerations regarding maternal perception of the firstborn. In Hellmuth J (ed): *Exceptional Infant.* New York, Brunner/Mazel, 1971.

Christensson K, Cabrera T, Christensson E, et al: Separation distress call in the human neonate in the absence of maternal body contact. *Acta Paediatr* 84:468-473, 1995.

Condon WS, Sander LW: Synchrony demonstrated between movements of the neonate and adult speech. *Child Dev* 45:456, 1974.

Dixon S, Snyder J, Holve R, Bromberger P: Behavioral effects of circumcision with and without anesthesia. *J Dev Behav Pediatr* 5:246-250, 1984.

Edelman AI, Kartz M: Olfactory recognition: A genetic or learned capacity. *J Dev Behav Pediatr* 13:126, 1992.

Eyer DE: *Mother-Infant Bonding: A Scientific Fiction.* New Haven, CT, Yale University Press, 1992.

Feldman W, Feldman M: The intelligence of breastfeeding. *Lancet* 347:1037, 1996.

Forsyth B, Canny P: Perceptions of vulnerability 3½ years after problems of feeding and crying in early infancy. *Pediatrics* 88:757, 1991.

Fraiberg S: *The Magic Years.* New York, Charles Scribner's Sons, 1959.

Goldin-Meadow S: Language development under atypical learning conditions. In Nelson K (ed): *Children's Language.* Hillsdale, NJ, Lawrence Erlbaum Associates, 1985.

Green M, Solnit AJ: Reactions to the threatened loss of a child: A vulnerable child syndrome. *Pediatrics* 34:58, 1964.

Izard C: Innate and universal facial expression: Evidence from developmental and cross-cultural research. *Psychol Bull* 115:288, 1994.

Kennell J: The time has come to reassess delivery room routines. *Birth* 21:49, 1994.

Kirya C, Werthmann MW: Neonatal circumcision and penile dorsal nerve block: A painless procedure. *J Pediatr* 96:998, 1978.

Klaus M, Kennell J: *Maternal-Infant Bonding.* St Louis, CV Mosby, 1976.

Klaus M, Kennell J, Klaus P: *Mothering the Mother: How a Doula Can Help You Have a Shorter, Easier and Healthier Birth.* Reading, MA, Addison-Wesley, 1993.

Korner A: The effect of the infant's state, level of arousal, sex and ontogenic stage on the care giver. In Lewis M, Rosenblum L (eds): *The Effect of the Infant on the Care Giver.* New York, John Wiley & Sons, 1974.

Kuhl PK, Williams KA, Lacerda F, et al: Linguistic experience alters phonetics perception in infants by six months of age. *Science* 255:606-608, 1992.

Lawrence R: *Breastfeeding: A Guide for the Medical Professional.* St Louis, CV Mosby, 1989.

Leon M: Touch and smell. In Field TM (ed): *Touch in Early Development.* Mahwak, NJ, Lawrence Erlbaum Associates, 1995.

Lewin R (ed): *Child Alive.* Garden City, NY, Anchor Press, 1977.

Lopez S: *The Effect of the Lullaby and Game Song on the Behavior of the Newborn* [doctoral dissertation]. LaJolla, CA, University of California–San Diego, Department of Music, 1991.

Lucas A, Morley R, Cole TJ, Gore SM: A randomized, multicenter study of human milk versus formula and later development in preterm infants. *Arch Dis Child Fetal Neonatal Ed* 70:F141-F146, 1994.

MacFarlane A: Olfaction. In *The Development of Social Preference in the Human Neonate.* Ciba Foundation Symposium No. 33, 1975.

Marean G, Werner L, Kuhl P: Vowel categorization by very young infants. *Dev Psychol* 28:396, 1992.

McKenna JJ: The potential benefits of infant-parent co-sleeping in relation to SIDS prevention: Overview and critique of epidemiological bedsharing studies. In Rognum TO (ed): *Sudden Infant Death Syndrome: New Trends in the '90s.* Oslo, Norway, Scandinavian University Press, 1995.

McKenna J, Moska S: Sleep and arousal, synchrony and independence among mothers and infants sleeping apart and together: An experiment in evolutionary medicine. *Acta Paediatr Scand* 397:94, 1994.

Melzoff AN, Moore MK: Imitation of facial and manual gestures by the human neonate. *Science* 198:75, 1977.

Mennella J, Beauchamp G: Early flavor experiences: When do they start? *Zero to Three* 14(2):1, 1993.

Mennella J, Beauchamp G: Maternal diet alters the sensory qualities of human milk and the nursling's behavior. *Pediatrics* 88:737, 1991.

Miranda SB: Visual abilities and pattern preferences of premature and full term infants. *J Exp Child Psychol* 10:139, 1970.

Nissen E, Lilia G, Matthiesen AS, et al: Effects of maternal pethidine on infants' developing breast feeding behavior. *Acta Paediatr* 84:140-145, 1995.

O'Driscoll K, Meagher D, Boylan P (eds): *Active Management of Labor.* St Louis, CV Mosby, 1993.

Parke R: *Fathers.* Cambridge, MA, Harvard University Press, 1981.

Piaget J, Inhelder B: *The Psychology of the Child.* New York, Basic Books, 1969.

Porter F, Wolf CM, Gold J, et al: Pain and pain management in newborn infants: A survey of physicians and nurses. *Pediatrics* 100:626-632, 1997.

Prechtl H, Beentema D: *The Neurological Examination of the Full Term Newborn Infant.* Philadelphia, JB Lippincott, 1975.

Prodromidis M, Field T, Arendt R, et al: Mothers touching newborns: A comparison of rooming-in versus minimal contact. *Birth* 22(4):196-200, discussion 201-203, 1995.

Righard L, Alda MO: Effect of delivery room routine on success of first breastfeed. *Lancet* 336:1105, 1990.

Self PA, Horowitz FD, Paden LY: Olfaction in newborn infants. *Dev Psychol* 7:349, 1972.

Selley WG, Ellis RE, Flack FC, Brooks WA: Coordination of sucking, swallowing and breathing in the newborn: Its relationship to infant feeding and normal development. *Br J Disord Commun* 25:311-327, 1990.

Stephan CW, Langlois JH: Baby beautiful: Adult attributions of infant competence as a function of infant attractiveness. *Child Dev* 55:576, 1984.

Sullivan RM, Taborsky-Barba S, Mendoza R, et al: Olfactory classical conditioning in neonates. *Pediatrics* 87:511-518, 1991

Thomasgard M, Meltz WP: The vulnerable child revisited. *J Dev Behav Pediatr* 16:47, 1995.

Varendi H, Porter RH, Winberg J: Does the newborn baby find the nipple by smell? *Lancet* 344:989, 1994.

Volpe JJ: *Neurology of the Newborn,* 3rd ed. Philadelphia, WB Saunders, 2002.

Walker M: Do labor medications affect breastfeeding? *J Hum Lact* 13:131, 1997.

Weber F, Woolridge M, Baum J: An ultrasonographic study of the organization of sucking and swallowing by newborn infants. *Dev Med Child Neurol* 28:19, 1986.

Yamauchi Y, Yamanouchi I: The relationship between rooming-in/not rooming-in and breastfeeding variables. *Acta Paediatr Scand* 79:1017, 1990.

Chapter 8

Achenbach TM, Howell CT, Aoki MF, Rauh VA: Nine-year outcome of the Vermont intervention program for low birth weight infants. *Pediatrics* 91:45-55, 1993.

Als H, Gilkerson L, Duffy F, et al: A three center, randomized, controlled trial of individualized developmental care for very low birth weight preterm infants: Medical, neurodevelopmental, parenting, and caregiving effects. *J Dev Behav Pediatr* 24:399-408, 2003.

Als H, Lawhon G, Duffy FH, et al: Individualized developmental care for the very low-birth-weight preterm infant. Medical and neurofunctional effects. *JAMA* 272:853-858, 1994.

Als H, Tronick E, Adamson L, Brazelton TB: The behavior of the full term yet underweight newborn infant. *Dev Med Child Neurol* 18:590-602, 1976.

American Academy of Pediatrics Task Force on Newborn and Infant Hearing: Newborn and infant hearing loss: Detection and intervention. *Pediatrics* 103:527, 1999.

Anderson GC: Current knowledge about skin-to-skin (kangaroo) care for preterm infants. *J Perinatol* 11:216, 1991.

Ardura J, Andres J, Aldana J, Revilla MA: Development of sleep-wakefulness rhythm in premature babies. *Acta Paediatr* 84:484-489, 1995.

Aucott S, Donohue PK, Atkins E, Allen MC: Neurodevelopmental care in the NICU. *Ment Retard Dev Disabil Res Rev* 8:298-308, 2002.

Bernal JF: Night waking in infants during the first fourteen months. *Dev Med Child Neurol* 15:760, 1973.

Bier JB, Oliver T, Ferguson AE, Vohr BR: Human milk improves cognitive and motor development of premature infants during infancy. *J Hum Lact* 18:361-367, 2002.

Bowlby J: *Attachment and Loss-Loss: Sadness and Depression*, vol 3. New York, Basic Books, 1980.

Chapieski ML, Evankovich KD: Behavioral effects of prematurity. *Semin Perinatol* 21:221, 1997.

Conde-Agudelo A, Diaz-Rossello JL, Belizan JM: Kangaroo mother care to reduce morbidity and mortality in low birthweight infants. *Cochrane Database Syst Rev*, issue 2. CD002771.DOI:10-1002/14651858, CD002771, 2003.

Cuisinier M, de Kleine M, Kollee L, et al: Grief following the loss of a newborn twin compared to a singleton. *Acta Paediatr* 85:339-343, 1996.

Dixon S, LeVine RA, Keefer C, et al: Perinatal circumstances and newborn outcome among the Gusii of Kenya: Assessment of risk. *Infant Behav Dev* 5:11, 1982.

Feldman F, Eidelman AI: Intervention programs for premature infants: How and do they affect development? *Clin Perinatol* 25:613, 1998.

Feldman R, Eidelman AI, Sirota L, Weller A: Comparison of skin-to-skin (kangaroo) and traditional care: Parenting outcomes and preterm infant development. *Pediatrics* 110:16-26, 2002.

Feldman R, Eidelman AI: Direct and indirect effects of breast milk on the neurobehavioral and cognitive development of premature infants. *Dev Psychobiol* 43:109-119, 2003.

Feldman R, Weller A, Sirota L, Eidelman AI: Skin-to-skin contact (kangaroo care) promotes self-regulation in premature infants: Sleep-wake cyclicity, arousal modulation, and sustained exploration. *Dev Psychol* 38:194-207, 2002.

Feldman R, Weller A, Sirota L, Eidelman AI: Testing a family intervention hypothesis: The contribution of mother-infant skin-to-skin contact (kangaroo care) to family interaction, proximity, and touch. *J Fam Psychol* 17:94-107, 2003.

Ferber SG, Kuint J, Weller A, et al: Massage therapy by mothers and trained professionals enhances weight gain in premature infants. *Early Hum Dev* 67:37-45, 2002.

Frischer L: The death of a baby in the infant special care unit. *Pediatr Clin North Am* 45:691, 1998.

Gorski PA: Premature infant behavioral and physiological responses to caregiving interventions in the intensive care nursery. In Call JD, Galenson E, Tyson R (eds): *Frontiers of Infant Psychiatry*. New York, Basic Books, 1983, pp 256-263.

Goubet N, Clifton R, Shah B: Learning about pain in preterm infants. *J Dev Behav Pediatr* 22:418-424, 2001.

Green M, Solnit AJ: Reactions to the threatened loss of a child: A vulnerable child syndrome. *Pediatrics* 34:58, 1964.

Gross SJ, Mettelman BB, Dye TD, Slagle TA: Impact of family structure and stability on academic outcome in preterm children at 10 years of age. *J Pediatr* 138:169-175, 2001.

Grunau RE, Weinbery J, Whitfield MF: Neonatal procedural pain and preterm cortisol response to novelty at 8 months. *Pediatrics* 114:e77-e84. URL: http://www.pediatrics.org/cgi/content/full/114/1/e77, 2004.

High PC, Gorski PA: Recording environmental influences on infant development in the intensive care nursery. In Gottfried AW, Gaiter JL (eds): *Infant Stress under Intensive Care*. Baltimore, University Park Press, 1985, pp 131-155.

Hille ETM, den Ouden AL, Bauer L, et al: School performance at nine years of age in very premature and very low birth weight infants: Perinatal risk factors and predictors at five years of age. Collaborative Project on Preterm and Small for Gestational Age (POPS) Infants in The Netherlands. *J Pediatr* 125:426-434, 1994.

Jacobs SE, Sokol J, Ohlsson A: The Newborn Individualized Developmental Care and Assessment Program is not supported by meta-analyses of the data. *J Pediatr* 140:699-706, 2002.

Jain A, Concato J, Leventhal JM: How good is the evidence linking breastfeeding and intelligence? *Pediatrics* 109:1044-1053, 2002.

Johnston CC, Stevens B, Pinelli J, et al: Kangaroo care is effective in diminishing pain response in preterm neonates. *Arch Pediatr Adolesc Med* 157:1084-1088, 2003.

Lickliter R: The role of sensory stimulation in perinatal development: Insights from comparative research for care of the high- risk infant. *J Dev Behav Pediatr* 21:437-447, 2000.

Lindemann E: Symptomatology and management of acute grief. *Am J Psychiatry* 101:141, 1944.

Long JG, Lucey JF, Philip AGS: Noise and hypoxemia in the intensive care nursery. *Pediatrics* 65:143, 1980.

Lozoff B, Brittenham GM, Trause MA, et al: The mother-newborn relationship: Limits of adaptability. *J Pediatr* 91:1-12, 1977.

Lucas A, Bishop NJ, King FJ, Cole TJ: Randomised trial of nutrition for preterm infants after discharge. *Arch Dis Child* 67:324-327, 1992.

Lucas A, Morely R, Cole TJ, et al: Breast milk and subsequent intelligence quotient in children born preterm. *Lancet* 339:261-264, 1992.

Messmer PR, Rodriguez S, Adams J, et al: Effect of kangaroo care on sleep time for neonates. *Pediatr Nurs* 23:408-414, 1997.

Mortensen EL, Michaelsen KM, Sanders SA, Reinisch JM: The association between duration of breastfeeding and adult intelligence. *JAMA* 287:2365-2371, 2002.

Mouradian L, Als H, Coster W: Neurobehavioral functioning of healthy preterm infants of varying gestational ages. *J Dev Behav Pediatr* 21:408-416, 2000.

Nyqvist KH, Lutes LM: Co-bedding twins: A developmentally supportive care strategy. *J Obstet Gynecol Neonatal Nurs* 27:450, 1998.

Page JM, Schneeweiss S, Whyte HE, Harvey P: Ocular sequelae in premature infants. *Pediatrics* 92:787-790, 1993.

Parke RD: *Fathers*. Cambridge, MA, Harvard University Press, 1981.

Pierrehumbert B, Nicole A, Muller-Nix C, et al: Parental post-traumatic reactions after premature birth: Implications for sleeping and eating problems in the infant. *Arch Dis Child Fetal Neonatal Ed* 88: F400-F404, 2003.

Richards A, Kelly E, Doyle L, Callanan C: Cognition, academic progress, behavior and self-concept at 14 years of very low birth weight children. *J Dev Behav Pediatr* 22:11-18, 2001.

Rivkees SA: Developing circadian rhythmicity in infants. *Pediatrics* 112:373-381, 2003.

Rojas MA, Kaplan M, Quevedo M, et al: Somatic growth of preterm infants during skin-to-skin versus traditional holding: A randomized, controlled trial. *J Dev Behav Pediatr* 24:163-168, 2003.

Schaal B, Hummel T, Soussignan R: Olfaction in the fetal and premature infant: Functional status and clinical implications. *Clin Perinatol* 31:261-285, 2004.

Senn TE, Andrews-Espy K: The effects of neurobehavioral assessment of feeding and weight gain in preterm infants. *J Dev Behav Pediatr* 24:85-88, 2003.

Simons SHP, van Dijk M, Anand KS, et al: Do we still hurt newborn babies? *Arch Pediatr Adolesc Med* 157:1058-1064, 2003.

Singer LT, Salvator A, Guo S, et al: Maternal psychological distress and parenting stress after the birth of a very low-birth-weight infant. *JAMA* 281:799-805, 1999.

Symington A, Pinelli J: Developmental care for promoting development and preventing morbidity in preterm infants. *Cochrane Database Syst Rev*, issue 4. CD001814.DOI:10-1002/14651858, CD001814, 2003.

Upahhyay A, Aggarwal R, Narayan S, et al: Analgesic effect of expressed breast milk in procedural pain in term neonates: A randomized, placebo-controlled, double-blind trial. *Acta Pediatr* 93:518-522, 2004.

Vance JC, Najman JM, Thearle MJ, et al: Psychological changes in parents eight months after the loss of an infant from stillbirth, neonatal death, or sudden infant death syndrome—a longitudinal study. *Pediatrics* 96:933-938, 1995.

Vickers A, Ohlsson VA, Lacy JB, Horsley A: Massage for promoting growth and development of preterm and/or low birth-weight infants. *Cochrane Database Syst Rev*, issue 2. CD000390.DOI:10-1002/14651858, CD000390, 2004.

Vohr BR, Msall ME: Neuropsychological and functional outcomes of very low birth weight infants. *Semin Perinatol* 21:202, 1997.

Wallerstedt C, Higgins P: Facilitating perinatal grieving between the mother and the father. *J Obstet Gynecol Neonatal Nurs* 25:389, 1996.

Weiss SJ, Wilson P, St John Seed M, Paul SM: Early tactile experience of low birth weight children: Links to later mental health and social adaptation. *Infant Child Dev* 10:93-115, 2001.

Weller A, Feldman R: Emotion regulation and touch in infants: The role of cholecystokinin and opioids. *Peptides* 24:779-788, 2003.

Westrup B, Bohm B, Lagercrantz H, Stjernqvist K: Preschool outcome in children born very prematurely and cared for according to the Newborn Individualized Developmental Care and Assessment Program (NIDCAP). *Acta Pediatr* 93:498-507, 2004.

Whitfield MF: Psychosocial effects of intensive care on infants and families after discharge. *Semin Neonatol* 8:185-193, 2003.

Whitfield MF, Grunau R, Holsti L: Extremely premature (£800 g) schoolchildren: Multiple areas of hidden disability. *Arch Dis Child Fetal Neonatal Ed* 77:F85, 1997.

Chapter 9

American Academy of Pediatrics: The transfer of drugs and other chemicals into human milk. *Pediatrics* 93:137, 1994.

American Academy of Pediatrics: The pediatrician's role in family support programs. *Pediatrics* 95:781, 1995.

American Academy of Pediatrics: Breastfeeding and the use of human milk. *Pediatrics* 100:1035, 1997.

American Academy of Pediatrics: The role of home visitation programs in improving health outcomes for children and families. *Pediatrics* 101:486, 1998.

Anisfeld E, Casper V, Nozyce M, Cunningham N: Does infant carrying promote attachment? An experimental study of the effects of increased physical contact on the development of attachment. *Child Dev* 61:1617-1627, 1990.

Barber V, Skaggs M: *The Mother Person.* New York, Schocken Books, 1975.

Barr R, McMullan SJ, Spiess H, et al: Carrying as colic therapy: A randomized controlled trial. *Pediatrics* 87:623-630, 1991.

Beardslee WR, Zuckerman BS, Amaro H, McAllister M: Depression among adolescent mothers: A pilot study. *J Behav Dev Pediatr* 9:62-65, 1988.

Beck CT: The effects of postpartum depression on child development: A meta-analysis. *Arch Psychiatr Nurs* 12:12, 1998.

Boer F, Dunn J: *Children's Sibling Relationships: Developmental and Clinical Implications.* Hillsdale, NJ, Lawrence Erlbaum Associates, 1992.

Bower TGR: The visual world of infants. *Sci Am* 215:80, 1966.

Brazelton TB: *Touchpoints: Your Child's Emotional and Behavioral Development.* Reading, MA, Addison-Wesley, 1992, pp 12-13.

Brazelton TB, Cramer BG: *The Earliest Relationship,* part III. Reading, MA, Addison-Wesley, 1990.

Brazelton TB, Koslowski B, Main M: The origins of reciprocity: The early mother/infant interaction. In Lewis M, Rosenblum L (eds): *The Effect of the Infant on Its Caregiver.* New York, John Wiley & Sons, 1974, p 59.

Briggs GG, Freeman RK, Yaffe SJ: *Drugs in Pregnancy and Lactation,* 5th ed. Baltimore, Williams & Wilkins, 1998.

Campbell SB, Cohen JF, Meyers T: Depression in first-time mothers: Mother-infant interaction and depression chronicity. Special Section: Parental Depression and Distress: Implications for Development. *Dev Psychol* 31:364-376, 1995.

Condon WS, Sander LW: Neonate movement is synchronized with adult speech. *Science* 183:99-101, 1974.

Cooper PH, Murray L: Postnatal depression. *BMJ* 20:316, 1998.

Cox, JL, Holden JM, Sagovsky R: Detection of post-natal depression: Development of the 10 item Edinburgh Post Natal Depression Scale. *Br J Psychiatry* 150:782-786, 1987.

Dixon S: Helping siblings adjust to the new baby. In Jellinek M, Patel BP, Froehle MC (eds): *Bright Futures in Practice: Mental Health,* vol 2, *Tool Kit.* Arlington, VA, National Center for Education in Maternal and Child Health, 2002.

Dixon SD, Yogman M, Tronick E, et al: Early infant social interaction with parents and strangers. *J Am Acad Child Psychiatry* 20:32-52, 1981.

Dunn J: Temperament, siblings, and the development of relationships. In Carey WB, McDevitt SC (eds): *Prevention and Early Intervention: Individual Differences As Risk Factors for Mental Health of Children.* New York, Brunner/Mazel, 1994, pp 50-58.

Dunn J, Kendrick C: *Siblings.* Cambridge, MA, Harvard University Press, 1982.

Dunn J, Kendrick C, MacNamee R: The reaction of first-born children to the birth of a sibling: Mothers' reports. *J Child Psychol Psychiatry* 22:1, 1981.

Dunn J, McGuire S: Sibling and peer relationships in childhood. *J Child Psychol Psychiatry* 33:67-105, 1992.

Dunn J, Plomin R: *Separate Lives: Why Siblings Are So Different.* New York, Basic Books, 1990.

Hetherington EM, Parke RD: Emotional development. In Hetherington EM, Parke RD (eds): *Child Psychology: A Contemporary Viewpoint.* New York, McGraw-Hill, 1979, pp 215-218.

Hill V, Eriks J: Turn-taking in the caregiver-infant interactional system. In Barnard K (ed): *Nursing Child Assessment Satellite Training: Learning Resource Manual.* Seattle, Washington: University of Washington, 1980, pp 44-49.

Klaus MH, Kennell JH, Klaus PH: *Bonding: Building the Foundations of Secure Attachment and Independence.* Reading, MA, Perseus Books, 1995.

Kuhl PK, Andruski JE, Chistovich IA, et al: Cross-language analysis of phonetic units in language addressed to infants. *Science* 277:684-686, 1997.

Maccoby E: *Patterns of Child Rearing.* Stanford, CA, Stanford University Press, 1976.

MacFarlane JA: Olfaction in the development of social preference in human neonates. In *Parent-Infant Interaction,* Ciba Foundation Symposium No. 33. New York, Elsevier, 1975, pp 103-133.

Mehler J, Dupoux E: *What Infants Know: The New Cognitive Science of Early Development.* Cambridge, MA, Blackwell, 1994.

Murray L, Cooper PJ: *Postpartum Depression and Child Development.* New York, Guilford Press, 1997.

Najonc RB, Markus GB: Birth order and intellectual development. *Psychol Rev* 82:74, 1975.

Parke RD: *Fatherhood.* Cambridge, MA, Harvard University Press, 1996.

Rice RL, Slater CJ: An analysis of group versus individual child health supervision. *Clin Pediatr (Phila)* 36:685, 1997.

Schanler RJ, Shulman RJ, Lau C, et al: Feeding strategies for premature infants: Randomized trial of gastrointestinal priming and tube-feeding method. *Pediatrics* 103:434-435, 1999.

Schubert HJP, Wagner ME, Shubert D: Child spacing effects: A comparison of institutionalized and normal children. *Dev Behav Pediatr* 4:262, 1983.

Seidman D: Postpartum psychiatric illness: The role of the pediatrician. *Pediatr Rev* 19:128, 1998.

Stern D: The infant's repertoire. In Stern D (ed): *The First Relationship: Infant and Mother.* Cambridge, MA, Harvard University Press, 1977.

Teti DM, Gelfand DM, Messinger DS, Isabella R: Maternal depression and the quality of early attachment: An examination of infants, preschoolers and their mothers. Special Section: Parental Depression and Distress: Implications for Development. *Dev Psychol* 31:364-376, 1995.

Tronick EZ, Als H, Adamson L: The infant's response to entrapment between contradictory messages in face-to-face interaction. *J Child Psychol Psychiatry* 7:1, 1978.

Walton GE, Bower NJA, Bower TGR: Recognition of familiar forms by newborns. *Infant Behav Dev* 15:265, 1992.

Weinberg MK, Tronick EZ: Maternal depression and infant maladjustment: A failure of mutual regulation. In Noshpity JD (ed): *Handbook of Child and Adolescent Psychiatry,* vol 1, *Infants and Preschoolers: Development and Syndromes.* New York, John Wiley & Sons, 1997.

Weiss JS: *Your Second Child.* New York, Summit Books, 1981.

Weissman MM, Gammon GD, John K, et al: Children of depressed parents. Increased psychopathology and early onset of major depression. *Arch Gen Psychiatry* 44:847, 1987.

Zuckerman B, Beardslee WR: Maternal depression: An issue for pediatricians. *Pediatrics* 79:110, 1987.

Chapter 10

Altemeier WA 3rd, O'Connor SM, Sherrod KB, Vietze PM: Prospective study of antecedents for nonorganic failure to thrive. *J Pediatr* 106:360-365, 1985.

American Academy of Pediatrics: Positioning and SIDS. *Pediatrics* 89:1120, 1992.

American Academy of Pediatrics: Breastfeeding and the use of human milk. *Pediatrics* 100:1035, 1997.

American Academy of Pediatrics: Changing concepts of sudden infant death syndrome: Implications for infant sleep environment and sleep position. *Pediatrics* 105:650, 2000.

Barr RG, Elias M: Nursing interval and maternal responsiveness: Effect on early infant crying. *Pediatrics* 81:529, 1988.

Barr RG, Hopkins B, Green JA: *Crying As a Sign, a Symptom, & a Signal: Clinical, Emotional and Developmental Aspects of Infant and Toddler Crying.* London, Cambridge Press, 2000.

Barr RG, Kramer MS, Pless IB, et al: Feeding and temperament as determinants of early infant crying/fussing behavior. *Pediatrics* 84:514-521, 1989.

Barr RG, McMullen SJ, Spiess H, et al: Carrying as colic "therapy": A randomized, controlled trial. *Pediatrics* 87:623-630, 1991.

Barr RG, Rotman A, Yaremko J, et al: The crying of infants with colic: A controlled empirical description. *Pediatrics* 90:14-21, 1992.

Boyce WT, Barr RG, Zeltzer LK: Temperament and the psychobiology of childhood stress. *Pediatrics* 90:483, 1992.

Brazelton TB: Crying in infancy. *Pediatrics* 29:579, 1962.

Brazelton TB: Nutrition during early infancy. In Susking RM (ed): *Textbook of Pediatric Nutrition.* New York, Raven Press, 1981.

Carey WB, McDevitt SC: *Coping with Children's Temperament: A Guide for Professionals.* New York, Basic Books, 1995.

Carey WB: Colic: Prolonged or excessive crying in young infants. In Levine MD, Carey WB, Crocker A (eds): *Developmental-Behavioral Pediatrics*, 3rd ed. Philadelphia, WB Saunders, 1999.

Cox JL, Holden JM, Sagovsky R: Detection of postnatal depression: Development of the 10 item Edinburgh Postnatal Depression Scale. *Br J Psychiatry* 150:782, 1987.

Davis BE, Moon RY, Sachs HC, Ottolini MC: Effects of sleep position on infant motor development. *Pediatrics* 102:1135-1140, 1998.

Eisenberg A, Murkoff HE, Hathaway SE: *What to Expect in the First Year*, 2nd ed. New York, Workman Publishing, 2003.

Evans RW, Fergusson DM, Allardyce RA, Taylor B: Maternal diet and infantile colic in breast fed infants. *Lancet* 1:1340-1342, 1981.

Ferber R: Sleeplessness in children. In Ferber R, Kryger M (eds): *Principles and Practices of Sleep Medicine in the Child*. Philadelphia, WB Saunders, 1995, pp 79-89.

Ferber R: *Solve Your Child's Sleep Problems*. New York, Fireside Books, 2004.

Fleming P, Blair PS, Bacon C, et al: Environments of infants during sleep and the risk of the sudden infant death syndrome: Results of 1993-1995 case control study for confidential enquiry into stillbirths and deaths in infancy. Confidential Enquiry into Stillbirths and Deaths Regional Coordinators and Researchers. *BMJ* 313:191-195, 1996.

Forsyth BWC: Colic and the effect of changing formulas: A double-blind multiple crossover study. *J Pediatr* 115:521, 1989.

Forsyth BWC, McCarthy PL, Leventhal JM: Problems of early infancy, formula changes, and mothers' beliefs about their infants. *J Pediatr* 106:1012, 1985.

Hunziker UA, Barr RG: Increased carrying reduces infant crying: A randomized controlled trial. *Pediatrics* 77:641, 1986.

Jakobsson I, Lindberg T: Cow's milk proteins cause infantile colic in breast fed infants: A double-blind crossover study. *Pediatrics* 71:268, 1983.

Jellinek MS: *Bright Futures in Practice: Mental Health*. Washington, DC, National Center for Education in Maternal and Child Health, 2002.

Kim J, Barr RG, Stein MT: Colic in newborns. *Pediatr Rev* 25:1-2, 2004.

Kramer MS, Barr RG, Dagenais S, et al: Pacifier use, early weaning, and cry/fuss behavior: A randomized controlled trial. *JAMA* 286:322-326, 2001.

Larson K, Ayllon T: The effects of contingent music and differential reinforcement on infant colic. *Behav Res Ther* 28:119, 1990.

Lozoff B: Influence of childhood sleep practices and problems. In Ferber R, Kryger M (eds): *Principles and Practices of Sleep Medicine in the Child*. Philadelphia, WB Saunders, 1995, pp 69-73.

Macknin ML, Medendorp SV, Maier MC: Infant sleep and bedtime cereal. *Am J Dis Child* 143:1066, 1989.

McKenna JJ: Cosleeping. In Carskadon MA (ed): *Encyclopedia of Sleep and Dreaming*. New York, MacMillan, 1993, pp 145-148.

Metcalf TJ, Irons TG, Sher LD, Young PC: Simethicone in the treatment of infant colic: A randomized, placebo-controlled, multicenter trial. *Pediatrics* 94:29-34, 1994.

National Center on Shaken Baby Syndrome: http://www.dontshake.com/.

Pershing J, James H, Swanson J, et al: Prevention and management of positional skill deformities in infants. *Pediatrics* 112:199-202, 2003.

Rosen D, Loeb L, Jura M: Differentiation of organic from nonorganic failure to thrive syndrome in infancy. *Pediatrics* 66:689, 1980.

Sander L, Julia H, Stechler G: Regulation and organization in early infant-caretaker interaction. In Robinson RJ (ed): *Brain and Early Behavior*. New York, Academic Press, 1969.

Shonkoff J, et al: *From Neurons to Neighborhood: The Science of Early Child Development*. National Research Council, National Academic Press, 2000.

Smith DW, et al: *Growth and Its Disorders.* Philadelphia, WB Saunders, 1976.

Spencer JAD, Moran DJ, Lee A, Talbert D: White noise and sleep induction. *Arch Dis Child* 65:135-137, 1990.

Stein MT, Colarusso CA, McKenna JT, Powers NG: Cosleeping (bedsharing) among infants and toddlers. *J Dev Behav Pediatr* 18:408-412, 1997.

Stein MT, Kessler DB, Hubbard E: Failure to thrive in a four-month-old nursing infant. *J Dev Behav Pediatr* 23:266-270, 2002.

Taubman B: Clinical trial of the treatment of colic by modification of parent-infant interaction. *Pediatrics* 74:998, 1984.

Wessel MA, Cobb JC, Jackson EB, et al: Paroxysmal fussing in infancy, sometimes called "colic." *Pediatrics* 14:421-435, 1954.

Whitten CF, Pettit MG, Fischhoff J: Evidence that growth failure from maternal deprivation is secondary to undereating. *JAMA* 209:1675, 1969.

Chapter 11

American Academy of Pediatrics: *Sleep Problems in Children and Adolescents.* Elk Grove Village, IL, American Academy of Pediatrics 2002.

Anders T, Sadeh A, Appareddy V: Normal sleep in infants and children. In Ferber R, Kryger M (eds): *Principles and Practice of Sleep Medicine in the Child.* Philadelphia, WB Saunders, 1995.

Anders TF, Eiben LA: Pediatric sleep disorders: A review of the past ten years. *J Am Acad Child Adolesc Psychiatry* 36:9-20, 1997.

Anders TF, Halpern LF, Hua J: Sleeping through the night: A developmental perspective. *Pediatrics* 90:554, 1992.

Bohlin G, Hagekull B, Rydell A: Attachment and social functioning: A longitudinal study from infancy to middle childhood. *Social Dev* 9:24-39, 2000.

Brazelton TB: *Touchpoints.* Reading, MA, Addison-Wesley, 1992.

Brazelton TB, Kowalski K, Main M: Early mother-infant reciprocity. In *Parent-Infant Interaction,* Ciba Foundation Symposium No 33. New York, Elsevier North-Holland, 1975, pp 137-154.

Campbell SB, Cohn JF, Meyers T: Depression in first-time mothers: Mother-infant interaction and depression chronicity. *Dev Psychol* 31:349, 1995.

Caudill W, Weinstein H: Maternal care and infant behavior in Japan and America. *Psychiatry* 32:12, 1969.

Chance P: *Learning through Play,* Pediatric Round Table Series No 3. Skillman, NJ, Johnson & Johnson Baby Products Co, 1979.

Cohn JF, Tronick EZ: Three month old infants' reactions to simulated maternal depression. *Child Dev* 54:185, 1983.

Dixon S, Vogman M, Tonick E, et al: Early infant interaction with parents and strangers. *J Am Acad Child Psychiatry* 20:32-52, 1981.

Dixon S, LeVine RA, Tonick E, et al: Mother-infant interaction among the Gusii of Kenya. In Field TM, Sostek AM, Vietze P, Liederman PH (eds): *Culture and Early Interactions.* Hillsdale, NY, Lawrence Erlbaum Associates, 1981.

Duhaime AC, Christian CW, Rorke LB, Zimmerman RA: Nonaccidental head injury in infants—The "shaken baby syndrome." *N Engl J Med* 338:1822-1829, 1998.

Ferber R: *Solve Your Child's Sleep Problems.* New York, Simon & Schuster, 1985.

Ferber R, Kryger M: *Principles and Practice of Sleep Medicine in the Child.* Philadelphia, WB Saunders, 1995.

Field T: Infants of depressed mothers. *Infant Behav Dev* 18:1, 1995.

Gibson EJ: Ontogenesis of the perceived self. In Neisser U (ed): *The Perceived Self: Ecological and Interpersonal Sources of Self Knowledge.* New York, Cambridge University Press, 1993.

Ginsburg H, Opper S: *Piaget's Theory of Intellectual Development*. Englewood Cliffs, NJ, Prentice-Hall, 1969.

Greenspan S: Clinical assessment of emotional milestones in infancy and early childhood. *Pediatr Clin North Am* 38:1371, 1991.

Greenspan S: *The Growth of the Mind and the Endangered Origins of Intelligence*. Reading, MA, Addison-Wesley, 1997.

Hamilton CE: Continuity and discontinuity of attachment from infancy through adolescence. *Child Dev* 71:694-698, 2000.

Hartman EL: *The Functions of Sleep*. New Haven, CT, Yale University Press, 1973.

Howard B, Wong J: Sleep disorders. *Pediatr Rev* 22(10):327-342, 2001.

Isabella RA: Origins of attachment: Maternal interactive behavior across the first year. *Child Dev* 64:605, 1993.

Lipsitt L: The pleasures and annoyances of infants: Approach and avoidance behavior of babies. In Lipsitt L, Reese HW, Bourne LE (eds): *Child Development*. Glenview, IL, Scott Foresman, 1978.

Lozoff B: Culture and family: Influences on childhood sleep practices and problems. In Ferber R, Kryger M (eds): *Principles and Practices of Sleep Medicine in the Child*. Philadelphia, WB Saunders, 1995.

Lozoff B, Wolf A, Davis N: Co-sleeping in urban families with young children in the United States. *Pediatrics* 74:171, 1984.

Madansky D, Edelbrock C: Cosleeping in a community sample of 2- and 3-year old children. *Pediatrics* 86:197, 1990.

NICHD: *Early Childcare and Children's Development prior to School Entry*. SRCD proceedings. Minneapolis, MN, April 2001.

Papousek H: Individual variability in learned response in human infants. In Robinson RJ (ed): *Brain and Early Behavior*. New York, Academic Press, 1969.

Parmelee AH, Wenner WH, Schulz HR: Infant sleep patterns: From birth to 16 weeks of age. *J Pediatr* 65:576, 1964.

Stein MT, Colarusso CA, McKenna JT, Powers NG: Cosleeping (bedsharing) among infants and toddlers. *J Dev Behav Pediatr* 18:408-412, 1997.

Stern D: Mother and infant at play. In Lewis M, Rosenblum L (eds): *The Effect of the Infant on Its Caregiver*. New York, John Wiley & Sons, 1974, pp 187-213.

Stern D: *The First Relationship: Infant and Mother*. Cambridge, MA, Harvard University Press, 1977.

Trotter S, Thoman E (eds): *Social Responsiveness of Infants*, Pediatric Round Table Series No 2. Skillman, NJ, Johnson & Johnson Baby Products Co, 1978.

Tureki S: *The Difficult Child*. New York, Bantam, 1989.

Zeanah CH: Disturbances of attachment in young children adopted from institutions. *J Dev Behav Pediatr* 21:230-236, 2000.

Zuckerman B, Beardslee WR: Maternal depression: A concern for pediatricians. *Pediatrics* 79:110, 1987.

Zuckerman B, Blitzer EC: Sleep disorders. In Gabel S (ed): *Behavioral Problems in Pediatrics*. New York, Grune & Stratton, 1981, pp 257-272.

Chapter 12

Bayley N: *Bayley Scales of Infant Development*. New York, Psychological Corp, 1993.

Bower TGR: Object perceptions in infants. *Perception* 1:15, 1972.

Bower TGR: *A Primer of Infant Development*. San Francisco, WH Freeman, 1977.

Bushnell EW, Boudreau JP: Motor development and the mind: The potential role of motor abilities as a determinant of aspects of perceptual development. *Child Dev* 64:1005, 1993.

Caplan PJ, Kinsborne M: Baby drops the rattle: Asymmetry of duration of grasp in infants. *Child Dev* 47:532, 1976.

Chamberlain HD: The inheritance of left-handedness. *J Hered* 19:557, 1928.

Clifton RK, Rochat P, Robin DJ, Berthier NE: Multimodal perception in the control of infant reaching. *J Exp Psychol Hum Percept Perform* 20:876-886, 1994.

Erhardt RP: *Developmental Hand Dysfunction: Theory, Assessment and Treatment.* Baltimore, RAMSCO, 1982.

Goldfield EC, Michel GF: Spaciotemporal linkage in infant interlimb coordination. *Dev Psychobiol* 19:259, 1986.

Gramza AE: Response to the manipulability of a play dyad. *Psychol Rep* 38:1107, 1976.

Lantz C, Melen K, Forsberg H: Early infant grasping involves radial fingers. *Dev Med Child Neurol* 38:668, 1996.

Mandell RJ, Nelson DL, Ceumak SA: Differential laterality of hand function in right-handed and left-handed boys. *Am J Occup Ther* 38:114, 1984.

Matthew A, Cook M: The control of reaching movements by young infants. *Child Dev* 61:1238, 1990.

Michel GF, Hawkins DA: Postural and lateral asymmetries in the ontogeny of handedness during infancy. *Dev Psychobiol* 19:247, 1986.

Newman C, Atkinson J, Braddich O: The development of reaching and looking preferences in infants to objects of different sizes. *Dev Psychol* 37:561-572, 2001.

Spencer JP, Verejiken B, Diedrich FJ, Thelan E: Posture and emergence of manual skills. *Dev Sci* 3:216-233, 2000.

Thelen E: Motor development: A new synthesis. *Am Psychol* 50:79-95, 1995.

Thelen E, Corbetta D, Kamm K, et al: The transition to reaching: Mapping intention and intrinsic dynamics. *Child Dev* 64:1058-1098, 1993.

Thelen E, Corbetta D, Spencer J: The development of reaching during the first year: The role of movement speed. *J Exp Psychol Hum Percept Perform* 22:1059-1076, 1996.

Thelen E, Smith LB: *A Dynamic Systems Approach to the Development of Cognition and Action.* Cambridge, MA, MIT Press, 1994.

Touwen BCL: The neurological development of prehension: A developmental neurologist's view. *Int J Psychophysiol* 19:115, 1995.

Twitchell TE: The automatic grasping responses of infants. *Neuropsychologia* 3:247, 1955.

VanStrien JW, Bouma A: Sex and familial sinistrality differences in cognitive abilities. *Brain Cogn* 27:137, 1995.

Vohr BR, Garcia-Coll CT: Neurodevelopmental and school performance of very low-birth-weight infants: A seven-year longitudinal study. *Pediatrics* 76:345, 1985.

vonHofsten C: Motor development as the development of systems. *Dev Psychol* 25:950, 1989.

Wang PL: Interaction between handedness and cerebral functional dominance. *Int J Neurosci* 11:35, 1980.

Chapter 13

Ainsworth MDS: *Infancy in Uganda: Infant Care and the Growth of Attachment.* Baltimore, Johns Hopkins Press, 1967.

Barnard K: *Nursing Child Assessment Feeding Scales (NCAST).* Seattle, University of Washington, 1978.

Bowlby J: *Attachment,* vol 1, New York, Basic Books, 1969.

Bowlby J: Separation: *Anxiety and Anger.* New York, Basic Books, 1969.

Bretherton I: The origin of the attachment theory: John Bowlby and Mary Ainsworth. *Dev Psychol* 28:759, 1992.

Fraiberg S: *The Magic Years.* New York, Charles Scribner's Sons, 1959.

Goin-DeCarie T: *The Infant's Reaction to Strangers.* New York, International Universities Press, 1974.

Grossman KE, Grossman K: The wider concept of attachment in cross cultural research. *Early Hum Dev* 33:31, 1990.

Isabella RA: Origins of attachment: Maternal interactive behavior across the first year. *Child Dev* 64:605, 1993.

Kagan J, Kearsley RB, Zelano P: *Infancy: Its Place in Human Development.* Cambridge, MA, Harvard University Press, 1978.

Leach P: *Your Growing Child,* 2nd ed. New York, Alfred A Knopf, 1989.

Lozoff B, Paludetto R, Lotz S: Transitional object use in the United States, Japan and Italy. Paper presented to the Ambulatory Pediatric Association, Carmel, CA, May 1985.

Lozoff B, Wolf A, Davis N: Cosleeping in urban families with young children in the United States. *Pediatrics* 74:171, 1984.

Madansky D, Edelbrock C: Cosleeping in a community of 2-3 year old children. *Pediatrics* 86:198, 1990.

Mahler M, Pine F, Bergman A: *The Psychological Birth of the Human Infant: Symbiosis and Individuation.* New York, Basic Books, 1975.

McKenna J, Mosko S, Richard C: Bedsharing promotes breastfeeding. *Pediatrics* 100:214, 1997.

Owen MT, Cox MJ: Marital conflict and the development of infant-parent attachment relationships. *J Fam Psychol* 11:152, 1997.

Pederson DR, Moran G: Expressions of the attachment relationship outside of the strange situation. *Child Dev* 67:915, 1996.

Rutter M: Separation experiences: A new look at an old topic. *J Pediatr* 95:147, 1995.

Sherman M, Hertzig M, Austrian R, Shapiro T: Treasured objects in school aged children. *Pediatrics* 68:379-386, 1981.

Spitz RA: The smiling response. Genet Psychol Monogr 34:57, 1946.

Sroufe LA, Egeland B, Kreulzer T: The fate of early experience following developmental change: Longitudinal approaches to individual adaptation in childhood. *Child Dev* 61:1363, 1990.

Stein MT: Common issues in feeding. In Levine MD, Carey WB, Crocker A (eds): *Developmental-Behavioral Pediatrics,* 3rd ed. Philadelphia, WB Saunders, 1999, pp 392-396.

Stein MT, Call J: Extraordinary changes in behavior in an infant after a brief separation. *J Dev Behav Pediatr* 19:424, 1998.

Stein MT, Colarusso CA, McKenna J: Cosleeping (bedsharing) among infants and toddlers. *J Dev Behav Pediatr* 18:408, 1997.

Telzrow R: Developmental considerations in infant feeding. In Howard RB, Herbold MH (eds): *Nutrition in Clinical Care.* New York, McGraw-Hill, 1982.

van Ijzendoorn MH, Goldenberg S, Kroonenberg PM, Frenkel OJ, et al: The relative effects of maternal and child problems on the quality of attachment: A meta-analysis of attachment in clinical samples. *Child Dev* 63:840-858, 1992.

van Ijzendoorn MT, Kroonenberg PM: Cross-cultural patterns of attachment: A meta-analysis of the strange situation. *Child Dev* 59:147, 1988.

Vaughn B, Egeland B, Sroufe LA, Waters E: Individual differences in infant-mother attachment at twelve and eighteen months: Stability and change in families under stress. *Child Dev* 50:971-975, 1979.

Waters E: The reliability and stability of individual differences in infant-mother attachment. *Child Dev* 49:483, 1978.

Winnicott DW: Transitional objects and transitional phenomena. In Winnecott DW (ed): *Collected Papers: Through Pediatrics and Psychoanalysis.* London, Tavistock Publications, 1958.

Chapter 14

Adelson E, Fraiberg S: Gross motor development of infants blind from birth. *Child Dev* 45:114, 1974.

American Academy of Pediatrics: The Doman-Delcato treatment of neurologically handicapped children. *Pediatrics* 70:810, 1982.

American Academy of Pediatrics: Injuries associated with infant walkers. *Pediatrics* 108:790-792, 2001.

American Academy of Pediatrics, Committee on Pediatric Aspects of Physical Fitness, Recreation and Sports: Swimming instructions for infants. *Pediatrics* 65:847, 1980.

American Academy of Pediatrics, Task Force on Infant Positioning and SIDS: Positioning and sudden infant death syndrome (SIDS): Update. *Pediatrics* 98:1216, 1996.

Bayley N: *Bayley Scales of Infant Development.* New York, Psychological Corp, 1969.

Bennett HJ, Wagner T, Fields A: Acute hyponatremia and seizures in an infant after a swimming lesson. *Pediatrics* 72:125, 1983.

Berger W, Quinlern J, Dietz V: Afferent and efferent control of stance and gait developmental changes in children. *Electroencephalogr Clin Neurophysiol* 66:244, 1987.

Brazelton TB: *Toddlers and Parents: A Declaration of Independence.* New York, Delacorte Press, 1974.

Burnett CN, Johnson EW: Development of gait in children: Parts I and II. *Dev Med Child Neurol* 13:196, 1971.

Chaplais JZ, MacFarlane IA: A review of four hundred and four late walkers. *Arch Dis Child* 59:512, 1984.

Chisholm JS: *Navajo Infancy.* New York, Aldine, 1983.

Clark JE, Phillips SJ: A longitudinal study of intralimb coordination in the first year of walking: A dynamical systems analysis. *Child Dev* 64:1143, 1993.

Clark JE, Whitall J, Phillips SJ: Human interlimb coordination: The first six months of independent walking. *Dev Psychobiol* 21:445, 1988.

Crouchman M: The effect of baby walkers on early locomotor development. *Dev Med Child Neurol* 28:757, 1986.

Davis BE, Moon RY, Sachs HC, Ottolini MC: Effects of sleep position on infant motor development. *Pediatrics* 102:1135-1140, 1998.

deGroot L, deGroot CJ, Hopkins B: An instrument to measure independent walking: Are there differences between preterm and full term infants? *J Child Neurol* 12:304, 1994.

Dennis W: Does culture appreciably affect patterns of infant behavior? *J Soc Psychol* 12:305, 1940.

Dixon S, Keefer C, LeVine R, et al: Perinatal circumstances and newborn outcome among the Gusii of Kenya: Assessment of risk. *Infant Behav Dev* 5:11-32, 1982.

Fraiberg SH: *The Magic Years.* New York, Charles Scribner's Sons, 1959.

Freis S, Klemms A, Muller K: Gait analysis by measuring ground reaction forces in children: Changes to an adaptive gait pattern between the ages of one to five years. *Dev Med Child Neurol* 39:228, 1997.

Gesell A, Thompson H: *The Psychology of Early Growth.* New York, Macmillan, 1938.

Glascoe, F, Altemeier WA, MacLean WE: The importance of parents' concerns about their child's development. *Arch Dis Child* 143:955, 1989.

Harriman AE, Lukosius PA: On why Wayne Dennis found Hopi infants retarded in age at onset of walking. *Percept Mot Skills* 55:79, 1982.

Hennessy M, Dixon S, Simon S: The development of gait: A study in African children ages one to five. *Child Dev* 55:844, 1984.

Holm V: A western version of the Doman-Delcato treatment of patterning for developmental disabilities. *West J Med* 139:553, 1984.

Hopkins B, Westra T: Maternal expectations of their infants' development: Some cultural differences. *Dev Med Child Neurol* 31:384, 1989.

Jaffe M, Kugelman A, Tirogh E, et al: Relationship between the parachute reactions and standing and walking in normal infants. *Pediatr Neurol* 11:38-40, 1994.

Majnemer A, Rosenblatt B: Reliability of parental recall of developmental milestones. *Pediatr Neurol* 10:304, 1994.

Marques-Bruna P, Grimshaw P: Reliability of gait parameters in children under two years of age. *Percept Mot Skills* 98:123-130, 2004.

McGraw M: *The Neuromuscular Maturation of the Human Infant.* New York, Hafner Press, 1945.

Preis S, Klenn S, Müller K: Gait analysis by measuring ground reaction forces in children: Changes to adaptive gait patterns between the ages of one to five years. *Dev Med Child Neurol* 39:228-233, 1997.

Ridenour MV: Infant walkers: Developmental tool or inherent danger? *Percept Mot Skills* 55:1201, 1982.

Sahler OJ, McAnarney ER: *The Child from Three to Eighteen.* St Louis, CV Mosby, 1981.

Steinwender G, Saraph V, Scheiber S, et al: Intrasubject repeatability of gait analysis data in normal and spastic children. *Clin Biomech* 15:134-139, 2000.

Sutherland DH: The evolution of clinical gait analysis. *Gait Posture* 21:447-461, 2005.

Thelan E: Motor development: A new synthesis. *Am Psychol* 50:79-91, 1985.

Thelen E, Bradshaw G, Ward JA: Spontaneous kicking in month old infants: Manifestation of a human central locomotor program. *Behav Neural Biol* 32:45, 1981.

Whitall J, Getchell N: From walking to running: Applying a dynamical systems approach to the development of locomotor skills. *Child Dev* 66:1541, 1995.

Wolff P: Theoretical issues in the development of motor skills. In Lewis M, Taft L (eds): *Developmental Disabilities: Theory, Assessment and Intervention.* New York, Spectrum Publications, 1981.

Wyke B: The neurological basis of movement: A developmental overview. In Holt K (ed): *Movement and Child Development.* London, Heinemann Medical Books, 1975.

Chapter 15

Ainsworth MDS: Infant-mother attachment. *Am Psychol* 34:932, 1979.

American Academy of Pediatrics: The short- and long-term consequences of corporal punishment, Part 2. *Pediatrics* 98:803, 1996.

American Academy of Pediatrics, Committee on Psychosocial Aspects of Child and Family Health: Policy statement on guidance for effective discipline. *Pediatrics* 101:723, 1998.

Baron-Cohen S, Allen J, Gillberg C: Can autism be detected at 18 months? The needle, the haystack and the CHAT. *Br J Psychiatry* 161:839-843, 1992.

Beers NS, Howard B: Managing temper tantrums. *Pediatr Rev* 24:70-71, 2003.

Brazelton TB: A child-oriented approach to toilet training. *Pediatrics* 29:121-128, 1962.

Brazelton TB, Christophersen ER, Frauman AC, et al: Instruction, timeliness, and medical influences affecting toilet training. *Pediatrics* 103:1353-1358, 1999.

Brazelton TB, Gatson RL, Howard RB: Developmental feeding issues. In Howard RB, Winter HS (eds): *Nutrition and Feeding of Infants and Toddlers.* Boston, Little, Brown, 1984.

Carey WB: Clinical use of temperament data in pediatrics. In Porter R, Collins GM (eds): *Temperament in Infants and Young Children,* Ciba Foundation Symposium No. 89. London, Pitman Books, 1982.

DeVries MW, deVries MR: Cultural relativity of toilet training readiness: A perspective from East Aftrica. *Pediatrics* 60:170-177, 1977.

Drabman RS, Jarvie B: Counseling parents of children with behavior problems: The use of extinction and time-out techniques. *Pediatrics* 59:78, 1977.

Eron LD: Research and public policy. *Pediatrics* 98:821, 1996.

Filipek PA, Pasquale JA, Baranek GT, et al: The screening and diagnosis of autistic spectrum disorders. *J Autism Dev Disord* 29:439-484, 1999.

Gordon T: *P.E.T.: Parent Effectiveness Training.* New York, Plume Books, 1975.

Graziano AM, Hamblen JL, Plante WA: Subabusive violence in child rearing in middle-class American families. *Pediatrics* 98:845, 1996.

Howard BJ: Advising parents on discipline: What works. *Pediatrics* 98:809, 1996.

Kagan J: *The Nature of the Child.* New York, Basic Books, 1984, pp 43-48.

Kanner L: Autistic disturbances of affective contact. *Nervous Child* 2:217-250, 1943.

Koegel RL, Koegel LK, McNerney E: Pivotal behaviors in the treatment of autism. *J Clin Child Psychol* 30:19-32, 2001

Larsen MA, Tentis E: The art and science of disciplining children. *Pediatr Clin North Am* 50:817-840, 2003.

Mahler M, Pine F, Bergman A: *The Psychological Birth of the Human Infant.* New York, Basic Books, 1975.

McCormick KF: Attitudes of primary care physicians toward corporal punishment. *JAMA* 267:3161, 1992.

Osterling J, Dawson G: Early recognition of children with autism: A study of first birthday home videotapes. *J Autism Dev Disord* 24:247-257, 1994.

Rapin I: The autistic spectrum disorders. *N Engl J Med* 347:302-303, 2002.

Roberts MW, Powers SW: Adjusting chair time-out enforcement procedures for oppositional children. *Behav Ther* 21:257, 1990.

Scarboro ME, Forehand R: Effects of two types of response-contingent time-outs on compliance and oppositional behavior of children. *J Exp Child Psychol* 19:252, 1975.

Sherman M, Hertzig M, Austrian R, Shapiro T: Treasured objects in school aged children. *Pediatrics* 68:379-386, 1981.

Showalter JE: The modification of behavior modification. *Pediatrics* 59:130, 1977.

Straus MA: Spanking and the making of a violent society. *Pediatrics* 98:837, 1996.

Vaughan VC, Litt IF: *Child and Adolescent Development: Clinical Implications.* Philadelphia, WB Saunders, 1990, p 204.

Wilson DR, Lyman RD: Time-out in the treatment of childhood behavior problems: Implementation and research issues. *Child Family Behav Ther* 4:5, 1982.

Winnicott DW: Transitional objects and transitional phenomena. In Winnicott DW: *Collected Papers.* London, Tavistock Publishing, 1958, pp 229-242.

Wissow LS, Roter D: Toward effective discussion of discipline and corporal punishment during primary care visits: Findings from studies of doctor-patient interaction. *Pediatrics* 94:587, 1994.

Chapter 16

Anglin J: Vocabulary development: A morphological analysis. *Monogr Soc Res Child Dev* 58:238, 1993.

Aram DM, Hall NE: Longitudinal follow-up of children with preschool communication disorders: Treatment implications. *School Psychol Rev* 18:487, 1989.

Bandura A (ed): *Psychological Modeling.* Chicago, Atherton, Aldine, 1971.

Bates E: Plasticity, localization and language development. In Borman SH, Fletcher JM (eds): *The Changing Nervous System: Neurobehavioral Consequences of Early Brain Disorders.* New York, Oxford University Press, 1999.

Bellugi U, Wang P: Williams syndrome: From cognition to brain to gene. In *Encyclopedia of Neuroscience.* Amsterdam, Elsevier Science, 1999, pp 214-247.

Berk LE: Private speech and self-regulation in children with impulse-control difficulties: Implications for research and practice. *J Cogn Educ Psychol* 2:1-21, 2001.

Bialystock E: *Bilingualism in Development: Language, Literacy and Cognition.* New York, Cambridge University Press, 2001.

Brown R: *A First language: The Early Stages.* Cambridge, MA, Harvard University Press, 1973.

Cazden CB: *Language in Early Childhood Education.* Washington, DC, National Association for the Education of Young Children, 1981.

Chomsky N: Formal discussion. In Bellugi U, Brown R (eds): *The Acquisition of Language. Monogr Soc Res Child Dev* 29(92):35, 1964.

Condon W, Sander L: Neonate movement is synchronized with adult speech: Interactional participation and language acquisition. *Science* 183:99, 1974.

Coplan J: Evaluation of the child with delayed speech or language. *Pediatr Ann* 14:203, 1985.

Coplan J, Gleason JR, Ryan R, et al: Validation of an early language milestone scale in a high-risk population. *Pediatrics* 70:677-683, 1982.

de Villiers PA, de Villiers JG: *Early Language.* Cambridge, MA, Harvard University Press, 1979.

Elliot J: *Child Language.* New York, Cambridge University Press, 1981.

Fenson L, Dale PS, Reznick JS, et al: Variability in early communicative development. *Monogr Soc Res Child Dev* 59(5):1-173, discussion 174-185, 1994.

Ferguson C: Baby talk in six languages. *Anthropology* 66:114, 1964.

Garvey C: *Children's Talk.* Cambridge, MA, Harvard University Press, 1984.

Glascoe F: Can clinical judgment detect children with speech-language problems? *Pediatrics* 87:317, 1991.

Grosjean F: *Life with Two Languages.* Cambridge, MA, Harvard University Press, 1982.

Kolvin I, Fundudis T: Speech and language disorders of childhood. In Apley J, Ounsted C (eds): *One Child.* London, William Heinemann Medical Books–Spastics International Medical Publications, 1982.

Levine M, Brooks R, Shonkoff JP: *A Pediatric Approach to Learning Disorders.* New York, John Wiley & Sons, 1980.

Mattys SL, Jusczyk PW: Phonotactic cues for segmentation of fluent speech by infants. *Cognition* 78:91-121, 2001.

Mills DL, Coffey-Corena S, Neville HJ: Language comprehension and cerebral specialization from 13-20 months. *Dev Neuropsychol* 13:397-445, 1997.

Nagy WE, Scott JA: Vocabulary processes, In Kamil ML, Mosenthal PB (eds): *Handbook of Reading Research,* vol 3. Mahwah, NJ, Lawrence Erlbaum Associates, 2000, pp 269-284.

Neville HJ, Bruer JT: Language processing: How experience affects brain organization. In Bailey DB, Bruer JT, Symors FJ, Lichtruan JW (eds): *Critical Thinking about Critical Periods.* Baltimore, Paul H Brookes, 2001, pp 151-172.

Pinker S: *The Language Instinct.* New York, Morrow, 1994.

Richardson S: The child with delayed speech. *Contemp Pediatr* 16:55, 1992.

Ringler NM: The development of language and how adults talk to children. *Infant Ment Health J* 2:71, 1981.

Snow CE: Mothers' speech to children learning language. *Child Dev* 43:549, 1972.

Super C, Harkness S: Why African children are so hard to test. In Adler LL (ed): *Cross Cultural Research at Issue.* New York, Ethos, 1978.

Thal D, Bates E: Language and communication in early childhood. *Pediatr Ann* 18:299, 1989.

Thal D, Reilly J, Seibert L, Jeffries R, Fenson J: Language Development in Children at risk for language impairment: Cross-population comparisons *Brain and Language* 88(2): 167-179, 2004.

Thal D, Reilly J (eds): Origins of language disorders. Special edition of *Dev Neuropsychol* 13, 1997.

Chapter 17

American Academy of Pediatrics: Media education. *Pediatrics* 104:341-343, 1999.

American Academy of Pediatrics: Children, adolescents and television. *Pediatrics* 107:423-426, 2001.

American Academy of Pediatrics: Media violence. *Pediatrics* 108:1222-1226, 2001.

Anders T, Eiben L: Pediatric sleep disorders: A review of the past 10 years. *J Am Acad Child Adolesc Psychiatry* 36:9, 1997.

Anderson CA, Bushman BJ: The effects of media violence on society. *Science* 295:2377-2379, 2002.

Anderson DR, Huston AC, Schmitt KL, et al: *Early Television Viewing and Adolescent Behavior.* Boston, Blackwell, 2001.

Bergan D, Mauer D: Symbolic play, phonological awareness and literacy skills at three age levels. In Roskos KA, Christie JF (eds): *Play & Literacy in Early Childhood: Research from Multiple Perspectives.* Mahwah, NJ, Lawrence Erlbaum Associates, 2000, pp 45-62.

Bettelheim B: *Uses of Enchantment.* New York, Random House, 1976.

Bruner J: Children at play. In Lewin R (ed): *Child Alive.* Garden City, NY, Anchor Press, 1975.

Bryant J, Zillman D (eds): *Media Effects: Advances in Theory and Research.* Hillsdale, NJ, Lawrence Erlbaum Associates, 1994.

Bushman BJ, Anderson CA: Media violence and the American public: Scientific facts versus media misinformation. *Am Psychol* 56:477-489, 2001.

Bushman BJ, Hussmann LR: Effects of televised violence on aggression, In Singer DG, Singer JL (eds): *Handbook of Children and the Media.* Thousand Oaks, CA, Sage, 2001, pp 223-254.

Chance P: *Learning through Play.* New Brunswick, NJ, Johnson & Johnson, 1979.

Christakis DA, Zimmerman FJ, Digiuseppe DL, McCarty CA: Early television exposure and subsequent attentional problems in children. *Pediatrics* 113:708-713, 2004.

Cole M, Cole S: *The Development of Children,* 3rd ed. New York, WH Freeman, 1996.

Comstock G, Paik H: *Television and the American Child.* New York, Academic Press, 1991.

Coon KA, Goldberg J, Rogers BL, Tucker KL: Relationships between use of television during meals and children's food consumption patterns. *Pediatrics* 107:E7, 2001.

Crespo CJ, Smit E, Trorano RP, et al: Television watching, energy intake and obesity in US children: Results from the Third N HANES, 1988-1994. *Arch Pediatr Adolesc Med* 155:360-365, 2001.

Elkind D: *The Hurried Child: Growing Up Too Fast Too Soon.* Reading, MA, Addison-Wesley, 1981.

Ferber R, Kryger M: *Principles and Practice of Sleep in the Child.* Philadelphia, WB Saunders, 1995.

Fraiberg S: *The Magic Years.* New York, Charles Scribner's Sons, 1959.

Goncu A: Development of inter-subjectivity in social pretend play. *Hum Dev* 36:185, 1993.

Guilleminault C (ed): *Sleep and Its Disorders in Children.* New York, Raven Press, 1987.

Haugland SW, Wright JL: *Young Children and Technology: A World of Discovery.* Boston, Allyn & Bacon, 1997.

Healy JM: Early television exposure and subsequent attentional problems in children [editorial]. *Pediatrics* 113:917-918, 2004.

High P, Hopman M, La Grasse L, Linn H: Evaluation of a clinic-based program to promote book sharing and bedtime stories among low-income urban families with young children. *Arch Pediatr Adolesc Med* 152:459, 1998.

Kohlberg L: Development of moral character and moral ideology. In Hoffman ML, Hoffman LW (eds): *Review of Child Development Research,* vol 1. New York, Russell Sage Foundation, 1974.

Konner M: Aspects of the developmental ethology of foraging people. In Blurton-Jones N (ed): *Ethological Studies of Child Behavior.* New York, University of Cambridge Press, 1972.

Lesser G: *Children and Television.* New York, Random House, 1974.

Lewis M, Rosenblum M (eds): *The Origins of Fear.* New York, John Wiley & Sons, 1975.

Li X, Atkins M: Early childhood computer experience and cognitive and motor development. *Pediatrics* 113:1715-1722, 2004.

Mendelsokn AL, Mogilner LN, Dreyer BP, et al: The impact of a clinic-based literacy intervention on language development in inner-city preschool children. *Pediatrics* 107:130-134, 2001.

Murphy B: *The Widening World of Childhood.* New York, Basic Books, 1962.

Mussen PH, Conger JJ, Kagan J: *Essentials of Child Development and Personality.* New York, Harper & Row, 1980.

National Center for Education Statistics: *Young Children's Access to Computers in the Home and in the School in 1999-2000* (NCES 2003-036). Washington, DC, US Department of Education, 2003.

Nicholes PM: *Children's Movies: A Critical Guide to the Best Films Available on Video and DVD*. New York, Hewey Hoyt, 2003.

Rideout VJ, Vandewater EA, Wartella EA: *Zero to Six: Electronics, Media in the Lives of Infants, Toddlers and Preschoolers*. Menlo Park, CA, Kaiser Family Foundation, 2003.

Robinson TN, Sapher M, Kraemer HC, et al: Effects of reducing television viewing on children's request for toys: A randomized controlled trial. *J Dev Behav Pediatr* 22:179-184, 2001.

Robinson TN, Wilde ML, Navractecy LC, et al: Effects of reducing children's television and video-game use on aggressive behavior: A randomized controlled trial. *Arch Pediatr Adolesc Med* 155:17-23, 2001.

Rutter M (ed): *Scientific Foundation of Developmental Psychiatry*. Baltimore, University Park Press, 1981.

San Luis NB, Stein MT: Lying, stealing and cheating. In Parker S, Zuckerman B (eds): *Behavioral-Developmental Pediatrics: A Handbook for Primary Care*, 2nd ed. Boston, Little, Brown, 2004.

Sege R, Dietz W: Television viewing and violence in children: The pediatrician as agent of change. *Pediatrics* 94:600, 1994.

Signorelli N: Television portrayals of women, and children's attitudes. In Berry GL, Asamen JK (eds): *Children and Television*. Newbury Park, CA, Sage, 1993.

Subrahmanyam K, Greenfield PM, Kraut RE, Gross EF: The impact of computer use on children's and adolescents' development. *Appl Dev Psychol* 22:7-30, 2001.

Surgeon General's Scientific Advisory Committee on Television and Growing Up: *The Impact of Televised Violence*. Washington, DC, US Government Printing Office, 1972.

Taras HL Sullis JF, Nader PR, Nelson J: Children's television-viewing habits and the family environment. *Am J Dis Child* 144:357-359, 1990.

Taras HL, Sullis JF, Patterson TL, et al: Television's influence on children's diet and physical activity. *J Dev Behav Pediatr* 10:176-180, 1989.

Taylor M: *Imaginary Companions and the Children Who Create Them*. New York, Oxford University Press, 1999.

Valkenburg PM, VanderVoort THA: Influence of TV on daydreaming and creative imagination: A review of the research. *Psychol Bull* 116:316, 1994.

Whitehurst G, Fischel JE: Practitioner review: early developmental language delay: what, if anything should the clinician do about it? *J Child Psych and Psychiatry* 35(4): 613-648, 1994.

Winnicott D: *Playing and Reality*. New York, Basic Books, 1971.

Wright JL, Shade DD (eds): *Young Children: Active Learners in a Technological Age*. Washington, DC, NAEYC, 2001.

Chapter 18

Bigler R, Liben L: A cognitive-development approach to racial stereotyping and reconstructive memory in Euro-American children. *Child Dev* 64:1507, 1993.

Crick N, Grotpeter N: Relational aggression, gender and social psychological adjustment. *Child Dev* 66:710, 1995.

Damon W, Hart D: *Self Understanding in Childhood and Adolescence*. New York, Cambridge University Press, 1988.

Dixon S: Gender identity: Early orientation to atypical behavior. In Rudolph A, Hoffman J, Rudolph C (eds): *Rudolph's Pediatrics*, 20th ed. Stamford, CT, Appleton & Lange, 1996.

Erikson E: *Childhood and Society*, 2nd ed. New York, WW Norton, 1963.

Freud S: *New Introductory Lectures on Psychoanalysis*. New York, WW Norton, 1965.

Hirschfield LA: Do children have a theory about race? *Cognition* 54:209-252, 1995.

Lorenz K: *On Aggression*. New York, Harcourt, 1963.

Pomerantz E, Ruble DN, Frey KS, Greulich F: Meeting goals and confronting conflict: Children's changing perceptions of social comparison. *Child Dev* 66:723-728, 1995.

Chapter 19

American Academy of Pediatrics: The inappropriate use of school "readiness" tests. *Pediatrics* 95:437, 1995.

American Academy of Pediatrics: Recommendations for preventive pediatric health care. *Pediatrics* 105:645-646, 2000.

Bandura A: *Cognitive Social Learning Theory.* Englewood Cliffs, NJ, Prentice-Hall, 1977.

Byrd RS, Weitzman M, Auinger MS: Increased behavior problems associated with delayed school entry and delayed school progress. *Pediatrics* 100:654, 1997.

Chamberlin RW, Nader PR: Relationship between nursery school behavior patterns and late school functioning. *Am J Orthopsychiatry* 41:597, 1971.

Comer JP: The Yale–New Haven primary prevention project: A follow-up study. *J Am Acad Child Psychiatry* 24:154, 1985.

Fierro-Cobas V, Chan E: Language development in bilingual children: A primer for pediatricians. *Contemp Pediatr* 18:79-98, 2001.

Individuals with Disabilities Act, Public Law No 101-476, 104 Stat 1146 (1990).

Lee VE, Brooks-Gunn J, Schnur E, Liaw FR: Are Head Start effects sustained? A longitudinal follow-up comparison of disadvantaged children attending Head Start, no preschool and other preschool programs. *Child Dev* 61(2):495-507, 1990.

Lesaux N, Siegel L: The development of reading in children who speak English as a second language. *Dev Psychol* 39:1005-1019, 2003.

Morrison FJ, Griffith EM, Alberts DM: Nature-nurture in the classroom: Entrance age, school readiness, and learning in children. *Dev Psychol* 33:254, 1997.

Paradise JL, Dollaghan CA, Campbell TF, et al: Otitis media and tympanostomy tube insertion during the first three years of life: Developmental outcomes at 4 years. *Pediatrics* 112:265, 2003.

Piaget J, Inhelder B: *The Psychology of the Child.* New York, Basic Books, 1968.

Prontnicki J, Taft L: Coordination problems: Clumsiness to major motor disorders. In Rudolph CD, Rudolph AM (eds): *Rudolph's Pediatrics*, 21st ed. New York, McGraw-Hill, 2003, p 481.

Rutter M: *Fifteen Thousand Hours: Secondary Schools and Their Effects on Children.* Cambridge, MA, Harvard University Press, 1979.

Shaywitz SE: Dyslexia. *N Engl J Med* 338:307, 1998.

Shore R: *Rethinking the Brain: New Insights into Early Development.* New York, Families and Work Institute, 1997.

Simpson GA, Fowler MG: Geographic mobility and children's emotional/behavioral adjustment and school functioning. *Pediatrics* 93:303, 1994.

Sturner R, Howard B: Preschool development 1: Communicative and motor aspects. *Pediatr Rev* 18: 291-301, 1997.

Taft LT, Barowsky EI: The clumsy child. *Pediatr Rev* 10:247, 1989.

Vohr BR, Cashore WJ, Bigsby R: Stresses and interventions in the neonatal intensive care unit. In Levine MD, Carey WB, Crocker AC (eds): *Developmental-Behavioral Pediatrics*, 3rd ed. Philadelphia, WB Saunders, 1999, pp 263-275.

Chapter 20

American Academy of Pediatrics: The classification of child and adolescent mental conditions in primary care. In *Diagnostic and Statistical Manual for Primary Care (DSM-PC), Child and Adolescent Version.* Elk Grove Village, IL, American Academy of Pediatrics, 1996.

American Academy of Pediatrics. Committee on Quality Improvement and Subcommittee on Attention-Deficit/Hyperactivity Disorder: Diagnosis and evaluation of the child with attention-deficit/hyperactivity disorder. *Pediatrics* 105:1158-1170, 2000.

American Academy of Pediatrics. Committee on Quality Improvement, Subcommittee on Attention-Deficit/Hyperactivity Disorder: Clinical practice guideline: Treatment of the school-age child with attention-deficit/hyperactivity disorder. *Pediatrics* 108:1033-1044, 2001.

American Academy of Pediatrics/National Initiative for Children's Healthcare Quality (NICHQ): *ADHD: Caring for Children with ADHD: A Resource Toolkit for Clinicians.* Chicago, American Academy of Pediatrics, 2004.

Barkley RA, Fischer M, Edelbrock CS, Smallish L: The adolescent outcome of hyperactive children diagnosed by research criteria: I: An 8-year prospective follow-up study. *J Am Acad Child Adolesc Psychiatry* 29:546-555, 1990.

Biederman J, Faraone S, Milberger S, et al: A prospective 4-year follow-up study of attention-deficit hyperactivity and related disorders. *Arch Gen Psychiatry* 53:437-446, 1996.

Conners CK: A teacher rating scale for use in drug studies with children. *Am J Psychiatry* 126:152, 1969.

Dworkin PH: School failure. In Parker S, Zuckerman B (eds): *Behavioral and Developmental Pediatrics: A Handbook for Primary Care.* Boston, Little, Brown, 1995, p 189.

Egger HL, Costello EJ, Angold A: School refusal and psychiatric disorders: A community study. *J Am Acad Child Adolesc Psychiatry* 42:797-807, 2003.

Eisenberg L: School phobia: A study in the communication of anxiety. *Am J Psychiatry* 114:712, 1958.

Elkind D: *Children and Adolescents: Interpretive Essays on Jean Piaget.* New York, Oxford University Press, 1974.

Feldman HM: Attention deficits. In *Gellis and Kagan's Current Pediatric Therapy*, 17th ed. Philadelphia, WB Saunders, 2002, pp 381-385.

Green M, Wong M, Atkins D: *Diagnosis of Attention Deficit/Hyperactivity Disorder*, Technical review 3 (AHCPR Publication No. 99-0050). Rockville, MD, US Department of Health and Human Services, Agency for Health Care Policy and Research, 1999.

Hobson RP: Piaget: On the ways of knowing in childhood. In Rutter M, Hersov L (eds): *Child and Adolescent Psychiatry: Modern Approaches.* Boston, Blackwell Scientific, 1985.

Jensen P, Arnold L, Richters J, et al: 14-month randomized clinical trial of treatment strategies for attention deficit hyperactivity disorder. *Arch Gen Psychiatry* 56:1073-1086, 1999.

Keefer CH: Separation difficulties: Clinging behaviors to school refusal. In Rudolf CD, Rudolf AM (eds): *Rudolph's Pediatrics*, 21st ed. New York, McGraw-Hill, 2003, pp 450-454.

Kinsbourne M, Caplan P: *Children's Learning and Attention Problems.* Boston, Little, Brown, 1979.

Levine MD: Attention and dysfunctions of attention. In Levine MD, Carey WB, Crocker AC (eds): *Developmental-Behavioral Pediatrics*, 3rd ed. Philadelphia, WB Saunders, 1999, pp 499-519.

Levine MD, Oberklaid F: Hyperactivity: Symptom complex or complex symptom? *Am J Dis Child* 134:409, 1980.

Lindsay RL: School failure/disorders of learning. In Bergman AB (ed): *20 Common Problems in Pediatrics.* New York, McGraw-Hill, 2001, pp 319-336.

MTA Cooperative Group: National Institute of Mental Health Multimodal Treatment Study of ADHD follow-up: 24-month outcomes of treatment strategies for attention-deficit/hyperactivity disorder. *Pediatrics* 113:754-761, 2004.

Mannuzza S, Klein R, Bessler A, et al: Adult psychiatric status of hyperactive boys grown up. *Am J Psychiatry* 155:493-498, 1998.

Miller A, Lee S, Raina P, et al: *A Review of Therapies for Attention-Deficit/Hyperactivity Disorder.* Ottawa, Ontario, Canadian Coordinating Office for Health Technology Assessment (CCOHTA), 1998.

Office of Special Education and Rehabilitation Services, U.S. Department of Education: *A Guide to the Individualized Education Program*, July 2000, www.ed.gov/offices/OSERS/OSEP/IEP_Guide.

Pelham WE, Wheeler T, Chronis A: Empirically supported psychosocial treatments for attention deficit hyperactivity disorder. *J Clin Child Psychol* 27:190-205, 1998.

Piaget J: *The Origins of Intelligence in Children.* New York, International Press, 1952.

Shaywitz S: *Overcoming Dyslexia. A New and Complete Science-Based Program for Overcoming Reading Problems at Any Level.* New York, Alfred A. Knopf, 2003.

Sleator EK, Ullman RK: Can the physician diagnose hyperactivity in the office? *Pediatrics* 67:13, 1981.

Stein M, Zentall S, Shaywitz S, Shaywitz B: Challenging case: A school-aged child with delayed reading skills. *J Dev Behav Pediatr* 20:381-385, 1999.

Stein MT, Duffner PK, Werry JS, Trauner DA: School refusal and emotional lability in a 6-year-old boy. *J Dev Behav Pediatr* 17:187-190, 1996.

Stein MT, Lounsbury B: A child with a learning disability: Navigating school-based services. *J Dev Behav Pediatr* 22:188-191, discussion 191-192, 2001.

Stein MT, Rapin I, Yapko D: Selective mutism. *J Dev Behav Pediatr* 22(Suppl):123-126, 2001.

Swanson JM, Kraemer HC, Hinshaw SP, et al: Clinical relevance of the primary findings of the MTA: Success rates based on severity of symptoms at the end of treatment. *J Am Acad Child Adolesc Psychiatry* 40:168-179, 2001.

Wender E: Hyperactivity. In Parker S, Zuckerman B: *Behavioral and Developmental Pediatrics: A Handbook for Primary Care.* Boston, Little, Brown, 1995.

Wender EH: Managing stimulant medication for attention-deficit/hyperactivity disorder. *Pediatr Rev* 22:183-190, 2001.

Van Zomeren AH, Brouwer WH: *Clinical Neuropsychology of Attention.* New York, Oxford University Press, 1994.

Chapter 21

Achenbach TM, Edelbrock C: *Manual for the Child Behavior Checklist and Revised Behavior Profile.* Burlington, VT, University of Vermont, 1983.

Alpert E, Freund K: *Partner Violence: How to Recognize and Treat Victims of Abuse—A Guide for Physicians.* Waltham, MA, Massachusetts Medical Society, 1992.

American Academy of Pediatrics: *Sports Medicine: Health Care for Young Athletes*, 2nd ed. Elk Grove Village, IL, American Academy of Pediatrics, 1991.

American Academy of Pediatrics: *Manual on Injury Prevention.* Elk Grove Village, IL, American Academy of Pediatrics, 1997.

America's Children: Key National Indicators of Wellbeing. Federal Interagency Forum on Child and Family Statistics, 2003.

Anthony E, Cohler B: *The Invulnerable Child.* New York, Guilford Press, 1987.

Appley J: *The Child with Abdominal Pains.* Boston, Blackwell Scientific, 1975.

Asher SR, Coie JD: *Peer Rejection in Children.* Cambridge, MA, Cambridge Press, 1990.

Asher S, Renshaw P, Hymel S: Peer relations and the development of social skills. In Moore S, Chess S, Thomas A (eds): *Temperament in Clinical Practice.* New York, Guilford Press, 1986.

Block J, Block J: The role of ego-control and ego-resiliency in the organization of behavior. In Collin WA (ed): *Minnesota Symposium on Child Psychology*, vol 13. Hillsdale, NJ, Lawrence Erlbaum Associates, 1979.

Boyle JT: Recurrent abdominal pain: An update. *Pediatr Rev* 18(9):310, 1997.

Breslau N: Does brain dysfunction increase children's vulnerability to environmental stress? *Arch Gen Psychiatry* 47:15, 1990.

Carey WB, McDevitt SC: *Coping with Children's Temperament.* New York, Basic Books, 1995.

Cooper C (eds): *The Young Child: Reviews of Research*, vol 3. Washington, DC, National Association for the Education of Young Children, 1982.

Dorn LD, Campo JC, Thato S, et al: Psychological comorbidity and stress reactivity in children and adolescents with recurrent abdominal pain and anxiety disorders. *J Am Acad Child Adolesc Psychiatry* 42:66-75, 2003.

Dworkin P: *Learning and Behavior Problems of School Children.* Philadelphia, WB Saunders, 1985.

Elkind D: *The Hurried Child: Growing Up Too Fast, Too Soon.* Reading, MA, Addison-Wesley, 1988.

Epps RP, Manley MW: A physician's guide to preventing tobacco use during childhood and adolescence. *Pediatrics* 88:140, 1991.

Erikson EH: *Childhood and Society,* 2nd ed. New York, WW Norton, 1963.

Frederick C: Children traumatized in small groups. In Eth S, Pynoos R (eds): *Post-traumatic Stress Disorders in Children.* Washington, DC, American Psychiatric Press, 1985.

Freud S: *Introductory Lectures in Psychoanalysis.* New York, WW Norton, 1965.

Garmezy N: Stressors of childhood. In Garmezy N, Rutter M (eds): *Stress, Coping and Development in Children.* New York, McGraw-Hill, 1998.

Heisel JS, Ream S, Raitz R, et al: The significance of life events as contributing factors in the diseases of children. 3. A study of pediatric patients. *J Pediatr* 83:119-123, 1973.

Hughes M, Zimin R: Children with psychogenic abdominal pain and their families: Management during hospitalization. *Clin Pediatr (Phila)* 17:569, 1978.

Janes CL, Hesselbrock VM: Problem children's adult adjustment predicted from teacher ratings. *Am J Orthopsychiatry* 48:300, 1978.

Kemper KJ: Parental drug, alcohol, and cigarette addiction. In Parker S, Zuckerman B (eds): *Behavioral and Developmental Pediatrics: A Handbook for Primary Care.* Boston, Little, Brown, 1995, pp 378-383.

Klin A, Volkmar FR, Sparrow SS (eds): *Asperger Syndrome.* New York, Guilford Press, 2000.

Kohlberg L: *Essays on Moral Development,* vol 1, *The Philosophy of Moral Development.* New York, Harper & Row, 1981.

Levine M: *A Mind at a Time.* New York, Simon & Schuster, 2002.

Levine M: *The Myth of Laziness.* New York, Simon & Schuster, 2003.

Levine MD: *Developmental Variation and Learning Disorders.* Cambridge, MA, Educators Publishing Service, 1993.

Levine MD, Oberklaid F, Meltzer L: Developmental output failure: A study of low productivity in school age children. *Pediatrics* 67:18, 1981.

Lewis BL, Khaw K: Family functioning as a mediating variable affecting psychosocial adjustment of children with cystic fibrosis. *J Pediatr* 101:636, 1982.

Ludwig S, Kornberg AE (eds): *Child Abuse: A Medical Reference.* New York, Churchill Livingstone, 1992.

Martin RP: Activity level, distractibility, and persistence: Critical characteristics in early schooling. In Kohnstamm GA, Bates JE, Rothbart MK (eds): *Temperament in Childhood.* New York, John Wiley & Sons, 1989, pp 451-461.

Murphy L, Moriarty A: *Vulnerability, Coping and Growth.* New Haven, CT, Yale University Press, 1976.

Mussen P, Conger J, Kagan J: *Child Development and Personality.* New York, Harper & Row, 1969.

Newacheck P, Taylor W: Prevalence and impact of childhood conditions. *Am J Public Health* 82:364, 1992.

Ollendick T, Oswald D, Francis G: Validity of teacher nominations in identifying aggressive, withdrawn and popular children. *J Clin Child Psychol* 18:221, 1989.

Osofsky JD: Community-based approaches to violence prevention. *J Dev Behav Pediatr* 18:405, 1997.

Perrin EC, Newacheck P, Pless IB, et al: Issues involved in the definition and classification of chronic health conditions. *Pediatrics* 91:787-793, 1993.

Piaget J: *The Origins of Intelligence in Children.* New York, International University Press, 1952.

Piaget J, Inhelder B: *The Psychology of the Child.* New York, Basic Books, 1968.

Putnam N: Revenge or tragedy: Do nerds suffer from a mild pervasive developmental disorder? In Feinstein S (ed): *Adolescent Psychiatry: Developmental and Clinical Studies.* Chicago, University of Chicago Press, 1990.

Pynoos R, Eth S: Children traumatized by witnessing acts of personal violence: Homicide, rape or suicide behavior. In Eth S, Pynoos R (eds): *Post-traumatic Stress Disorders in Children.* Washington, DC, American Psychiatric Press, 1985.

Rosenthal R, Jacobson L: *Pygmalion in the Classroom*. New York, Holt, Rinehart & Winston, 1968.

Routh D, Ernst A: Somatization disorder in relatives of children and adolescents with functional abdominal pain. *J Pediatr Psychol* 9:427, 1984.

Rutter M, Tizard J, Whitmore K: *Education, Health and Behavior*. London, Longman Group, 1970.

Samuels S: *Enhancing Self-concept in Early Childhood: Theory and Practice*. New York, Human Sciences Press, 1977.

Sarnoff C: *Latency*. New York, Aronson, 1976.

Schaefer C: *Childhood Encopresis and Enuresis: Causes and Therapy*. New York, Van Nostrand Reinhold, 1979.

Schechter N, Berde C, Yaster M: *Pain in Infants, Children and Adolescents*, 2nd ed. Baltimore, Lippincott, Williams & Wilkins, 2002.

Singer DC, Singer JL, Zuckerman DM: *Using TV to Your Child's Advantage*. Reston, VA, Acropolis Books, 1990.

Spivak H: Bullying: Why all the fuss? *Pediatrics* 112:1421-1422, 2003.

Stein MT, Rappaport L, Frazer CH, Zeltzec L: Recurrent abdominal pain. *J Dev Behav Pediatr* 22(Suppl): S133-S137, 2001.

Stein MT, Klin A, Miller K, et al: When Asperger syndrome and a nonverbal learning disability look alike. *J Dev Behav Pediatr* 25:190-195, 2004.

Stein RE, Gortmaker SL, Perrin EC, et al: Severity of illness: Concepts and measurement. *Lancet* 2: 1506-1509, 1987.

Strasburger VC: Children, adolescence and television. *Pediatr Rev* 13:144, 1992.

Subrahmanyam K, Kraut RE, Greenfield PM, Gross EF: The impact of home computer use on children's activities and development. *Future Child* 10:123-144, 2000.

Tanguay PB: *Nonverbal Learning Disabilities at School: Educating Students with NLD, Asperger Syndrome and Related Conditions*. Jessica Kingsley Publishing, 2002.

van der Wal MF, de Wit CAM, Hirasing RA: Psychosocial health among young victims and offenders of direct and indirect bullying. *Pediatrics* 111:1312-1317, 2003.

Werner E, Smith R: An epidemiologic perspective on some antecedents and consequences of childhood mental health problems and learning disabilities. *J Am Acad Child Psychiatry* 18:292, 1979.

Williams S, Steiner H: Childhood trauma. In Klykylo W, Kay J, Rube D (eds): *Clinical Child Psychiatry*. Philadelphia, WB Saunders, 1998.

Wolraich ML: *Disorders of Development and Learning: A Practical Guide to Assessment and Management*. St Louis, CV Mosby, 1996.

Chapter 22

Abassi V: Growth and normal puberty. *Pediatrics* 102:507, 1998.

American Academy of Pediatrics, Committee on Practice and Ambulatory Medicine: Recommendations for preventive pediatric health care. *Pediatrics* 105:645, 2000.

American Medical Association: *Guidelines for Adolescent Preventive Services (GAPS), Recommendations Monograph*. American Medical Association, Chicago, 1997.

American Medical Association: *Physician Firearm Safety Guide*. American Medical Association, 1998.

Anderson SE, Dallal GE, Must A: Relative weight and race influence average age at menarche: Results from two nationally representative surveys of US girls studied 25 years apart. *Pediatrics* 111:844-850, 2003.

Bearman P, Bruckner H: *Power in Numbers: Peer Effects on Adolescent Girls' Sexual Debut and Pregnancy*. Washington, DC, National Campaign to Prevent Teen Pregnancy, 1999.

Black JL, Nader PR: Academic achievement. In Friedman SB, Fisher M, Schonberg SK (eds): *Comprehensive Adolescent Health Care*. St Louis, Quality Medical, 1992.

Bright Futures: Guidelines for Health Supervision for Infants, Children, and Adolescents, 2nd ed, revised. Washington, DC, Georgetown University, 2002.

Britto MT, Garrett JM, Dugliss MA, et al: Risky behavior in teens with cystic fibrosis or sickle cell disease: A multicenter study. *Pediatrics* 101:250-256, 1998.

Copeland KC: Variations in normal sexual development. *Pediatr Rev* 8(2):18, 1986.

Dittus PJ, Jaccard J: Adolescents' perceptions of maternal disapproval of sex: Relationship to sexual outcomes. *J Adolesc Health* 26:268, 2000.

Elkind D: Cognitive structure and adolescent experience. *Adolescence* 2:427, 1967.

Elkind D: Understanding the young adolescent. *Adolescence* 13:127, 1978.

English A, Kenney K: *State Minor Consent Laws: A Summary*, 2nd ed. Chapel Hill, NC, Center for Adolescent Health & the Law, 2003.

Erikson EH: *Identity, Youth and Crisis*. New York, WW Norton, 1968.

Felice ME: Adolescence. In Levine MD, Carey WB, Crocker AC (eds): *Developmental-Behavioral Pediatrics*, 2nd ed. Philadelphia, WB Saunders, 1992.

Fisher M: Adolescent health assessment and promotion in office and school settings. *Adolesc Med* 10: 71-86, 1999.

Freud S: The transformation of puberty. In Esman AH (ed): *Psychology of Adolescence*. New York, International Universities Press, 1975, pp 86-99.

Fujii CM, Felice ME: Physical growth and development: Current concepts. *Prim Care* 14:1, 1987.

Garn SM: Physical growth and development. In Friedman SB, Fisher M, Schonberg SK (eds): *Comprehensive Adolescent Health Care*. St Louis, Quality Medical, 1992.

Goldenring JM, Rosen DS: Getting into adolescent heads: An essential update. *Contemp Pediatr* 21:64, 2004.

Grunbaum JA, Kann L, Kinchen SA, et al: Youth risk behavior surveillance, United States, 2001. *MMWR Surveill Summ* 51(4):1-62, 2002.

Hamburg BA: Psychosocial development. In Friedman SB, Fisher M, Schonberg SK (eds): *Comprehensive Adolescent Health Care*. St Louis, Quality Medical, 1992.

Herman-Giddens ME, Slora EJ, Wasserman RC, et al: Secondary sexual characteristics and menses in young girls seen in office practice: A study from the pediatric research in office settings network. *Pediatrics* 99:505-512, 1997.

Herman-Giddens ME, Wang L, Koch G: Secondary sexual characteristics in boys—estimates from the National Health and Nutrition Examination Survey III, 1988-1994. *Arch Pediatr Adolesc Med* 155: 1022-1028, 2001.

Joffe A, Blythe MJ: *Adolescent Medicine: Handbook of Adolescent Medicine, State of the Art Reviews*, vol 14, No 2. Philadelphia, Hanley & Belfus, June 2003.

Kaplowitz PB, Slora EJ, Wasserman RC, et al: Earlier onset of puberty in girls: Relation to increased body mass index and race. *Pediatrics* 108:347-353, 2001.

Kulin HE, Muller J: The biological aspects of puberty. *Pediatr Rev* 17(3):75, 1996.

Ladd GW: Peer relationships. In Friedman SB, Fisher M, Schonberg SK (eds): *Comprehensive Adolescent Health Care*. St Louis, Quality Medical, 1992.

Litt IF: Pubertal and psychosocial development: Implications for pediatricians. *Pediatr Rev* 16(7):243, 1995.

Mansbach JM, Gordon CM: Demystifying delayed puberty. *Contemp Pediatr* 18(4):43, 2001.

Marshall WA, Tanner JM: Variations in the pattern of pubertal changes in boys. *Arch Dis Child* 45:13, 1970.

Midyett LK, Moore WV, Jacobsen JD: Are pubertal changes in girls before age 8 benign? *Pediatrics* 111: 47-51, 2003.

National Center on Addiction and Substance Abuse at Columbia University (CASA): *2002 CASA National Survey of American Attitudes on Substance Abuse VII: Teens, Parents, and Siblings*. New York, QEV Analytic, 2002.

Neinstein LS, Kaufman FR: Abnormal growth and development in adolescence. In Neinstein LS (ed): *Adolescent Health Care: A Practical Guide*, 3rd ed. Baltimore, Williams & Wilkins, 1996.

Piaget J: The intellectual development of the adolescent. In Caplan G, Levovici S (eds): *Adolescence: Psychosocial Perspective.* New York, Basic Books, 1969.

Reiter EO, Lee PA: Have the onset and tempo of puberty changed? *Arch Pediatr Adolesc Med* 155:988, 2001.

Robinson KL, Jelljohann SK, Price JH: Predictors of sixth graders engaging in sexual intercourse. *J Sch Health* 69:369-375, 1999.

Rosenthal SL, Von Ranson KM, Cotton S, et al: Sexual initiation: Predictors and developing trends. *Sex Transm Dis* 28:527-532, 2001.

Sandler AD, Levine MD: Learning and attention deficit disorders. In Friedman SB, Fisher M, Schonberg SK (eds): *Comprehensive Adolescent Health Care.* St Louis, Quality Medical, 1992.

Santelli JS, Kaiser J, Hirsch L, et al: Initiation of sexual intercourse among middle school adolescents: The influence of psychosocial factors. *J Adolesc Health* 34:200-208, 2004.

Stone LJ, Church J: Pubescence, puberty, and physical development. In Esman AH (ed): *Psychology of Adolescence.* New York, International Universities Press, 1975.

Tanner JM: *Growth at Adolescence,* 2nd ed. Boston, Blackwell Scientific, 1962.

Vanoss Marin B, Coyle KK, Gomez CA, et al: Older boyfriends and girlfriends increase risk of sexual initiation in young adolescents. *J Adolesc Health* 27:409, 2000.

Weiner IB: Distinguishing healthy from disturbed adolescent development. *J Dev Behav Pediatr* 11:151, 1990.

Women's Sports Foundation Report: *Sport and Teen Pregnancy.* East Meadow, NY, Women's Sports Foundation, 1998.

Wu T, Mendola P, Buck GM: Ethnic differences in the presence of secondary sex characteristics and menarche among US girls; the Third National Health and Nutrition Examination Survey, 1988-1994. *Pediatrics* 110:752-757, 2002.

Chapter 23

Abma JC, Chandra A, Mosher WD, et al: Fertility, family planning, and women's health: New data from the 1995 National Survey of Family Growth. *Vital Health Stat 23* 19:1-114, 1997.

Abma J, Driscoll A, Moore K: Young women's degree of control over first intercourse: An explanatory analysis. *Fam Plann Perspect* 30:12, 1998.

American Academy of Pediatrics: *Substance Abuse: A Guide for Health Professionals.* Elk Grove Village, IL, American Academy of Pediatrics, 1988.

American Academy of Pediatrics Committee on Adolescence: Adolescent pregnancy—current trends and issues: 1998. *Pediatrics* 103:516, 1999.

American Academy of Pediatrics Committee on Adolescence: Contraception and adolescents. *Pediatrics* 104:1161, 1999.

American Academy of Pediatrics Committee on Adolescence: Care of the adolescent sexual assault victim. *Pediatrics* 107:1476, 2001.

American Academy of Pediatrics Committee on Adolescence: Policy statement—identifying and treating eating disorders. *Pediatrics* 111:204, 2003.

American Academy of Pediatrics, Committee on Injury and Poison Prevention and Committee on Adolescence: The teenage driver. *Pediatrics* 98:987, 1996.

American Academy of Pediatrics, Committee on Practice and Ambulatory Medicine: Recommendations for preventive pediatric health care. *Pediatrics* 96:373, 1995.

American Psychiatric Association: *Diagnostic and Statistical Manual of Mental Health Disorders,* 4th ed (DSM-IV). Washington, DC, American Psychiatric Association, 1994.

Arias E, Anderson RN, Kang HC, et al: Deaths: Final data for 2001. *Natl Vital Stat Rep* 52(3):1, 2003.

Black JL: Adolescents with learning problems. *Prim Care* 14:203, 1987.

Blum RW, Rinehart PM: *Reducing the Risk: Connections That Make a Difference in the Lives of Youth.* Minneapolis, MN, Center for Adolescent Health and Development, University of Minnesota, 1998.

Cagampang HH, Barth RP, Korpi M, et al: Education Now and Babies Later (ENABL): Life history of a campaign to postpone sexual involvement. *Fam Plann Perspect* 29(3):109, 1997.

Casey BJ, Giedd JN, Thomas KM: Structural and functional brain development and its relation to cognitive development. *Biol Psychol* 54:241, 2000.

Centers for Disease Control and Prevention: *Tracking the Hidden Epidemics: Trends in STDs in the United States.* Atlanta, Centers for Disease Control and Prevention, 2000.

Centers for Disease Control and Prevention: Trends in sexual risk behaviors among high school students—United States, 1991-2001. *MMWR Morb Mortal Wkly Rep* 51(38):856-859, 2002.

Centers for Disease Control and Prevention: *Sexually Transmitted Disease Surveillance, 2002.* Atlanta, Centers for Disease Control and Prevention, 2003.

Cohen M, Friedman SB: Nonsexual motivation of adolescent sexual behavior. *Med Aspects Hum Sex* 9:31, 1975.

Cromer BA, Frankel ME, Keder LM: Compliance with breast self-examination instruction in healthy adolescents. *J Adolesc Health Care* 10:105, 1989.

Darroch JE, Singh S: *Why Is Teenage Pregnancy Declining? The Roles of Abstinence, Sexual Activity, and Contraceptive Use. Occasional Report No. 1.* New York, Alan Guttmacher Institute, 1999.

Dietz WH: Health consequences of obesity in youth: Childhood predictors of adult disease. *Pediatrics* 101:518S, 1998.

East PL, Felice ME: *Adolescent Pregnancy and Parenting—Findings from a Racially Diverse Sample.* Mahway, NJ, Lawrence Erlbaum Associates, 1996.

Elkind D: Egocentrism in adolescence. *Child Dev* 38:1025, 1967.

Ensign J, Santelli J: Shelter-based homeless youth. *Arch Pediatr Adolesc Med* 151:817, 1997.

Ensign J, Santelli J: Health status and services use: Comparison of adolescents at a school-based clinic with homeless adolescents. *Arch Pediatr Adolesc Med* 152:20, 1998.

Frankowski BL, American Academy of Pediatrics Committee on Adolescence: Sexual orientation and adolescents. *Pediatrics* 113:1827, 2004.

Garofalo R, Wolf RC, Wissow LS, et al: Sexual orientation and risk of suicide attempts among a representative sample of youth. *Arch Pediatr Adolesc Med* 153:487, 1999.

Gates GJ, Sonenstein FL: Heterosexual genital sexual activity among adolescent males, 1988 and 1995. *Fam Plann Perspect* 32:295, 2000.

Gogtay N, Giedd JN, Hayashi KM, et al: Dynamic mapping of human cortical development during childhood through early adulthood. *Proc Natl Acad Sci U S A* 101:8174, 2004.

Griesemer BA: Ergogenic aids elevate health risks in young athletes. *Pediatr Ann* 32:733, 2003.

Grunbaum JA, Kann L, Kinchen S, et al: Youth Risk Behavior Surveillance—United States, 2003. *MMWR Surveill Summ* 53(2):1-96, 2004.

Henshaw SK: Unintended pregnancy in the United States. *Fam Plann Perspect* 30:24, 1998.

Henshaw SK: *U.S. Teenage Pregnancy Statistics with Comparative Statistics for Women Aged 20-24.* New York, Alan Guttmacher Institute, 2004.

Irwin CE, Shafer MA: Adolescent sexuality: Negative outcomes of a normative behavior. In Rogers DE, Ginzbert E (eds): *Adolescents at Risk: Medical and Social Perspectives.* Boulder, CO, Westview Press, 1992.

James DC: Coping with a new society: The unique psychosocial problems of immigrant youth. *J Sch Health* 67(3):98, 1997.

Johnston LD, O'Malley PM, Bachman JG, et al: *Monitoring the Future National Results on Adolescent Drug Use: Overview of Key Findings, 2003* (NIH Publication No. 04-5506). Bethesda, MD, National Institute on Drug Abuse, 2004.

Kirby D: *No Easy Answers—Research Findings on Programs to Reduce Teen Pregnancy.* Washington, DC, National Campaign to Prevent Teen Pregnancy, 1997.

Kirby D, Korpi M, Barth RP, et al: The impact of the Postponing Sexual Involvement curriculum among youths in California. *Fam Plann Perspect* 29(3):100, 1997.

Klein JF, Berry CC, Felice ME: The development of a testicular self-examination instructional booklet for adolescents. *J Adolesc Health Care* 11:235, 1990.

Knight JR: Adolescent substance use: Screening, assessment, and intervention. *Contemp Pediatr* 14(4):45, 1997.

Koester MC: Making the preparticipation athletic evaluation more than just a "sports physical." *Contemp Pediatr* 20(9):85, 2003.

Kohlberg L, Gilligan C: The adolescent as a philosopher: The discovery of the self in a post-conventional world. In Kagan J, Coles R (eds): *12 to 16: Early Adolescence.* New York, WW Norton, 1972.

Kreipe RE: Eating disorders among children and adolescents. *Pediatr Rev* 16(10):370, 1995.

Krowchuk DP, Kreiter SR, Woods CR, et al: Problem dieting behaviors among young adolescents. *Arch Pediatr Adolesc Med* 152:884, 1998.

Luster T, Small SA: Sexual abuse history and number of sexual partners among female adolescents. *Fam Plann Perspect* 29(5):204, 1997.

Must A, Strauss RS: Risks and consequences of childhood and adolescent obesity. *Int J Obes* 23(Suppl 2): S2-S11, 1999.

National Adolescent Health Information Center, UCSF: Fact sheet: Out-of-home youth-foster care, incarcerated, homeless/runaways adolescents. *Adolescent Fact File.* San Francisco, National Adolescent Health Information Center, August 1996.

Nelson JA: Gay, lesbian, and bisexual adolescents: Providing esteem-enhancing care to a battered population. *Nurse Pract* 22(2):94, 1997.

Offer D, Ostrow E, Howard K: Adolescence: What is normal? *Am J Dis Child* 143:731, 1989.

Ozer EM, Brindis CD, Millstein SG, et al: *America's Adolescents: Are They Healthy?* San Francisco, National Adolescent Health Information Center, 1997.

Park A: What makes teens tick? *Time,* May 10:p 57, 2004.

Piaget J: The intellectual development of the adolescent. In Caplan G, Lebovici S (eds): *Adolescence: Psychological Perspectives.* New York, Basic Books, 1969.

Putting What Works to Work—A Project of the National Campaign to Prevent Teen Pregnancy: American opinion on teen pregnancy and related issues 2003. *Science Says* 7:February, 2004.

Radkowsky M, Siegel LJ: The gay adolescent: Stressors, adaptations, and psychosocial interventions. *Clin Psychol Rev* 17:191, 1997.

Raj A, Silverman JG, Amaro H: The relationship between sexual abuse and sexual risk among high school students: Findings from the 1997 Massachusetts youth risk behavior survey. *Maternal Child Health J* 4:125, 2000.

Remafedi G: Homosexual youth: A challenge to contemporary society. *JAMA* 258:222, 1987.

Remafedi G, Resnick M, Blum R, et al: Demography of sexual orientation in adolescents. *Pediatrics* 89: 714, 1992.

Resnick MD, Bearman PS, Blum RW, et al: Protecting adolescents from harm. Findings from the National Longitudinal Study on Adolescent Health. *JAMA* 278:823, 1997.

Rich LM, Kim SB: Employment and the sexual and reproductive behavior of female adolescents. *Perspect Sexual Reprod Health* 34(3):127, 2002.

Rosenberg ML, Martinez R: Graduated licensure: A win-win proposition for teen drivers and parents. *Pediatrics* 98:987, 1996.

Santelli JS, Abma J, Ventura S, et al: Can changes in sexual behaviors among high school students explain the decline in teen pregnancy rates in the 1990s? *J Adolesc Health* 35(2):80, 2004.

Schoen C, Davis K, Scott Collins K, et al: *The Commonwealth Fund Survey of the Health of Adolescent Girls.* New York, The Commonwealth Fund, 1997.

Schwartz DF: Violence. *Pediatr Rev* 17(6):197, 1996.

Sheslow D, Hassink S, Wallace W, et al: The relationship between self-esteem and depression in obese children. *Ann N Y Acad Sci* 699:289, 1993.

Slyper AH: The pediatric obesity epidemic: Causes and controversies. *J Clin Endocrinol Metab* 89:2540, 2004.

Stashwick C: When you suspect an eating disorder. *Contemp Pediatr* 13(11):124, 1996.

Stock JK, Bell MA, Boyer DK, et al: Adolescent pregnancy and sexual risk-taking among sexually abused girls. *Fam Plann Perspect* 29(5):200, 1997.

Szilagyi M: The pediatrician and the child in foster care. *Pediatr Rev* 19(2):39, 1988.

Troiden R: Homosexual identity development. *J Adolesc Health Care* 9:105, 1988.

Ventura SJ, Mathews TJ, Hamilton BE: Births to teenagers in the United States, 1940-2000. *Natl Vital Stat Rep* 49(10):1-23, 2001.

Weiner IB: Distinguishing healthy from disturbed adolescent development. *J Dev Behav Pediatr* 11:151, 1990.

Wolraich ML, Felice ME, Drotar D (eds): *The Classification of Child and Adolescent Mental Diagnoses in Primary Care.* Elk Grove Village, IL, American Academy of Pediatrics, 1996.

Wonderlich SA, Brewerton TD, Jocic Z, et al: Relationship of childhood sexual abuse and eating disorders. *J Am Acad Child Adolesc Psychiatry* 36:1107, 1997.

Yanovski JA: Pediatric obesity. *Rev Endocr Metab Dis* 2:371, 2001.

Zimmer-Gembeck MJ: The development of romantic relationships and adaptations in the system of peer relationships. *J Adolesc Health* 31:216, 2002.

Chapter 24

American Academy of Pediatrics: Homosexuality and adolescence. *Pediatrics* 92:631, 1993.

American Academy of Pediatrics: *Guidelines for Health Supervision, III.* Elk Grove Village, IL, American Academy of Pediatrics, 1997.

American Academy of Pediatrics Committee on Substance Abuse: Role of the pediatrician in the prevention and management of substance abuse. *Pediatrics* 91:1010, 1993.

American Psychiatric Association: *Diagnostic and Statistical Manual of Mental Disorders,* 4th ed (DSM-IV). Washington, DC, American Psychiatric Association, 1994.

Anderson B, Farrow J: Incarcerated adolescents in Washington state: Health services and utilization. *J Adolesc Health* 22:363, 1998.

Bass CA, Jungkind DL, Silverman NS, Bondi JM: Clinical evaluation of a new polymerase chain reaction assay for detection of *Chlamydia trachomatis* in endocervical specimens. *J Clin Microbiol* 31:2648-2653, 1993.

Brewer N, Lowry R, Kann L, et al: Trends in sexual behaviors among high school students—United States, 1991-2001. *MMWR Morb Mortal Wkly Rep* 51:856-859, 2002.

Elster AB, Kuznets NJ (eds): *AMA Guidelines for Adolescent Preventive Services.* Baltimore, Williams & Wilkins, 1994.

Ernol FKE, Innala SM, Whitan FL: Biological explanation, psychological explanation and tolerance of homosexuals: A cross-national analysis of beliefs and attitudes. *Psychol Rep* 65:1003, 1989.

Friedman LS, Stronin L, Hingson R: A survey of attitudes, beliefs, behaviors and knowledge about AIDS and HIV testing by adolescents and young adults enrolled in alcohol and drug treatment. *J Adolesc Health Care* 14:442, 1993.

Friedman RC, Downey JI: Homosexuality. *N Engl J Med* 331:933, 1996.

Futterman D, Hein K, Reuben N, et al: Human immunodeficiency virus–infected adolescents: The first 50 patients in a New York City program. *Pediatrics* 91:730-735, 1993.

Garl MH, Brookmeyer R: Methods for projecting course of the acquired immunodeficiency syndrome epidemic. *J Natl Cancer Inst* 80:900, 1988.

Goldenring JM, Cohen E: Getting into adolescents' heads. *Contemp Pediatr* 5:75, 1988.

Grunbaum JA, Kann L, Kinchen S, et al: Youth risk behavior surveillance—United States, 2001. *MMWR Surveill Summ* 51(4):1-62, 2002.

Johnston L, O'Malley P, Bachman J: *National Survey Results on Drug Use from the Monitoring the Future Study, 1975-1995*. Rockville, MD, National Institutes on Drug Abuse, 1995.

Kinsey AC, Pomeroy WB, Martin CE: *Sexual Behavior in the Human Male*. New York, WB Saunders, 1948.

Kinsey AC, Pomeroy WB, Martin CE: *Sexual Behavior in the Human Female*. New York, WB Saunders, 1953.

Koob GF, Bloom FE: Cellular and molecular mechanisms of drug dependence. *Science* 242:715, 1988.

Marrazzo JM, White CL, Krekeler B, et al: Community based urine screening for *Chlamydia trachomatis* with a ligase chain reaction assay. *Ann Intern Med* 127:796-803, 1997.

McNeely CA, Nonnemaker JM, Blum RW: Promoting school connectedness: Evidence from the National Longitudinal Study of Adolescent Health. *Sch Health* 72(4):138-146, 2002.

Morey MA, Friedman LS: Health care needs of homeless adolescents. *Curr Opin Pediatr* 5:395, 1993.

O'Connor PG, Schottenfeld RS: Patients with alcohol problems. *N Engl J Med* 338:592, 1998.

Pennbridge J, MacKenzie R, Swofford A: Risk profile of homeless pregnant adolescents and youth. *J Adolesc Health* 12:534, 1991.

Rawitscher LA, Saitz R, Friedman LS: Adolescents' preferences regarding human immunodeficiency virus (HIV)-related physician counseling and HIV testing. *Pediatrics* 96:52, 1995.

Remafedi G: Adolescent homosexuality: Psychological and medical implications. *Pediatrics* 79:331, 1987.

Remafedi G, Farrow JA, Deiswas RW: Risk factors for attempted suicide in gay and lesbian youth. *Pediatrics* 87:879, 1991.

Robertson LM, Middleman AB: Knowledge of health insurance coverage by adolescents and young adults attending a hospital-based clinic. *J Adolesc Health Care* 22:439, 1998.

Rogers PD, Adger H Jr: Alcohol and adolescents. *Adolesc Med* 4:295-304, 1993.

Rosenberg PS, Biggar RJ: Trends in HIV incidence among young adults in the United States. *JAMA* 279:1894, 1998.

Ryan RC, Futterman D: Lesbian and gay youth: Care and counseling. *Adolesc Med* 8:207-374, 1997.

Schuckit MA: Genetics and the risk for alcoholism. *JAMA* 254:2614, 1985.

Snyder HN, Sickmond M: *Juvenile Offenders and Victims: 1999 National Report*. Washington, DC, Office of Juvenile Justice and Delinquency Prevention, 1999. www.ojjdp.ncjrs.org.

Stevens-Simon C, Parson J, Montgomery C: What is the relationship between postpartum withdrawal from school and repeat pregnancy and adolescent mothers? *J Adolesc Health Care* 7:191, 1986.

Turner CF, Ku L, Rogers SM, et al: Adolescent sexual behavior, drug use and violence: Increased reporting with computer survey technology. *Science* 280:867-873, 1998.

Wheeler K, Malmquist J: Treatment approaches in adolescent chemical dependency. *Pediatr Clin North Am* 34:437, 1987.

Chapter 25

American Academy of Pediatrics: Issues of confidentiality in adoption: The role of the pediatrician. *Pediatrics* 93:339, 1994.

American Academy of Pediatrics: Family pediatrics. *Pediatrics* 111(Suppl):1541, 2003.

American Academy of Pediatrics, Committee on Early Childhood, Adoption, and Dependent Care: Families and adoption: The pediatrician's role in supporting communication. In *Policy Reference Guide of the American Academy of Pediatrics*. Elk Grove Village, IL, American Academy of Pediatrics 1997.

American Medical Association: Violence: A compendium. *JAMA*, American Medical News and Specialty Journals of the American Medical Association, 1992.

Ames EW: *The Development of Romanian Orphanage Children Adopted to Canada*. Burnaby, British Columbia, Canada, Simon Fraser University, 1997.

Anderson JZ, White GD: An empirical investigation of interaction and relationship patterns in functional and dysfunctional nuclear families and stepfamilies. *Fam Process* 25:407, 1986.

Anthony EJ: Children at risk for psychosis growing up successfully. In Anthony EJ, Cohler B (eds): *The Invulnerable Child.* New York, Guilford Press, 1987.

Bassuk EL, Rubin L: Homeless children: A neglected population. *Am J Orthopsychiatry* 57:279, 1987.

Block JH, Block J: The role of ego-control and ego-resiliency in the organization of behavior. In Collins WA (ed): *Development of Cognition, Affect and Social Relations: The Minnesota Symposia on Child Psychology,* vol 3. Hillsdale, NJ, Lawrence Erlbaum Associates, 1980.

Bowlby J: Loss: Sadness and depression. In Bowlby, J: *Attachment and Loss,* vol 3. New York, Basic Books, 1980.

Brooks-Gunn J, Duncan GJ: The effects of poverty on children. *Future Child* 7(2):55-71, 1997.

Bryner KB: The Amish way of death: A study of family support systems. In Moos RH (ed): *Coping with Life Crises: An Integrated Approach.* New York, Plenum Press, 1986.

Cohen GJ: Helping children and families deal with divorce and separation. *Pediatrics* 110:1019-1023, 2002.

Dubowitz H, Feigelman S, Zuravin S, et al: The physical health of children in kinship care. *Am J Dis Child* 146:603-610, 1992.

Edelman MW, Mihaly L: Homeless families and the housing crisis in the United States. *Child Youth Services Rev* 11:91, 1989.

Ganong LH, Coleman M: The effects of remarriage on children: A review of the empirical literature. *J Appl Fam Child Studies* 33:389, 1984.

Garbarino J, Seves J, Schellenbach C: Families at risk for destructive parent-child relations in adolescence. *Child Dev* 55:174, 1984.

Garmezy N: Children under stress: Perspectives on antecedents and correlates of vulnerability and resistance to psychopathology. In Rabin AI, (ed): *Further Explorations in Personality.* New York, John Wiley & Sons, 1981.

Gold M, Perrin EC, Futterman D, Friedman SB, et al: Children of gay or lesbian parents. *Pediatr Rev* 15:354-358, 1994.

Heatherington EM, Cox M, Cox R: Long-term effects of divorce and remarriage on the adjustment of children. *J Am Acad Child Psychiatry* 24:518, 1985.

Herndon A, Combs LG: Stepfamilies as patients. *J Fam Pract* 15:917, 1982.

Hoyt LA: Anxiety and depression in young children of divorce. *J Clin Child Psychol* 19:26, 1999.

Johnson JR, Kline M, Tschann JM: Ongoing postdivorce conflict: Effects on children of joint custody and frequent access. *Am J Orthopsychiatry* 59:576, 1989.

Kappelman MM, Black J: Children of divorce: The pediatrician's responsibility. *Pediatr Ann* 9:48, 1980.

Kellam S, Ensminger M, Turner R: Family structure and the mental health of children. *Arch Gen Psychiatry* 34:1012, 1977.

Lazarus RS: *Psychological Stress and the Coping Process.* New York, McGraw-Hill, 1966.

Lewis FM, Woods NF, Hough EE, Bensley LS: The family's functioning with chronic illness in the mother: The spouse's perspective. *Soc Sci Med* 29:1261-1269, 1989.

Mahler MS, Pine F, Bergman A: *The Psychological Birth of the Human Infant: Symbiosis and Individuation.* New York, Basic Books, 1975.

Maslow AH: *Motivation and Personality,* 2nd ed. New York, Harper & Row, 1970.

Murphy LB, Moriarty AE: *Vulnerability, Coping and Growth.* New Haven, CT, Yale University Press, 1976.

National Center for Children with Poverty: *Low Income Children in the United States.* New York, Columbia University, 2003.

O'Connor TG, Rutter M: The English and Romanian adoptees study team: Attachment disorder behavior following severe deprivation: Extension and longitudinal follow-up. *Am Acad Child Adolesc Psychiatry* 39:703-712, 2000.

Papernow Q: *Becoming a Stepfamily: Patterns of Development in Remarried Families.* San Francisco, Jossey-Bass, 1993.

Patterson CJ: Children of lesbian and gay parents. *Adv Clin Child Psychol* 19:235, 1997.

Patterson GR: Stress: A change agent for family process. In Garmezy N, Rutter M (eds): *Stress, Coping and Development in Children.* Baltimore, Johns Hopkins University Press, 1988.

Perrin EC: *Sexual Orientation in Children and Adolescents: Implications for Health Care.* New York, Kluwer Academic/Plenum, 2002.

Radovanic H: Parental conflict and children's coping styles in litigating separated families: Relationships with children's adjustment. *J Abnorm Child Psychol* 21:697, 1993.

Rutter M: Families. In Rutter M (ed): *Helping Troubled Children.* New York, Brunner-Mazel, 1975.

Rutter, M, Andersen-Wood L, Beckett C, et al: Quasi-autistic patterns following severe early global privation. *J Child Psychol Psychiatry* 40:537-549, 1999.

Sameroff AJ, Barocas R, Seifer R: The early development of children born to mentally ill women. In Watt NF, Anthony EJ, Wynne LC: *Children at Risk for Schizophrenia: A Longitudinal Perspective.* New York, Cambridge University Press, 1984.

Schor ED: Foster care. *Pediatr Clin North Am* 35:1241, 1988.

Sokoloff B: Adoption and foster care: The pediatrician's role. *Pediatr Rev* 1:57, 1979.

Sorosky AD, Baran A, Pannor R: *The Adoption Triangle.* New York, Doubleday, 1978.

Spock B: *Dr. Spock's Baby and Child Care,* 7th ed. New York, Pocket Books, 1998, pp 685-688.

Stein MT: Challenging case: The use of family drawings by children in pediatric practice. *J Dev Behav Pediatr* 18:334, 1997.

Stein MT, Dillar L, Resnikoff R: ADHD, divorce, and parental disagreement about the diagnosis and treatment. *J Dev Behav Pediatr* 21:53-57, 2000.

Stein MT, Faber S, Berger S, Kilman G: International adoption: A four-year-old child with unusual behaviors adopted at six-months of age. *J Dev Behav Pediatr* 24:63-69, 2003.

Stein MT, Perrin E, Potter J: A difficult adjustment to school: The importance of family constellation. *J Dev Behav Pediatr* 23:171-174, 2002.

Van Ryn M, Burke J: The effect of patient race and socio-economic status on physicians' perceptions of patients. *Soc Sci Med* 50:813, 2000.

Visher EB, Visher JS: Stepfamilies are different. *J Fam Ther* 7:9, 1985.

Wallerstein JS: Separation, divorce and remarriage. In Levine MD, Carey WB, Crocker AC (eds): *Developmental-Behavioral Pediatrics,* 3rd ed. Philadelphia, WB Saunders, 1999, pp 149-161.

Wallerstein JS, Johnston JR: Children of divorce: Recent findings regarding long term effects and recent studies of joint and sole custody. *Pediatr Rev* 11:197, 1990.

Wallerstein J, Kelly J: *Surviving the Breakup: How Children and Parents Cope with Divorce.* New York, Basic Books, 1980.

Werner EE, Smith RS: *Vulnerable but Invincible: A Longitudinal Study of Resilient Children and Youth.* New York, McGraw-Hill, 1982.

Wessel MA: The pediatrician and adoption. *N Engl J Med* 262:446, 1960.

Chapter 26

American Academy of Pediatrics: The assessment and management of acute pain in infants, children, and adolescents. *Pediatrics* 108:787-793, 2001.

Azarnoff P: Parents and siblings of pediatric patients. *Curr Probl Pediatr* 14:1, 1984.

Bergman AB, Stamm SJ: The morbidity of cardiac nondisease in school children. *N Engl J Med* 276:1008, 1967.

Bibale R, Walsh M: Development of children's concept of illness. *Pediatrics* 66:912, 1980.

Coleman WL: *Family-Focused Behavioral Pediatrics.* Philadelphia, Lippincott Williams & Wilkins, 2001.

Coleman WL, Howard BJ: Family-focused behavioral pediatrics: Clinical techniques for primary care. *Pediatr Rev* 16:448, 1995.

Dingle JH, Badger BF, Jordan WS Jr: *Illness in the Home: A Study of 25,000 Illnesses in a Group of Cleveland families.* Cleveland, OH, Western Reserve University, 1964.

Kemper KJ, Forsyth BW, McCarthy PL: Persistent perceptions of vulnerability following neonatal jaundice. *Am J Dis Child* 144:238, 1990.

Kharasch S, Saxe G, Zuckerman B: Pain treatment: Opportunities and challenges. *Arch Pediatr Adolesc Med* 157:1054, 2003.

Klineman A, Eisenberg L, Good B: Culture, illness and care. *Ann Intern Med* 88:251, 1978.

Lefcourt HM: *Locus of Control: Current Trends in Theory and Research.* Hillsdale, NJ, Lawrence Erlbaum Associates, 1976.

Mahler M: *The Psychological Birth of the Human Infant: Symbiosis and Individuation.* New York, Basic Books, 1975.

Olness KN, Kohen DP: *Hypnosis and Hypnotherapy with Children*, 3rd ed. New York, Guilford Press, 1996.

Parmelee AH: Childhood illness as a source of psychological growth, unpublished presidential address, Society for Research in Child Development, 1985.

Parmelee AJ Jr: Illness and the development of social competence. *J Dev Behav Pediatr* 18:120, 1997.

Perrin EC, Gerrity PS: There's a demon in your belly: Children's understanding of concepts regarding illness. *Pediatrics* 67:841, 1981.

Perrin EC, Nowacheck P, Pless IB, et al: Issues involved in the definition of chronic health conditions. *Pediatrics* 91:787-793, 1993.

Perrin JM: Chronic illness. In Levine MD, Carey WB, Crocker AC (eds): *Developmental-Behavioral Pediatrics*, 3rd ed. Philadelphia, WB Saunders, 1999, pp 335-345.

Peterson L, Shigetomi C: The use of coping techniques to minimize anxiety in hospitalized children. *Behav Ther* 12:1, 1981.

Reis EC, Roth EK, Syphan JL, et al: Effective pain reduction for multiple immunization injections in young infants. *Arch Pediatr Adolesc Med* 157:1115-1120, 2003.

Robertson J: *Young Children in Hospital*, 2nd ed. London, Tavistock, 1970.

Rutter M: Separation experiences: A new look at an old topic. *J Pediatr* 95:147, 1979.

Siegel LJ, Peterson L: Stress reduction in young dental patients through coping skills and sensory information. *J Consult Clin Psychol* 48:785, 1980.

Stein MT, Coleman WL, Epstein RM: "We've tried everything and nothing works": Family centered pediatrics and clinical problem solving. *J Dev Behav Pediatr* 18:117, 1997.

Stein MT, Flores G, Graham EA, et al: Cultural and linguistic determinants in the diagnosis and management of development delay in a 4-year-old. *J Dev Behav Pediatr* 23:371, 2002.

Sugarman LI: Hypnosis: Teaching children self-regulation. *Pediatr Rev* 17:5, 1996.

Thompson RH, Vernon DTA: Research on children's behavior after hospitalization: A review and synthesis. *J Dev Behav Pediatr* 14:28, 1993.

Valadian I, Stuart HC, Reed RB: Studies of illness of children followed from birth to 18 years. *Monogr Soc Res Child Dev* 26:9, 1961.

Vernon DTA, Blake BA: *The Psychological Responses of Children to Hospitalization and Illness: A Review of the Literature.* Springfield, IL, Charles C Thomas, 1965.

Visintainer MA, Wolfer JA: Psychological preparation for surgical pediatric patients: The effects on children's and parents' stress responses and adjustment. *Pediatrics* 56:187, 1975.

Zeltzer LK, Dolgin MJ, LeBaron S, LeBaron C: A randomized, controlled study of behavioral intervention for chemotherapy distress in children with cancer. *Pediatrics* 88:34-42, 1991.

Zeltzer LK, Jay SM, Fisher DM: The management of pain associated with pediatric procedures. *Pediatr Clin North Am* 36:1, 1989.

Chapter 27

Aguilara DC: *Crisis Intervention: Theory and Methodology.* St Louis, CV Mosby, 1974.

Blubond-Langer M: Meanings of death to children. In Feifel H (ed): *New Meanings of Death.* New York, McGraw-Hill, 1977.

Bowlby J: Grief and mourning in infancy and early childhood. *Psychoanal Study Child* 15:9, 1960.

Children's Defense Fund: *Annual Report: The State of America's Children.* Washington, DC, Children's Defense Fund, 1993.

Duggal HS, Berezkin G, John V: PTSD and TV viewing of the World Trade Center. *J Am Acad Child Adolesc Psychiatry* 41:494-495, 2002.

Fairbrother G, Stuber J, Galeo S, et al: Unmet need for counseling services by children in New York City after the September 11 attacks on the World Trade Center: Implications for pediatricians. *Pediatrics* 113:1367-1374, 2004.

Fox S: *Good Grief: Helping Groups of Children When a Friend Dies.* Boston, New England Association for the Education of Young Children, 1988.

Geltman PL, Augustyn M, Barnett E, et al: War trauma experience and behavioral screening of Bosnian refugee children resettled in Massachusetts. *J Dev Behav Pediatr* 21:255-261, 2002.

Good Grief Program: *Books and Videos on Loss for Children and Adolescents: An Annotated Bibliography.* Boston, 1996, The Good Grief Program, One Boston Medical Center Place, Boston, MA 02118.

Groves BM, Zuckerman B, Marans S, Cohen DJ: Silent victims: Children who witness violence. *JAMA* 269:262-264, 1993.

Honig AS: Stress and coping in young children. *Young Children* 41(4):51-63, 41(5):47-59, 1986.

Hurt H, Malnued E, Brodsky NL, Giannetta J: Exposure to violence: Psychological and academic correlates in child witnesses. *Arch Pediatr Adolesc Med* 155:1351-1356, 2001.

Kastenbaum RJ: *Death, Society, and Human Experience,* 4th ed. New York, MacMillan, 1977.

Kemper KJ, Kelleher KJ: Family psychosocial screening: Instruments and techniques. *Child Health* 4:325, 1996. Public domain access: http//www.pedstest.com/links/resources.html.

Kliman G: Death: Some implications in child development and child analysis. *Adv Thanatol* 4:43, 1980.

Kreicbergs U, Valdimarsdottir U, Onelov E, et al: Talking about death with children who have severe malignant disease. *N Engl J Med* 351:1175-1186, 2004.

Laraque D, Boscareno JA, Battista A, et al: Reactions and needs of tri-state area pediatricians after the events of September 11: Implications for children's mental health services. *Pediatrics* 113:1357-1366, 2004.

Margolin G, Gordis EB: The effects of community violence on children. *Annu Rev Psychol* 51:445-479, 2000.

Marsh Schlesinger J, Lee E: Mourning in different cultures. In Walsh F, McGoldrick M (eds): *Living beyond Loss: Death in the Family.* New York, WW Norton, 1991.

McFarlene JM, Groff JY, O'Brien J, Watson K: Behaviors of children who are exposed and not exposed to intimate partner violence: An analysis of 330 Black, White and Hispanic Children. *Pediatrics* 112:202-207, 2003.

Nagy M: The child's theories concerning death. *J Genet Psychol* 73:3, 1948.

National Association for the Education of Young Children: *When Disaster Strikes: Helping Young Children Cope.* Washington, DC, National Association for the Education of Young Children, 1996.

Pedlener I, Grand R: The 9/11 terror attacks: Emotional consequences persist for children. *Contemp Pediatr* 9:43, 2002.

Rando T: *Grief, Dying and Death.* Champaign, IL, Research Press, 1984, p 155.

Saravay B: Short-term play therapy with two preschool brothers following sudden paternal death. In Webb NB (ed): *Play Therapy with Children in Crisis: A Casebook for Practitioners.* New York, Guilford Press, 1991.

Schonfeld DJ: Supporting children after terrorist events: Potential roles for pediatricians. *Pediatr Ann* 32:182-187, 2003.

Schuler ME, Nair P: Witnessing violence among inner-city children of substance-abusing and non–substance-abusing women. *Arch Pediatr Adolesc Med* 155:342-346, 2001.

Silverman PR: *Never Too Young to Know: Death in Children's Lives.* New York, Oxford University Press, 2000.

Spinetta JJ: The dying child's awareness of death: A review. *Psychol Bull* 81:256, 1974.

Taylor L, Zuckerman B, Harik V, Groves BM: Witnessing violence by young children and their mothers. *J Dev Behav Pediatr* 5:120-123, 1994.

Terr LC: *Too Scared To Cry: Psychic Trauma in Childhood.* New York, Harper & Row, 1990.

Vermeiren R, Schwab-Stone M, Deboutte D, et al: Violence exposure and substance use in adolescents: Findings from three countries. *Pediatrics* 111:535-540, 2003.

Wagman Borowsky I, Ireland M: Parental screening for intimate partner violence by pediatricians and family physicians. *Pediatrics* 110:509-516, 2002.

Webb NB (ed): *Helping Bereaved Children: A Handbook for Practitioners.* New York, Guilford Press, 1993.

Wolfe L: Should parents speak with a dying child about impending death? *N Engl J Med* 351:1251-1253, 2004.

Chapter 28

Blumenthal D: The future of quality measurement and management in a transforming health care system. *JAMA* 278:1622, 1997.

Lamp JM, Howard PA: Guiding parents' use of the Internet for newborn education. MCN Am J Matern Child Nurs 24:33, 1999.

Rippen H: Criteria for assessing the quality of health information on the Internet. At http://www.mitretek.org/hiti/showcase/documents/criteria.html.

Silberg W, Lunberg G, Musacchio R: Assessing, controlling and assuring the quality of medical information on the Internet. *JAMA* 277:1244, 1997.

Index

Note: Page numbers followed by f refer to figures; page numbers followed by t refer to tables; page numbers followed by b refer to boxes.

A